MYELINATION AND DEMYELINATION

ADVANCES IN EXPERIMENTAL MEDICINE AND BIOLOGY

Recent Volumes in this Series

Volume 93
IMMUNITY TO BLOOD PARASITES OF ANIMALS AND MAN
Edited by Louis H. Miller, John A. Pino, and John J. McKelvey, Jr.

Volume 94
OXYGEN TRANSPORT TO TISSUE – III
Edited by I. A. Silver, M. Erecińska, and H. I. Bicher

Volume 95
ACID PROTEASES: Structure, Function, and Biology
Edited by Jordan Tang

Volume 96
HORMONE RECEPTORS
Edited by David M. Klachko, Leonard R. Forte, and John M. Franz

Volume 97
PHARMACOLOGICAL INTERVENTION IN THE AGING PROCESS
Edited by Jay Roberts, Richard C. Adelman, and Vincent J. Cristofalo

Volume 98
IMMUNOBIOLOGY OF PROTEINS AND PEPTIDES • I
Edited by M. Z. Atassi and A. B. Stavitsky

Volume 99
THE REGULATION OF RESPIRATION DURING SLEEP AND ANESTHESIA
Edited by Robert S. Fitzgerald, Henry Gautier, and Sukhamay Lahiri

Volume 100
MYELINATION AND DEMYELINATION
Edited by Jorma Palo

Volume 101
ENZYMES OF LIPID METABOLISM
Edited by Shimon Gatt, Louis Freysz, and Paul Mandel

Volume 102
THROMBOSIS: Animal and Clinical Models
Edited by H. James Day, Basil A. Molony, Edward E. Nishizawa, and
Ronald H. Rynbrandt

Volume 103
HOMEOSTASIS OF PHOSPHATE AND OTHER MINERALS
Edited by Shaul G. Massry, Eberhard Ritz, and Aurelio Rapado

MYELINATION AND DEMYELINATION

Edited by
Jorma Palo
University of Helsinki, Finland

PLENUM PRESS • NEW YORK AND LONDON

Library of Congress Cataloging in Publication Data

Symposium on Myelination and Demyelination:
  Recent Chemical Advances, Helsinki, Finland, 1977.
  Myelination and demyelination.

  (Advances in experimental medicine and Biology; v. 100)

  "Proceedings of the Symposium on Myelination and Demyelination: Recent Chemical
Advances held in Helsinki, Finland, August 29-31, 1977."
  Includes index.
  1. Demyelination—Congresses. 2. Myelin—Congresses. I. Palo, Jorma. II. Title. [DNLM:
1. Myelin sheath—Physiology—Congresses. 2. Demyelination—Congresses. 3. Multiple
sclerosis—Etiology—Congresses. WL102.5 S989m]
RC347.S93 1977   616.8'34   78-4067
ISBN 0-306-32700-7

Proceedings of the Symposium on Myelination
and Demyelination: Recent Chemical Advances
held in Helsinki, Finland, August 29—31, 1977

© 1978 Plenum Press, New York
A Division of Plenum Publishing Corporation
227 West 17th Street, New York, N.Y. 10011

Printed in the United States of America

Preface

A satellite symposium entitled "Myelination and Demyelination: Recent Chemical Advances" was held in Helsinki from August 29 to 31, 1977, after the Sixth International Meeting of the International Society for Neurochemistry (ISN) in Copenhagen.

Myelin is a nervous tissue structure that is most suitable as a subject of biochemical investigation. It is easy to isolate in a highly purified form, is rather stable even after death, and is affected by a variety of neurological and other diseases. Its lesions are particularly important in the study of multiple sclerosis, a disease which is relatively prevalent in Finland and has therefore been of interest to a great many Finnish scientists.

The first half of this book is concerned with the biochemical composition and molecular organization of myelin, the second half with the experimental and clinical aspects of demyelination. The comments given after each of the presentations at the symposium were not recorded as such, but each author was requested to modify his or her paper accordingly.

The editing and publication of this book would not have been possible without the excellent efforts and co-operation of my wife, Mrs. L.-M. Palo, acting as general secretary and later as editorial secretary of the symposium. As Organizing Committee Chairman, I would also like to thank the members of the Committee: Dr. M. Haltia, Dr. E. Kivalo, Dr. T. Kosunen, Dr. M. Panelius, and especially Dr. P. Riekkinen, a member of the Program Committee of the ISN. I would like to express my appreciation for the financial support received from the following sponsors: Ministry of Education, The Academy of Finland, University Foundation of the University of Turku, City of Helsinki, Ciba-Geigy, Orion Corporation, Apolab, Kodak, Medilab, and Farmos Group, Ltd. Finally, I would like to thank Dr. A. Salmi for organizing the discussion on "The Possible Viral Etiology of Multiple Sclerosis" and collecting short summaries from each of the participants.

It is my hope that this book will be yet another milestone on the long road toward the final discovery of the causes of multiple sclerosis and other diseases of that all too vulnerable part of the nervous system, the myelin sheath.

Jorma Palo
Helsinki
January, 1978

Contents

Introduction and Comments   1
   Elizabeth Roboz Einstein

I. MYELINATION

Biochemistry

Biosynthesis of Myelin and Neurotoxic Factors
        in the Serum of Multiple Sclerosis
        Patients   19
   A. N. Davison and M. I. Sabri

Lipid and Fatty Acid Composition of Human
        Cerebral Myelin during Development   27
   Lars Svennerholm and Marie T. Vanier

Enzymic Studies on Glial and Neuronal Cells
        During Myelination   43
   Helmut Woelk and Rosemarie Jahrreiss

Regional Developmental and Fractional Studies on
        Myelin and Other Carbonic Anhydrases
        in Rat CNS   55
   Victor Sapirstein, Michael Trachtenberg,
   Marjorie B. Lees, and Omanand Koul

Studies of Isolated, Maintained Oligodendroglia:
        Biochemistry, Metabolism, and In
        Vitro Myelin Synthesis   71
   Shirley E. Poduslo

Studies of Myelin Proteins in Human
        Peripheral Nerve   95
   Keiichi Uyemura, Masaru Suzuki, and
   Kunio Kitamura

Protein Heterogeneity in Rat CNS Myelin
        Subfractions   117
    T. V. Waehneldt

The Preparation and Analysis of Myelin from
        Small Quantities of Central
        Nervous Tissue: Regional Studies
        of the Quaking Mouse   135
    G. E. Fagg, T. V. Waehneldt, and V. Neuhoff

Studies on the Action of Myelin Basic Protein
        (MBP) in Rat Brain   147
    C. G. Honegger, W. Bucher, and H. P. von Hahn

In Vivo Incorporation of ^{32}P into Myelin Basic
        Protein from Normal and Quaking Mice   159
    Jean-Marie Matthieu and Adrien D. Kuffer

Abnormal Myelin Maturation In Vitro: The Role
        of Cerebrosides   171
    Keith Bradbury

Retardation of Brain Myelination by
        Malnourishment and Feeding Low
        Protein Irradiated Diet in Rats   179
    Mohammad Habibulla and Hema Krishnan

                    Molecular Organization

The Molecular Architecture of Myelin:
        Identification of the External
        Surface Membrane Components   189
    Joseph F. Poduslo

Conformation of Myelin Basic Protein and
        Its Role in Myelin Formation   207
    B. E. Chapman, L. T. Littlemore, and
    W. J. Moore

Cross-Linking of Lipid Bilayers by Central
        Nervous System Myelin Basic Protein:
        Aggregation of Free and Vesicle-
        Bound Protein   221
    Ross Smith

Molecular Organisation in Central Nerve
        Myelin   235
    A. J. Crang and M. G. Rumsby

Covalent Probe Investigations with Isolated
        Central Nerve Myelin Preparations   249
    A. J. Crang, Jacqueline Grainger, and
    M. G. Rumsby

On the Accessibility and Localisation of
        Cerebrosides in Central Nervous
        System Myelin   263
    Christopher Linington and Martin G. Rumsby

II. DEMYELINATION

Experimental Demyelination

Autoimmunity in Multiple Sclerosis: Do We
        Have an Experimental Model?   277
    Marian W. Kies

Molecular Bases for the Difference in the
        Potency of Myelin Basic Protein
        from Different Species in Lewis Rats   289
    George A. Hashim

Comparison of the Rat and Mouse Encephalitogenic
        Determinants   303
    K. T. Burgess, C. C. A. Bernard, and
    P. R. Carnegie

The Action of Trypsin on Central and Peripheral
        Nerve Myelin   307
    E. H. Eylar and M. W. Roomi

Clearance of Myelin Basic Protein from Blood
        of Normal and EAE Rabbits   329
    L. F. Eng, Y.-L. Lee, K. Williams,
    G. Fukayama, B. Gerstl, and M. Kies

Basic Protein Hydrolysis in Lymphocytes of
        Lewis Rats with Experimental
        Allergic Encephalomyelitis   347
    Marion Edmonds Smith

Neutral Proteinases Secreted by Macrophages
        Degrade Basic Protein: A Possible
        Mechanism of Inflammatory Demyelination   365
    William T. Norton, Wendy Cammer, Barry R. Bloom,
    and Saimon Gordon

Virus Infection in Demyelinating Diseases 383
    V. ter Meulen and H. Wege

Early and Late CNS-Effects of Corona
        Virus Infection in Rats 395
    K. Nagashima, H. Wege, and V. ter Meulen

A Search for the "Multiple Sclerosis Virus" -
        Lack of Effect of Brain Extracts on
        Myelin Development in Chickens,
        Mice, and Rats 411
    N. R. Sims, C. C. A. Bernard, L. Horvath,
    I. R. Mackay, and P. R. Carnegie

Plasmalogenase Is Elevated in Early Demyelinating
        Lesions 423
    Lloyd A. Horrocks, Sheila Spanner, Rita Mozzi,
    Sheung Chun Fu, Robert A. D'Amato, and
    Steven Krakowka

Effect of Diphtheritic Demyelination on Axonal
        Transport in the Sciatic Nerve and
        Subsequent Muscle Changes in the
        Chicken 439
    Antony D. Kidman, William de C. Baker, and
    H. Jane Sippe

Myelin Deficiency in Experimental Phenylketonuria:
        Contribution of the Aromatic Acid
        Metabolites of Phenylalanine 453
    Yen Hoong Loo, Joseph Scotto, and
    Henryk M. Wisniewski

Peripheral Nerves as Target Tissue of the
        Immune Response in EAN. A Neurochemical
        and Morphological Study 471
    G. K. Molnár and P. J. Riekkinen

Biochemical Studies of CNS and PNS in Human and
        Experimental Diabetes 479
    J. Palo, Edith Reske-Nielsen, and P. Riekkinen

The Effect of Intoxication with Alkylnitrosourea
        Derivatives on Cerebral Myelin 487
    M Wender, Z. Adamczewska-Goncerzewicz,
    O. Mularek, and B. Zgorzalewicz

Clinical Demyelination

Cellular and Humoral Responses to Myelin
        Basic Protein in Multiple
        Sclerosis: A Dichotomy   501
    William Sheremata, Denise D. Woods, and
    Mario A. Moscarello

Cerebrospinal Fluid Myelin Basic Protein
        and Multiple Sclerosis   513
    Steven R. Cohen, Mary Jane Brune,
    Robert M. Herndon, and Guy M. McKhann

Proteolytic Activity in CSF   521
    P. T. Richards and M. Louise Cuzner

The Immune Response in Human Demyelinating
        Diseases   529
    Hans Link

Isoelectric Focusing and Isotachophoresis for
        Investigation of CSF and Serum
        Proteins in Demyelinating and
        Infectious Neurological Diseases   545
    K. G. Kjellin and Å. Siden

Proliferating Cells in Demyelinating States   561
    M. I. Reunanen, J. Ilonen, and
    K. Järvenpää

Topographic Analysis of MS and Control Brains   569
    M. Röyttä, H. Frey, P. Riekkinen,
    and U. K. Rinne

Biochemical Study on Myelin in
        Adrenoleukodystrophy   585
    Tadashi Miyatake, Toshio Ariga,
    Tetsushi Atsumi, and Yoshiaki Komiya

Metabolic Studies of Adrenoleukodystrophy   601
    Tadashi Ogino, Herbert H. Schaumburg,
    Kunihiko Suzuki, Yasuo Kishimoto, and
    Ann E. Moser

The Possible Viral Etiology of Multiple Sclerosis

Virological Aspects of Multiple Sclerosis   623
    V. ter Meulen

The Role of Viruses in the Pathogenesis of
        Demyelinative Disorder 625
   William Sheremata

Jejunal Viral Antigen in Multiple Sclerosis
        and Amyotrophic Lateral Sclerosis 627
   Albert W. Cook, Louis P. Pertschuk,
   Jagdish K. Gupta, and Dong S. Kim

Aspects of the Viral Antibody Response in
        Multiple Sclerosis 633
   B. R. Ziola and A. A. Salmi

Autoimmunity to Receptors as a Possible Cause
        of Multiple Sclerosis 637
   P. R. Carnegie

Immunoglobulins in Multiple Sclerosis 639
   Hans Link

Summary of the General Discussion on the Possible
        Viral Etiology of Multiple Sclerosis 641
   A. Salmi

Index 643

INTRODUCTION AND COMMENTS

Elizabeth Roboz Einstein

Department of Physiology, Institute of Human Development
University of California
Berkeley, California, U.S.A.

As the first speaker at the Symposium, I take the opportunity
to thank the organizers of that meeting, and especially Dr. J. Palo
and Mrs. L.-M. Palo for all the arrangements they made. I am sure
that all the participants share my sentiments when I say that it
was a privilege to meet in the historically significant and archi-
tecturally magnificent Finlandia Hall.

Because of time restrictions, the manuscripts of the presentations at the Symposium could not be made available to me. In the
process of recollecting the papers after several weeks - rather,
months - the memory plays some tricks. We tend to remember those
papers which are in the same line as our own, whether they be con-
firmatory or contradictory. My task was made easier by our editor,
Dr. J. Palo, who advised me to relate some of the papers presented
at Helsinki to my own.

My comments are restricted to four topics which appeared on
the agenda of the Symposium. I discussed these in the framework
of other important contributions in that particular field, compared different approaches to the problem, and pointedly asked
questions whose answers depend on future research. At the end I
have taken up the problem of basic versus applied research, con-
cluding that there is no strict division between the two.

I believe that a certain need is being filled with my "mini"
Introduction and Comments, since no discussion of the presentations
is being published in this volume.

With this in mind, I have narrowed down my discussion to four
studies from the Symposium, which I will discuss in light of my
own and other pertinent studies. These studies are the following:
1) Degradation of the basic protein by proteolytic enzymes.
2) Suppression of experimental allergic encephalomyelitis
   (EAE).

1

3) The presence of central nervous system (CNS) proteins in the
cerebrospinal fluid (CSF).
4) Discussion and criticism of the methods used for the determination of proteins in the CSF.

DEGRADATION OF THE BASIC PROTEIN BY PROTEOLYTIC ENZYMES

The pathological aspect involving the myelin, with emphasis on
the proteolysis, was explored by the speakers. This recalls two
events of ten years ago which were the catalysts of a number of
publications following this line. One was when we prepared the
acid proteinase from brain tissue and used it for digestion of the
purified encephalitogen, as reported in the proceedings of the
Locarno meeting held in 1967 (18). A gradual degradation of the
encephalitogen occurred, and after five hours a faster-moving, well-
defined peptide appeared. The polypeptide was later isolated and
found to be active (9).

The other event was at a symposium devoted to lipids in multiple
sclerosis (MS), when Dr. P. Riekkinen and I called attention to the
changes which occur in proteins. Before this time, only histological
reports had been published, mainly from the laboratory of Dr. C.M.W.
Adams. The results showed that the proteolytic activity is increased around active plaques of MS; however, according to Adams
(1), the histochemical detection does not permit accurate cellular
localization of the enzyme(s) involved. Later we carried out joint
research with Dr. Adams on the same MS brain specimen, divided into
half, he using histochemical and we biochemical techniques. The
values we obtained for acid proteinase and the electrophoretic
pattern revealed that the changes are most pronounced in specimen
around histologically well-defined plaques (17). The breakdown of
the basic protein may be observed in electrophoresis in the form of
polypeptides, but the extent of degradation of the basic protein is
not the same in all MS brains. In one particular MS brain the basic
protein must have been completely degraded not only in and around
the plaque, but also in the tissue distant from the plaque (17).
In another study (14), a direct numerical relationship could be
established between the basic protein and acid proteinase expressed
by an arbitrary formula. As expected, the higher the acid proteinase,
the lower the basic protein.

In the process of demyelination, the proteolytic and lipolytic
enzymes break up the myelin lamellae. No prior role in the sequence
of events has been established between the two, although there is
an indication that the lipids protect the myelin basic protein from
degradation (34). It may well be that lipolysis accelerates dis-
sociation of the myelin constituents, although this has not been
proven. Another alternative is that lipolysis and proteolysis take
place simultaneously.

At the Helsinki Symposium, the group from the University of
Turku (Röyttä et al.) extended their studies beyond acid proteinase

to acid phosphatase, 2',3'-cyclic nucleotide-3'-phosphohydrolase
(CNP-ase), β-glucuronidase and leucine aminopeptidase. All enzymes
except CNP-ase were elevated in the demyelinated area. In the
studies, the basic protein was absent in two MS cases but in three
it was present; this agrees with our overall findings. The fibrillar
acidic protein GFA was seen in plaque area. This could be expected,
since Eng et al. (23) found that this protein is increased in MS
brain, although present at a lower level in normal brain.

In EAE, degradation of the myelin has also been demonstrated.
I should interject here that many investigators do not consider EAE
a counterpart and ideal model for MS. Without getting into the pro
and contra arguments, I recall Dr. M.W. Kies´ excellent presentation
at the Symposium. According to Dr. M.W. Kies, the analogy between
EAE and MS is weak, mainly because cells and antibodies sensitized
to basic protein in the peripheral blood have not been demonstrated
in MS. We may add to this that neither has been in the CSF. Most
importantly, in contrast to EAE, where the disease can be transferred in the form of lymphoid cells taken from sensitized donors
(in this case rats), MS cannot be transferred to animals (41).

The role of proteolytic enzymes in demyelination was reported
first by histochemical studies (4, 32). As far as demyelination in
EAE is concerned, the degradation obviously depends not only on
proteolytic but also on lipolytic enzymes. There is about a 25%
increase in phospholipase A of mitochondrial origin (69). However,
lipid breakdown was not on the program, and therefore I shall not
discuss it here.

Most of the work on proteolytic enzymes in EAE has been carried
out on acid proteinase, using monkey brain (44). An increase of
acid proteinase was found parallel with decrease of basic protein,
similar to the finding in MS. Here in EAE one can assume that the
acid proteinase derives from inflammatory cells which cloister
around the blood vessels in the affected area.

Other proteinases with an optimum closer to neutral pH 6.5
have been investigated (31, 49). In the study of Govindarajan (31),
in which I participated, neutral proteinase was included besides
the acid proteinase and was assayed routinely. Seven monkey brain
specimens were used, some with HNB-treated basic protein. This
preparation injected into monkey is active (44), in contrast to
guinea-pig, where it is inactive.

The proteolytic activity in the spinal cord of rats with acute
EAE was measured (7). As control, rats injected only with Freund´s
adjuvant were used. The pH measurements were carried out through
the range 2.0-8.0 and there was higher proteolytic activity in the
lymph nodes than in the spinal cord. Smith (48) examined the lymph
nodes (both popliteal and inguinal) in rat and monkey and found an
increase in cathepsin A although there was no basic protein in the
inoculum. Since lymphoid cells are produced in vivo only by antigen
stimulation (39), the antigen here appears to be one of the components of the killed tubercle bacilli. This increase due to
Freund´s adjuvant was considered to be non-specific. In the

Helsinki presentation using a larger number of samples, Smith found
significant differences in the proteolytic activity in the lymphocytes of the lymph nodes between those injected only with Freund´s
adjuvant and those with complete inoculum. Dr. Smith concluded that
high activity at neutral pH of the lymphocytes from lymph node may
be the first step in myelin destruction of EAE.

In the context of the proteolytic enzymes, a recent publication
of Marks et al. (36) should be mentioned. Although the experiments
were extended to four different morphological variants of EAE, only
the regular EAE is pertinent to my discussion. There was a 2-3.5
fold increase in cathepsins A and C (both exopeptidases with maximal
activity at pH 5.5). Cathepsin A is a dipeptidylaminopeptidase which
removes N-terminal dipeptide from the protein. It may be mentioned
that Barrett (3) proposed that the expression "cathepsin" should be
abandoned from exopeptidases and used only for endopeptidases.

Besides CNS and the lymph nodes, another source for the proteolytic enzymes in EAE was considered by Dr. W.T. Norton at this
symposium. He proposed as a result of his studies that macrophages
activated by a reaction of T-lymphocytes with an antigen (in this
particular case with the encephalitogen) may initiate the destruction
of the myelin. This was based on the work of Unkeless et al.(60), who
reported that macrophages secrete neutral proteinase including a
plasminogen activator which is stimulated by macrophages.

The important question is: where do increased proteolytic enzymes originate in MS and EAE? We know that the normal brain contains acid proteinase besides a number of other proteases and pep-
tidases. The studies of Sammeck and Brady (46) indicate that
catabolic enzymes originate in the close vicinity of the myelin.
In inflammatory conditions these enzymes apparently may originate
elsewhere. As we learned from the papers presented at the Symposium
and from other studies, there are multiple potential sources which
supply us with proteolytic enzymes activated in EAE and MS. These
are be believed to be lysosomes endogeneous to CNS (20, 35), the
lymphocytes originating from the lymph nodes (Smith, at this Symposium), and macrophages activated by the reaction of T-lymphocytes
with the basic protein (Norton, at this Symposium).

Concerning the extent of participation of neutral and acid
proteinase in the breakdown of the basic protein, no final definite
picture emerged. The brain itself has a low level of basic proteinase and as a matter of fact, of all tissues examined, the brain has
the lowest level (59). Would this shift the emphasis to the neutral
proteinase originating outside CNS from the lymph nodes (Smith) or
from macrophages (Norton)?

A further question: is there interplay between endopeptidases
such as cathepsin D and some exopeptidases? Does it remain a limited
proteolysis? In vitro experiments using acid proteinase (cathepsin
D) prepared from nervous tissue and the basic myelin protein as
substrate, we found that after incubation for 5 h three faster-
moving peptides appear; after 24 h, only two remained without any
trace of the basic protein (20). The electrophoretic pattern in

some cases of MS brain tissue was similar to the pattern obtained
in vitro. This would suggest limited proteolysis: however, how do
we account for those admittedly rare cases where no fast-moving
polypeptides originating in the basic protein could be observed?
Do we have a limited proteolysis, or do other enzymes take over
after the endoenzyme (cathepsin D) cleaves the phenylalanine-phenyl-
alanine bond, thereby making it accessible to exopeptidases?

Complete protein hydrolysis needs the synergistic action of
different cathepsins (30). Do we have in MS a complete breakdown in
some cases and not in other cases? According to Barrett (3), who
did the most extensive work on cathepsin D, one may assume that
after an endopeptidase such as cathepsin D acts upon the protein,
the process opens the way for exopeptidases. This might be the case
in MS. Besides the assumed mobilized enzymes endoeneous to CNS,
do the enzymes from mitochondrial subfraction of the lymph nodes
(Smith) and from macrophages via plasminogen activator (Norton) work
in succession? Norton's impressive theory notwithstanding, one might
also consider direct action of proteolytic enzymes present in the
macrophages. There are a number of proteolytic enzymes in the activated macrophage (68). The authors prepared almost pure macrophages and found cathepsins A, B, C and D; nevertheless, the action
of all these enzymes produced incomplete proteolysis. The nature
of the substrate plays a decisive role in the breakdown. In the
case of the basic protein, structural features characterized by unfolded conformation make it suitable for an easy breakdown (11, 26).

Some of the questions at the Symposium have been answered. The
nature of the basic protein provides the proper target. The sources
for the enzyme are glial cells, lymphocytes and macrophages. Participation of many enzymes in degradation has been reported, but the
manner of activation has not been solved. It may well be that cAMP,
which is shown to play a definite role in regulating lysosomal,
neutral proteinase and lymphocyte reactivity, is significantly involved in the process. The answer to this question remains the task
of the future. Only then can we hope to undertake the reversal of
the myelin degradation process in MS (personal communication with
Dr. J. Clausen).

SUPPRESSION OF EAE

Of great interest is the possible adaptation of some of the
results obtained from research with experimental allergic encephalomyelitis to multiple sclerosis. Admittedly the connection of EAE
to MS is limited to similar pathology, increase of acid proteinase
and the result of this, degradation of the basic protein. There is
a resemblance of inflammatory lesions in monkey with EAE and MS.
The distinction between the two conditions may be considered a
variation in the tempo of the pathogenic process (42). The essential
difference between the two is that we cannot transfer MS with

lymphoid cells as we can EAE (41). Most importantly, in contrast
to the experimental disease, we and probably others had MS in mind
when we started the suppression experiments in animals. That EAE
may be suppressed with the basic encephalitogenic protein given
without Freund's adjuvant has been demonstrated in several laboratories (2, 13) including ours (19). Our aim was to use in suppression experiments a non-encephalitogenic protein. For this
purpose a basic protein preparation from a seven-week-old human
brain was used. This gave only partial protection; not all guinea-
pigs survived. However, those which survived and were reinjected
with the encephalitogen in Freund's adjuvant did not develop EAE.

Greater success was obtained with the basic protein modified
through tryptophan with 2-hydroxy-5-nitrobenzylbromide (HNBr) (10).
The HNBr protein, which is non-encephalitogenic in guinea-pigs,
suppressed EAE in all the treated animals (15). Similar results
were obtained by Swanborg (53). The conclusion may be reached from
these experiments that the basic protein of the myelin has two
sites: one required for activity in guinea-pig with prerequisite
of intact tryptophan in position 116 of the protein, and the other
suitable for protection where the tryptophan is not required. For
more details see review by Rauch and Einstein (43), Eylar (24) and
Carnegie and Dunkley (8).

The concept that certain residue of the protein is essential
for encephalitogenicity while others may induce a variety of immune
responses has been strengthened by the studies of Bergstrand (5, 6).
I should mention that the peptide of 9 amino acids containing
tryptophan is encephalitogenic in guinea-pig (64), yet this nonapeptide does not inhibit EAE (54). A contrasting finding related
to nonapeptide appeared in the papers of the Ukrainian Academy of
Sciences (57). According to these authors, the treatment with the
synthetic nonapeptide is effective, but only if EAE is produced with
the same peptide, and not when induced with the complete intact
encephalitogenic protein. These findings strengthen the unrelated-
ness of the encephalitogenicity and cellular immunity. Furthermore,
since in the induction and inhibition different determinants are
involved, this, according to Swanborg (55) suggests that the non-
encephalitogenic portion of the molecule induces tolerance through
stimulation of suppressor T-lymphocytes and this interferes with
the disease-inducing effector lymphocytes. This topic has been
discussed in the Symposium by Dr. Kies with a somewhat different
conclusion, namely that only the intact encephalitogenic protein is
protective. A similar opinion was expressed in less certain terms
by Eylar (25) at a Symposium on MS. When asked by one of the
participants, "Would you not want to treat human patients with an
inactivated basic protein?" his answer was, "No, because I suspect
if you modify the site of the encephalitogen, you will not get the
suppression."

An early report by Svet-Moldavskaja and Svet-Moldavskij (51)
is pertinent here: they assumed that the mature brain has two
"factors": one which induced EAE, and another which protects against

it. Svet-Moldavskij (52) went further and suggested that for the
preparation of rabies vaccine immature animals, where the myelination
is not complete (consequently is not encephalitogenic),should be
used. I do not know whether this advice has been followed by the
Soviet health authorities.

In deciding whether to use the unaltered encephalitogenic
protein or its "detoxified" form, which in this case is equivalent
with the preparation chemically made non-encephalitogenic, the
following should be considered: a number of cases with post-
encephalomyelitis due to treatment with rabies vaccine has been
reported (47). Furthermore, when I was doing research at the Pasteur
Institute in Bangkok in 1962, a large number of persons bitten by
rabid dogs were vaccinated and some developed postvaccinal encephalomyelitis and were treated at the University Hospital affiliated with
the Pasteur Institute. Blood samples were taken from 12 persons
before and after the fourteenth vaccination. The delayed hypersensitivity test was performed, with basic protein, before on 12
and after on 10 persons (2 declined to give blood after the last
vaccination). Irrespective of whether postvaccinal encephalomyelitis
developed, the skin test was positive for all vaccinated persons,
the redness disappearing in about 8 days (I myself have taken the
test). We made a short report at the World Federation in Japan
(38), the main point of which I wish to emphasize: the vaccine does
not have Freund´s adjuvant. We may assume that this is the same
compound in postvaccinal encephalomyelitis, namely the basic protein
of the myelin, and we know that the injection of this produces EAE.
We may consider rabies postvaccinal encephalomyelitis the human
counterpart of the experimental disease EAE.

We still have a long way to go before any treatment may be
proposed for MS. Besides the unsettled relationship between human
demyelinating disease and EAE which is fundamental to the problem,
the difficulty of proposing treatment with modified non-encephalitogenic basic protein is that the activity of the modified protein
depends on the species injected. The HNBr protein which is inactive
yet suppresses EAE in guinea-pig (15) is active in rabbit (16) and
monkey (42).

There are several regions with different strengths in the
encephalitogenic protein. The tryptophan region, which is most
effective in guinea-pig, may be reduced from 9 amino acid residues
to five (66). The activity also depends on the adjuvant. From a
certain peptide P2-1, 15 μg is required when the conventional
inoculum is used, but only 5 μg when B pertussis is used (65).

It is not known which amino acid residue is important for the
activity in human, and consequently which amino acid should be
blocked in order to inactivate it. At the present time, therefore,
we cannot make plans to use in some form the basic protein for
amelioration of the symptoms of MS.

THE PRESENCE OF CNS PROTEINS IN THE CSF

Studies on the blood-CSF barrier in relation to immune response have been carried out in the past (29) but not on the CNS-CSF barrier evidenced by the exit of proteins from CNS into CSF. In this context I am referring to proteins endogeneous to CNS; the gamma globulin which may be synthetized in the brain (58) does not belong to the particular group I wish to discuss here. It has been recognized that there is no "absolute" blood-CSF barrier; likewise the CNS-CSF barrier does not represent absolute, but rather graded impermeability. It was assumed that the brain-CSF barrier does not permit secretion of large molecules such as proteins into the CSF. However, one reason for not being able to detect CNS proteins in the fluid is that the fluid is constantly removed and proteins remaining in a low concentration could not be demonstrated with the techniques available in the past. (We applied as large a volume as 50 ml CSF concentrate, lyophilized, on polyacrylamide gel electrophoresis but no band indicating a CNS protein could be detected in the pattern.)

With the introduction of the very sensitive radioimmunoassay, which detects proteins at nanogram level, three CNS proteins have been recently demonstrated in the fluid. The presence of glial fibrillary acidic (GFA) protein was found in the CSF using 2-sites immunoradiometric assay (I.R.M.A.) by Eng et al. (22). Their technique consists essentially of two steps: 1) a reaction of soluble unknown antigen with a solid-phase antibody, and 2) reaction product combined with labeled antibody. The range of detection was 0.22-220 µg (nanogram). GFA is increased in plaque of MS brain but is not specific for a particular disease (23). Another protein, S-100, was also demonstrated in the fluid (37). These authors used a microcomplement fixation test with monospecific S-100 antiserum to detect the presence of S-100 in the CSF of MS and of non-neurological patients, who served as controls. The outcome was that a number of CSF from MS patients exhibited an increased level of S-100, however, in other neurological diseases with destruction of brain tissue, the fluid had also an increased level of S-100.

A recent report (12 and at the Symposium) of finding basic myelin protein in the CSF has not only theoretical but also practical significance. The basic myelin protein appeared in the CSF of MS patients. Another investigator reported a fragment of the basic protein (67). This investigator's polypeptide represents a 43-88 amino acid residue. Both investigators employed the technique of radioimmunoassay where the basic protein is labeled with [125]I. The methods described by the two groups are similar except that Cohen et al. (12) measured displacement of whole basic protein from antibody, whereas Whitaker (67) measured displacement of a fragment of 43-88 amino acid residue which he calls EP-P1. Cohen et al. used, besides immunochemical, a molecular filtration technique. The molecular sieve indicated the presence of a whole molecule. Yet the investigations leave the door open to the possibility that both

forms, the intact protein and its degradation product, are present
in the CSF. High concentration of proteolytic enzyme has been demonstrated in MS brain. It may well be that the encephalitogen,
after it is reduced in size, crosses the barrier and enters the
CSF (18). The theoretical aspect of basic protein presence in the
CSF relates to the diffusion of a large molecule from the nervous
tissue by transport across a cerebral arteriole, strengthening the
concept of relative barrier.

From a practical point of view it is important that the method
of radioimmunoassay, as applied by these investigators, may be used
for unconcentrated fluid and because it has great sensitivity, one
can measure as little as 2 µg (nanograms) of basic protein. It is
of diagnostic significance that the level rises in exacerbation and
is lower in remission. Consequently it may be considered an index
of active demyelination. In contrast, the previous diagnostic tests
for MS using cultured lymphocytes, the demyelinating properties of
the sera and the increased gamma-globulin in the CSF do not reveal
changes in the clinical conditions of the patient, however Olsson
and Link (40) reported differences. We, on the other hand, found
at the beginning of MS a continuous increase of gamma-globulin
with aggravation of the disease, but no decrease with improvement.
IgG remained high in remission (56).

Another test which also appears to be promising was reported
by Dr. M.L. Cuzner at the Symposium. It measures proteolytic enzyme
activity in the fluid. Richards and Cuzner developed a sensitive
assay for quantitative determination of proteolytic enzyme in the
CSF as measured at acid and neutral pH. First they separated the
cells from the supernatant and used for the enzyme assay ^{125}I-basic
protein as substrate. The authors found in the inflammatory cells
very active neutral proteinase, but in the supernatant the neutral
proteinase was found to be negligible. In contrast, acid proteinase was high. The authors concluded from these findings that if
neutral proteinase plays a role, it is only in the early stages of
MS. The sensitive assay for quantitative determination of proteolytic enzyme in the CSF was used for the fluid of MS patients in
stable and relapsing condition; some differences were found.

As far as the source of the proteolytic enzyme is concerned,
according to Oehmichen (39), small lymphocytes are found even in
normal CSF. In normal condition probably the enzymes could not be
measured, but in pathological conditions the lymphoid cells are
increased and as a consequence the proteolytic enzymes are elevated
and measurable, as Cuzner´s results have shown.

DISCUSSION AND CRITICISM OF THE METHODS USED FOR THE DETERMINATION
OF PROTEINS IN CSF

A few recently developed procedures for the determination of
CSF proteins have been presented in Helsinki and in larger numbers
at the Copenhagen Congress of the International Society for Neuro-

chemistry during the Workshop arranged by Dr. A. Lowenthal. The
aim of the Workshop was to improve the existing techniques for sensitivity and accuracy, and to correlate the data obtained from various
neurological diseases with the normal.

At Helsinki, separation of CSF proteins by isoelectric focusing
was discussed by Dr. Å. Sidén of Dr. K.G. Kjellin's group from Karolinska Hospital, Stockholm. Sidén presented data on the application
of electrofocusing to MS. This is a relatively new method and may
be used on polyacrylamide gel, either in cylinder, slab, or on
Sephadex thin-layer. The principle of the technique, briefly described is the following: the proteins move in pH gradients until
the isoelectric pH is reached; at this point they concentrate.
Although isoelectric focusing is considered to be one of the most
sensitive techniques for detection and separation of various proteins
(61, 62), its application to CSF is beset with some serious problems.

I had the privilege of having been invited by Dr. K.G. Kjellin
to his laboratory to observe the technique of isoelectric focusing,
in use there already for several years. (I am not listing their
contributions to the field, since their paper will be published in
this book.) Although in certain neurological diseases the visual
pattern appears to be different from normal, its interpretation is
not easy to accomplish. The gamma-globulin region consists of five
or more extremely close bands. In some but not all MS cases, the
bands vary greatly. The technical difficulty with the method is
that the carrier Ampholine, which consists of many ampholytes,
contributes to the colored background, thereby interfering with the
stained proteins. Apparently this difficulty has been overcome by
Felgenhauer, who did a special study on electrofocusing (28). Together with Dr. S.N. Vinogradow (of Wayne State University) they
synthesized ampholytes and with these non-commercial ampholytes
the colored background was reduced (63). It is important that the
artifacts be completely eliminated and afterwards the numerous protein bands be identified.

To facilitate the identification of the proteins which appear
in isoelectric focusing, the technique of crossed immunoelectrofocusing was devised by Stibler (50). It is a two-dimensional
technique combining isoelectric focusing with rocket immunoelectrophoresis. It may well be that this technique together with a recently developed one (27) which utilized a two-dimensional system
consisting of electrophoresis on agarose gel and acrylamide gel,
will reveal some proteins which do not originate in the serum. They
already found two heterogeneous groups of proteins in the normal CSF:
one characterized by low molecular weight and the other by fast-
moving proteins which are not present in the serum. However, these
techniques are still in the developmental stage and the problem of
whether these proteins originate in the CNS has not been satisfac-
torily settled.

One of the participants of the Symposium questioned the advantage of these new techniques over the more conventional methods
used presently in clinical laboratories. I myself am not convinced

that these are suitable at present as diagnostic aids. For this
purpose we need well-defined, identified proteins which can be
measured quantitatively and visualized in form of oligoclonal IgG
(33). On the other hand, there is a possibility that by the use
of these very same micro-techniques new proteins of the CSF may be
discovered.

A micro-method for the preparation of myelin, utilizing a very
small quantity of brain tissue, was presented at the Symposium by
Dr. G.E. Fagg et al. The technique has been described in detail (45)
and was found by Fagg et al. to be useful for the isolation of
myelin from discrete regions of the brain. One microgram of wet
tissue was sufficient for the separation of the proteins on polyacrylamide gel. This type of microtechnique may be useful also for
the separation of the CSF proteins.

It is not the intent of this short introductory chapter to
evaluate the various techniques available for the determination of
gamma-globulin in the CSF; however, mention should be made of a
method which not only serves the purpose of determining the gammaglobulin but also isolating it. The technique requires only 0.5 ml
of fluid and utilizes the molecular sieving action of DEAE Sephadex
A-50 on a specially constructed microcolumn (21). After the chromatographic treatment, the gamma-globulin is free of all other proteins present in the fluid.

Investigation of the CSF best illustrates an overlapping between
basic and applied research. Dr. A.N. Davison in an excellent
article (published as the Newsletter of the International Brain
Research Organization, April 1977) speaks about mission-oriented
and pure research. I am taking his statement out of context: he
was not speaking specifically about CSF but rather in general terms.
He said that in the opinion of many, applied research lacks the
scientific merit of pure research and has a lower prestige. I
believe that the statement may be applied (with great injustice,
may I add) to research on CSF. Davison goes on further, saying
that one should support and encourage those working on applied
problems. As I see it, in the case of CSF that would mean working
out procedures which may be useful not only in differential diagnosis and in helping to unravel the nature of neurological disease
but, if possible, in discovering new proteins and establishing
their physiological role. This certainly would embrace basic and
applied research.

REFERENCES

1. Adams, C.W.M., Research on Multiple Sclerosis, C. Thomas,
   Springfield, Ill. (1971).
2. Alvord, E.C., Shaw, C.M., Hruby, S. and Kies, M.W., Encephalitogen induced inhibition of experimental allergic encephalomyelitis: prevention, suppression and therapy, Ann. N. Y. Acad.
   Sci. 122 (1965) 333-345.

3. Barret, A.J., Lysosomal and related proteinases, in Proteases and Biological Control (E. Reich, D.B. Riffkin and E. Shaw, eds.) Cold Spring Harbor Conferences on Cell Proliferation, vol. 2 (1975) pp. 467-801.

4. Benetato, G.E., Gabrielescu, E. and Boros, I., The biochemistry of cerebral proteases in experimental allergic encephalomyelitis, Rev. Roumaine. Physiol. 2 (1965) 379-384.

5. Bergstrand, H., Localization of antigenic determinants on bovine encephalitogenic protein, Eur. J. Biochem. 27 (1972) 126.

6. Bergstrand, H., Encephalitogenic activity in rabbits of the C terminal region of bovine basic myelin protein. Localization to two different regions. FEBS Letts. 3 (1975) 195-198.

7. Buletza, G.F. and Smith, M.E., Enzymic hydrolysis of myelin basic protein and other proteins in CNS and lymphoid tissue from normal and demyelinating rats, Biochem. J. 156 (1976) 627-633.

8. Carnegie, P.R. and Dunkley, P.R., Basic proteins of central and peripheral nervous system myelin, Adv. Neurochem. 1 (1975) 95-135.

9. Chao, L.P. and Einstein, E.R., Isolation and characterization of an active fragment from enzymatic degradation of encephalitogenic protein, J. Biol. Chem. 243 (1968) 6050-6058.

10. Chao, L.P. and Einstein, E.R., Localization of the active site through chemical modification of the encephalitogenic protein, J. Biol. Chem. 245 (1970) 6397-6403.

11. Chao, L.P. and Einstein, E.R., Physical properties of the encephalitogenic protein: molecular weight and conformation, J. Neurochem. 17 (1970) 1121-1132.

12. Cohen, S.R., Herndon, R.M. and McKhann, G.M., Radioimmunoassay of myelin basic protein in spinal fluid, New Engl. J. Med. 293 (1976) 1455-1457.

13. Driscoll, B.F., Kies, M.W. and Alvord, E.C., Successful treatment of experimental allergic encephalomyelitis (EAE) in guinea pigs with homologous myelin basic protein, J. Immunol. 112 (1974) 392-397.

14. Einstein, E.R., Acid proteinase activity in multiple sclerotic brain in multiple sclerosis, in Multiple Sclerosis: Progress in Research (E.J. Field, T.M. Bell and P.R. Carnegie, eds.) Academic Press, New York (1972) pp. 105-110.

15. Einstein, E.R., Chao, L.P. and Csejtey, J., Suppression of EAE by chemically modified encephalitogen, Immunochemistry 9 (1972) 1013-1019.

16. Einstein, E.R., Chao, L.P., Csejtey, J., Kibler, R.F. and Shapira, R., Species specificity in response to tryptophan modified encephalitogen, Immun. Chem. 9 (1972) 73-84.

17. Einstein, E.R., Csejtey, J., Dalal, K.B., Adams, C.W.M., Bayliss, O.B. and Hallpike, J.F., Proteolytic activity and basic protein loss in and around multiple sclerosis plaques. Combined biochemical and histochemical observations, J.

Neurochem. 19 (1972) 653-662.

18. Einstein, E.R., Csejtey, J., Davis, W.J., Lajtha, A. and Marks, N., Enzymatic degradation of encephalitogenic protein, Int. Arch. Allergy 36 (1969) 363-375.

19. Einstein, E.R., Csejtey, J., Davis, W.J. and Rauch, H.C., Protective action of the encephalitogen and other basic proteins in experimental allergic encephalomyelitis, Immunochemistry 5 (1968) 567-575.

20. Einstein, E.R., Csejtey, J. and Marks, N., Degradation of encephalitogen by purified acid proteinase, FEBS Letts. 1 (1968) 191-195.

21. Einstein, E.R., Richard, K.A. and Kwa, G.B., Determination of gamma globulin in the cerebrospinal fluid by quantitative chromatography, J. Lab. Clin. Med. 68 (1966) 120-130.

22. Eng, L.F., Lee, Y.L. and Miles, L.E.M., 2-site immunoradiometric assay for glial fibrillary acidic protein in human cerebral spinal fluid, Fifth International Meeting of the ISN, Barcelona (1975) p. 302.

23. Eng, L.F., Vanderhaegen, J.J., Bignami, A. and Gerstl, B., An acidic protein isolated from fibrous astrocytes, Brain Res. 28 (1971) 351-354.

24. Eylar, E.H., Experimental allergic encephalomyelitis and multiple sclerosis, in Multiple Sclerosis Immunology, Virology and Ultrastructure (F. Wofgram, G.E. Ellison, J.G. Stevens and J.M. Andrews, eds.) Academic Press, New York (1972) pp. 449-486.

25. Eylar, E.H., Discussion to Experimental allergic encephalomyelitis and multiple sclerosis, in Multiple Sclerosis Immunology, Virology and Ultrastructure (F. Wolfgram, G.E. Ellison, J.G. Stevens and J.M. Andrews, eds.) Academic Press, New York (1972) p. 480.

26. Eylar, E.H. and Thompson, M., Allergic encephalomyelitis: the physiochemical properties of the basic protein encephalitogen from bovine spinal cord, Arch. Biochem. Biophys. 129 (1969) 468-479.

27. Felgenhauer, K. and Hagedorn, D., Evaluation of CSF proteins by two-dimensional mapping technique, Sixth International Meeting of the ISN, Copenhagen (1977) p. 338.

28. Felgenhauer, K. and Pak, S.J., Detection of ampholine patterns, Ann. N.Y. Acad. Sci. 209 (1973) 147-153.

29. Felgenhauer, K., Schliep, G. and Rapic, N., Evaluation of the blood-CSF barrier by protein gradients and the humoral immune response within the central nervous system, J. Neurol. Sci. 30 (1976) 113-128.

30. Goettlich-Riemann, W., Young, J.O. and Tappel, A.G., Cathepsin D, A and B and the effect of pH in the pathway of protein hydrolysis, Biochim. Biophys. Acta 243 (1971) 137.

31. Govindarajan, K.R., Rauch, H.C., Clausen, J. and Einstein, E.R., Changes in cathepsins B-1 and D-1, neutral proteinase and

2',3'-cyclic nucleotide 3'-phosphohydrolase activities in monkey brain with experimental allergic encephalomyelitis, J. Neurol. Sci. 23 (1974) 295-306.

32. Kerekes, M.F., Feszt, T. and Kovacs, A., Catheptic activity in the cerebral tissue of the rabbit during EAE, Experientia 21 (1965) 42-46.

33. Link, H., Oligoclonal immunoglobulin G in multiple sclerosis brain, J. Neurol. Sci. 16 (1972) 103-114.

34. London, Y. and Vossenberg, F.G.A., Specific interaction of central nervous system myelin basic protein with lipids, Biochim. Biophys. Acta 478(1973) 478-490.

35. Marks, N., Grynbaum, A. and Lajtha, A., The breakdown on myelin-bound protein by intra and extracellular proteases, Neurochem. Res. 1 (1976) 93-111.

36. Marks, N., Grynbaum, A. and Levine, S., Proteolytic enzymes in ordinary, hyperacute, monocytic and passive transfer forms of experimental allergic encephalomyelitis, Brain Res. 123 (1977) 147-157.

37. Murazio, M., Massaro, A. and Michetti, F., A brain specific protein (S-100) in cerebrospinal fluid of multiple sclerosis patients, Proc. Int. Soc. Neurochem. 6 (1977) 324.

38. Nakao, A., Einstein, E.R. and Dharmaraksa, S., Relationship between experimental allergic encephalomyelitis and rabies postvaccinal encephalomyelitis, First Asian and Oceanian Congress of Neurology, Tokyo, Japan (1962) p. 129.

39. Oehmichen, M., Cerebrospinal Fluid Cytology, W.B. Saunders, Philadelphia (1976).

40. Olsson, J.E. and Link, H., Immunoglobulin abnormalities in multiple sclerosis. Relation to clinical parameters. Exacerbations and remissions. Arch. Neurol. 28 (1973) 392.

41. Paterson, P.Y., Transfer·of allergic encephalomyelitis in rats by means of lymph node cells, J. Exp. Med. 111 (1960) 119.

42. Rauch, H.C. and Einstein, E.R., Induction and suppression of experimental allergic encephalomyelitis in the non-human primate, J. Neurol. Sci. 23 (1974) 99-116.

43. Rauch, H.C. and Einstein, E.R., Specific brain proteins: A biochemical and immunological review, in Reviews of Neuroscience, vol. 5 (S. Ehrenpreis and I.J. Kopin, eds.) Raven Press, New York (1974) pp. 283-343.

44. Rauch, H.C., Einstein, E.R. and Csejtey, J., Enzymatic degradation of myelin basic protein in central nervous system lesions of monkeys with experimental allergic encephalomyelitis, Neurobiology 3 (1973) 195-205.

45. Ruchel, R., Mesecke et al., Microelectrophoresis in continuous polyacrylamide gradient gels, Hoppe-Seyler's Z. Physiol. Chem. 355 (1974) 997-1020.

46. Sammeck, R. and Brady, R.O., Studies of the catabolism of myelin basic proteins of the rat in situ and in vitro, Brain Res. 42 (1972) 441-453.

47. Shiraki, H. and Otani, S., Clinical and pathologic features of rabies postvaccinal encephalomyelitis in man, in Allergic Encephalomyelitis (M.W. Kies and E.C. Alvord, eds.) C. Thomas, Springfield, Ill. (1965).

48. Smith, M.E. and Rauch, H.C., Metabolic activity of CNS proteins in rats and monkeys with experimental allergic encephalomyelitis, J. Neurochem. 23 (1974) 775-785.

49. Smith, M.E., Sedgewick, M. and Tagg, J.S., Proteolytic enzymes and experimental demyelination in the rat and the monkey, J. Neurochem.23 (1974) 465-471.

50. Stibler, H., Crossed immunoelectrofocusing for identification of normal and abnormal CSF proteins, J. Neurol. Sci. 32 (1977) 331-336.

51. Svet-Moldavskaja, I.A. and Svet-Moldavskij, G.J., Acquired resistance to experimental allergic encephalomyelitis, Nature 181 (1958) 1536-1537.

52. Svet-Moldavskij, G.J., Andjaparidze, O.G., Unanov, S.S. et al. Allerginfree antirabies vaccine, Bull. Wld. Hlth. Org. 32 (1965) 47-57.

53. Swanborg, R.H., Antigen-induced inhibition of experimental allergic encephalomyelitis. I. Inhibition in guinea pigs injected with non-encephalitogenic modified myelin basic protein, J. Immunol. 109 (1972) 540.

54. Swanborg, R.H., Antigen-induced inhibition of experimental allergic encephalomyelitis. Localization of an inhibitory site distinct from major encephalitogenic determinant of myelin basic protein, J. Immunol. 114 (1975) 191-194.

55. Swanborg, R.H., Maintenance of immunologic self tolerance by nonimmunogenic forms of antigen, Clin. Exp. Immunol. 26 (1976) 597-600.

56. Takuomi, H., Shoichkiro, K. et al., Changes of cerebrospinal fluid protein during course of demyelinating disease, Annual Report of the Ministry of Health and Welfare, Demyelinating Disease Research Committee, Japan 1976, p. 71.

57. Terletskaya, Ja., Belik, Ja. V., Kozulina, E.P. et al., Effectiveness of experimental allergic encephalomyelitis treatment in guinea pigs with myelin basic protein and encephalitogenic synthetic peptide, Papers of the Ukrainian Academy of Sciences, Series "B" Geology, Geophysics, Chemistry and Biology, No. 10, Kiev, 1976.

58. Tourtellotte, W.W., On cerebrospinal immunoglobulin (IgG) quotients in MS and other diseases. A review and a new formula to estimate the amount of IgG synthesized per day by the CNS, J. Neurol. Sci. 10 (1970) 279-304.

59. Umana, C.R., Protein degradation at neutral pH. Possible enzymic and control mechanisms. Proc. Soc. Exp. Biol. Med. 138 (1971) 31-38.

60. Unkeless, J.C., Gordon, S. and Reich, E., Secretion of plasminogen activator by stimulated macrophages, J. Exp. Med. 139 (1974) 834-850.

61. Vesterberg, O., Isoelectric focusing of protein, in Methods in Enzymology, vol. 22 (J. Jacoby, ed.) Academic Press, New York (1971) pp. 389-412.

62. Vesterberg, O. and Svensson, H., Isoelectric fractionation, analysis and characterization of ampholyte in natural pH gradient, Acta Chem. Scand. 20 (1966) 820-834.

63. Vinogradow, S.N., Lowenkron, S., Andonian, M.R. et al., Synthetic ampholytes for isoelectric focusing of proteins, Biochem. Biophys. Res. Commun. 54 (1973) 501-506.

64. Westall, F.C., Robinson, A.B., Caccam, J., Jackson, J. and Eylar, E.H., Essentail chemical requirement for induction of allergic encephalomyelitis, Nature 229 (1971) 22-24.

65. Westall, F.C. and Thompson, M., Encephalitogenic regions for the Lewis rat within the myelin basic protein, Immun. Commun. (1977) 13-21.

66. Westall, F.C. and Thompson, M., Further definition of the encephalitogenic region for guinea pigs, Immun. Commun. 6 (1977) 23-31.

67. Whitaker, J., Myelin encephalitogenic protein fragments in cerebrospinal fluid of persons with multiple sclerosis, Neurology 27 (1977) 911-920.

68. Wiener, E. and Curelaru, Z., The intracellular distribution of cathepsins and other acid hydrolases in mouse peritoneal macrophages, J. Reticuloendothel. Soc. 17 (1975) 319.

69. Woelk, H., Kanig, K. and Peiler-Ichikawa, Phospholipid metabolism in experimental allergic encephalomyelitis, J. Neurochem. 23 (1974) 745-750.

MYELINATION

Biochemistry

BIOSYNTHESIS OF MYELIN AND NEUROTOXIC FACTORS IN THE SERUM

OF MULTIPLE SCLEROSIS PATIENTS

A.N. Davison and M.I. Sabri

Department of Neurochemistry, Institute of Neurology
    The National Hospital
Queen Square, London WC1N 3BG, U.K.

SUMMARY

The in vitro synthesis of myelin proteins has been studied by measuring the incorporation of $[^3H]$ lysine in developing rat brain slices. This incorporation system has been used to assay potentially gliotoxic and myelinolytic agents. A reduced incorporation of the labelled amino acid into myelin proteins occurs in the presence of anti-myelin anti-serum and anti-basic protein anti-serum. Diphtheria toxin has been found to inhibit the synthesis of myelin basic and proteolipid protein in the white matter slices of developing rats. Recent experiments with serum samples from multiple sclerosis patients in exacerbation suggest the presence of a factor which interferes with the synthesis of myelin in white matter slices.

INTRODUCTION

An understanding of the mechanism of myelination and the exact role of the myelin-formative cell is of importance not only in our knowledge of membrane biosynthesis but also for an appreciation of the pathogenesis of the demyelinating diseases. Infective agents, such as viruses, may affect neurons as well as glia and it is, therefore, necessary to determine the participation of the different cell types in such diseases as multiple sclerosis (MS) (16).
    Myelination. In the central nervous system (CNS) myelination is heralded by the migration and accumulation of cytoplasmic lipid droplets and dense rough endoplasmic reticulum in the oligodendroglial cells (7). Electron microscopic studies on the

morphological sequence of myelination in the CNS and time lapse
cinematography indicate that the myelin sheath is an extension of
the glial plasma membrane (7). It seems likely that myelin precursors are synthesized by the endoplasmic reticulum and that their
cisternae, together with intermediary-fragments of the myelin formative cell membrane, can be isolated in the microsomal fraction
from developing brain. Higher microsomal phosphohydrolase activity
and increased myelin basic protein have been observed in different
areas of the developing rat brain in parallel with myelin synthesis
(2). Apparently the high molecular weight (Wolfgram) protein is
synthesized on the endoplasmic reticulum of the formative cell and
then found on the outer myelin membrane or interperiod line (Mandel,
P. et al., private communication). There is other evidence to
suggest a precursor-product relationship between the microsomal
membrane and myelin. On purification of the myelin from the developing rodent brain a "myelin-like" fraction can be isolated
which, from its composition and metabolism, may be the extended
plasma membrane of the formative cell (6, 15). Thus the compact
myelin has increased galactocerebroside content and decrease in the
high molecular-weight protein in comparison to the "myelin-like"
fraction. During development an increase occurs in the smaller
basic protein concentration and after an initial increase no change
in proteolipid protein. It is of interest that proteolipid protein
synthesis lags behind that of the basic and high molecular-weight
proteins (3). Both proteolipid protein and ethanolamine phospholipid enters myelin sequentially, after components are inserted
randomly. Myelin lipid synthesis still continues after inhibition
of protein formation (4), suggesting that, at least, sulphatide,
phosphatidyl choline and phosphatidyl ethanolamine do not enter the
myelin membrane synchronously with newly-formed protein. The subsequent metabolism of the sheath is still a matter of debate (see
for example 5, 9, 14).

    The oligodendroglial cell and myelination. It has been con-
cluded that oligodendroglial cells are the site of synthesis of
myelin, although there is only a little evidence that the glial
membrane and myelin are chemically identical. Thus, isolated human
oligodendroglia contain myelin proteins but with a higher basic:
proteolipid protein ratio than is found in myelin (10). The question still exists, therefore, as to whether or not oligodendrocytes are the only cells supporting myelin synthesis. It has been
suggested that neurons also play an important part in the biogenesis
of at least some myelin components. Studies of Giorgi et al. (8)
in the rabbit optic pathway, in which radioactive precursor was
injected directly into the eye, have been interpreted as indicating
neuronal synthesis of myelin proteins and their further transport
along the optic nerve fibres. These results have been challenged
recently by Autilio-Gambetti et al. (1) and Prensky et al.(13)
who concluded that neurons do not significantly contribute to the
synthesis of myelin proteins in rabbits. There may be an explanation for the apparent discrepancy. Myelin and oligodendrocytes

have been found in rabbit retinae (17) and the preparation in vitro
can be used to synthesize myelin basic and proteolipid proteins.
This is probably due to the presence of oligodendrocytes for rat
retinae, which do not have myelinated fibres, failed to synthesize
these myelin proteins.

EXPERIMENTAL STUDIES AND DISCUSSION

We have applied some of the techniques mentioned above to
study oligodendroglial activity by measuring myelin synthesis. The
incorporation of labelled amino acid (e.g. $[^3H]$ lysine) into the protein of white matter slices from the pons of young rat brain has
been examined. Myelin fraction proteins are then separated and
specific radioactivity determined as cpm/mg protein. Proteolipid
and high molecular weight myelin proteins had about twice the
specific activity of the encephalitogenic basic protein (Table 1)
as also reported by Pellkofer and Jatzkewitz (11) The system we
used first is sensitive to puromycin but not to aiptheria toxin.
When slices were prepared from mice fed with 0.5% cuprizone in the
diet, incorporation of $[^3H]$ lysine into myelin protein was decreased
by about 33% but incorporation into total protein was unaffected.
We were able to confirm the observation made by Pellkofer and Jatzkewitz (11) that when incubated with 5% anti-basic protein rabbits´
sera there was decreased incorporation of radioactive lysine into
myelin basic protein but in acute EAE we found inhibition of total
white matter protein synthesis. In Jatzkewitz´s experiments spinal
cord protein synthesis was not affected but the rabbits were killed
35 days after inoculation. Although in the presence of human
control serum there was reduced uptake of amino acid in comparison
to slices maintained in Ringer solution alone this inhibition could
be reproduced simply by incubation precursor with albumin (Table 2).

Table 1. In vitro incorporation of $[^3H]$ lysine into myelin proteins
in rat white matter (pons).

Myelin fraction	Standard incubation medium (cpm per mg/ protein)	+ Puromycin (1mM final con- centration)
Total white matter protein	7260	710
Myelin basic protein	2290	1145
Proteolipid protein	4350	1170
Wolfgram protein	4190	770

Table 2. Incorporation of $[^3H]$ lysine into white matter slice protein. The effects were studied of normal serum, albumin and serum from paralysed guinea pigs 13 days after administration of Freund's adjuvant and myelin basic protein (100 µg).

Medium	(N)	Cpm per mg/protein
Kreb's ringer	(3)	90,173±7,270
Normal serum	(3)	55,272±5,600
Serum (EAE)	(3)	37,714±6,100
Albumin (75 mg/ml)	(3)	50,394±1,700

Table 3. The effect of MS serum on the incorporation of $[^3H]$ lysine into rat brain slice protein. Sera were incubated for 2 h with isotope and slices of pons from developing rat brain.

	Cpm per mg/protein
Normal control serum	11,072±2,140 (3)
MS serum - remission	14,050±3,150 (3)
MS serum - relapse (same patient)	7,640±1,250 (3)

Additional inhibition of total white matter protein synthesis was found in some cases of MS patients in exacerbation (Table 3). In a patient with circulating antimyelin antibody there was marked inhibition of myelin basic and proteolipid protein, but not of total white matter protein (Table 4).

In order to minimize these non-specific effects our experiments were repeated by preincubating the slices with the test serum for 1 h. The slices were then washed and suspended in fresh Ringer containing $[^3H]$ lysine and the preparation was incubated for 2 h at 37°C. Under these conditions (Table 5) diphtheria toxin had an inhibitory effect. This may be because a finite period of incubation is necessary to allow for the polypeptide B to interact with the outer surface membrane and so facilitate the intracellular action of the second toxic moiety (polypeptide A). Pleasure et al. (12) also found an incubation period of 1 h for an inhibitory effect of diphtheria on peripheral nerve protein synthesis.

In more recent experiments, therefore, serum samples from controls and MS patients in exacerbation with added complement were routinely pre-incubated for 1 h. The slices were washed and re-suspended in Ringer with added $[^3H]$ lysine. Incorporation was measured into myelin proteins. Preliminary experiments suggest only small amounts of complement dependent antibody in some MS patients during an exacerbation which interferes with the synthesis of total white matter protein and myelin protein by the intact glia of the white matter slice. Dr. I. Grundke-Iqbal has reported that

Table 4. Effect of antimyelin antiserum on the incorporation of $[^3\text{H}]$lysine in white matter proteins. Slices from the pons of 19-day-old rats were incubated with 10% antiserum for 2 h at 37°C.

	White matter slices cpm per mg/protein		Cell free system cpm per mg/protein	
	Total proteins	Myelin basic protein + proteolipid protein	Total proteins	Myelin basic protein + proteolipid protein
Control serum	9,058±230	460	4,358±234	200
Antimyelin antiserum	11,926±150	252	3,895±330	136

myelinotoxicity remains after IgG is removed from active MS sera.
Thus the unexpected result of our initial study is that the serum
of animals with acute allergic encephalomyelitis and serum from
some but not all patients with a relapse of MS contain a factor
which inhibits incorporation of lysine into total white matter and
myelin protein. This non-selective inhibition is seen on incubation
with diphtheria and puromycin. Anti-myelin, anti-basic protein,
antiserum and cuprizone, however, appear to act selectively on
myelin protein synthesis.

Table 5. Effect of diphtheria toxin on the incorporation of $[^3H]$
lysine in developing rat brain slices. Slices from the pons of 18-
day-old rats were preincubated with toxin for 2 h at 37°C before
adding $[^3H]$lysine in the incubation medium.

	Total proteins cpm per mg/protein	Myelin proteins
Kreb's ringer (3)	50,806±2,667	208,160±4,160
Diphtheria toxin (3)	23,768±1,890	84,200±1,780

REFERENCES

1. Autilio-Gambetti, L., Gambetti, P. and Shafer, B., Glial and
   neuronal contribution to proteins and glycoproteins recovered
   in myelin fractions, Brain Res.84 (1975) 336-340.
2. Banik, N.L. and Smith, M.E., Protein determinants of myelination
   in different regions of developing rat central nervous system,
   Biochem. J. 162 (1977) 247-302.
3. Benjamins, J.A., Guarnieri, M., Miller, K., Sonneborn, M. and
   McKhann, G.M., Sulphatide synthesis in isolated oligodendroglial
   and neuronal cells, J. Neurochem. 23 (1974) 751-758.
4. Benjamins, J.A., Herschkowitz, N., Robinson, J. and McKhann,
   G.M., The effects of inhibitors of protein synthesis on incorporation of lipids into myelin, J. Neurochem. 18 (1971)
   729-738.
5. Benjamins, J.A. and Smith, M.E., Metabolism of myelin, in
   Myelin (P. Morell, ed.) Plenum Press, New York and London
   (1977) pp. 233-265.
6. Burton, R.M. and Burton, K.T., Comments on the biosynthesis of
   CNS myelin membranes: Surface proteins labelled with Iodine-
   125, in Myelination and demyelination: Recent chemical advances, Satellite symposium of the ISN, Helsinki, August 1977.
7. Davison, A.N., Myelinogenesis, in Myelin, Neurosci.Res. Prog.
   Bull. 9,Pt. 4 (1971) pp. 465-470.

8. Giorgi, P.P., Karlsson, J.O., Sjöstrand,J. and Field, E.J.,
    Axonal flow and myelin protein in the optic pathway, Nature
    New Biol. 244 (1973) 121-124.
9. Hofteig, J.H. and Druse, M.J., Metabolism of three subfractions
    of myelin in developing rats, Life Sci. 18 (1976) 543-552.
10. Iqbal, K., Grundke-Iqbal, I. and Wisniewski, H.M., Oligodendro-
    glia from human autopsied brain: bulk isolation and some chemi-
    cal properties, J. Neurochem.28 (1977) 707-716.
11. Pellkofer, R. and Jatzkewitz, H., Alteration of myelin bio-
    synthesis in slices of rabbit spinal cord by antiserum to myelin
    basic protein and by puromycin, J. Neurochem. 27 (1976) 351-
    354.
12. Pleasure, D.E., Feldmann, B. and Prockop, D.J., Diphtheria
    toxin inhibits the synthesis of myelin proteolipid and basic
    proteins by peripheral nerve in vitro, J. Neurochem. 20 (1973)
    81-91.
13. Prensky, A.L., Fujimoto, K. and Agrawal, H.C., Are myelin pro-
    teins synthesized in retinal ganglia cells? J. Neurochem. 25
    (1975) 883-887.
14. Sabri, M.I., Bone, A.H. and Davison, A.N., Turnover of myelin
    and other structural proteins in the developing rat brain,
    Biochem. J. 142 (1974) 499-507.
15. Waehneldt, T.V., Protein heterogeneity in CNS myelin subfrac-
    tions, in Myelination and demyelination: Recent chemical ad-
    vances, Satellite symposium of the ISN, Helsinki, August 1977.
16. Wisniewski, H.M., Immunopathology of demyelination in auto-
    immune diseases and virus infections, Br. Med. Bull. 33 (1977)
    54-59.
17. Wisniewski, H.M. and Bloom, B.R., Experimental allergic optic
    neuritis (EAON) in the rabbit, J. neurol. Sci. 24 (1975) 257-
    263.

LIPID AND FATTY ACID COMPOSITION OF HUMAN CEREBRAL MYELIN

DURING DEVELOPMENT

Lars Svennerholm and Marie T. Vanier[+]

Department of Neurochemistry, Psychiatric Research
Centre, University of Göteborg, St. Jörgens Hospital
S-42203 Hisings Backa, Sweden

SUMMARY

A development study of major lipid fatty acids in human brain
myelin was undertaken and compared to those in cerebral white matter
of the same region. The myelin was isolated from 23 subjects at
ages from newborn to old age. The proportions of cholesterol and
galactolipids increased in myelin during the first 6 months of age
and up to 2 years of age in cerebral white matter. During the same
periods the individual phospholipids also showed marked variations.
Serine phosphoglycerides and especially sphingomyelins increased,
and choline phosphoglycerides decreased.

The fatty acid patterns of ethanolamine phosphoglycerides (EPG)
and sphingomyelins underwent the largest maturation changes. The
proportions of saturated fatty acids in EPG diminished rapidly with
a corresponding increase of monoenoic acids. Fatty acids of the
linoleic acid series showed a peak between 4 months and 12 months
of age, and then their proportion slowly diminished to old age.
The fatty acid changes in serine phosphoglycerides were much less
pronounced than in EPG but of similar type. In sphingomyelin the
proportion of saturated long-chain fatty acids diminished while the
proportion of monoenoic acids increased - this increase continued
at least to the age of 15 years. The same fatty acid changes
occurred in cerebrosides and sulfatides as in the sphingomyelins,
but they were less pronounced.

The fatty acid changes during development were much more pronounced in white matter than in myelin but already from 1-2 years

---

[+] Present address: Department of Biochemistry, Faculty of Medicine,
University of Lyon, B.P. 12, F-69600-Oullins, France.

of age the lipids of myelin and white matter had the same patterns
- in the galactolipids from 2 months of age.

The individual variations of the lipid fatty acid patterns
were small except for at the youngest ages and the variations found
for this period might depend on the difficulties in determining the
gestational age.

INTRODUCTION

The changes in lipid composition of human myelin with maturation have been the object for a number of studies (8, 11, 19),the
most systematical by Fishman et al. (10). The fatty acid composition of adult myelin lipids has been assayed by Clausen and Berg-
Hansen (4) and by Woelk and Borri (31). No previous systematic
study of the fatty acid composition of the major myelin lipids
during maturation is on record, although such data would be very
valuable for the study of various metabolic, inflammatory or
nutritive diseases in childhood. The most frequently quoted investigation on myelin fatty acids is that by O'Brien and Sampson
(20) but their material consisted of myelin from only four brains.
The present study of myelin lipids completes a series of papers
from this laboratory reporting the fatty acid composition of the
major lipid classes in normal human brain and their variation with
age (22, 25-29).

EXPERIMENTAL

Tissues. Human brains from 23 subjects, from newborn to old
ages, were obtained from the Department of Forensic Medicine within
48 h of death. Most of the infants had died a sudden death of unknown cause and the children and adults in accidents or from acute
respiratory or cardiac diseases. None of the subjects had any
previous history of neurologic or psychiatric disease and all had
normal body and brain weights. The brain had no gross abnormalities.
Cerebral white matter was dissected from the semiovale centre from
all brain samples, and from cerebellum and brain stem in selected
individuals. Part of the tissue was spared for direct lipid analysis, the remaining being used for myelin isolation, performed in
most cases without any freezing of the sample.

Isolation of myelin. Varying amounts of cerebral white matter
were used as starting material according to the age: 30 g from new-
borns, 10-15 g between 1-3 months of age, 5 g between 3-6 months of
age, 2 g at 12 months of age, and 1 g from older children and adults.
Norton's procedure (16) as described by Norton and Poduslo (17) was
used. A 5% homogenate of white matter was used from neonatal up to
3-month-old brains and a 1% homogenate from older brains. All preparations were performed in a Spinco L 65 B ultracentrifuge, using
a swinging bucket SW 27.2 rotor. Portions of 20 ml homogenate

in 0.32 M sucrose were layered over 18 ml 0.85 M sucrose on each of
six tubes and the tubes centrifuged at 75,000 g for 30 min. In
only one respect was the original procedure modified: the final
myelin pellet was washed in 0.156 M KCl instead of water to remove
the sucrose.

    Quantitative determinations. The lipids were extracted with
chloroform-methanol 1:1, v/v (30). On the lipid extract, phosphorus
was assayed with a modified Fiske-Subbarow method (27), cholesterol
with a ferric chloride method (5) and galactolipids with an orcinol
procedure (24). Cerebrosides and sulfatides were separated by thin-
layer chromatography on Silica Gel G with chloroform-methanol-water-
acetic acid 70:30:3:1, v/v, as developing solvent. The two fractions
were scraped off and their galactose content measured.The determination of the molar percentage of individual phospholipids was performed after separation by thin-layer chromatography (25) by phosphorus assay on each fraction. Ethanolamine phosphoglycerides
plasmalogens were assayed by a procedure adopted in our laboratory
(14). All fatty acid determinations were performed by gas-liquid
chromatography of the methyl esters on 15% diethylene-glycolsucci-
nate polyester (DEGS) columns on a Perkin-Elmer chromatograph model
900. The methyl esters of the phosphoglycerides were prepared by
alkaline methanolysis (25) and those of the sphingolipids by acidic
methanolysis (26). All values were expressed in relative molar
concentrations. The composition of the major lipid classes of
myelin was expressed as the ratio component: total phospholipids.

    Protein was assayed with the Lowry procedure (15) with serum
albumin as standard, and with a gravimetric method: the myelin was
lyophilized and dried to constant weight over phosphorus pentoxide.
After hydration of the myelin, the lipids were extracted by chloroform-methanol and the sample processed as described by Norton and
Poduslo (17).

                              RESULTS

    Myelin was at first studied from three regions, the semiovale
centre of cerebrum, the white matter of cerebellum and the brain
stem. As illustrated by some of the findings obtained in a 2-
month-old infant (Table 1), myelin from the semiovale centre is
much less mature with regard to lipid composition and fatty acid
patterns than myelin from either of the two other areas. Since
the onset and rate of myelination vary in different areas of the
brain, any developmental study must be based on analysis of samples
from similar anatomical regions, and we thus selected myelin from
the semiovale centre for systematical investigation.

    Protein determinations. The total protein concentration was
determined with the Lowry method in portions of all the myelin
specimens, but repeated analysis revealed a range of variation
often exceeding 10%, and the procedure was therefore abandoned
in favour of a gravimetric determination. The protein content of

Table 1. Lipid composition and fatty acid patterns of ethanolamine
phosphoglycerides in myelins of semiovale centre of cerebrum, cerebellum and brain stem in a 2-month-old infant.

	Semiovale centre	Cerebellum	Brain stem
		Lipid ratio	
Lipid			
Phospholipids	1.00	1.00	1.00
Cholesterol	0.75	0.87	0.90
Cerebrosides	0.17	0.33	0.33
Fatty acids of ethanolamine			
phosphoglycerides		Molar percentage	
16:0	7.0	6.7	6.4
18:0	25.2	7.7	7.3
18:1	9.6	30.4	30.1
20:1	0.4	6.7	7.6
20:3(n-6)	1.6	3.5	3.8
20:4(n-6)	16.6	12.2	11.7
22:4(n-6)	15.0	17.9	20.1
22:5(n-6)	5.4	2.0	2.4
22:6(n-6)	16.7	7.9	6.6

myelin was measured by the latter method in brains ranging from 2
months to 46 years of age. Total protein constituted 29 to 32%
of the dry myelin weight, and did not vary significantly with age.

Lipid compositions. Changes with age of the lipid composition
of human cerebral myelin are shown in Fig. 1 a, and corresponding
results obtained for white matter from the same brain region in
Fig. 1 b. All values are given in molar ratios, phospholipid being
taken as unit.

The same trends were observed in myelin and in white matter,
but they followed different courses. In the early phases of myelination, the proportion of galactolipids and that of cholesterol were
much higher in myelin than in white matter, but already from 12
months of age they were only slightly higher in myelin. The
galactolipid/phospholipid ratio continued to be higher in myelin
than in white matter until the age of 20 years, after which age
no difference was observed. The cholesterol content of myelin
exceeded that of white matter also at the highest ages. The lipid
composition reached the adult pattern at about 5 years of age and
the mean phospholipid/cholesterol/cerebroside/sulfatide ratio in
adult myelin was 1.00/1.23/0.44/0.12 compared to 1.00/0.86/0.18/
0.07 at the age of 10 days and 1.00/1.00/0.32/0.09 at 2.5 months
of age.

The proportions of the individual phospholipid classes of
myelin changed with age. Choline phosphoglycerides diminished from
35% to 25% (molar percentage of total phospholipid), ethanolamine
phosphoglycerides remained constant around 40%, serine phospho-

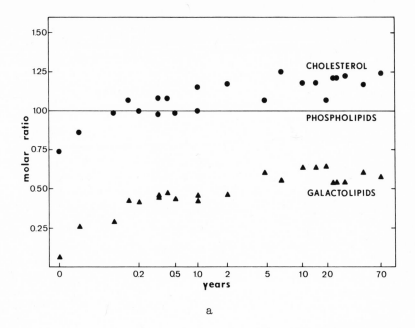

a

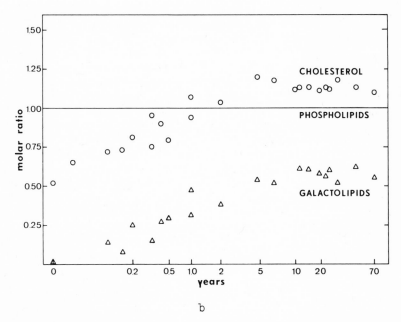

b

Fig. 1.   The molar ratio of cholesterol ● ○, phospholipids, and galactolipids ▲ △ , in cerebral myelin (a) and white matter (b) with ageing.

glycerides increased from 14 to 18%, and sphingomyelin from 10% to
18%. The adult pattern was reached at about five years of age.
The percentage of ethanolamine phosphoglycerides in plasmalogen form
was determined in a small number of brains, and constituted 78-82%
after 2 years of age.

Fatty acid compositions of phosphoglycerides. Among the
phosphoglycerides, the fatty acid patterns of the ethanolamine
phosphoglycerides showed the largest changes (Fig. 2). The proportion of saturated fatty acids diminished rapidly, and there was
a corresponding increase of the monoenoic fatty acids. There were
only two major saturated fatty acids, stearic and palmitic acids.
The latter was constant, while stearic acid diminished from 30%
to less than 10%, a level reached by 5 years of age. The monoenoic
acids continued to increase throughout life, oleic acid from 25%
and eicosaenoic acid from 4% to 9%. A direct inverse relation
between saturated and monoenoic acids was modified by the changes
in the proportion of polyunsaturated fatty acids. Already from 2
months of age, myelin contained only about 5% of fatty acids of
the linolenic acid series, but the fatty acids of the linoleic acid
series constituted a large fraction. The latter group of fatty
acids reached a peak around the age of one year, then a constant
decrease was observed. The proportion of arachidonic acid, 20:4
(n-6), diminished from 15% at birth to 8-9% from puberty. The predominating polyunsaturated fatty acid of myelin and white matter,
22:4(n-6), increased from 15% at birth to a peak of about 25%
between 4 months and 12 months of age, whereafter it diminished to
17-19% in myelin of adult cerebrum. Docosapentaenoic acid, 22:5
(n-6), constituted about 2% in myelin from the youngest children,
but diminished to less than 1% after one year of age.

Similar fatty acid changes occurred in the ethanolamine
phosphoglycerides from white matter, although their timing was delayed: the pattern already observed after 2 months of age in myelin
was not reached before the age of 1-2 years in the white matter.
The fatty acid compositions of ethanolamine phosphoglycerides were
similar in myelin and in white matter, but the proportion of
monoenoic acids was higher and that of saturated acids lower in
myelin than in white matter.

The fatty acid patterns of the serine phosphoglycerides (Fig.
3) underwent similar but less pronounced changes than those of
ethanolamine phosphoglycerides. The most prominent event was the
increase of monoenoic acids, which involved both 18:1 and 20:1,
although the latter only reached a proportion of 5%. The increase
of monoenoic acids continued at least to 30 years, while the
saturated and polyunsaturated fatty acids decreased. There was
only a small diminution of the proportion of saturated fatty acids,
but the polyunsaturated fatty acids diminished from 15% to less
than 8%. The fatty acids of the linoleic acid series, 20:4(n-6)
and 22:4(n-6) both decreased to about the same extent, while the
proportion of fatty acids of the linoleic acid series was small
(approx. 1-2%) and constant throughout the period studied.

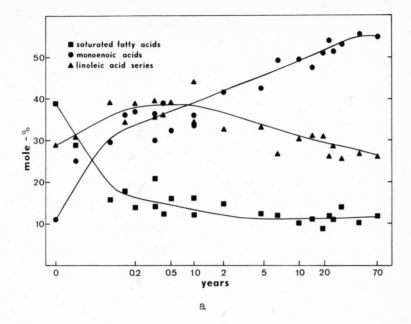

a

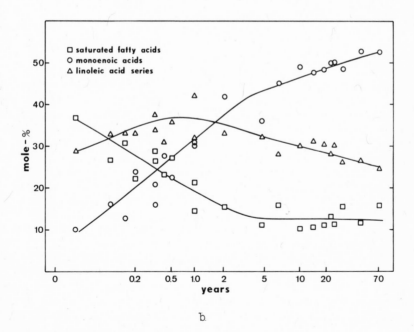

b

Fig. 2.   The fatty acid composition of ethanolamine phosphoglycerides of cerebral myelin (a) and white matter (b).

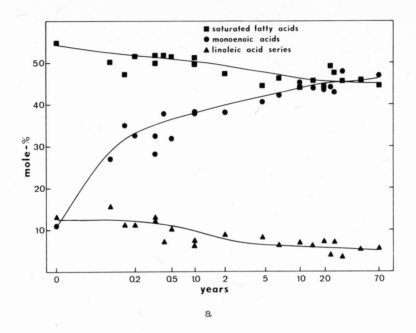

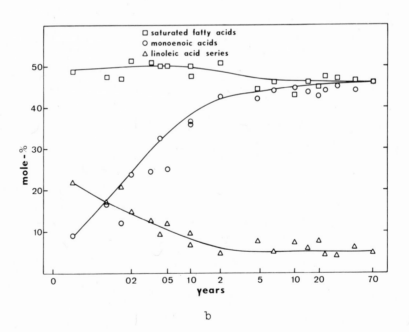

Fig. 3. The fatty acid composition of serine phosphoglycerides of cerebral myelin (a) and white matter (b).

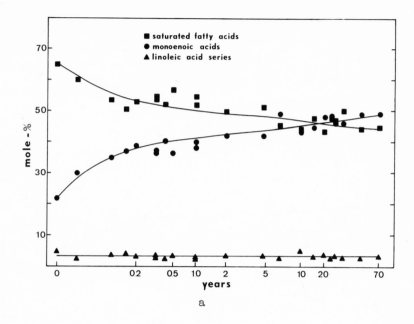

a

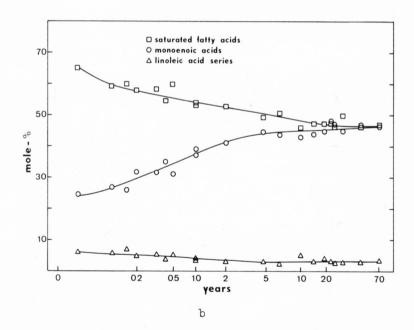

b

Fig. 4. The fatty acid composition of choline phosphoglycerides of cerebral myelin (a) and white matter (b).

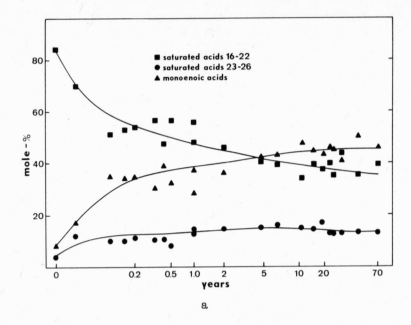

a

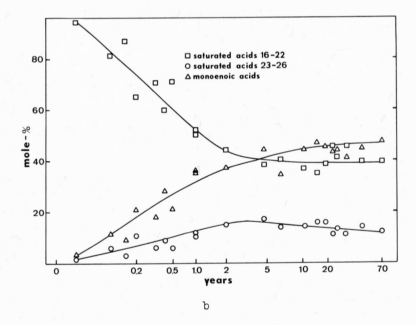

b

Fig. 5.   The fatty acid composition of sphingomyelins of cerebral myelin (a) and white matter (b).

From ten years of age there was no significant difference in the fatty acid patterns of myelin and white matter.

In the choline phosphoglycerides (Fig. 4), the proportions of polyunsaturated fatty acids were small and constant during the whole period, and the proportions of saturated fatty acids diminished to the same extent as those of monoenoic acids increased. These changes continued also at the highest ages. Myelin had during the whole period significantly higher proportion of monoenoic acids than white matter.

<u>Fatty acid compositions of sphingolipids.</u> The other lipid, besides ethanolamine phosphoglycerides, which varied substantially in its fatty acid pattern during development, and also showed large differences between cerebral white matter and myelin during an early period, was sphingomyelin (Fig. 5). In myelin the proportion of saturated long-chain (C_{16}-C_{22}) fatty acids diminished, while that of the saturated very long-chain (C_{23}-C_{26}) fatty acids was constant. The proportion of monoenoic fatty acids increased from the newborn to 45% in the adults – the increase continued at least to puberty. Only three monoenoic acids constituted more than 1%: 24:1, 25:1, and 26:1. The highest proportion of 24:1 and 26:1 was reached at about 15 years of age, but 25:1 was higher in the two oldest brains, where its proportion was 7%. From two years of age the fatty acid compositions were the same in the sphingomyelins of white matter and of myelin.

The fatty acid patterns of cerebrosides (Fig. 6) and sulfatides were the same in cerebral white matter and in myelin except for the children below 2 months of age. Before this age the proportion of 18:0 was slightly higher, and 24:0 slightly lower, in white matter than in myelin. The same fatty acid changes with age occurred in cerebrosides and sulfatides. The proportion of saturated fatty acids diminished and that of monoenoic acids increased. These changes continued to at least puberty and the proportions of 25:1, 23h:1, and 25h:1 increased to the oldest ages studied.

DISCUSSION

Previous investigations have shown rather large changes in the lipid composition of brain myelin isolated from various animal species during development (1-3, 6, 7, 9, 12, 13, 16, 18). Although differences in the magnitude of the changes have been found, all published results agree qualitatively, showing an increase in the relative proportion of the galactolipids and a decrease in that of the phospholipids. The content of cholesterol has been considered to increase in several studies (9, 12), but was reported to be constant by Norton and Poduslo (18). Earlier studies of myelin isolated from human brain (8, 11, 19, 21) have given incomplete and somewhat controversial data because of a limited number of brains studied and a less advanced technique for the isolation of myelin.

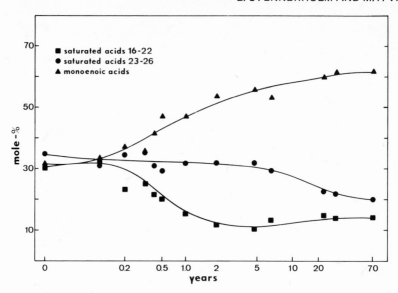

Fig. 6.   The fatty acid composition of cerebrosides in cerebral myelin.

Fishman and coworkers'(10) study of human myelin showed results which differed considerably from those obtained in the previous investigations of myelin of small animals. They studied eleven brains ranging from neonatal to adult age, and found no significant change in the relative concentration of cholesterol and galactolipids and only a slight decrease of phospholipids in myelin during maturation.

Our results for the lipid composition of cerebral myelin are very similar to those reported by Fishman et al. (10) except for their results for the newborn brain. Fishman et al. (10) considered their results not to show any significant change in the relative concentration of cholesterol and galactolipids but a modest decrease of phospholipids. We have studied a larger material of myelin and it is obvious from our study that the proportions of cholesterol and particularly galactolipids increase during maturation - the increase being most pronounced before 3-months of age. Nevertheless, the lipid composition of the myelin from the newborn brain found by them is dubious. They might have isolated the myelin from a more mature area than the frontal lobe, since we have confirmed in our human brains the previous results in rat brain that chemical maturity begins in the hindbrain and proceeds rostrally (21).

Despite the small discrepancies discussed, the values for the lipid content of the myelin were very small (67%) and the proportion of the major phospholipid classes was almost identical in the two studies. Therefore, we consider that the fatty acid patterns presented here were obtained on myelin samples with a representative composition of major lipids for the age.

There has been a serious lack of data on the normal fatty acid composition of the myelin lipids during development. The values reported by O'Brien and Sampson (20) on myelin from a 10-month-old infant, two children aged 6 and 9 years and an adult have long been used. Very large variations between the fatty acid patterns of the lipids isolated from white matter and myelin as well as from the different brains – especially the two children – were found. In our study, the fatty acid compositions of the different lipids during maturation showed only moderate changes. Ethanolamine phosphoglycerides and sphingomyelins varied most, and are therefore the most sensitive indicators of delayed or disturbed myelination. A direct correlation was always observed between the findings in white matter and myelin during infancy, and it was remarkable that already from two years of age, white matter and myelin had similar fatty acid patterns.

This similarity between the findings in white matter and myelin implied that the moderate but definite changes of the fatty acid compositions previously found in white matter (22, 24, 26) were also observed in myelin after the major lipid classes had reached an adult pattern, i.e. after 5 years of age. Age changes of the same type have earlier been reported for phosphoglycerides and sphingolipids in myelin of human (13) and monkey brain (23).

In ethanolamine phosphoglycerides the proportion of monoenoic acids continued to increase on the expense of the polyunsaturated fatty acids of the linoleic acid series and in the sphingolipids on the expense of the very long chain (C_{23}-C_{26}) saturated fatty acids. An increased proportion of monoenoic acids with ageing was also found in the other phosphoglycerides and glycosphingolipids of human myelin.

REFERENCES

1. Agrawal, H.C., Banik, N.L., Bone, A.H., Davison, A.N., Mitchell, R.F. and Spohn, M., The identity of a myelin-like fraction isolated from developing brain, Biochem. J. 126 (1970) 635-642.
2. Agrawal, H.C., Trotter, J.L., Mitchell, R.F. and Burton, R.M., Criteria for identifying a myelin like fraction from developing brains, Biochem. J. 136 (1973) 1117-1119.
3. Banik, N.L. and Davison, A.N., Enzyme activity and composition of myelin and subcellular fractions in the developing rat brain, Biochem. J. 115 (1969) 1051-1062.
4. Clausen, J. and Berg-Hansen, I., Myelin constituents of human central nervous system, Acta Neurol. Scand. 46 (1970) 1-17.
5. Crawford, N., An improved method for the determination of free and total cholesterol using the ferric chloride reaction, Clin. Chim. Acta 3 (1958) 357-367.

6. Cuzner, M.L. and Davison, A.N., The lipid composition of rat brain myelin and subcellular fractions during development, Biochem. J. 106 (1968) 29-34.

7. Dalal, K.B. and Einstein, E.R., Biochemical maturation of the central nervous system I. Lipid changes, Brain Res. 16 (1969) 441-451.

8. Eng, L.F., Chao, F.-C., Gerstl, B., Pratt, D. and Tavaststjerna, M.G., The maturation of human white matter myelin. Fractionation of the myelin membrane proteins, Biochemistry 7 (1967) 4455-4465.

9. Eng, L.F. and Noble, E.P., The maturation of rat brain myelin, Lipids 3 (1968) 157-162.

10. Fishman, M.A., Agrawal, H.C., Alexander, A., Golterman, J. Martenson, R.E. and Mitchell, R.F., Biochemical maturation of human central nervous system myelin, J. Neurochem. 24 (1975) 689-694.

11. Gerstl, B., Eng, L.F., Hayman, R.B. and Tavaststjerna, On the composition of human myelin, J. Neurochem. 14 (1967) 661-670.

12. Horrocks, L.A., Composition of mouse brain myelin during development, J. Neurochem. 15 (1968) 483-488.

13. Horrocks, L.A., Composition and metabolism of myelin phosphoglycerides during maturation and aging, Progress in Brain Res. 40 (1973) 383-395.

14. Karlsson, I., Effects of different dietary levels of essential fatty acids on the fatty acid composition of ethanolamine phosphoglycerides in myelin and synaptosomal plasma membranes, J. Neurochem. 25 (1975) 101-107.

15. Lowry, O.H., Rosebrough, N.J., Farr, A.L. and Randall, R.J., Protein measurement with the Folin phenol reagent, J. Biol. Chem. 193 (1951) 265-275.

16. Norton, W.T., Recent developments in the investigations of purified myelin, in Adv. Exp. Med. Biol., Chemistry and brain development (R. Paoletti and A.N. Davison, eds.) Vol. 13 (1972) Plenum Press, New York, pp. 327-337.

17. Norton, W.T. and Poduslo, S.E., Myelination in rat brain: method of myelin isolation, J. Neurochem. 21 (1973) 749-757.

18. Norton, W.T. and Poduslo, S.E., Myelination in rat brain: changes in myelin composition during brain maturation, J. Neurochem. 21 (1973) 759-773.

19. O'Brien, J.S. and Sampson, E.L., Lipid composition of the normal human brain: gray matter, white matter and myelin, J. Lipid Res. 6 (1975) 537-566.

20. O'Brien, J.S. and Sampson, E.L., Fatty acid and fatty aldehyde composition of the major brain lipids in normal human gray matter, white matter and myelin, J. Lipid Res. 6 (1965) 545-551.

21. Smith, M.E., A regional survey of myelin development: some compositional and metabolic aspects, J. Lipid Res. 14 (1973) 541-551.

22. Ställberg-Stenhagen, S.K. and Svennerholm, L., Fatty acid com-
    position of human brain sphingomyelins: normal variation with
    age and changes during myelin disorders, J. Lipid Res. 6 (1965)
    146-155.
23. Sun, G.Y. and Samorajski, T., Age differences in the acyl group
    composition of phosphoglycerides in myelin isolated from the
    brain of the rhesus monkey, Biochim. Biophys. Acta 316 (1973)
    19-27.
24. Svennerholm, L., The quantitative estimation of cerebroside
    in nervous tissue, J. Neurochem. 1 (1956) 42-53.
25. Svennerholm, L., Distribution and fatty acid composition of
    phosphoglycerides in normal human brain, J. Lipid Res. 9
    (1968) 570-579.
26. Svennerholm, L. and Ställberg-Stenhagen, S., Changes in the
    fatty acid composition of cerebrosides and sulfatides of
    human tissue with age, J. Lipid Res. 9 (1968) 215-225.
27. Svennerholm, L. and Vanier, M.-T., The distribution of lipids
    in the human nervous system II. lipid composition of human
    foetal and infant brain, Brain Res. 49 (1972) 458-468.
28. Svennerholm, L. and Vanier, M.-T., The distribution of lipids
    in the human nervous system III. Fatty acid composition of
    phosphoglycerides of human foetal and infant brain, Brain Res.
    50 (1973) 341-351.
29. Svennerholm, L. and Vanier, M.-T., The distribution of lipids
    in the human nervous system IV. Fatty acid composition of major
    sphingolipids of human infant brain, Brain Res. 55 (1973)
    413-423.
30. Vanier, M.-T., Holm, M., Öhman, R. and Svennerholm, L.,
    Developmental profiles of gangliosides in human and rat brain,
    J. Neurochem. 18 (1971) 581-592.
31. Woelk, H. and Borri, P., Lipid and fatty acid composition of
    myelin purified from normal and MS brains, Europ. Neurol. 10
    (1973) 250-260.

ENZYMIC STUDIES ON GLIAL AND NEURONAL CELLS DURING MYELINATION

Helmut Woelk and Rosemarie Jahrreiss

Einheit für Neurobiochemie der Universitäts-
Nervenklinik Erlangen, 852 Erlangen, and
Universitäts-Nervenklinik der Universität des
Saarlandes
665 Homburg/Saar, G.F.R.

SUMMARY

The formation of ethanolamine plasmalogen from labelled
1-alkyl-2-acyl-sn-glycero-3-phosphorylethanolamine was studied in
neurons and glial cells of the developing rat brain. It was found
that the conversion of the ether to the enol-ether bond of the
1-alkyl moiety by the neuronal and glial desaturase system requires
unsaturated fatty acids at the 2 position of the substrate. There
is almost no difference between the activity of the neuronal and
glial desaturase during the period of active myelination, whereas
the neuronal cell fraction of the adult rats displays a threefold
higher enzyme activity as compared to the glial cells.

Evidence for the involvement of a microsomal electron transport system in the enzymic conversion of alkylacyl-glycero-3-
phosphorylethanolamine to ethanolamine plasmalogen was obtained
by using specific antibodies against NADH-cytochrome b_5 reductase.
Cytochrome b_5 stimulated the biosynthesis of ethanolamine
plasmalogen.

Abbreviations used:
GPC, sn-glycero-3-phosphorylcholine; GPE, sn-glycero-3-phosphoryl-
ethanolamine; GPS, sn-glycero-3-phosphorylserine.

INTRODUCTION

Experimental evidence has been forwarded during the last years for marked differences in phospholipid metabolism between glial- and neuronal cell-enriched fractions. The neuronal cell bodies were found to possess a much higher rate of base-exchange for both serine and ethanolamine than the glial cell-enriched fraction (6) and Freysz et al. (5) showed in their extensive investigation on the kinetics of the biosynthesis of phospholipids in neurons and glial cells, isolated from rat brain cortex, that neuronal phospholipids had a faster turnover than glial phospholipids. Recently, we obtained indirect evidence for a faster turnover of glycerophosphatides in neurons than in glial cells, since neurons contained a considerably higher phospholipase A_1 and A_2 activity when compared to the glial cell-enriched fraction (11).

There is only little information on the mechanism of the biosynthesis of ethanolamine plasmalogen (1-alk-1'-enyl-2-acyl-sn-glycero-3-phosphorylethanolamine) by brain cells. In the brain tissue ethanolamine plasmalogen reaches particularly high values accounting for approximately 80% of total ethanolamine phosphatides in the myelin sheath. Investigation of plasmalogen biosynthesis in intact cells has led to conflicting opinions regarding the aliphatic precursor of the alkenyl moiety. The postmitochondrial fraction of Ehrlich ascites cells and preputial gland tumors can synthesize ethanolamine plasmalogens from the long chain fatty alcohols and dihydroxyacetone phosphate (10) or 1-alkyl-2-acyl-sn-glycero-3-phosphate (1). It appears to be well established that one mechanism by which 1-alk-1'-enyl-2-acyl-sn-glycero-3-phosphorylethanolamine can be formed involves dehydrogenation of the 1-alkyl moiety and that cytochrome b_5 participates into the reaction (8).

EXPERIMENTAL

Preparation of glia and neurons from rat and rabbit brain.
The neuronal and glial fractions were prepared from young and adult Wistar rats and from white rabbits weighing about 1,5 kg. The animals were anaesthetized with sodium pentobarbitone and killed by intracardiac perfusion of Ringer solution. The whole brain was removed quickly, weighed and sliced. The procedure employed for the preparation and identification of neurons and glia was essentially by the methods of Blomstrand and Hamberger (2, 3) and Goracci et al. (6) as indicated elsewhere (11).

The neuronal fraction contained more than 90% of neuronal cell bodies, freed for the greater part of their axonal processes and with very little contamination by glial cells. The glial cell-enriched fraction contained about 90% glial cells. Endothelial cells and free nuclei were the main contaminants of both cell

fractions. The purity of the neuronal and glial cell suspensions
was further assessed by using the base-exchange enzymic system as
a marker for the neuronal cell bodies (6). Using serine and
ethanolamine as nitrogeneous bases, neuronal/glial ratios of about
3 to 4 were found for the base-exchange activity.

Oligodendroglia were obtained by the method of Poduslo and
Norton (9).

Subcellular fractionation of the cell-enriched preparations.
Neuronal and glial microsomes were obtained as described in detail
by Goracci et al. (6). The microsomes displayed 88% of the glucose-
6-phosphatase activity and 91% of the NADPH:cytochrome c oxidore-
ductase activity of the whole cell homogenate.

Substrates. 1-[^{14}C]alkyl-2-acyl-GPE (substrate A) was prepared
from the brain phospholipids after intracerebral injection of
1-[^{14}C]hexadecanol (52 µCi/µmole/animal) into 14 day-old-rats.
Twenty-four hours after the administration of the labelled alcohol,
the animals were sacrificed and the brain ethanolamine phosphoglycerides purified. In order to remove the 1-alk-1'-enyl portion,
the ethanolamine phosphoglycerides were subjected to mild acid
hydrolysis according to a modified Dawson's procedure (4). 1,2-
Diacyl-GPE was removed with the use of purified lipase from porcine
pancreas. The method is based on the selective deacylation by
lipase action at the 1 position of the 1,2-diacyl compounds of
naturally occurring phosphatide mixtures, containing 1,2-diacyl-,
alkenyl-acyl- and alkylacyl-glycerophosphatides. The final preparation of 1[^{14}C]alkyl-2-acyl-GPE (specific activity of 4,2 µCi/
µmole) was obtained by silicic acid or Florisil column chromatography.

[^{14}C]-labelled 1-alkyl-2-acyl-GPE (substrate B) was prepared
from 14-day-old rats after intracerebral injection of 1-[^{14}C]
acetate. Twenty-four hours after the administration of the labelled
precursor the rats were sacrificed, the brain lipids extracted and
the ethanolamine phosphoglycerides purified. The 1-alk-1'-enyl-2-
acyl portion (ethanolamine plasmalogen) of the [^{14}C]-labelled
ethanolamine phosphoglycerides was transformed into the corresponding
acylalkyl-compound by catalytic hydrogenation. In order to remove the
the remaining plasmalogens, the ethanolamine phosphoglycerides were
subjected to mild acid hydrolysis according to a modified Dawson's
procedure (4). The phosphoglyceride mixture, containing 1,2 diacyl-
and 1-alkyl-2-acyl-GPE, was purified by means of column chromatography on Florisil.

1-[^{14}C]alkyl-GPE was obtained by silicic acid column chromatography after removing the fatty acids from the 2 position of
1-[^{14}C]alkyl-2-acyl-GPE with phospholipase A_2 from Naja naja venom.
The labelled 1,2-diacyl-, 2-acyl-1-alk-1'-enyl- and 2-acyl-1-alkyl
glycerophosphatides, used for the measurement of the phospholipase
A_2 activity, were prepared and checked as described previously (13).
Hydrolysis of the phosphoglycerides, which differed in the radical
at the 1 position and were labelled at the 2 position with different
fatty acids, by phospholipase A_2 from naja naja venom, showed that
the radioactivity was almost exclusively recovered in the fatty

acids freed from the substrates, indicating that specific incorporation of the labelled fatty acids into the 2 position of the phosphoglycerides had occurred. Hydrolysis of the 1,2-diacyl-glycero-
phosphatides, labelled at the 1 position, by phospholipase A_2 from
crotalus atrox venom, showed that 94-96% of the radioactivity was
recovered in the lyso-compounds, indicating that specific incorporation of the labelled fatty acids into the 1 position of the
lyso derivatives had occurred.

RESULTS

The formation of ethanolamine plasmalogen from $1-[^{14}C]$ alkyl-
2-acyl-sn-GPE (prepared from brain tissue after injection of
$1-[^{14}C]$ hexadecanol) and $[^{14}C]$-labelled 1-alkyl-2-acyl-GPE (prepared from brain tissue after injection of $[^{14}C]$ acetate and catalytic
hydrogenation of the plasmalogen portion) has been studied in
neurons and glial cells of the developing rat brain (Table 1).
As can be seen from Table 1, $1-[^{14}C]$ alkyl-2-acyl-GPE is a much
better substrate for the formation of ethanolamine plasmalogen
by the neuronal and glial desaturation system than the corresponding hydrogenated glycerophospatide. It appears that the conversion
of the ether to the enol-ether bond of the 1-alkyl moiety by the
neuronal and glial desaturation system requires unsaturated fatty
acids at the 2 position of the substrate. Furthermore, there is
almost no difference between the activity of the neuronal and glial
desaturase during the period of active myelination, whereas the
neuronal cell fraction of the adult rats displays a threefold
higher enzyme activity as compared to the glial cells. With increasing age of the animals a decrease in the desaturase activity
can be observed. The decrease is much more pronounced in glia
than in neurons (Table 1).

The dehydrogenation of the 1-alkyl moiety requires a reduced
pyridine nucleotide (NADH or NADPH) and is strongly inhibited by
KCN, but not by CO/O_2. Further evidence for the involvement of a
microsomal electron transport system in the enzymic conversion of
$1-[^{14}C]$ alkyl-2-acyl-GPE to ethanolamine plasmalogen was obtained
by using specific antibodies against NADH-cytochrome b5 reductase.
Table 2 clearly demonstrates the inhibition of plasmalogen formation
by adding increasing amounts of antibody against NADH-cytochrome b5
reductase to the incubation system. On the other hand, addition
of cytochrome b5 stimulated the biosynthesis of ethanolamine
plasmalogen from the corresponding alkyl-ether by oligodendroglial
microsomes (Table 3). In order to investigate whether Piracetam
(2-oxo-pyrrolidine-1-acetamide) has some effect on the biosynthesis
of ethanolamine plasmalogen, the animals were injected i.p. for 10
days with increasing amounts of the nootropic substance. Table 4
shows that the effect of Piracetam on the formation of ethanolamine
plasmalogen resembles the action of cytochrome b5 on the dehydrogenation of the 1-alkyl moiety as shown in Table 3.

Table 1. Formation of ethanolamine-plasmalogen from the corresponding 1-alkyl-2-acyl-sn-glycero-3-phosphorylethanolamine in neurons and glial cells of the rat brain during myelination.

Age	A			B		
	Neurons	Glia	Neuronal/glial ratio	Neurons	Glia	Neuronal/glial ratio
14 days	2.11	2.05	1.03	0.31	0.33	0.94
21 days	1.23	0.84	1.46	0.28	0.22	1.27
Adult	0.91	0.36	2.53	0.12	0.05	2.40

Each incubation mixture contained in a total volume of 0.25 ml 0.1 M Tris/HCl buffer, pH 7.1: 15 nmoles of 1-[^{14}C]alkyl-2-acyl-sn-GPE (substrate A) or [^{14}C]-labelled 1-alkyl-2-acyl-sn-GPE (hydrogenated substrate, B), NaF (12 mM), ATP (10 mM), NADP$^+$ (2 mM), glucose-6-P (6 mM), MgCl$_2$ (4 mM), glucose-6-P-dehydrogenase (0.41 U), GSH (2 mM) and 325 to 480 µg of glial or neuronal protein. The substrates were added as a sonicated dispersion in 0.15% Tween 80. Incubations were carried out for 60 min at 37°C in a shaking water bath. Values are expressed as nmol ethanolamine-plasmalogen formed x mg^{-1} prot. x h^{-1}.

Table 2. Influence of anti NADH-cytochrome b5 reductase on the formation of ethanolamine-plasmalogen from 1-[14C]alkyl-2-acyl-sn-glycero-3-phosphorylethanolamine by oligodendro-glial microsomes of 20-day-old rats.

Antibody against NADH-cytochrome b5 reductase (mg)	Control globulin (mg)	Ethanolamine-Plasmalogen formed in the presence of				Ratio antibody-microsomal protein
		Antibody globulin (nmol)	Inhibition (%)	Control globulin (nmol)	Inhibition (%)	
-	-	1.42				
2.0	2.0	0.98	31.3	1.26	10.8	4.0
4.0	4.0	0.80	43.8	1.13	20.4	8.0
8.0	8.0	0.37	74.5	1.10	22.5	16.0
10.0	10.0	0.22	82.2	1.14	19.7	20.0

Each incubation mixture contained in a total volume of 1.0 ml 0.1 M Tris/HCl buffer, pH 7.1: 60 nmoles of 1-[14C]alkyl-2-acyl-GPE, NaF (12 mM), ATP (10 mM), NADH (2 mM), glucose-6-P (6 mM), MgCl2 (4 mM), glucose-6-P-dehydrogenase (1.64 U), GSH (2 mM), 0.3 ml of the 100,000 x g supernatant, 498 µg microsomal protein and antibody or control globulin as indicated. The substrates were added as a sonicated dispersion in 0.15% Tween 80. Incubations were carried out for 60 min at 37°C in a shaking water bath.

Both substances enhance the formation of ethanolamine plasmalogen from 1-$[^{14}C]$ alkyl-2-acyl-GPE (Tables 3 and 4).

In another series of experiments exogenously added glycerophosphatides, specifically labelled either in the 1 or in the 2 position, were used to measure the activity of phospholipase A_2 from the neuronal-enriched cell fraction of the rabbit. As can be seen from Table 5 the enzyme hydrolysed the 1,2-diacyl-glycerophosphatides more rapidly than the acylalkyl- and acylalkenyl-compounds. Choline plasmalogen and the corresponding alkyl-derivative were cleaved at almost similar rates by the phospholipase A_2. Among the various 1,2-diacyl-glycerophosphatides, the neuronal phospholipase A_2 preferred phosphatidylcholine as a substrate, whereas phosphatidylserine was hydrolysed less actively. Table 5 shows, furthermore, that norepinephrine, injected into the lateral ventricle of the rabbit brain, stimulated the hydrolysis of the various glycerophosphatide substrates.

Table 3. Effect of cytochrome b_5 on the formation of ethanolamine-plasmalogen from 1-$[^{14}C]$ alkyl-2-acyl-sn-glycero-3-phosphoryl-ethanolamine by oligodendroglial microsomes of 20-day-old rats.

Addition	Concentration (mg/mg of micr. protein)	Ethanolamine-Plasmalogen formed (nmol/mg protein/h)	Difference (%)
–	–	2.94	–
Control IG	1.8	2.78	– 6
Cytochrome b_5	0.5	3.85	+ 31
	1.2	4.49	+ 53
	3.6	5.67	+ 93
	4.5	6.23	+ 112

Incubation conditions as in Table 2.

Table 4. Influence of Piracetam on the formation of ethanolamine-plasmalogen from 1-[^{14}C]alkyl-2-acyl-sn-glycero-3-phosphoryl-ethanolamine by neuronal microsomes of 20-day-old rats.

Piracetam (mg/kg/day)	Ethanolamine-plasmalogen formed (nmol/mg protein/h)	Increase (%)
–	2.96	–
60	3.87	30.7
80	4.56	54.0
100	5.76	94.6
120	6.02	103.3
140	6.12	108.7

The incubation conditions were as described in Table 2 with the exception that instead of oligondendroglial microsomes neuronal microsomal protein was used. The animals were pretreated for 10 days with the dose of Piracetam.

DISCUSSION

The present results have shown that the microsomal 1-alkyl-2-acyl-GPE desaturation reaction is catalyzed by a membrane-bound multicomponent desaturase system requiring the supply of reducing equivalents from pyridine nucleotides. It may be supposed that in the desaturase reaction, which transforms the alkyl-ether to the enol-ether moiety, a cyanide sensitive factor (CSF) is operating as the terminal oxidase as it has been proposed for the oxidative conversion of stearoyl-CoA to oleoyl-CoA (7). The use of various specific inhibitors including antisera against NADH-cytochrome b5 reductase indicate the role of microsomal flavoproteins in the supply of reducing equivalents from NADPH or NADH to the cyanide sensitive factor. Cytochrome b5 seems to be functional as an electron carrier between the flavoproteins and the CSF.

1-alkyl-2-acyl-GPE with unsaturated fatty acids at the 2 position served as a good substrate for plasmalogen synthesis, whereas 1-alkyl-GPE was transformed to the corresponding plasmalogen only after the addition of CoA to the incubation system, indicating that the dehydrogenation of the 1-alkyl moiety only occurs on the intact phospholipid molecule.

The observation that norepinephrine stimulates the hydrolysis of glycerophosphatides by phospholipase A2 (Table 5) could suggest that phospholipase A2 might be concerned in the molecular changes taking place in membranes during synaptic transmission. In an investigation on the incorporation of ^{32}P into the phospholipids

Table 5. Hydrolysis of different glycerophosphatides by neuronal phospholipase A_2.

Substrates	Phospholipase A_2 [nmol/(mg × h)]	Norepinephrine[a] phospholipase A_2 [nmol/(mg × h)]	Difference[b] (%)
1-[^{14}C]stearoyl-2-acyl-sn-GPC	48.7	73.9	51.7
1-[^{14}C]stearoyl-2-acyl-sn-GPE	39.6	61.3	54.7
1-[^{14}C]stearoyl-2-acyl-sn-GPS	20.3	33.2	63.5
1-Alk-1'-enyl-2-[^{14}C]linoleoyl-sn-GPC	18.5	27.8	50.2
1-Alkyl-2-[^{14}C]linoleoyl-sn-GPC	17.8	27.2	52.8

Each incubation mixture contained in a total volume of 1.0 ml: 0.1 M sodium acetate buffer, pH 5.4; 1.0 μmol of the glycerophosphatide substrate; 3 mg of sodium taurocholate and varying amounts of neuronal protein (ranging from 248 to 524 μg). Incubation at 37°C for 1 h. For details, see Experimental. Each figure represents the average of five experiments; SEM was less than 8%.

[a] The animals were injected intraventricularly with 100 μg of L-norepinephrine (for details, see Experimental.

[b] Per cent of increase in activity of norepinephrine experiments, as compared to controls.

of neuronal- and glial cell-enriched fractions, Woelk <u>et al.</u> (12)
presented experimental evidence that norepinephrine, injected into
the lateral ventricle of rabbit brain, increased the incorporation
of ^{32}P into phosphatidylinositol of both glial and neuronal cell
bodies, but had no effect on the specific radioactivity of glial
and neuronal ethanolamine plasmalogen and sphingomyelin. The
labelling of phosphatidylcholine was slightly inhibited by
norepinephrine in the glial cell-enriched fraction, whereas with
neurons no inhibition could be observed (12). On the basis of
these observations it was concluded that increased incorporation
of the label into phosphatidic acid and phosphatidylinositol may
occur in neurons which respond to the neurotransmitter with
excitation, whereas inhibition of ^{32}P incorporation into phosphatidylcholine may be connected with inhibitory transmission (12).

REFERENCES

1. Blank, M.L., Wykle, R.L. and Snyder, F., Enzymic synthesis of
    ethanolamine plasmalogens from an O-alkyl glycerolipid,
    <u>FEBS Lett.</u>18 (1971) 92-94.
2. Blomstrand, C. and Hamberger, A., Protein turnover in cell-
    enriched fractions from rabbit brain, <u>J. Neurochem.</u> 16 (1969)
    1401-1407.
3. Blomstrand, C. and Hamberger, A., Amino acid incorporation <u>in
    vitro</u> into protein of neuronal and glial cell-enriched
    fractions, <u>J. Neurochem.</u> 17 (1970) 1187-1195.
4. Dawson, R.M.C., A hydrolytic procedure for the identification
    and estimation of individual phospholipids in biological
    samples, <u>Biochem. J.</u> 75 (1960) 45-53.
5. Freysz, L., Bieth, R. and Mandel, P., Kinetics of the bio-
    synthesis of phospholipids in neurons and glial-cells isolated
    from rat brain cortex, <u>J. Neurochem.</u> 16 (1969) 1417-1424.
6. Goracci, G., Blomstrand, C., Arienti, G., Hamberger, A. and
    Porcellati, G., Base-exchange enzymic system for the synthesis
    of phospholipids in neuronal and glial cells and their sub-
    fractions: a possible marker for neuronal membranes, <u>J. Neuro-
    chem.</u> 20 (1973) 1167-1180.
7. Oshino, N. and Omura, T., Immunochemical evidence for the
    participation of cytochrome b$_5$ in microsomal stearoyl-CoA
    desaturation reaction, <u>Arch. Biochem. Biophys.</u>157(1973) 395-404.
8. Paltauf, F., Prough, R.A., Masters, B.S.S. and Johnston, J.M.,
    Evidence for the participation of cytochrome b$_5$ in plasmalogen
    biosynthesis, <u>J. Biol. Chem.</u> 249 (1974) 2661-2662.
9. Poduslo, S.E. and Norton, W.T., Isolation and some chemical
    properties of oligodendroglia from calf brain, <u>J. Neurochem.</u>
    19 (1972) 727-736.
10. Snyder, F., Blank, M.L. and Wykle, R.L., The enzymic synthesis
    of ethanolamine plasmalogens, <u>J. Biol. Chem</u>. 246 (1971) 3639-
    3645.

11. Woelk, H., Goracci, G., Gaiti, A., Porcellati, G., Phospho-
    lipase A_1 and A_2 activities of neuronal and glial cells of the
    rabbit brain, Hoppe Seyler's Z. Physiol. Chem. 354 (1973)
    729-736.
12. Woelk, H., Kanig, K., Peiler-Ichikawa, K., Phospholipid
    metabolism in experimental allergic encephalomyelitis: Activity
    of mitochondrial phospholipase A_2 of rat brain towards speci-
    fically labelled 1,2-diacyl-, 1-alk-1'-enyl-2-acyl- and 1-alkyl-
    2-acyl-sn-glycero-3-phosphorylcholine, J. Neurochem. 23 (1974)
    745-750.
13. Woelk, H., Porcellati, G., Subcellular distribution and kinetic
    properties of rat brain phospholipases A_1 and A_2. Hoppe
    Seyler's Z. Physiol. Chem. 354 (1973) 90-100.

REGIONAL DEVELOPMENTAL AND FRACTIONAL STUDIES ON MYELIN AND OTHER CARBONIC ANHYDRASES IN RAT CNS

Victor Sapirstein[1], Michael Trachtenberg[2],
Marjorie B. Lees[1] and Omanand Koul[1]
[1]Department of Biochemistry, The Eunice Kennedy Shriver
Center, Waltham, Mass. 02154, and the Department of
Biological Chemistry, Harvard Medical School,
Boston, Mass. 02115; [2]Department of Neurology,
Boston Veteran's Administration Hospital,
South Huntington Avenue, Boston, Mass. 02130, U.S.A.

SUMMARY

Myelin carbonic anhydrase (CA) was studied with respect to
its development in various brain regions and light and heavy myelin
(LM and HM). The data indicate that the specific activity of myelin
CA has a clear neuraxial distribution, increasing rostrally. The
absolute activities and relative distribution are invariant with
age; this suggests the CA activity in myelin is independent of
stage and degree of myelination. The studies on HM and LM illustrate
that HM, like total myelin, has a constant CA activity during development. In contrast, LM although equal to HM at 14 days, progressively decays to an adult level which is one-fourth that of HM.
The distribution of CA in myelin was further investigated by comparing the activity in myelin with that present in the SN_4 fraction.
The activity in this latter fraction, which is derived from heavy
myelin, was found to be 2.2 times higher than that in the myelin
fraction. Thus, in the adult there exists an almost ten-fold range
of activities among the various myelin fractions, $SN_4 > HM > LM$.
This may indicate a segregation of activity towards the outer
lamellae. This segregation may have physiological importance in
that it is this region of the sheath which should be integrally involved in control of myelin edema. Evidence indicates that there
is an interaction of chloride with the enzyme, and maybe the primary
ion moved by CA in order to initiate an osmotic flux out of the
sheath. The interaction of chloride with the enzyme is dependent
on the CA complex with the membrane in that solubilization and

partial (60-fold) purification results in a preparation which is
refractory to anions.

INTRODUCTION

Carbonic anhydrase (carbonate hydrolyase, EC. 4.2.1.1., CA) is
a ubiquitous enzyme associated with both acid base balance and
fluid and ion movements in a variety of tissues (9, 24). CA has
been implicated in at least two brain pathologies: seizure (14, 26)
and edema (6). In the latter, a potassium-stimulated uptake of
chloride and fluid is mediated by CA and is localized to glia (6)
(astrocytes) (13). These observations are supported by histochemical and microdissection demonstrations that the enzyme is concentrated in neuroglia, specifically in astrocytes (5, 12, 18, 19,
28). As a consequence the presence of CA has been used as a glial
marker (34, 37). CA has been found in purified myelin and has been
identified in this membrane histochemically (19). In myelin the
enzyme may play a similar role to that described above and thus
be implicated in mechanisms controlling hydration. Such processes
may be important during maturation when a compaction of the myelin
sheath and a decrease in its water content occurs. Specific toxic
agents have been shown to induce edema and vacuolization of myelin
(11, 17) and this process has been shown to be reversible (15)
suggesting that active mechanisms exist for maintaining the low
water content of myelin.
An age-related differential sensitivity along the neuraxis to
seizures, spreading depression and myelin vacuolization has been
recognized (29, 33, 36). These differences indicate that both
regional and developmental factors should be considered in assessing the role of CA in the CNS. Several groups have studied the
regional and developmental pattern of brain CA but some of the
data are conflicting (2, 20, 29, 30). Furthermore, the studies
were limited to the total CA. The present study was undertaken to
examine the regional and developmental distribution of the soluble,
membrane-bound and myelin portions of brain CA. The distribution
of enzyme markers within myelin itself (3, 39) has prompted us to
examine CA in myelin subfractions such as light and heavy myelin
and the microsome-free myelin-like fraction of Waehneldt, SN_4
(38).

EXPERIMENTAL

Thirty-six female Long-Evans rats (ages 16, 37, 75 and 90
days) were each transcardially perfused with oxygenated, heparinized
phosphate buffered saline. The brain and spinal cord were removed,

quickly cooled to $4^{\circ}C$ and dissected into four regions. Each region was either analyzed immediately or frozen and stored at $-70^{\circ}C$. Samples from four to six animals were combined, depending on their ages. The four regions studied were: spinal cord (SC) consisting of cervical, thoracic and lumbosacral portions; lower brain stem (LBS) consisting of mesencephalon, pons and medulla oblongata; cerebellum (CB) consisting of cortex, deep nuclei and peduncles; and upper brain stem (UBS) consisting of subcortical telencephalic nuclei and white matter, and diencephalon, i.e. forebrain sine cortex.

A 10% tissue homogenate in 0.32 M sucrose containing 2 mM EDTA was prepared. The soluble fraction was obtained by centrifugation of the homogenate at 110,000 x g for 75 min in a Beckman L265 ultra-centrifuge. EDTA was incorporated into the homogenization medium since preliminary studies showed that in the absence of EDTA low and inconsistent values for CA activity were obtained in the soluble fraction. The term total CA activity refers to the enzyme activity in the homogenate. Membrane-bound CA was calculated as the difference between the CA activity in the homogenate and the activity in the soluble fraction.

Myelin was isolated by the procedure of Norton and Poduslo (31) with two modifications: a 10% tissue homogenate (w/v) was prepared and the homogenization medium contained 2 mM EDTA. Purified myelin was washed three times with deionized water to remove sucrose and was resuspended in 0.1% dithiothreitol prior to assay. The extent of contamination of myelin with the soluble fraction was determined by measurement of lactic dehydrogenase activity (4). By this criterion, less than 0.8% contamination with soluble fraction was present in the myelin.

Light and heavy myelin were prepared from cerebral hemispheres of Sprague Dawley rats of 14, 20, 30, and 90 days of age essentially by the procedure of Agrawal et al. (1). Light myelin was defined as the material floating above 0.55 M sucrose and heavy myelin as the material floating on 0.75 M sucrose. All fractions were re-cycled on discontinuous gradients to ensure homogeneity. The SN_4 and corresponding myelin fraction, prepared with the procedure described by Waehneldt and Mandel (38), were supplied by Dr. Thomas Waehneldt.

CA was assayed at $4^{\circ}C$ using a micromodification of the Maren (29) technique. One unit of activity was defined as that enzyme activity which produced a 50% decrease in the time required for a fixed pH change as compared to an uncatalyzed preparation. One unit of activity is equivalent to 1 Wilbur-Anderson unit based on values reported for human carbonic anhydrase C (Sigma Chemical Co., St. Louis, Mo.). Protein was determined by the procedure of Lowry (22) as modified by Lees and Paxman (21). All analyses were carried out in triplicate.

Table 1. Distribution of carbonic anhydrase activities (units/g wet wt.) in the 90-day-old rat.

Region	Total	Soluble	Membrane-bound	Membrane-bound %
Upper brain stem	2,380	1,000	1,380	58.0
Lower brain stem	1,666	674	992	59.6
Cerebellum	1,042	625	417	40.0
Spinal cord	412	143	269	64.3

Carbonic anhydrase activity was measured by the method of Maren (23). Total refers to activity in the homogenate, soluble to activity in the 110,000 x g supernatant. Activity in the membrane-bound fraction was calculated as the difference between the total and the soluble fractions. Tissue from 4 rats was pooled for each analysis; assays were carried out in triplicate (reproducibility approx. ± 5%).

RESULTS

Table 1 shows the CA activity in different regions of the central nervous system of the 90-day-old rat. A progressive increase is observed in the CA activity (units/g fresh tissue) in the homogenates from spinal cord regions to the upper brain stem. Individual regions of the spinal cord (cervical, thoracic and lumbrosacral) were initially studied but no differences were found; the data from the various cord regions were therefore pooled. Despite the similarity in the anatomical level and embryological origin of cerebellum and lower brain stem, appreciable differences between their CA activities are evident.

Separation of the tissue into membrane-bound and soluble fractions reveals the same rostro-caudal distribution of CA as was observed in the homogenate. In the soluble fraction, however, the CA activity in the cerebellum is equal to that in the lower brain stem. As a consequence, the membrane-bound fraction from the cerebellum accounts for only 35-40% of the total activity whereas, for all other regions, the membrane fraction accounts for 60% of the activity.

A distinct component of the membrane-bound enzyme is the myelin-associated CA. Table 2 shows that this fraction exhibits the same general rostral increase in activity as do other fractions. However, it differs from the regional distribution of the total membrane-bound CA in that the specific activities of the myelin enzyme from lower brain stem and cerebellum are essentially equivalent. Based on the yield of myelin obtained by Norton and Poduslo (32) we estimate that in the upper and lower brain stem and in the spinal cord the myelin CA accounts for 7-10% of the membrane-bound activity. However, the myelin enzyme from cerebellum accounts

Table 2. Specific activity of brain carbonic anhydrases (units/mg protein) as a function of age.

Region	37 Days			90 Days		
	Total	Soluble	Myelin	Total	Soluble	Myelin
Upper brain stem	10.6	28.35	11.4	23.8	53.7	12.4
Lower brain stem	8.8	20.5	5.4	17.5	37.4	6.5
Cerebellum	5.9	18.4	5.6	11.0	33.6	6.8
Spinal cord	2.5	ND	2.0	4.3	9.3	2.1

Values are from brain regions derived from 4 rats of the specified ages. Assays were performed in triplicate (reproducibility approx. $\pm$ 5%). ND = not determined.

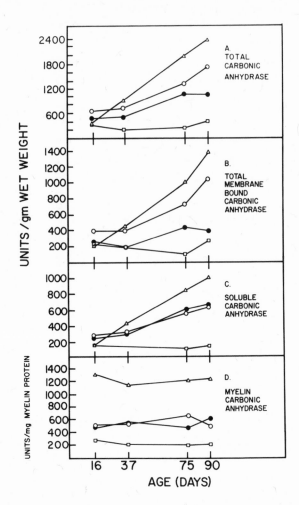

Fig. 1. Carbonic anhydrase activity in different regions of the CNS at different ages. Fractions are defined in Experimental section. Material from 4 animals was pooled to obtain data at 37, 75, and 90 days; 6 animals were used at 16 days. A-C, activity expressed as units/gram wet weight, D activity expressed as units/ mg myelin protein. Upper brain stem (△) ; lower brain stem (O); Cerebellum (●) and spinal cord (▢).

for 20% of the activity of the membrane-bound fraction. This
regional distribution is unchanged when myelin is isolated in the
presence of 2 mM EDTA, a procedure which releases significant
amounts of CA from other brain membrane fractions. Furthermore,
assay of myelin fractions in the presence of Triton X-100 (0.5%)
+ dithiothreitol (0.1%) did not change the absolute activities.
     The developmental changes in total CA activity associated with
different regions of the nervous system are shown in Fig. 1A. The
regional pattern present at 16 days is distinguished by very low
activity in upper brain stem indicative of its latent development.
Second, the lower brain stem CA activity is relatively elevated,
possibly associated with the early maturation of cardiovascular
respiratory and other vegetative control centers. With the exception
of spinal cord, which showed adult enzyme levels at 16 days, the
CA activity of each region increased with age. The enzyme activity
in the homogenate exhibits the adult regional distribution at 37
days. By 75 days of age the cerebellum seems to reach maximal CA
activity while upper and lower brain stem activities continue to
increase. Partition of the tissue activity into membrane bound and
soluble fractions (Fig. 1B and C) reveals a similar developmental
pattern as was manifest for the total activity.

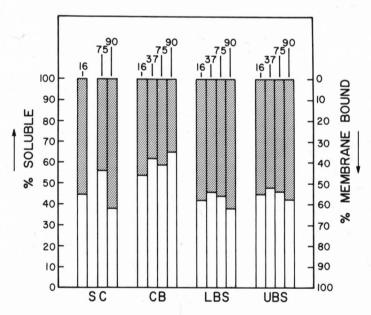

Fig. 2. The relative distribution of carbonic anhydrase in the
soluble and total membrane fractions from rats of 16, 37, 75 and
90 days postnatal. Fractions were prepared as described in
Experimental. Brain regions from 6 animals were pooled for the
determinations on the 16-day-old rats; 4 animals were pooled for
other ages.

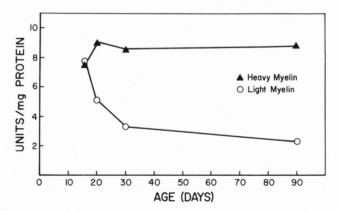

Fig. 3. Carbonic anhydrase activity in light and heavy myelin as
a function of age. All assays were performed in triplicate with
mean values reported.

      The low activity of membrane-bound CA in cerebellum relative
to lower brain stem noted in the adult is evident at all ages,
while the level of the soluble enzyme in these regions is equal
through 90 days of development. These patterns of regional and
age dependent CA activity, expressed as units/g wet weight, are
maintained when the data are expressed as specific activities (units/
g protein) (Table 2). The specific activities of both the total
and soluble enzymes (and therefore the membrane-bound fraction)
double between 37 and 90 days of age. Figure 2 illustrates that,
regardless of age, approximately 55-60% of the total enzyme is
membrane-bound for all regions except cerebellum where 40% of the
CA is consistently membrane-bound.
      The regional distribution of the myelin enzyme is similar to
other CA fractions at 90 days. However, the developmental pattern
of myelin CA is distinguished from the other CA populations in that
its specific activity is invariant with age (Fig. 1D and Table 2).
Even in myelin from upper brain stem, the adult specific activity
is observed at 16 days at a time when the homogenate and total
membrane-bound CA in this region are extremely low. Myelin CA is
therefore independent of the stage and degree of myelination.
      The age dependency of myelin carbonic anhydrase in light and
heavy myelin fractions was also investigated (Fig. 3). At 14 days
the enzyme activity in the two myelin fractions is equal. The
activity in the light myelin shows a marked decrease with age whereas
that in the heavy myelin remains essentially constant. Consequently
at 90 days there exists a 4-fold difference in activity between
light and heavy myelin. The lower activity observed in this series
of experiments as compared with those reported above is attributed
to the use of deionized water in the former experiments.
      Preliminary results on the activity of carbonic anhydrase in
the SN_4 fraction in the adult rat reveals a 2.2-fold greater

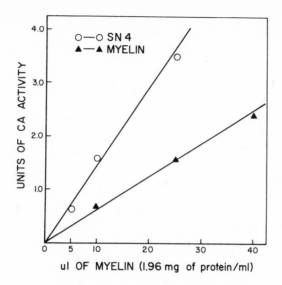

Fig. 4. Relative carbonic anhydrase activity in myelin and the SN$_4$ fraction. SN$_4$ and myelin were prepared as described in Experimental and lyophilized. The material was resuspended in 0.1% DTT in a glass-teflon homogenizer and assayed. The relative activity was calculated from the ratio of the respective slopes.

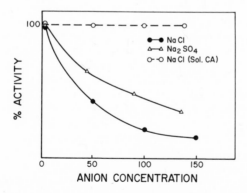

Fig. 5. Effect of anions on myelin carbonic anhydrase. Myelin was resuspended in 0.1% DTT and incubated with aliquots of concentrated salt solutions. Correction was made for dilution (10%). The solubilized enzyme was prepared according to Sapirstein and Lees (35).

activity than in the bulk myelin fraction (Fig. 4). Thus in the
adult an almost 10-fold gradient of activity exists with SN_4 >
heavy myelin ▷ light myelin.

The effects of anions on myelin carbonic anhydrase was examined
(Fig. 5). The enzyme shows a marked sensitivity to chloride which
is concentration dependent and anion specific: 50% inhibition of
the enzyme is achieved with approximately 50 mM Cl^- while over twice
as much SO_4 is necessary for an equivalent effect. The effect of
chloride, however, appears to asymptote before complete inhibition.
Solubilization and partial purification (60-fold) of the myelin
enzyme yields a preparation which is no longer sensitive to chloride.
The inability to achieve total inhibition and the insensitivity of
the enzyme after partial purification suggest that the anion effect
may be mediated via another myelin component.

DISCUSSION

The data presented in this paper demonstrate a clear neuraxial
distribution of myelin, soluble, membrane-bound and the total CA
activity. The results obtained for the enzyme activity of the
homogenate in the present study agree well with several previous
reports. The data are consistent with the developmental results of
Ashby and Schuster (2) which showed a progressive, almost linear,
increase in activity between 14 and 45 days in cerebellum-lower
brain stem. Our respective studies differ only in that we measured
these areas separately and extended the age to 90 days. Koul and
Kanungo (20) also examined developmental changes in total CA activity. Although they do not make a direct comparison between cerebellum and cerebral medulla (equivalent to upper brain stem in the
present study; Koul, personal communication) their values show a
ratio of 1:2 for cerebellum:upper brain stem and are thus in close
agreement with our results. Their data on age differences in these
regions are also consistent with the values reported here.

Another developmental study with which some valid comparisons
can be made is that of Nair and Bau (29, 30). They reported an
early truncation of spinal cord CA activity at approximately 18
days, which compares with our results showing full expression of
CA activity in spinal cord by 16 days. They also reported a relatively high value at early ages for lower brain stem which again
is similar to the results obtained in the present study. However,
the work of Nair and Bau conflicts with our study with respect to
the activity in the caudate nucleus. This structure is part of
our upper brain stem which we find is high in CA activity; in a
separate study we found the CA activity in the caudate to be relatively high (Trachtenberg and Sapirstein, in preparation). At
present we cannot reconcile this discrepancy.

Our conclusion from the present study is that a high percentage
of membrane-bound CA occurs in all areas of the CNS. The average

percentage of membrane-bound activity is close to that calculated
from the results of Cammer et al. (8) and Yandrasitz et al.(40)
both of whom report only about 45% of the CA activity recoverable
in the soluble fraction. These results are in contrast to findings
in other tissues, including kidney (25) where only 5-10% is membrane
bound. This suggests that the membrane bound enzyme may play a
distinct and important role in CA mediated phenomena in brain. The
soluble enzyme has been associated with acid-base regulation (24)
and as such may be responsible for maintaining the low CO_2 tension
necessary for the unimpeded function of neurons (14). The brain-
specific, potassium-stimulated CA dependent uptake of chloride and
fluid by astrocytes (6, 13) suggests that the membrane-bound form
may be important in these translocation processes. These supposi-
tions are strengthened by the correlation of the activities of the
respective enzyme fractions with the developmental and neuraxial
susceptibility to seizures and spreading depression (26, 27, 33).
If the soluble and membrane-bound forms prove to serve distinct
functions, control over their relative distribution becomes an important issue. The results reported here indicate that the soluble
and membrane-bound CA, of which the myelin enzyme is only a small
part, exhibit very similar developmental patterns. In fact, the
relative distribution of the enzyme is invariant with age in all
regions studied. The data presented on their development therefore
suggest that their appearance is coextensive and they may derive
developmentally from a common enzyme pool. The data of Koul and
Kanungo (20) on CA activity relative to protein and DNA suggest
that after 28 days of age the increase in CA is largely a result of
glial (astrocyte) differentiation and not cell proliferation. They
report that CA activity increases 4.5-fold with respect to protein
while it increases almost 20-fold with respect to DNA. Thus, close
to 80% of the increase in CA is a correlate of differentiated growth
and only 20% of new cell body formation. Our data, illustrating
the parallel development of soluble and membrane-bound CA, suggest
that the increase in CA is a concomitant of differentiation of the
whole cell and not just a consequence of the laying-down of differentiated membrane.

The development of the myelin enzyme stands in contrast to
that of the soluble and total membrane-bound CA. Specifically the
myelin CA activity is fully expressed by 16 days of age and the
relative regional activity is invariant with age. These data illustrate that the regional variation of myelin CA is not just a consequence of the different CA levels in a given region, since at 16
days when total membrane-bound spinal cord CA is equal to that in
upper brain stem, the myelin enzyme from these regions exhibits a
ratio of activities of 1:6. Thus, the myelin enzyme appears to be
under a separate developmental control and is independent of the
stage and degree of myelination. As noted above, the other enzyme
populations exhibit increased activities which correlate with differentiation. The myelin isolated at any point in development

represents a differentiated oligodendroglial membrane. Thus, although the myelin membrane at 16 days of age is still maturing, the membrane has been committed to differentiation and with respect to CA is fully differentiated.

The functions of this enzyme in myelin are still a matter for speculation. The association of CA with water movement in other brain compartments as well as in other tissues suggests a similar role for this protein in myelin. The regional distribution of the myelin enzyme correlates well with the effects of triethyltin (TET) on myelin integrity. TET, which causes a vacuolization and edema of myelin, was shown by Smith (36) to exert its most severe effect in spinal cord which is lowest in myelin CA while forebrain myelin, which is high in CA activity, is comparatively refractory to this toxic agent. Sapirstein (unpublished results) has found that TET does not inhibit CA in vitro even at a molar excess of 10^4, suggesting the edema is not due to a direct effect on the enzyme. It may, however, derive from an ionic imbalance resulting from other cytotoxic effects. One possibility is that TET and perhaps hexachlorophene promote an ion and fluid influx into myelin (7, 8; Cammer and Norton, personal communication). The resulting fluid accumulation may be minimized or prevented by the action of the myelin CA. The early developmental appearance of CA in this membrane suggests the possibility that the enzyme plays an important role in the dehydration of myelin associated with maturation.

The results on the distribution of carbonic anhydrase in different myelin fractions indicates that in the adult this enzyme is asymmetrically distributed. There exists a 10-fold difference in activity between SN_4 and light myelin. The difference in CA activity between SN_4 and the myelin is consonant with the distribution of 2',3'-cyclic nucleotide 3'-phosphohydrolase activity in these fractions, as described by Waehneldt (39).

The myelin enzyme seems to interact with chloride ions in an anion specific manner, as measured by a decrease in CO_2 hydration. This may represent an association with an anion transport system. The effect of chloride, however, is not the same as is observed with the B isozyme from the red blood cell. Firstly, the soluble B isozyme interacts directly with chloride, while the chloride effect on the myelin enzyme appears to be indirect. Secondly, the anion effect on the B isozyme occurs via a mechanism which is the same as the sensitivity to imidazole (16); the myelin enzyme whether membrane-bound or solubilized appears to be refractory to imidazole.

Acknowledgements. This investigation was supported by U.S. Public Health Service National Institution of Health Grant NS 13649 and Veterans Administration Project No. 8519.

REFERENCES

1. Agrawal, H.C., Trotter, T.H., Mitchell, R.F. and Burton, R.M., Metabolic studies on myelin: evidence for a precursor role of

   a myelin subfraction, Biochem. J. 140 (1974) 99-109.

2. Ashby, W. and Schuster, E.M., Carbonic anhydrase in the brain
   of the new born in relation to functional maturity, J. Biol.
   Chem. 184 (1950) 109-116.

3. Benjamins, J., Miller, K. and McKhann, G.M., Myelin subfractions
   in developing rat brain: Characterization and sulphatide metabolism, J. Neurochemistry 20 (1973) 1589-1603.

4. Bergmeyer, H.U., Bernt, E. and Ness, B., Lactic dehydrogenase,
   in Methods of Enzymatic Analysis (H.U. Bergmeyer, ed.) Academic
   Press, New York (1965) pp. 736-741.

5. Bhattacharjee, J., Developmental changes of carbonic anhydrase
   in the retina of the mouse: A histochemical study, Histochem.
   J. 8 (1976) 63-70.

6. Bourke, R.S., Kimelberg, H.K., West, C.R. and Bremer, A.M.,
   The effect of HCO_3 on the swelling and ion uptake of monkey
   cerebral cortex under conditions of raised extracellular
   potassium, J. Neurochem. 25 (1975) 323-328.

7. Cammer, W., Rose, A.L. and Norton, W.T., Biological and
   pathological studies of myelin in hexachlorophene intoxication,
   Brain Res. 98 (1975) 547-559.

8. Cammer, W., Fredman, T., Rose, A.L. and Norton, W.T., Brain
   carbonic anhydrase: Activity in isolated myelin and the effect
   of hexachlorophene, J. Neurochem. 27 (1976) 165-171.

9. Carter, M.J., Carbonic anhydrase: Isozymes, properties, distribution and functional significance, Biol. Rev. 47 (1972)
   465-513.

10. Davison, A.N., Myelinogenesis: Chemical aspects, Neurosciences
    Res. Prog. Bull. 9, No. 4 (1971) 465-470.

11. Eto, Y., Suzuki, K. and Suzuki, K., Lipid composition of rat
    brain myelin in triethyl tin-induced edema, J. Lipid. Res. 72
    (1971) 570-579.

12. Giacobini, E., A cytochemical study of the localization of
    carbonic anhydrase in the nervous system, J. Neurochem. 9 (1962)
    169-177.

13. Gill, T.H., Young, O.M. and Tower, D.B., The uptake of ^{36}Cl
    into astrocytes in tissue culture by a potassium-dependent
    saturable process, J. Neurochem. 23 (1974) 1011-1018.

14. Gray, W.D. and Rauh, C.E., Mechanism of the anticonvulsant
    action of acetazoleamide, a carbonic anhydrase inhibitor, J.
    Pharmacol. Exp. Ther. 163 (1968) 431-438.

15. Hirano, A., Edema damage, Neurosciences Res. Prog. Bull. 9, No.
    4 (1971) 493-496.

16. Kannan, K.K., Petef, M., Fridborg, K., Cid-Dresdner, A.   and
    Lovgren, S., Structure and function of carbonic anhydrases:
    Imidazole binding to human carbonic anhydrase B and the mechan-
    ism of action of carbonic anhydrases, FEBS. Lett. 73 (1977)
    115-119.

17. Kimbrough, R.D. and Gaines, T.B., Hexachlorophene effects on
    the rat brain, Archs. Envir. Hlth. 23 (1971) 114-118.

18. Korhonen, L.K., Näätänen, E. and Hyyppä, M., A histochemical
     study of carbonic anhydrase in some parts of the mouse brain,
     Acta Histochem. 18 (1964) 336-347.
19. Korhonen, L.K. and Hyyppä, M., Histochemical localization of
     carbonic anhydrase activity in the spinal and coeliac ganglia
     of the rat, Acta Histochem. 26 (1967) 75-79.
20. Koul, O. and Kanungo, M.S., Alterations in carbonic anhydrase
     of the brain of rats as a function of age, Exp. Geront. 10
     (1975) 273-278.
21. Lees, M.B. and Paxman, S., Modification of the Lowry procedure
     for the analysis of proteolipid protein, Anal. Biochem. 47
     (1972) 184-192.
22. Lowry, O.J., Rosebrough, N.J., Farr, A.L. and Randall, R.J.,
     Protein measurement with the Folin phenol reagent, J. Biol.
     Chem. 193 (1951) 265-275.
23. Maren, T.H., A simplified micromethod for the determination of
     carbonic anhydrase and its inhibitions, J. Pharmacol. Exp. Ther.
     130 (1960) 26-29.
24. Maren, T.H., Carbonic anhydrase: Chemistry, physiology, and
     inhibition, Physiolog. Rev. 47 (1967) 595-781.
25. McKinley, D.N. and Whitney, P.L., Particulate carbonic an-
     hydrase in homogenates of human kidney, Biochem. Biophys. Acta
     445 (1976) 780-790.
26. Millichap, J.G., Development of seizure patterns in newborn
     animals: Significance of brain carbonic anhydrase, Proc. Soc.
     Exp. Biol. (N.Y.) 97 (1958) 606-611.
27. Millichap, J.G., Woodbury, D.M. and Goodman, L.S., The anti-
     convulsant action of carbon dioxide: interaction with reserpine
     and inhibitors of carbonic anhydrase, J. Pharmacol. Exp. Ther.
     115 (1955) 251-258.
28. Musser, G.L. and Rosen, S., Localization of carbonic anhydrase
     activity in the vertebrate retina, Exp. Eye Res. 15 (1973)
     105-119.
29. Nair, V. and Bau, D., Effects of prenatal X-irradiation on the
     ontogenesis of acetylcholin-esterase and carbonic anhydrase
     in rat central nervous system, Brain Res. 16 (1969) 383-394.
30. Nair, V. and Bau, D., Studies on the functional significance
     of carbonic anhydrase in C.N.S. , Brain Res. 31 (1971) 185-
     193.
31. Norton, W.T. and Poduslo, S., Myelination in rat brain:method
     of myelin isolation, J. Neurochem. 21 (1973) 749-757.
32. Norton, W.T. and Poduslo, S., Myelination in rat brain:
     changes in myelin composition during brain maturation, J. Neuro-
     chem. 21 (1973) 749-757.
33. Ochs, S., Nature of spreading depression in neural networks,
     Intl. Rev. Neurobiol. 4 (1962) 1-69.
34. Rose, S.P.R. and Sinha, A.K., Bulk separation of neurons and
     glia: a comparison of techniques, Brain Res. 33 (1971) 205-
     217.

35. Sapirstein, V. and Lees, M.B., Isolation and characterization of myelin carbonic anhydrase, Tran. Intl. Soc. Neurochem. 8 (1977) 571.

36. Smith, M.E., Studies on the mechanism of demyelination: triethyl tin-induced demyelination, J. Neurochem. 21 (1973) 357-372.

37. Tower, D.B. and Young, O.M., The activities of butyryl-cholinesterase and carbonic anhydrase, the rate of anaerobic glycolysis, and the question of a constant density of glial cells in cerebral cortices of various mammalian species from mouse to whale, J. Neurochem. 20 (1973) 269-278.

38. Waehneldt, T.V., Isolation of rat brain myelin, monitored by polyacrylamide gel electrophoresis of dodecyl sulfate-extracted proteins, Brain Res. 40 (1975) 419-436.

39. Waehneldt, T.V., Ontogenetic study of a myelin derived fraction with 2',3'-cyclic-nucleotide 3'-phosphohydrolase activity higher than that of myelin, J. Biochem. 151 (1975) 435-437.

40. Yandrasitz, J.R., Ernst, S.A. and Salganicoff, L., The sub-cellular distribution of carbonic anhydrase in homogenates of perfused rat brain, J. Neurochem. 27 (1976) 707-715.

STUDIES OF ISOLATED, MAINTAINED OLIGODENDROGLIA:

BIOCHEMISTRY, METABOLISM, AND IN VITRO MYELIN SYNTHESIS

Shirley E. Poduslo

Johns Hopkins University School of Medicine,
    Department of Neurology
Baltimore, Maryland 21205, U.S.A.

SUMMARY

Oligodendroglia can be isolated in bulk from dissected white
matter of lamb or bovine brain. Studies of the composition of the
whole cell and of glial subfractions were performed to detect
similarities to mature myelin. With care isolated oligodendroglia
can now be maintained in culture for three to four days. While in
culture the cells elaborate a form of glial myelin which has characteristics of both the intact cell and of mature myelin. Glial
myelin reacts with both the antiserum to oligodendroglial surface
components and with antiserum to galacto-cerebroside; it increases
in amount with time in culture; if various radiolabeled substrates
are added to the cells in culture, the glial myelin has both lipids
and proteins which are extensively radiolabeled; the glial myelin
has both basic protein and 2',3'-cyclic AMPase associated with it.
Thus this model system may be an excellent system for studying
myelin assembly in vitro.

INTRODUCTION

Myelination in the central nervous system is a well studied
phenomenon. Both the morphology and biochemistry of events occurring in brain during the initial stages of myelin production, and
the chemical characterization of the end product, myelin, have been
thoroughly investigated. However, very little is known about the
cell that produces myelin, the oligodendroglial cell. Until recently it has not been possible to purify this cell type from brain
tissue, a very complex tissue composed of several cell types, all
with long, highly branched, intimately intertwined processes.

With current methods for the bulk isolation of cells from brain,
oligodendroglia can be obtained as a homogeneous population of
cells (6, 12). Once oligodendroglia are isolated, they are very
fragile cells that tend to lyse upon the slightest manipulation.
However, techniques have now been established to maintain these
cells as suspensions in tissue culture (4, 10) which enables one
to study the metabolic properties of oligodendroglia in vitro
(5, 10).

This chapter will summarize our studies with isolated and
maintained oligodendroglia. Included are:
  I. Properties of isolated oligodendroglia:,
  II. Properties of the plasma membranes and myelin from isolated
      oligodendroglia;
  III. Preparation of myelin subfractions in an attempt to isolate
      a glial plasma membrane fraction from calf or fetal calf
      brain;
  IV. Metabolic properties of oligodendroglia maintained in
      culture;
  V. Preparation of antiserum specific to oligodendroglial sur-
      face components;
  VI. In vitro synthesis of myelin.

EXPERIMENTAL

Bulk isolation of oligodendroglia. Cells are routinely isolated using sterile conditions with all manipulations performed in
a laminar flow hood. The cell medium contains 5% glucose, 5%
fructose, 1% albumin in a 10 mM KH_2PO_4:NaOH buffer, pH 6.0; all
sucrose, trypsin, and trypsin inhibitor solutions are dissolved in
cell medium, brought to a pH of 6.0, sterilized by filtration, and
cooled (12). Corpus callosum and centrum semiovale areas of lamb,
calf or bovine brain white matter are dissected free of gray matter,
minced, and incubated in a 0.1% trypsin solution at $37^\circ C$ for 90 min.

The softened tissue is cooled, comparable amounts of trypsin
inhibitor added, and the tissue washed several times. The tissue
is then dissociated in 0.9 M sucrose by passage through a series
of screens, first a single layer of nylon, followed by a double
layer of nylon, and then finally three times through stainless
steel screens of 74 μm. The cell suspension is layered onto discontinuous sucrose gradients consisting of 0.9 M, 1.35 M, and 1.55
M sucrose. After centrifugation at 3,300 x g for 15 min, the top
layers are discarded and the 1.55 M sucrose layer is collected as
the glial layer.

The yield of oligodendroglia is 15-30 x 10^6 cells per gram
wet weight of white matter; the variability in yield depends on the
age of the tissue obtained as well as the activity of the trypsin
used during isolation. It has been found that the isolated cells
retain residual trypsin activity which is assessed using a

spectrophotometric assay (11). The assay involves following the
amount of hydrolysis of an artificial substrate, BAEE (N-benzoyl-
L-arginine ethyl ester HCl) by monitoring a change in absorption
at 253 nm (7). The residual trypsin activity can be eliminated
by washing the cells in a fetal calf serum which is compatible
with the cells (see below).

Preparation for tissue culture. Oligodendroglia obtained from
the sucrose gradients are diluted slowly with cell medium containing
5% fetal calf serum, pH 6.0 (10). After centrifugation (1,000 rpm
for 10 min), the cells are gently suspended and washed in 5% fetal
calf serum in cell medium, first at pH 6.5 and then at pH 6.8, with
centrifugation at 800 rpm for 10 min each time. For tissue culture
studies, the cells are suspended in cell medium at pH 7.0, and
Dulbecco's enriched tissue culture medium is slowly added. After
10 min at 4°C, the cells are gently swirled, causing the two mediums
to intermix, and are recentrifuged. The cells are then carefully
suspended in enriched tissue culture medium and transferred to
culture bottles. Normally a yield of 6 x 10^8 oligodendroglia are
obtained from 40 grams wet weight of white matter; the cells are
divided into 4 tissue culture bottles, each containing 25 ml of
tissue culture medium. This tissue culture medium consists of
Dulbecco's high glucose medium (final glucose concentration, 0.6%),
5% fructose, 0.001% insulin, 1% antibiotics, 0.1% fungizone,
0.3% PIPES buffer, and 5% fetal calf serum, at pH 7.0. The cells
are maintained in a water jacketed incubator at 37°C in a 10%
CO_2:90% air flow through it.

Effects of trypsin and fetal calf serum. There is considerable
variation in the quality of trypsin obtained from different companies
and even in different batches from the same company. We have found
that some batches of trypsin are unsuitable for cell isolation.
Optimal conditions for each batch are established   by testing
various concentrations to determine which gives the maximal number
of intact cells. Thus once a suitable lot of trypsin is found,
large quantities are purchased; the dry powder is divided into small
vials which are stored at -70°C. Thereafter the trypsin is thawed
only once when used.

The reaction of cells isolated from brain to different lots of
fetal calf serum is also unpredictable. In fact some lots of serum
have been found to be actually toxic to cells, causing either cell
clumping and lysis or complete disintegration. For evaluation of
fetal calf serum, various batches are obtained from several companies; brain slices from 10-day-old rats are placed in tissue
flasks in enriched tissue culture medium with different lots of 20%
serum. After one week in culture, those exhibiting extensive cell
growth are noted. The corresponding sera from these cultures are
next tested by washing isolated cells from brain in 5% fetal calf
serum. With noncompatible serum neurons tend to fragment, while
oligodendroglia clump and lyse. Cellular intactness after washing
is therefore used as an index for the suitability of fetal calf

serum. All fetal calf serum is heat-inactivated at 56°C for 30
min and then stored at 4° prior to use. We have found that serum
stored longer than six months is frequently unusable.

  Maintenance of isolated oligodendroglia. Bulk isolated oligodendroglia can now be maintained as cell suspensions in tissue
culture for two to three days. The cells remain intact and viable
during this time. Isolated oligodendroglia are fragile and must
be manipulated with care during the washing procedures prior to
tissue culture. Cells at pH 7.0 also tend to aggregate into large
clusters. At first these cell clumps were discarded by filtration
through glass wool (since we assumed they were lysed cells); this
considerably reduced the yield of cells for culture. It was found,
however, upon careful examination of the cell aggregates by phase
microscopy that intact cells predominated. Consequently these cell
aggregates are also transferred into culture and frequently they
are dispersed after 24 hours. (Aggregation does not occur with rat
neurons isolated by a similar technique; thus, oligodendroglia may
have unique surface properties.)

  The cells are rigorously monitored for both intactness and
bacterial or yeast contamination while they are in culture. Intactness is assessed using phase microscopy, preferably at 400-800 X
magnification. Intact cells are round and glowing with little
evidence of a visible nucleus. If the nucleus is visible or acent-
ric, if the cells appear granular or the cytoplasm is vacuolated,
the cells are not healthy, even though they may still be intact.
With these cells the levels of incorporation of radioactive precursors are greatly reduced. With fragmented or lysed cells, the
levels of incorporation are barely detectable.

  Yeast or bacterial contamination of cell culture is assessed
by placing aliquots onto slants of Sabouraud dextrose modified agar
and heart infusion agar (both from Difco Laboratories, Michigan)
and then incubating for one to four days. The cell cultures are discarded if there is any evidence of yeast or bacterial growth. Yeast
and oligodendroglia are similar in size, but can be distinguished
by using a phase microscope at 400 or 800 X magnification. The
lower magnification usually found with inverted microscopes used
for tissue culture studies is not adequate for this distinction.
Since tissue is obtained from the abbatoir, contamination by yeast
is a major problem.

  Isolation of oligodendroglial plasma membranes and attached
myelin processes. Oligodendroglia isolated in bulk are homogenized
in a solution of 5 mM KCl, 5 mM $MgCl_2$, 0.25 M sucrose and 10 mM
Tris-HCl, pH 6.5 (8). The nuclei are removed and washed twice.
The combined supernatant fractions and washes are layered onto discontinuous sucrose gradients consisting of 1 M, 0.85 M and 0.5 M
sucrose (each dissolved in the buffered salts solution). The
gradients are centrifuged at 75,000 x g for 15 h and two layers are
obtained, a myelin and a plasma membrane layer. These two fractions
are concentrated and relayered onto separate continuous sucrose

gradients, generated from 0.32 M and 0.85 M sucrose over a cushion of 1 M sucrose. (These sucrose solutions are dissolved in water.) The continuous gradients are centrifuged at 75,000 x g for 4 h. This results in a light myelin layer at 0.5 M, a heavy myelin layer at 0.7 M, and a plasma membrane layer on 1 M sucrose. There is a pellet of subcellular organelle membranes.

Preparation of myelin subfractions from bovine and fetal calf white matter. Light and heavy myelin, as well as a third fraction of heavier density (which will be called a myelin-like fraction) were purified from both calf and fetal calf brain tissue. The myelin subfractions from calf white matter were prepared by a modification of our original myelin isolation procedure. The two low speed osmotically shocked supernatant solutions above the crude myelin pellets were combined, concentrated, and subjected to a final continuous sucrose gradient generated from 0.85 M sucrose and 0.5 M sucrose over a cushion of 1 M sucrose. Centrifugation of this continuous gradient at 70,000 x g for 15 h produced a light myelin layer on 0.5 M sucrose, with a myelin-like fraction on 1 M sucrose. If the osmotically shocked crude myelin pellets were subjected to similar continuous sucrose gradients, three layers were obtained: a light flocculent myelin layer at 0.5-0.6 M sucrose, followed closely by a thick heavy myelin layer at 0.6-0.7 M sucrose, and a myelin-like layer on 1 M sucrose. Thus three subfractions of myelin can be obtained from calf white matter: light myelin, heavy myelin, and a myelin-like fraction.

For fetal calf tissue, which contained very little white matter, no low speed centrifugations for the osmotic shock treatments were performed. The final sucrose gradients were continuous gradients similar to those described for calf. A 5-month fetal calf brain gave only one "myelin" band at 0.6 M sucrose and a myelin-like layer. A 6.5-month fetal calf brain sample gave the light and heavy myelin and a myelin-like sample, similar to more mature tissue.

RESULTS AND DISCUSSION

I. Biochemical Properties of Isolated Oligodendroglia.

Morphology. Oligodendroglia are isolated as a homogeneous population of round cells of 8-10 μm. Occasionally after isolation the cells retain a tiny process, as noted with phase microscopy (Fig. 1). On electron micrographs the cells exhibit a darkly stained round nucleus with a narrow rim of dense cytoplasm (14). The cytoplasm is rich in ribosomes and mitochondria as well as the characteristic microtubules. The cell processes are loosely packed myelin lamellae directly associated with the plasma membrane of the cell.

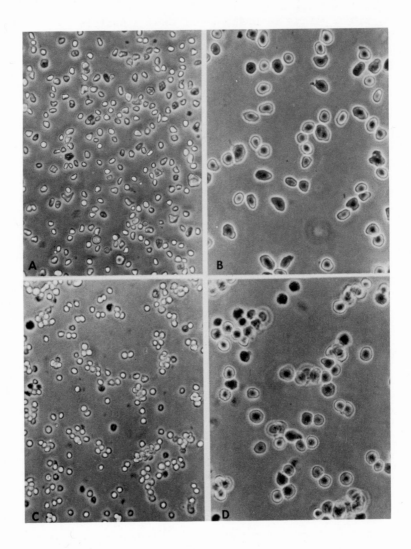

Fig. 1. Phase micrographs of lamb oligodendroglia isolated in bulk as described in the text. A and B: after isolation. C and D: after maintenance in culture for 24 h. Magnification: A and C, X 150; B and D, X 400.

Lipid composition. Oligodendroglia isolated in bulk from calf brain white matter are 29.5% lipid on a dry weight basis, consisting of 62% phospholipids, 14% cholesterol, and 10% galactolipids (12). The galactolipids are 7.3% cerebrosides and 1.5% sulfatide. Of the total phospholipids, 29.4% is phosphatidylcholine, 14.0% ethanolamine-phosphatides, 7.1% sphingomyelin, 4.7% phosphatidyl-serine, and 4.1% phosphatidylinositol. The ganglioside NANA (N-acetyl neuraminic acid) is 0.074% of dry weight. As indicated on Table 1, the lipid composition does differ from that of isolated rat neurons or rat astrocytes (13).

Table 1.   Comparison of three isolated cell types from brain.

	Rat neurons	Rat astrocytes	Bovine oligodendroglia
Total lipid, % of dry weight	24.1	38.9	29.5
Ganglioside NANA, % of dry wt.	0.069	0.18	0.074
Lipids, % of total lipid wt.			
Cholesterol	10.6	14.0	14.1
Total galactolipids	2.1	1.8	9.9
Cerebrosides	–	–	7.3
Sulfatides	–	–	1.5
Total phospholipids	72.3	70.9	62.2
Phosphatidylcholine	39.9	36.3	29.4
Ethanolaminephosphatides	18.2	20.1	14.0
Sphingomyelin	3.2	3.7	7.1
Phosphatidylserine	3.9	5.2	4.7
Phosphatidylinositol	4.9	3.5	4.1
RNA, pg/cell	24.2	29.1	1.95
DNA, pg/cell	8.18	11.2	5.14
DNA/RNA	0.34	0.38	2.6
Yield, 10^6 cells/g fresh tissue	17	3.5	11.4

II. Biochemical Properties of Purified Oligodendroglial Plasma Membranes and Glial Myelin.

Morphology and purity. Electron microscopy of the subfractions reveals a distinct difference between the glial myelin and the glial plasma membranes (8). The myelin layer consists of concentric whorls of lamellar rings and vesicles with the lamellar structures

having dark osmiophilic lines and lighter intraperiod lines, which
resemble less compacted myelin obtained from an immature animal.
The plasma membrane fraction is a homogeneous preparation of vesicles of various sizes and with adequate preservation, the triple
layered appearance of plasma membranes as observed in situ can be
seen. No contaminating organelles such as mitochondria or nuclei
are seen in either fraction.

The plasma membrane marker enzymes, Na^+, K^+-ATPase and 5'-
nucleotidase, are enriched in the plasma membrane fraction, but
are also active in the myelin fraction, indicating its close association with the plasma membrane (8). Likewise the myelin marker
enzyme, 2',3'-cyclic nucleotide 3'-phosphohydrolase (2',3'-cyclic
AMPase) exhibits high activity in glial myelin, but is also present
in the plasma membrane fraction (see Table 2).

Table 2. Specific activity of plasma membrane markers.

	Oligodendroglial Plasma membranes	Myelin	Oligodendroglial Whole cell
Na^+, K^+-ATPase*	9.8	6.3	1.6-3.2
5'-Nucleotidase*	8.6	5.0	1.2
2',3'-Cyclic AMPase*	117.5	275.5	36.6

*μmol Pi/mg prot/hour

Marker enzymes for subcellular organelles are present at marginal levels in these two fractions. Of the total found in the
intact cells, 7% of the acid phosphatase (a marker for lysosomes),
6% of the glucose-6-phosphatase (for microsomes) and 7% of the
thiamine pyrophosphatase (for Golgi apparatus and endoplasmic
reticulum) are present in the plasma membranes. The glial myelin
has 5,4, and 3%, respectively, of each. Neither cytochrome c
reductase or monoamine oxidase are present in glial myelin, but 2.5%
of the latter enzyme (a marker for mitochondrial outer membranes) is
present in the plasma membranes. Less than 2.5% of the RNA-P or
DNA-P is found in either fraction.

Lipid and protein composition. Glial myelin is 75% soluble in
organic solvents but only 60% of the dry weight is lipid. The lipids
consist of 24% cholesterol, 22% galactolipids, and 54% phospholipids
based on percentage of total lipids (Table 3). The plasma membranes
are 54% soluble in chloroform:methanol (C:M) with 43% total lipids,
which are composed of 20% cholesterol, 15% galactolipids, and 65%
phospholipids. The glial myelin has a higher mole ratio of galacto-
lipids/phosphatidylcholine and cholesterol/phospholipids, indicating

a composition differing from that of the whole cell. Thin layer
chromatography of the ganglioside fractions shows the presence of
the four major gangliosides, as well as G_{D3}, disialosyl lactosyl
ceramide, which is commonly found in bovine white matter. Gangliosides are associated with both the plasma membranes and the glial
myelin subfractions.

Table 3. Composition of oligodendroglial subcellular fractions.

	Myelin	Plasma membranes	Whole cell
% Dry weight			
C:M soluble	74.6	54.4	33.8
C:M insoluble	19.4	42.6	62.6
Gangliosides	0.5	0.5	0.4
% Total lipid			
Cholesterol	24.3	19.9	16.1
Galactolipids (Gal L)	22.1	14.8	11.4
Cerebrosides	18.2	11.7	9.6
Sulfatides	3.3	2.5	1.7
Phospholipids	53.7	65.2	72.5
Ethanolaminephosphatides (PE)	10.8	9.5	17.6
Phosphatidylcholine (PC)	22.0	32.5	36.4
Sphingomyelin	6.7	6.9	5.4
Phosphatidylinositol	2.4	3.8	4.9
Phosphatidylserine	7.6	6.5	5.3
Mole ratios			
PE/PC	0.56	0.32	0.53
Gal L/PC	0.95	0.43	0.29
Cholesterol/Phospholipids	0.91	0.62	0.45
Cerebrosides/Sulfatides	5.8	4.5	5.8

(Average of 3 experiments)

After disc gel electrophoresis of solubilized proteins, patterns were produced which had a predominance of high molecular
bands in both fractions. Glial myelin has bands corresponding to
the major myelin proteins, proteolipid protein and basic protein.
In contrast, the plasma membranes only have a protein band corresponding to the location of proteolipid protein. Staining the
plasma membranes for glycoproteins indicates the presence of several
bands of high molecular weight.

III.   Biochemical Properties of Myelin Subfractions from Calf
and Fetal Calf Brains.

This investigation was started for several reasons:
(a) To determine if an oligodendroglial plasma membrane fraction can be purified from whole tissue;
(b) To determine if the myelin-like fraction was indeed a
glial plasma membrane fraction;
(c) Finally it was hoped that comparisons of different myelin
subfractions would reveal possible stages in myelination as well as
any relationships between developing oligodendroglial plasma membranes and glial myelin. Thus light and heavy myelin and a fraction
of heavier density, designated as the myelin-like fraction, were
isolated from calf and from fetal calf brains at 5 months and 6.5
months of gestation. All of the samples were examined morphologically and were analyzed for lipids and proteins.
When preparing the subfractions of myelin, we were surprised
to find that light myelin was obtained from the osmotically shocked
low speed supernatant fraction which is usually discarded. Whether
this low speed supernatant fraction or the crude myelin pellets were
used to prepare light myelin, the solubility and lipid compositions
were the same.
Morphology and purity of calf myelin subfractions. An ultrastructural examination of light and heavy myelin from calf brain
revealed primarily multilamellar vesicles, with light myelin having
fewer lamellae per vesicle than heavy myelin. No recognizable
organelles such as mitochondria or nuclei were observed. The calf
myelin-like fraction, on the other hand, contained a heterogeneous
mixture of vesicles, amorphous dense material, and scattered multilamellar structures resembling myelin. Figures with a triple
layered appearance typical of plasma membranes were common, as well
as organelles resembling mitochondria and endoplasmic reticulum.
Much of the densely staining material, however, could not be identified.
Table 4 indicates the purity of the subfractions. Na^+, K^+-
ATPase and 5'-nucleotidase were both present in heavy myelin,
whereas only 5'-nucleotidase activity was found in light myelin.
Recycling the myelin fractions did not lower the enzyme activities.
The myelin associated enzyme (2',3'-cyclic AMPase) was present in
similar amounts in both myelin subfractions. The low levels of
other marker enzymes indicate little contamination by lysosomes,
mitochondria, or microsomes.
The heterogeneity found on the electron micrographs was emphasized by the diverse enzymatic activities present in the myelin-like
fraction. Increased levels of the plasma membrane marker enzymes,
as well as those indicating the presence of lysosomes, mitochondria,
the Golgi apparatus, endoplasmic reticulum, and nucleic acid-con-
taining particles were found. The unusual finding, however, was the
high level of the myelin related enzyme (2',3'-cyclic AMPase), some
three times the level normally found in myelin.

Table 4. Specific activity of subcellular organelle marker enzymes of calf myelin fractions.

	Light myelin	Heavy myelin	Myelin-like
5'-Nucleotidase*	4.33	1.54	4.61
Na^+, K^+-ATPase*	nd	0.54	7.04
2',3'-Cyclic AMPase*	250	243	813
Acid phosphatase*	nd	nd	0.16
Monoamine oxidase**	nd	nd	0.61
Glucose 6-phosphatase*	0.22	0.19	0.54
Thiamine pyrophosphatase*	0.04	0.04	0.21
RNA-P***	nd	9.29	311.25
DNA-P***	4.39	8.25	236.74

*μmoles Pi/mg prot/h; **units/mg prot/min; ***ng/mg dry wt; nd = not detected.

Morphology of fetal calf myelin subfractions. Electron micrographs of the 5-month fetal "myelin" fraction showed membranous vesicles, some with a pentalaminar structure. The 5-month fetal myelin-like fraction consisted of variously sized vesicles and many densely staining bodies. The 6.5-month fetal myelin subfractions on the other hand, had both light myelin with pentalaminar vesicles and heavy myelin with typical multilamellar structures. The myelin-like fraction of the 6.5-month fetus was similar to the younger 5-month fetal sample.

Lipids of the bovine myelin subfractions. Calf and 6.5-month fetal calf light and heavy myelin (Table 5) had similar solubility properties in chloroform:methanol and similar lipid compositions which confirm previous reports (2). As expected, however, the 5-month fetal "myelin" had different properties; it was only 58% soluble in organic solvents and consisted of 27% cholesterol, only 11% galactolipids, but a high concentration of phospholipids, 63%. In addition, both sets of the fetal myelin samples had consistently higher levels of gangliosides than those from calf. The thin layer chromatographic pattern of gangliosides was similar in all of the subfractions, although the actual amounts differed. It was surprising that G_{D3} was absent from all the samples, since it is present in both oligodendroglial myelin and plasma membranes.

In Table 6 the average values for lipids are expressed as mole ratios with cholesterol taken as 100. The similarities between light and heavy myelin are again noted as well as the differences between the myelin and myelin-like fractions. Moreover, changes that occur during development are clearly shown, such as the increase in galactolipids with the corresponding decrease in phospholipids, especially in phosphatidylcholine, with increasing age.

Table 5. Composition of bovine myelin subfractions.

| | Light myelin | | Heavy myelin | | | Myelin-like | | | Oligodendroglial | |
| | | | | | | | | | Myelin | Plasma membrane |
	6.5[a]	Calf[c]	5[a]	6.5[a]	Calf[c]	5[a]	6.5[a]	Calf[c]	Calf[d]	Calf[d]
Age	6.5[a]	Calf[c]	5[a]	6.5[a]	Calf[c]	5[a]	6.5[a]	Calf[c]	Calf[d]	Calf[d]
Brain weight (g)	85	300	53	85	300	53	85	300		
Yield (mg/10 g wet wt.)	4	355	1.2	18	573	7	12	17		
% of dry weight										
C:M soluble solids	91.0	94.4	57.5	88.0	96.7	56.0	59.4	58.5	74.6	54.4
C:M insoluble residue	3.8	1.7	38.1	8.4	1.5	39.4	37.4	41.4	19.4	42.6
Upper phase solids	5.2[b]	4.0	4.4	3.7[b]	1.9	4.6[b]	3.3[b]	0.1	6.0	3.1
Total protein	15.7[b]	23.5		29.5[b]	32.5	48.9[b]	47.5[b]	58.2	36.2	54.4
Total lipid	84.3[b]	72.6		70.5[b]	65.9	51.1[b]	52.5[b]	41.7	57.8	42.5
% of lipids										
Cholesterol	27.5	27.9	26.6	27.3	28.2	25.6	25.7	26.6	24.3	19.9
Galactolipids	24.4	27.4	10.9	20.3	24.7	2.7	9.8	21.8	22.1	14.8
Cerebrosides	19.4	20.8		15.9	19.8	2.3	8.7	18.6	18.2	11.7
Sulfatides	4.9	6.7		4.5	4.8	0.5	1.2	3.2	3.3	2.5
Total phospholipids	48.2	44.8	62.5	52.4	47.2	71.8	64.5	51.6	53.7	65.2
Phosphatidylethanolamine	16.2	17.4		17.3	19.0	16.0	17.8	15.5	10.8	9.5
Phosphatidylcholine	16.3	9.5		18.4	11.6	37.1	29.3	19.8	22.0	32.5
Sphingomyelin	5.1	6.8		4.5	6.0	5.0	4.9	7.9	6.7	6.9
Phosphatidylinositol	0.7	0.4		1.1	1.3	2.3	1.8	1.0	2.4	3.8
Phosphatidylserine	7.4	7.4		8.7	6.8	8.0	8.4	5.3	7.6	6.5
Unknown phospholipids	2.5	3.4		2.5	2.7	3.4	2.5	2.1	4.3	6.0
% of dry weight										
Gangliosides	0.25	0.09	2.12	0.31	0.04	0.94	0.86	0.32	0.52	0.49

a - Fetus, months of gestation; b - Calculated; c - Average of two preparations; d - Average of three preparations.

Table 6. Mole ratios+ of bovine myelin subfractions.

	Light myelin			Heavy myelin		Myelin-like			Oligodendroglial Myelin	Oligodendroglial Plasma membrane
Age	6.5ᵃ	Calf	5ᵃ	6.5ᵃ	Calf	5ᵃ	6.5ᵃ	Calf	Calf	Calf
Cholesterol	100	100	100	100	100	100	100	100	100	100
Total galactolipid (GL)	41	43	18	34	40	5	18	38	41	33
Cerebrosides	32	35		27	33	5	15	33	35	27
Sulfatides	7	10		7	7	1	2	5	6	6
Ratio: Cerebroside/ Sulfatide	4.60	3.57		3.80	4.80	5.0	7.5	6.6	5.80	4.50
Total phospholipid (PL)	87	82	117	96	84	141	124	97	110	162
Phosphatidylethanolamine (PE)	31	32		34	36	33	36	30	24	25
Phosphatidylcholine (PC)	28	21		32	19	70	54	36	43	77
Sphingomyelin	8	11		8	11	9	9	14	13	17
Phosphatidylinositol	1	1		1	1	5	3	1	5	8
Phosphatidylserine	13	13		15	11	15	15	9	14	13
Ratio: PE/PC	1.10	1.53		1.04	1.86	0.48	0.67	0.84	0.56	0.32
Ratio: GL/PC	1.45	2.07		1.04	2.07	0.07	0.33	1.04	0.95	0.43
Ratio: Cholesterol/PL	1.15	1.22	0.85	1.04	1.20	0.71	0.81	1.03	0.91	0.62

+ Mole ratios x 100, based on cholesterol=1. a - Fetus, months of gestation.

Proteins of the bovine myelin subfractions. Polyacrylamide
disc gel electrophoresis of the proteins from the light and heavy
myelin fractions from calf brain and 6.5-month fetal calf brain
produced similar patterns in agreement with previous studies. The
calf myelin-like fraction consisted of many high molecular weight
proteins, as well as several intermediate bands in the area corresponding to proteolipid protein, and a band with a mobility similar
to that of basic protein. The 5-month fetal "myelin" and myelin-
like fractions consisted of only high molecular weight proteins.

The myelin-like subfraction. The myelin-like fraction is
heterogeneous and heavily contaminated with membranes from subcellular organelles, as well as plasma membranes and possibly myelin.
The mole ratio of cholesterol:phospholipids:cerebrosides was 100:
141:5 in the 5-month fetal, 100:124:18 in the 6.5-month fetal and
100:97:38 in the calf myelin-like fractions. These changes may
reflect different types of contamination during isolation. Other
investigators have found similar changes in the myelin-like fraction
from rat brain; i.e. ratios of 100:191:2 were reported for 16-day-
old rats (1), and 100:164:13 in the adult rat (3). Another study
of 15-day-old rats gave a ratio of 100:120:12 (3). High molecular
weight proteins are consistently found, but basic and proteolipid
proteins may or may not be present.

How does this heterogeneous myelin-like fraction compare to
purified glial plasma membranes? Both the lipid and protein profiles differ from the plasma membranes. The myelin-like fraction
has different ratios of phospholipids, higher levels of cholesterol
and gangliosides, but lacks G_{D3}. It also has much higher levels of
the myelin-related enzyme (2',3'-cyclic AMPase), about seven times
the level found in plasma membranes. It is possible that this
fraction contains both axolemma and glial plasma membranes, as well
as contaminating subcellular organelle membranes. To date we have
not been able to isolate a purified glial plasma membrane fraction
from whole tissue.

A scheme for myelination. The properties of the glial plasma
membrane, glial myelin, and calf myelin are compared in Fig. 2 with
respect to both morphology and chemical composition. It is possible
to detect a pattern in the composition of each which may reflect the
process of myelination in the developing animal. For example, a
comparison of the lipids shows increasing cholesterol and galactolipids, and decreasing phospholipids, from the plasma membranes to
glial myelin to calf myelin. These changes are accompanied by
changes in protein patterns; i.e. basic and proteolipid protein increase as myelin matures with a concomitant decrease in high molecular weight proteins.

IV. Metabolic Properties of Oligodendroglia Maintained in
Culture.

Oligodendroglia maintained in culture (Fig. 1) actively syn-

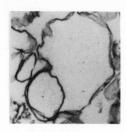
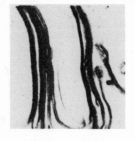
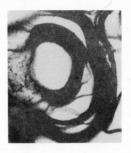

Oligodendroglial Plasma Membranes	Oligodendroglial Myelin	Calf Myelin
56% soluble in C:M	79% soluble in C:M	98% soluble in C:M
20% cholesterol	24% cholesterol	30% cholesterol
15% galactolipid	22% galactolipid	23% galactolipid
65% phospholipid	54% phospholipid	47% phospholipid
33% PC	22% PC	12% PC
10% PE	11% PE	18% PE
G_{D_3} +	G_{D_3} +	G_{D_3} -
PLP ±	PLP +	PLP +
	Basic +	Basic +

Fig. 2. Myelination

the size a variety of lipids and proteins <u>in vitro</u>. For this study, various radioactive precursors are added to the cells maintained in the enriched tissue culture medium which includes 5% fetal calf serum. No attempt is made to remove endogenous unlabeled substrate from the medium which means there is usually a several fold dilution of the precursor both by unlabeled substrates and by the large volume, 25 ml, in which the cells are maintained. After a specified time in culture, the cells are washed carefully, to keep them intact, and then are extracted in either organic solvents for lipid studies or detergents for protein studies. Radiolabeled products are quantitated by scintillation counting of lipids on thin layer chromatograms, (which are identified by co-migration with known lipid standards) or by scintillation counting of proteins on polyacrylamide gels.

    <u>Lipid synthesis.</u> <u>In vitro</u>, oligodendroglia actively synthesize the lipids which are predominant in brain and especially those enriched in myelin (10). For example, (Table 7), with $[^3H]$ or $[^{14}C]$galactose, all the lipids exhibit radioactivity, with cerebro-

sides showing high levels of incorporation. With acetic acid as
precursor, cholesterol has the most radioactivity. With glycerol,
the phospholipids predominate, especially phosphatidylcholine.
[^{35}S] sodium sulfate is incorporated primarily into sulfatides.

Table 7. Incorporation of radiolabeled precursors into lipids
synthesized by oligodendroglia in vitro.

	I [^{3}H] Galactose	II [^{3}H] HOAc	III [^{3}H] Glycerol	IV [^{14}C] Galactose	V [^{35}S] Na$_2$SO$_4$
Material at origin	95	95	202	85	–
Phosphatidyl serine and -inositol	3,093	442	726	216	–
Sphingomyelin	269	1,743	3,397	141	–
Phosphatidylcholine	1,553	3,973	7,541	70	–
Sulfatides		1,062	792	57	431
Phosphatidylethanolamine	2,103	1,694	2,056	498	–
Cerebrosides-OHFA	42,949	2,327	126	1,183	–
Cerebrosides-NFA			66	1,103	–
Cholesterol	1,271	34,606	1,438	922	–

Oligodendroglia were maintained in tissue culture flasks as described. The following conditions were used: I – 50 µCi
[^{3}H]galactose (specific activity 1-5 Ci/mole) for 1 day with approximately 0.35 mg of cell protein per flask. II – 50 µCi [^{3}H]acetic
acid, sodium salt (specific activity 500 mCi/mmole) for 18 h with
0.7 mg cell protein per flask. III – 50 µCi [^{3}H]glycerol (specific
activity 200 mCi/mmole) for 24 h with 1 mg cell protein per flask.
IV – 5 µCi [^{14}C]galactose (specific activity 50 mCi/mmole) for 2
days with 1 mg cell protein per flask. V – 500 µCi [^{35}S]sodium
sulfate (specific activity 10-1000 mCi/mmole sulfur) for 2 days
with 1 mg of cell protein per flask.
     Duplicate flasks were used for each time point. The cells
were removed from the flasks, and washed twice. They were then extracted for lipids with 0.1 mg of myelin lipid added as carrier.
After thin layer chromatography, the lipids were visualized with I$_2$
vapor, scraped into scintillation vials, and counted in a scintillation counter. The results are in DPM/mg protein.

Synthesis of lipids continues during 48 h in culture; the level
of synthesis almost doubles in each 24 h period. However, turnover
of certain lipids is becoming evident during 48 h. If the precursor
is added after the cells have been maintained in culture for 24 h,
and the cells are analyzed after an additional 24 h, the same level
of synthesis is detected on the second day as on the first day,
indicating that the cells remain viable in culture. Fragmented or
broken cells exhibit almost no incorporation. In the presence of
increasing amounts of KCN (6.5 mM - 76 mM), the incorporation of
[^{3}H]galactose into cerebrosides and other lipids is greatly reduced. The cells remain intact during these investigations.

It was necessary to adjust the quantity of cells used to detect
optimal synthesis of each lipid. For example, 0.1-0.2 mg of cell
protein per flask was sufficient to demonstrate active synthesis of
cerebroside; 1 mg of cell protein was slightly inhibitory. However
1 mg of cell protein was necessary to demonstrate the radiolabeling
of sulfatides with [^{35}S]sodium sulfate which was obviously very
much diluted by the tissue culture medium as well as the intracellular pools.

Synthesis of proteins. To study protein synthesis, isolated
oligodendroglia are maintained as suspension cultures for 2 days in
the presence of radiolabeled amino acids, such as [^{3}H]proline. The
cells are then washed and extracted with detergent. The soluble
proteins are then subjected to disc gel electrophoresis on 10% or
15% polyacrylamide gels; the gels are fixed, stained with Coomassie
blue, destained, sliced, and solubilized for scintillation counting.

As observed from Fig. 3 a spectrum of proteins is synthesized
by these glial cells, similar to the spectrum of lipids. However,
the proteins are less easily identified. Mostly high molecular
weight proteins are produced with this amino acid precursor, with
no detectable differences in the quantities produced. It is dis-
appointing that, thus far, we have been unable to demonstrate the
synthesis of either of the myelin-specific proteins, proteolipid
protein or basic protein. The possibility exists that these myelin
specific proteins have properties in the intact cell different from
those in isolated myelin, which may account for our inability to
detect them. Alternatively, these proteins may only be produced
during active myelin synthesis.

V. Preparation of Antiserum Specific to Oligodendroglial
Surface Components.

Two sera have been produced; one specific to rat neurons and
the other to lamb oligodendroglia, isolated in bulk from normal
brain. The specificities of the antisera were determined both by
immunofluorescence of the respective target cells and by absorptions
of the antisera by isolated cell populations from different tissues.
Only the antiserum specific to oligodendroglial surface components
(9) will be described here.

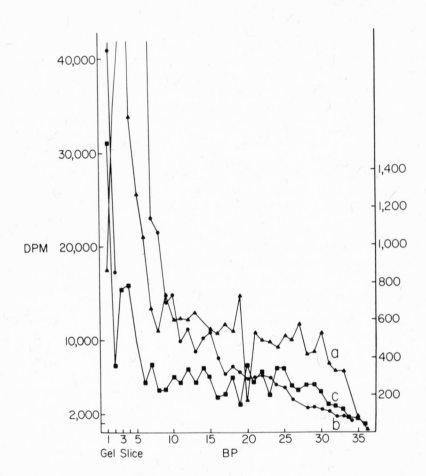

Fig. 3. Profile of radiolabeled proteins on 15% polyacrylamide gels (after disc gel electrophoresis) obtained from isolated oligo-dendroglia after exposure to [^{3}H]proline. Results are in DPM/mg protein. a. Calf cells, detergent (SDS) extract of whole cells; b. Lamb cells, detergent extraction of chloroform:methanol-insoluble residue; c. Lamb cells, detergent extraction of ether:ethanol-insoluble residue. The right axis is used for c.

The antiserum was produced in rabbits by subcutaneous injections in Freund's complete adjuvant of bulk isolated, washed oligodendroglia. Glia suspended in PBS were used for repeat injections at two week intervals for three injections. After the final set, the rabbits were bled, the serum was collected, heat-inactivated at 56°C for 30 min, and stored at -20°C in small vials.

The antiserum was tested for antibody activity by indirect immunofluorescence with suspensions of target cells maintained overnight. The cells were not fixed during this procedure. The antiserum was absorbed at room temperature for 30 min with cells dissociated from lamb liver, lamb red cells, isolated neurons, astrocytes, or oligodendroglia, or purified myelin. After centrifugation, the antiserum was removed and subsequently assessed for antibody activity.

With the use of maintained lamb oligodendroglia as the target cell and the antiserum produced to oligodendroglia, the glial cells exhibit bright green surface fluorescence at the titrations indicated in Table 8. Similar results were obtained with oligodendroglia isolated from calf or human brain. No surface fluorescence was observed when the antiserum was absorbed with isolated oligodendroglia. However, absorptions with rat neurons, lamb liver or red cells, lamb brain gray matter, or lamb myelin did not alter the surface fluorescence of the glial cells. Negative results were obtained with controls of conjugate alone, nonimmune rabbit serum, or antiserum without conjugate.

Based on immunofluorescence, the antiserum did not contain antibodies against any of the components used during the cell isolation (trypsin, albumin, fetal calf serum), since such antiserum would be expected to bind in a similar manner with all three cell types. This was not observed. Moreover, myelin does not appear to share the same surface components with oligodendroglia, since repeated absorptions with myelin did not change the specificity of the antiserum. This is in accord with the difference found in the biochemical compositions of oligodendroglial plasma membranes and myelin.

Recently we have had the opportunity to use our maintained cells to test antisera prepared by other investigators. Dr. Maurice Rapport has prepared antiserum against galactocerebroside, which at titrations of 1:200 reacts in patches with the oligodendroglial surface. However, there is no reaction if the antiserum is absorbed with either isolated oligodendroglia or isolated myelin. Dr. Melitta Schachner has prepared antiserum to bovine corpus callosum which also reacts with the surface of maintained oligodendroglia. Antiserum to basic protein, prepared by Dr. Steven Cohen, does not react with maintained oligodendroglia, although serum from rabbits with experimental allergic encephalomyelitis does.

Serum from multiple sclerosis patients and normal controls was obtained through the clinic at the Johns Hopkins Medical School. Over 75 different sera were tested. All of the sera from multiple sclerosis patients reacted with oligodendroglia but half of the

Table 8. Immunofluorescent staining of lamb oligodendroglia with antiserum to lamb oligodendroglia.

Treatment of antiserum	Fluorescence with antiserum diluted		
	1:80	1:160	1:270
None	+	+	+
Absorbed with:			
Liver	+	+	+
Liver and red blood cells	+	+	+
Gray matter	+	+	+
Rat myelin	+	+	+
Lamb myelin	+	+	+
Oligodendroglia	–	–	–

Aliquots of antiserum were sequentially absorbed with lamb liver and red blood cells as indicated in the text. Separate 0.1 ml unabsorbed aliquots were absorbed with 10X volume of dissected lamb brain gray matter; 1,2 mg of rat myelin protein; 1.56, 3.12, and 6.24 mg of lamb myelin protein; and 250 and 490 x 10^6 isolated lamb oligodendroglia. The results shown were the same for each concentration; titrations were the same before and after absorptions. +, positive surface fluorescence; –, no surface fluorescence.

Table 9. Incorporation of [³H]galactose into lipids of oligodendroglial plasma membranes and glial myelin.

Time in culture	6 h		1 day		2 days	
	Glial myelin	Plasma membranes	Glial myelin	Plasma membranes	Glial myelin	Plasma membranes
Material at origin	173	125	249	137	665	322
Phosphatidylserine and -inositol	67	62	932	451	2098	821
Sphingomyelin	80	31	3605	819	1475	338
Phosphatidylcholine	520	93	466	451	1163	789
Sulfatides	227	47	1911	1052	2285	1031
Phosphatidylethanolamine	906	280	10847	5285	5234	2576
Cerebrosides – OHFA	933	218	35976	21169	42160	21304
Cerebrosides – NFA	1040	109	19876	14299	12420	7842
Cholesterol	2186	498	3947	1366	3863	3221
DPM/mg protein						

Ratio: Myelin/Plasma Membranes

Time	6 h	1 day	2 days
Origin	1.4	1.8	2.1
Phosphatidylserine and -inositol	1.1	2.1	2.6
Sphingomyelin	2.6	4.4	4.4
Phosphatidylcholine	5.6	1.0	1.5
Sulfatides	4.8	1.8	2.2
Phosphatidylethanolamine	3.2	2.1	2.0
Cerebrosides – OHFA	4.3	1.7	2.0
Cerebrosides – NFA	9.5	1.4	1.6
Cholesterol	4.4	2.9	1.2

controls reacted as well. Thus, this reaction may be nonspecific, but is under further investigation.

VI. Myelin Synthesis in vitro.

Isolated oligodendroglia are free of contamination by myelin and only occasionally retain tiny processes. Once the cells are in tissue culture medium, however, they frequently project very thin filamentous processes. After 24 h in culture some of the cells have membranous rounded protrusions emanating from them. During the next 24-48 h, many cells have these membranous whorls which also increase in size, some of them becoming the same size as the cell. The cells remain intact and round during this time.

In an immunofluorescent assay with oligodendroglia in culture for 48 h, both the cells and the attached membranous whorls exhibit bright green surface fluorescence when reacted with either the antiserum to oligodendroglia or that to cerebrosides. Thus these newly formed membranous whorls ("glial myelin") have characteristics of both myelin and oligodendroglia.

To investigate this phenomenon further, cells in culture for 24 and 48 h were homogenized and both the plasma membranes and glial myelin fractions were purified. The myelin layer obtained from the sucrose gradients increased from cells in culture during 24 to 48 h, indicating the cells were indeed producing a form of myelin.

If $[^3H]$ galactose is added to oligodendroglia for various times, and the cells are then washed, homogenized, and plasma membranes and glial myelin prepared, the results presented in Table 9 are obtained.

For these experiments the glial myelin and plasma membranes were only subjected to one gradient during the preparation and were not further purified. From these data it is evident that both the glial myelin and plasma membranes have radioactivity associated with all the lipids, the radioactivity incorporated into the lipids increases with time in culture, and the glial myelin has a higher specific activity than the plasma membranes. No precursor product relationship is evident in this set of experiments. Experiments with other radiolabeled precursors give similar results. With $[^3H]$ acetic acid, cholesterol exhibits the most radioactivity and the incorporation into cholesterol increases with time in culture. With $[^3H]$glycerol the phospholipids, especially phosphatidylcholine, have the most radioactivity; with $[^{35}S]$sodium sulfate, sulfatides are exclusively radiolabeled.

If culture times are extended to 3 or 4 days, both light and heavy myelin can be purified from the cells. The amounts of radioactivity associated with each lipid in all three subfractions of glia are actively being assessed. It is apparent that each lipid is synthesized at different rates and assembled into glial myelin at different times.

If oligodendroglia are maintained with [^{3}H]proline and the glial subfractions purified and subjected to disc gel electrophoresis, the radioactivity associated with each protein can be determined. The plasma membranes seem to have a spectrum of proteins with radioactivity as in the intact cell. However, evidence of synthesis of proteins migrating to similar positions on gels as mature myelin proteins is apparent in both light and heavy myelin.

With the use of a more sensitive radioimmunoassay, it is possible to detect changes in basic protein, as glial subfractions are compared. More basic protein is associated with the plasma membranes (0.65 μg/mg protein) than with the intact cells (0.19 μg/mg protein). However, light (5.7 μg/mg protein) and heavy myelin (3.3 μg/mg protein) have the highest levels of basic protein. The amount of basic protein associated with the glial myelin also increases between one and two days in culture (this assay was performed by Dr. Steven Cohen). A highly sensitive assay for the myelin-associated enzyme (2',3'-cyclic AMPase) shows that the membranes have 80% of the activity of light and heavy myelin in which the level of activity is similar to that in mature myelin (these assays were performed by Dr. Terry Sprinkle).

Thus oligodendroglia appear to produce myelin in tissue culture. The glial myelin has properties similar to more mature myelin as well as properties of the intact cell.

Acknowledgements. Special thanks go to the collaborative efforts of Dr. W.T. Norton at the Albert Einstein Medical School in New York where this study was started and to Dr. G.M. McKhann at Johns Hopkins Medical School in Maryland where this research continues. In New York this research was supported by U.S. Public Health Service Grants NS 02476 and NS 03356 and the Multiple Sclerosis Society. In Maryland it is supported by funds from John A. Hartford Foundation, PHS Grants NS 10920, 08719, and 02491, and the Multiple Sclerosis Society.

REFERENCES

1. Agrawal, H.C., Banik, N.L., Bone, A.H., Davison, A.N., Mitchell, R.F. and Spohn, M., The identity of a myelin-like fraction isolated from developing brain, Biochem. J. 120 (1970) 635-642.
2. Autilio, L.A., Norton, W.T. and Terry, R.D., The preparation and some properties of purified myelin from the central nervous system, J. Neurochem. 11 (1964) 17-27.
3. Banik, N.L. and Davison, A.N., Enzyme activity and composition of myelin and subcellular fractions in the developing rat brain, Biochem. J. 115 (1969) 1051-1062.
4. Fewster, M.E. and Blackstone, S., In vitro study of bovine oligodendroglia, Neurobiology 5 (1975) 316-328.

5. Fewster, M.E., Ihrig, T. and Mead, J.F., Biosynthesis of long
    chain fatty acids by oligodendroglia isolated from bovine
    white matter, J. Neurochem. 25 (1975) 207-213.
6. Fewster, M.E., Scheibel, A.B. and Mead, J.F., The preparation
    of isolated glial cells from rat and bovine white matter,
    Brain Res. 6 (1967) 401-408.
7. Keil, B., Trypsin, in The Enzymes 13 (P.D. Boyer, ed.) Academic
    Press, N.Y. (1971) pp. 249-275.
8. Poduslo, S.E., The isolation and characterization of a plasma
    membrane and a myelin fraction derived from oligodendroglia of
    calf brain, J. Neurochem. 24 (1975) 647-654.
9. Poduslo, S.E., McFarland, H.F. and McKhann, G.M., Antiserums
    to neurons and to oligodendroglia from mammalian brain, Science
    197 (1977) 270-272.
10. Poduslo, S.E. and McKhann, G.M., Synthesis of cerebrosides by
    intact oligodendroglia maintained in culture, Neuroscience
    Letters 5 (1977) 159-163.
11. Poduslo, S.E. and McKhann, G.M., Maintenance of neurons isolated
    in bulk from rat brain: Incorporation of radiolabeled sub-
    strates, Brain Res. 132 (1977) 107-120.
12. Poduslo, S.E. and Norton, W.T., Isolation and some chemical
    properties of oligodendroglia from calf brain, J. Neurochem.
    19 (1972) 727-736.
13. Poduslo, S.E. and Norton, W.T., Isolation of specific brain
    cells, in Methods in Enzymology 35 (S.P. Colowick and N.O.
    Kaplan, eds.) Academic Press, N.Y. (1975) pp. 561-579.
14. Raine, C.S., Poduslo, S.E. and Norton, W.T., The ultrastructure
    of purified preparations of neurons and glial cells, Brain
    Res. 27 (1971) 11-24.

STUDIES ON MYELIN PROTEINS IN HUMAN PERIPHERAL NERVE

Keiichi Uyemura, Masaru Suzuki and Kunio Kitamura

Department of Physiology, Saitama Medical School

Moroyama, Irumagun, Saitama, Japan

SUMMARY

The myelin fraction from human peripheral nerve was prepared. Two basic protein fractions (BF-P2 and PB) were isolated from acid extracts of the myelin fraction and three glycoproteins(BR-PO, PASII and Y protein) were purified from its acid-insoluble residue. In biochemical analysis the human BF-P2 protein (M.W.13,000) showed similar but not identical properties to bovine BF-P2 protein. The PB fraction was suggested to include the encephalitogenic CNS-BP (M.W.18,000) and another, new protein of similar molecular weight.

Both the human BR-PO protein (M.W.28,000) and PASII protein (M.W.13,000) showed similar biochemical properties to the corresponding myelin proteins of bovine peripheral nerve, while they both are clearly different from other myelin proteins. Close relationship between the BR-PO protein and the Y protein (M.W.22,000) was suggested by amino acid analysis.

Injection of the myelin fraction of bovine peripheral nerve with the complete adjuvant produced EAN while the CNS-BP induced

---

Abbreviations used: CNS - Central nervous system; PNS - Peripheral nervous system; CNS-BP - Encephalitogenic basic protein (M.W. 18,000) in CNS myelin; FLPL - Folch-Lees type proteolipid in CNS myelin; BF-P2 protein - Basic protein (M.W.13,000) in PNS myelin; BR-PO protein - Glycoprotein (M.W.28,000) in PNS myelin; PASII protein - Glycoprotein (M.W.13,000) in PNS myelin; Y protein - Glycoprotein (M.W.22,000) in PNS myelin; SDS - Sodium dodecyl sulfate; PAS - Periodic acid-Shiff; EAN - Experimental allergic neuritis; EAE - Experimental allergic encephalomyelitis.

EAE in laboratory animals. However, all three purified proteins,
BF-P2, BR-PO and PASII, from bovine peripheral nerve myelin were
inactive in inducing demyelinating diseases.

INTRODUCTION

Recent studies revealed that the biochemical properties of
myelin proteins of the PNS are greatly different from those of the
CNS (2, 16, 20, 31), in spite of their morphological similarities.
However, there has been considerable confusion about the nature and
composition of the myelin proteins of PNS as reviewed by Carnegie
et al.(9).
In relation to neurological diseases of PNS, biochemical
studies on myelin proteins of human PNS are interesting and important projects. Only a few studies, however, have been reported on
myelin proteins in human PNS (1, 21, 26). We reported previously
the purification procedures and biochemical properties of basic
proteins and glycoproteins of pig and bovine PNS myelin (16, 17,
27-31). The purpose of the present study was to isolate and
characterize the basic proteins and glycoproteins of human PNS
myelin and to compare them with those of bovine PNS myelin which
were reported previously.

EXPERIMENTAL

Preparation of myelin fractions. Human spinal roots and spinal
cords were obtained from patients who died from non-neurological
diseases. All samples were dissected at autopsies within several
hours after death. The nerve samples were stored at -80°C until
biochemical analysis. Myelin fractions were prepared from human
intradural spinal roots and from the spinal cords by the method
described by Uyemura et al. (31) with minor modifications (0.85 M
sucrose solution was used instead of 0.80 M for homogenization of
the tissues). Crude myelin fractions were obtained at interphase
layers between 0.32 M and 0.85 M sucrose after density gradient
centrifugation at 65,000 g for 60 min. The layers were resuspended
in 0.85 M sucrose and recentrifuged. Final interphase layers were
washed with 0.24 M sucrose once, homogenized in distilled water in
order to release axoplasm by osmotic shock at 0°C and then centrifuged at 10,000 g for 10 min. After dialysis of the pellets, the
samples were lyophilized and were used as the myelin fractions of
PNS (spinal roots) and of CNS (spinal cords) for further analysis.
For electron microscopic examination, the pellets of myelin fragments
were fixed in 2% glutaraldehyde-0.1 M phosphate buffer for 120 min
and in 1% osmium tetraoxide-0.1 M phosphate buffer for 90 min suc-
cessively. After dehydration, the blocks were embedded in Epon
812 resin according to the procedure described by Luft (19).

Electron micrographs were made with a JEM-100C electron microscope.

Isolation of myelin basic proteins. The acid extracts and residue of the myelin fraction of human PNS were obtained by treatment of the fraction with 0.03 N HCl (pH 2.0) as described previously (17). The acid extracts of the myelin fraction were dialysed, concentrated, then applied on Sephadex G-75 column and eluted with 0.03 N HCl containing 0.15 M NaCl.

CNS-BP protein was purified with a similar method from a human CNS myelin fraction.

Isolation of myelin glycoproteins. The acid residue of the myelin fraction was dissolved in 20 vol. of chloroform-methanol (2:1, v/v) per wet weight, adjusted to pH 7.0 and centrifuged to obtain the insoluble material. This procedure was repeated again and the lipid-free precipitate thus obtained was solubilized in 10% SDS-0.1 M phosphate buffer (pH 7.2). After incubation for 1 h at 45°C, the sample was applied on a Sephadex G-200 column and eluted with 2% SDS-0.1 M phosphate buffer as described previously (16).

Polyacrylamide gel electrophoresis. The electrophoresis on 15% polyacrylamide gels at pH 4.3 was carried out according to the method of Reisfeld et al. (22). For SDS polyacrylamide gel electrophoresis at pH 7.2, the method of Shapiro et al. (23) was used with some modifications (16). The gels were stained with Coomassie brilliant blue R250 for proteins and periodic acid-Shiff (PAS) reagent for glycoproteins, respectively, according to the methods of Fairbanks et al.(12).

Amino acid analysis. About 1 mg of protein sample was hydrolysed in 1 ml of constant boiling HCl at 110°C for 22 h in an evacuated sealed tube. Amino acid analysis was carried out with a JEOL JLC-6AH automatic amino acid analyser as previously described (17).

Immunodiffusion. The anti-bovine BF-P2 protein antibody was prepared in rabbits (27). The agar gel immunodiffusion test was carried out on microscope slides coated with 0.85% agarose containing 76.5 mM Tris-120 mM NaCl buffer (pH 7.4) with 0.01% thiomersalum. The center well contained 10 µl of antibovine BF-P2 protein antibody solution (50 mg/ml) and the peripheral well contained 10µl of the sample in physiological saline. Precipitin lines appeared within 24 h and were developed maximally by 48 h at room temperature, at which time the plates were photographed.

Antigenic activity to induce demyelinating disease. The inoculum consisted of 1 part (by volume) of antigen solution (500 µg protein) and 1 part of Freund's complete adjuvant. The mixture was given intradermally once in each footpad of a test animal (guinea pig of 300-400 g body weight). All animals were sacrificed either when neurological symptoms developed or at 30 days after inoculation. Symptoms developed usually between 14-20 days after inoculation. Brains, spinal cords, Gasserian ganglia, dorsal ganglia and sciatic nerves of test animals were dissected and fixed in 10% formalin for at least 3 days. Sections were stained with luxol fast

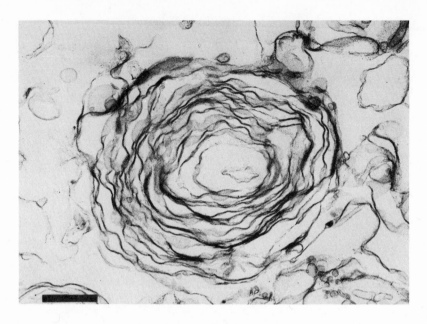

a

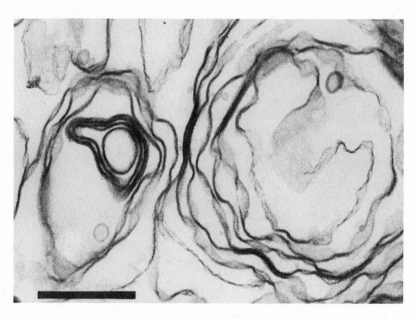

b

Fig. 1-a and 1-b. Electron micrographs of the myelin fraction from human PNS. Scales represent 0.5 μm.

blue and hematoxylin-eosin. The histological changes were examined
to confirm the diagnosis of demyelinating diseases, EAN (33) in the
PNS and EAE (18) in the CNS.

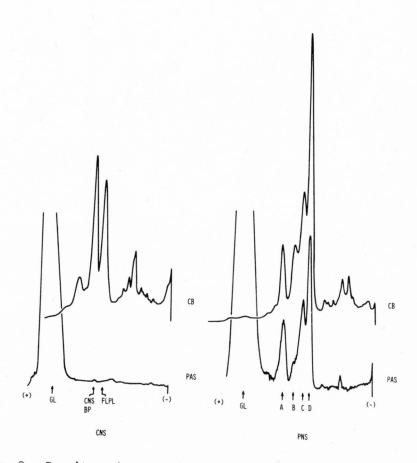

Fig. 2. Densitomeric comparison of myelin proteins from human PNS
and CNS in 1% SDS-10% polyacrylamide gel electrophoresis. Samples
were dissolved in 0.1 M sodium phosphate buffer, pH 7.2, containing
1% SDS, 1% 2-mercaptoethanol and 0.01% Malachite green. The gels
were stained with Coomassie blue (CB) or with PAS reagent. The CB
stained gels were scanned at 550 nm (reference: 460 nm), while the
gels stained with PAS were scanned at 550 nm (reference: 475 nm)
with a Dual-wavelength TLC scanner CS-900 (Shimazu). Each gel
contained 20 μg of protein for CB staining and 40 μg for PAS staining, respectively. GL: Glycolipids.

RESULTS

The myelin fraction from human PNS. Electron micrographs of
the myelin fraction of human PNS are shown in Fig. 1-a and 1-b.
The fraction consisted predominantly of isolated myelin lamellae.
Nuclei and mitochondria were completely absent, and contamination
with axonal membranes was very small.

Myelin proteins of human PNS showed four distinct bands (A,
B, C, D) with protein staining and three PAS positive bands (A, C,
D) in SDS polyacrylamide gel electrophoresis (Fig. 2). In human
PNS myelin, relatively denser bands of B and C than those of bovine
PNS myelin were characteristically observed. On the other hand,
proteins of human spinal cord myelin showed two main bands, CNS-
BP (18) and FLPL (13, 32) with one minor fast migrating band and
several bands in high molecular weight region with protein staining.
All these bands were PAS negative. Relative mobility of CNS-BP
was identical with that of the band B of PNS myelin. The FLPL
band of the CNS myelin migrated just between the bands C and D of
the PNS myelin. The mobility of the band A corresponded well to a
minor fast migrating band of the CNS myelin. These results suggest
that the bands A and D contain similar proteins as the BF and BR
proteins reported by us (16, 17, 30, 31) and the P2 and PO proteins
reported by Eylar´s group (2, 4-6, 14), respectively. As the band
A was PAS positive, it was also considered to contain a glycoprotein,
PASII, recently reported by us (16).

Electrophoretical patterns of the acid extracts and residue of
human PNS myelin revealed that the bands C and D were not extract-
able with acid and that all three PAS positive bands remained in
the residue (Fig. 3). It should be noted that the band A from acid
residue was both PAS and protein stainable while the band A from
acid extracts was protein stainable but PAS negative. Accordingly,
the former corresponded to a glycoprotein, PASII, and the latter
to a basic protein, BF-P2, respectively. An attempt to purify basic
proteins from acid extracts and glycoproteins of the acid residue
of human PNS myelin was made. Purification procedures of myelin
proteins of human PNS are summarized in the flowsheet (Table 1).

Isolation of basic proteins from human PNS myelin. The
chromatographic pattern of acid extracts of the PNS myelin fraction
on Sephadex G-75 column is shown in Fig. 4. Three peaks, PA, PB
and PC were obtained. The PB and PC fractions were collected. In
SDS electrophoresis, both the PB and PC fraction showed a single
band which migrated in an identical position with that of CNS-BP
(M.W. 18,000) and that of BF-P2 (M.W. 13,000), respectively (Fig.
5-a). In a 12.5% polyacrylamide gel electrophoresis at pH 4.3,
however, the PB fraction migrated to form two similar bands in the
region of CNS-BP although the PC fraction showed a single band
(Fig. 5-b). Relative mobility of the slow migrating band of the
PB fraction was identical with that of CNS-BP (Fig. 6). The faster
migrating band of the PB fraction was different from CNS-BP.

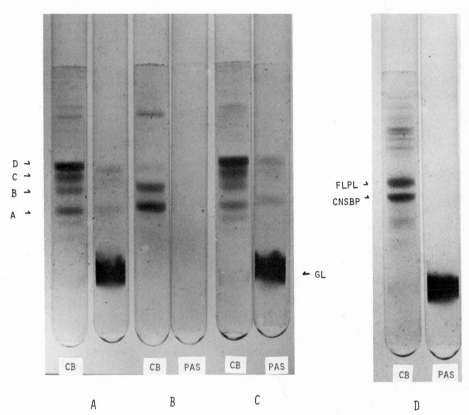

Fig. 3. Electrophoretic comparison of acid soluble and acid insoluble proteins of human peripheral nerve myelin. A: whole PNS
myelin proteins; B: acid extracts of PNS myelin; C: acid insoluble proteins of PNS myelin; D: whole CNS myelin proteins.
Each gel contained 20 µg of protein for CB staining and 40 µg
for PAS staining, respectively.

        This band seemed not to be a degradation product of CNS-BP
included in the PNS myelin because such a band was not detectable
when CNS-BP was obtained by a similar method from human spinal
cord. Attempts to further separate these bands from the PB fraction
were unsuccessful.
        When the relative mobility of the PC fraction-human BF-P2
protein was compared to that of the bovine BF-P2 protein in a 15%
polyacrylamide gel electrophoresis at pH 4.3, the human protein migrated slightly faster than the bovine one.(Fig. 7). These findings
indicated that the human BF-P2 protein was similar to but not
identical with the bovine BF-P2 protein.

Table 1

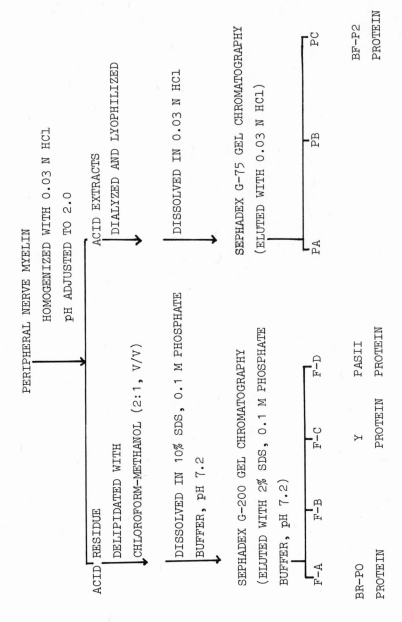

Immunological study of human BF-P2 protein. Tests between the
human and bovine BF-P2 protein and anti-bovine BF-P2 antibody showed
the converging arc of a homologous reaction (Fig. 8). On the
other hand, no precipitin line was observed between the PB fraction
and the antibody. Accordingly, the immunological determinant of
the human BF-P2 protein was revealed to be identical with that of
the bovine BF-P2 protein.

Amino acid analysis of basic proteins of human PNS myelin.
Amino acid compositions of the human PB fraction, BF-P2 protein,
CNS-BP and bovine BF-P2 protein are compared in Table 2. The human
BF-P2 protein showed, as a whole, a quite similar amino acid composition to the bovine BF-P2 protein with slight differences in
Gly, Val and Lys contents. From these results of both electrophoretical and immunological analysis it can be concluded that the
human BF-P2 protein certainly is of the similar type of protein
as the bovine BF-P2. The human PB fraction had a similar amino
acid pattern as the human CNS-BP. As this fraction contained a
protein band which migrated in an identical position with CNS-BP
in two types of electrophoresis, we considered that the human PNS
myelin might also contain the same protein as CNS-BP. However,
significant differences were observed in their Ser, Glu, Gly, Cys
and Arg contents. These discrepancies may indicate that the amino
acid composition of the other component of the PB fraction is different from CNS-BP.

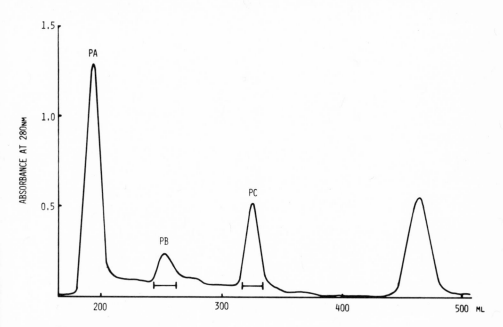

Fig. 4. Sephadex G-75 gel chromatography of acid soluble proteins
from human PNS myelin. Acid soluble proteins (80 mg) were applied
on a column (2.64 x 90 cm) and eluted with 0.03 N HCl containing
0.15 M NaCl at 4°C. Flow rate = 30 ml/h.

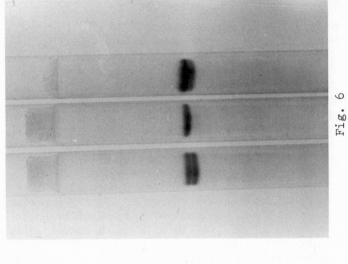

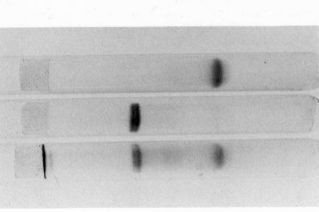

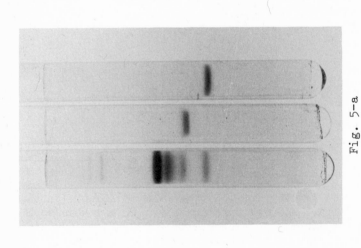

Fig. 5-a   Fig. 5-b   Fig. 6

Fig. 5-a. SDS polyacrylamide gel electrophoresis of the basic protein fractions from gel filtration. From left to right: whole PNS myelin (20 μg of protein), PB fraction (2.5 μg), and PC fraction (2.5 μg).

Fig. 5-b. Polyacrylamide gel electrophoresis (pH 4.3) of the basic protein fractions from gel filtration. From left to right: acid extracts of human PNS myelin (20 μg), PB fraction (5 μg), and PC fraction (2.5 μg).

Fig. 6. Electrophoretical comparison of the PB fraction and CNS-BP at pH 4.3. From left to right: the PB fraction (5.0 μg), CNS-BP (2.5 μg), and the mixture of the PB fraction and CNS-BP.

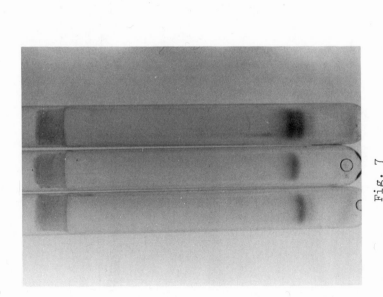

Fig. 7

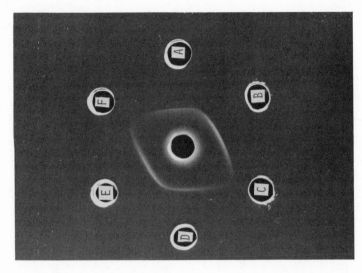

Fig. 8

Fig. 7. Electrophoretical comparison of human and bovine BF-P2 proteins at pH 4.3. From left to right: human BF-P2 protein (2.5 μg), bovine BF-P2 protein (2.5 μg), and mixture of the two proteins.

Fig. 8. Immunodiffusion of basic proteins of human PNS myelin(peripheral wells) against anti-bovine BF-P2 protein antibody (center well). A and D: bovine BF-P2 protein; B and E: human BF-P2 protein; C and F: human PB fraction; A, B and C: 3 μg protein each; D, E and F: 1.5 μg protein each.

Table 2. Amino acid composition (moles/100 moles) of myelin basic proteins.

Amino acid*	PB fraction (3)	Human BF-P2 protein (5)	CNS-BP**	Bovine BF-P2 protein*** (6)
Aspartic acid	7.9±0.3	9.4±0.2	6.4	9.8±0.2
Threonine	5.3±0.1	9.7±0.3	4.7	9.7±0.4
Serine	9.2±0.6	7.2±0.3	11.1	6.1±0.2
Glutamic acid	7.5±0.6	11.0±0.6	5.2	10.3±0.1
Proline	6.6±0.2	2.4±0.4	7.0	2.0±0.1
Glycine	12.8±1.1	9.5±0.2	15.2	7.5±0.1
Alanine	8.6±0.3	5.0±0.2	7.0	4.2±0.1
Cysteine	0.4±0.1	0.5±0.3****	0	0.3±0.4****
Valine	4.4±1.2	6.3±0.6	2.3	7.9±0.2
Methionine	1.4±0.2	2.3±0.1	1.1	2.4±0.1
Isoleucine	2.0±0.1	4.4±0.4	2.3	5.2±0.1
Leucine	6.3±0.2	7.2±0.4	4.7	8.0±0.2
Tyrosine	2.7±0.3	2.2±0.3	2.3	1.5±0.1
Phenylalanine	4.6±0.3	4.3±0.4	5.2	4.0±0.1
Histidine	5.9±0.1	1.5±0.2	5.8	0
Lysine	7.6±0.5	11.7±0.6	7.0	14.7±0.6
Arginine	6.9±1.0	5.5±0.2	11.1	5.6±0.2

Values are given as mean ± SD for several determinations. The numbers of determinations are shown in parentheses. *Tryptophan was not determined; **Data of Carnegie (1971); ***Data of Kitamura et al. (1975); ****About two moles/mole protein were detected after performic acid oxydation.

Table 3. Amino acid composition (moles/100 moles) of myelin glycoproteins.

Amino acid*	Human			Bovine**	
	BR-PO protein	Y protein	PASII protein	BR-PO protein	PASII
Aspartic acid	8.9	9.1	7.7	8.4	6.6
Threonine	5.6	5.4	6.9	6.2	6.8
Serine	7.5	6.9	10.2	6.8	10.2
Glutamic acid	8.8	8.4	8.9	8.4	8.5
Proline	4.1	4.6	2.2	3.7	2.0
Glycine	9.9	10.3	7.1	10.1	8.4
Alanine	5.9	5.2	6.8	6.4	6.8
Cysteine	0.5	1.4	1.4	0.9	1.0
Valine	8.7	9.2	6.9	8.6	8.0
Methionine	1.3	0.9	1.8	1.2	2.4
Isoleucine	4.3	5.1	6.4	4.3	4.8
Leucine	7.2	7.2	13.0	7.5	11.1
Tyrosine	4.8	5.5	3.8	5.5	3.7
Phenylalanine	3.6	4.3	6.3	3.6	6.3
Histidine	3.0	3.2	3.3	3.1	2.8
Lysine	7.7	6.4	4.0	8.7	6.6
Arginine	8.3	7.0	3.3	6.8	4.0

*Tryptophan was not determined. **Data of Kitamura et al. (16).
Values are given as the mean of two different determinations.

Isolation of glycoproteins of human PNS myelin. The delipidated acid residue of the human PNS myelin fraction was applied to a
Sephadex G-200 column and eluted with 2% SDS solution (Fig. 9). The
different parts of the two peaks, F-a, F-b, F-c and F-d (Fig. 9),
contained the following proteins: pure BR-PO, mainly BR-PO, mixture
of BR-PO and Y, and mainly PASII, respectively. Each subfraction
obtained from the gel chromatography was purified with rechromato-
graphy. Each of the purified BR-PO, Y and PASII proteins thus obtained showed a single band in SDS electrophoresis (Fig. 10). The
molecular weights of BR-PO, Y and PASII proteins were determined
as 28,000, 22,000 and 13,000, respectively.
    Amino acid compositions of glycoproteins in human PNS myelin.
Amino acid compositions of the purified glycoproteins are shown in
Table 3. The human BR-PO protein showed a very similar amino acid
pattern to that of bovine BR-PO protein. Similarity between the
patterns of human and bovine PASII proteins was also demonstrated
while obvious differences were noticed between the amino acid compositions of the BR-PO, BF-P2, PASII, CNS-BP and FLPL proteins.
The Y protein had a similar amino acid composition as BR-PO.
    Antigenic activities of myelin proteins to induce demyelinating
disease. The antigenic activities of the PNS myelin proteins to
produce demyelinating diseases, EAN and EAE, in laboratory animals
were examined. The results are summarized in Table 4. Since lesions
usually appear in the dorsal ganglia or Gasserian ganglia at an
early stage of EAN, these regions were histologically examined in

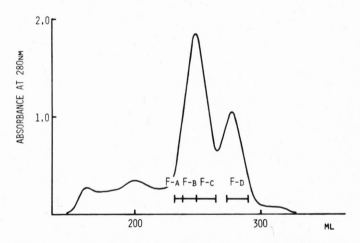

Fig. 9. Gel chromatographic profiles of acid insoluble proteins of
human PNS myelin on Sephadex G-200 column. 70 mg of the proteins
were dissolved in 3 ml of 0.1 M phosphate buffer, pH 7.2, containing 10% SDS and applied on a column (2.64 x 90 cm) equilibrated
and eluted with 0.1 M phosphate buffer containing 2% SDS. Flow
rate = 10 ml/h.

detail. Injection of 500 μg protein of the bovine PNS myelin induced EAN findings at a high rate while the same amounts of injected CNS-BP caused EAE findings without histological lesions in
the PNS. However, injections of the purified proteins of the PNS
myelin, such as BF-P2, BR-PO and PASII, had no or mild activities
to induce demyelination.

DISCUSSION

The human PNS myelin contains four fundamental protein components, two basic proteins BF-P2 and CNS-BP, and two glycoproteins,
BR-PO and PASII. The corresponding proteins of rabbit and bovine
PNS myelin have been studied independently by Eylar (2-6, 14) and
our groups (10, 15-17, 27-31). In addition, a third glycoprotein,
Y, was newly purified and the existence of a basic protein resembling CNS-BP was suggested (14).

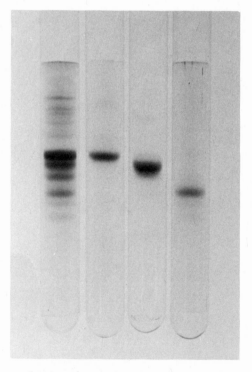

Fig. 10. SDS polyacrylamide gel electrophoresis of the purified
glycoproteins from human PNS myelin. From left to right: whole
myelin proteins of human PNS (30 μg), the BR-PO protein (5 μg),
the Y protein (10 μg), and the PASII protein (5 μg) with CB
staining.

Table 4. Antigenic activities to induce demyelinating disease in guinea pigs.

Antigen	No. of animals tested	No. with histological lesions of severity*							
		in PNS				in CNS			
		0	+	++	+++	0	+	++	+++
CNS-BP**	27	26	1	0	0	4	4	8	11
PNS Myelin	18	2	0	0	16	17	1	0	0
BF-P2***	7	7	0	0	0	7	0	0	0
BR-P0****	18	16	1	1	0	16	0	0	2
PASII****	5	4	1	0	0	5	0	0	0

*0: no lesions
+: mild, cell infiltration
++: moderate; mild demyelination
+++: severe; severe demyelination
**: purified from bovine CNS myelin
***: purified from bovine PNS myelin

As to the basic proteins, the BF-P2 protein is the major protein of the PNS myelin in man as well as in other species, such as ox and rabbit. This protein was newly purified from the pig PNS by our group (30) and was found to be widely distributed in mammals except guinea pig (14, 27). Recent studies revealed that the spinal cords of ox and rabbit also contained considerable amounts of the BF-P2 protein although it was almost absent from other tissues, such as brain, liver, kidney and muscle of rabbit by immunological tests (15, 27). As the SDS electrophoretical pattern of myelin proteins of human spinal cord also showed a minor protein band (PAS negative) in the position of M.W. 13,000, we considered that the human spinal cord also contained BF-P2. It is true that the BF-P2 protein is the main basic protein of PNS myelin, as CNS-BP is in the CNS myelin. However, the BF-P2 protein is also found in the spinal cord myelin, just as CNS-BP is found in the PNS myelin. Therefore, we cannot conclude that CNS-BP is restricted to the CNS or that BF-P2 is restricted to the PNS.

The presence of CNS-BP in the rabbit PNS myelin was reported by Brostoff and Eylar (3). Our previous reports also suggested that bovine PNS myelin contained CNS-BP (17, 30). Furthermore, biochemical analysis of the BP fraction indicated that human PNS myelin contained considerable amounts of CNS-BP. In electrophoretical analysis at pH 4.3, a protein band different from CNS-BP was observed in the PB fraction. On the basis of electrophoretical and amino acid analysis it was suggested that this protein was not a degradation product of CNS-BP but a new protein. As we have not yet obtained the purified protein from the PB fraction we cannot show definitive differences between them.

Some reports had indicated before that the major protein of the PNS myelin was a glycoprotein (11, 25, 34). Recently, Eylar's (4) and our group (16) independently purified a major glycoprotein, BR-PO, from rabbit or bovine PNS myelin. Bovine BR-PO protein contained a single carbohydrate chain (glucosamine:mannose:fucose: galactose:sialic acid = 2.6:2.7:0.8:1.0:0.8/mole) and Ile as the aminoterminal residue (16). A peptide containing a carbohydrate chain of bovine BR-PO protein was isolated recently by us and its amino acid sequence was found to be the following: Gly-Asp-Asn (Carbohydrate chain)-Gly-Thr (Kitamura et al., unpublished data). We also purified the PASII protein as a pure glycoprotein (glucosamine:mannose:fucose:galactose:glucose = 2.1:1.5:0.3:0.8:0.8/ mole) with an aminoterminal residue, Met (16). These two kinds of glycoproteins were found to be specific to the PNS myelin in various species (29). The third glycoprotein, Y, which is also obtained in a pure form, showed similarity to the ER-PO protein in its amino acid composition and the same amino-terminal amino acid, Ile, as bovine and human BR-PO protein (unpublished data). This Y protein may be a degradation product of the BR-PO protein because the molecular weight of Y (22,000) was less than that of the BR-PO protein (28,000).

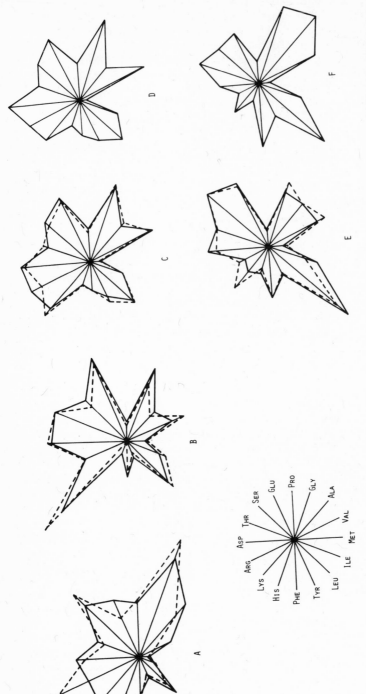

Fig. 11. Stardiagrams of amino acid compositions of myelin proteins. Molar percentage of each amino acid is shown as a distance from the center of the star; equimolar proportions are shown in the key to the lines.
A) ————: Human PB fraction, – – – – : Human CNS-BP, B) ———— : Human BF-P2 protein, – – – – : Bovine BF-P2 protein, C) ———— : Bovine BR-PO protein, – – – – : Bovine BR-PO protein, D) ———— : Human Y protein, E) ———— : Human PASII protein, – – – – : Bovine PASII protein, F) ————: FLPL (32).

The amino acid compositions of the CNS and PNS myelin proteins
are shown as their stardiagrams in Fig. 11. It is evident that the
amino acid compositions of the BR-PO, BF-P2 and PASII proteins of
human PNS myelin are similar to those of the corresponding proteins
of bovine myelin. The differences between the CNS-BP, FLPL, BF-P2,
BR-PO and PASII proteins are clearly demonstrated. As the amino
acid composition of the PASII protein is quite different from the
BF-P2 protein in spite of their similar molecular weights, it is
certain that the PASII protein is not a glycosylated derivative of
the BF-P2 protein. The PASII protein is also unlikely to be a
degradation product of the BR-PO protein as judged from the results
of carbohydrate and amino acid analysis. It is interesting that the
stardiagram of PASII protein has, as a whole, some similarities,
such as low basic and high hydrophobic amino acid contents, to that
of FLPL. This may suggest functional similarity of the two proteins
in the CNS and PNS myelin.

Polarities, the sum of the residue mole percentages of polar
amino acids (7), in human CNS-BP, FLPL, BF-P2, BR-PO, PASII and Y
proteins were 51.3, 33.7, 56.0, 49.8, 44.3 and 46.3, respectively.
Considering solubilities and polarities of each protein, FLPL is a
typical "integral" type protein (24) in the myelin membrane of CNS
while CNS-BP is a "peripheral" protein (24). Among the PNS myelin
proteins, the BF-P2 protein is a "peripheral" protein. On the
other hand, the three glycoproteins, BR-PO, PASII and Y, were rather
of the "integral" type. Investigation of the arrangement of these
glycoproteins in the PNS myelin membrane is also interesting.

The PNS myelin, as a whole, was reported not to induce EAE but
EAN in experimental animals (2, 31). However, injection of each
single protein component, purified from the bovine PNS myelin,
failed to induce demyelinating diseases. Further immunological
studies are now in progress in our laboratory to clarify the mechanism to induce EAN in experimental animals.

Acknowledgements. We are grateful to Dr. Matsuyama and Dr.
Ishikara, Department of Neuropathology, Tokyo Metropolitan Institute
for Neurosciences, for histological examination. This study was
supported in part by grants from the Ministry of Education, Japan.

REFERENCES

1. Ansari, K.A. and Komanduri, V., Human myelin basic proteins:
    A comparison of proteins from six different anatomic sites,
    Neurology 24 (1974) 94-98.
2. Brostoff, S., Burnett, P., Lampert, P. and Eylar, E.H.,
    Isolation and characterization of a protein from sciatic nerve
    myelin responsible for experimental allergic neuritis, Nature
    New Biol. 235 (1972) 210-212.
3. Brostoff, S.W. and Eylar, E.H., The proposed amino acid sequence
    of the P1 protein of rabbit sciatic nerve myelin, Arch. Biochem.
    Biophys. 153 (1972) 590-598.

4. Brostoff, S.W., Karkhanis, Y.D., Carlo, D.J., Reuter, W. and Eylar, E.H., Isolation and partial characterization of the major proteins of rabbit sciatic nerve myelin, Brain Res. 86 (1975) 449-458.

5. Brostoff, S.W., Sacks, H., Dal Canto, M., Johnson, A.B., Raine, C.S. and Wisniewski, H., The P2 protein of bovine root myelin: Isolation and some chemical and immunological properties, J. Neurochem. 24 (1975) 1037-1043.

6. Brostoff, S.W., Sacks, H. and Dipaola, C., The P2 protein of bovine root myelin: Partial chemical characterization, J. Neurochem. 24 (1975) 289-294.

7. Capaldi, R.A. and Vanderkooi, G., The low polarity of many membrane proteins, Proc.Nat. Acad. Sci. U.S.A. 69 (1972) 930-932.

8. Carnegie, P.R., Amino acid sequence of the encephalitogenic basic protein of human myelin, Biochem. J. 123 (1971) 57-67.

9. Carnegie, P.R.and Dunkley, P.R., Basic proteins of central and peripheral nervous system, in Advances in Neurochemistry Vol. 1 (B.W. Agranoff and M.H. Aprison, eds.) (1975) pp. 96-135.

10. Deibler, G.E., Kies, M.W. and Uyemura, K., Structural studies on basic protein isolated from peripheral nerve myelin, Trans. Am. Soc. Neurochem. 6 (1975) 85.

11. Everly, J.L., Brady, R.O. and Quarles, R.H., Evidence that the major protein in rat sciatic nerve myelin is a glycoprotein, J. Neurochem. 21 (1973) 329-334.

12. Fairbanks, G., Steck, T.L. and Wallach, D.F.H., Electrophoretic analysis of the major polypeptides of human erythrocyte membrane, Biochemistry 10 (1971) 2606-2617.

13. Folch-Pi, J. and Lees, M., Proteolipides, a new type of tissue lipoproteins, J. Biol. Chem. 191 (1951) 807-817.

14. Greenfield, G., Brostoff, S., Eylar, E.H. and Morell, P., Protein composition of myelin of the peripheral nervous system, J. Neurochem. 20 (1973) 1207-1216.

15. Kies, M.W., Deibler, D.E., Kramer, A., MacPherson, C.F. and Uyemura, K., Immunological and chemical similarities between PNS and CNS basic protein, Abstr., 5th Int. Meet. Int. Soc. Neurochem. (1975) p. 419.

16. Kitamura, K., Suzuki, M. and Uyemura, K., Purification and partial characterization of two glycoproteins in bovine peripheral nerve myelin membrane, Biochim. Biophys. Acta 445 (1976) 806-816.

17. Kitamura, K., Yamanaka, T. and Uyemura, K., On basic proteins in bovine peripheral nerve myelin, Biochim. Biophys. Acta 379 (1975) 582-591.

18. Laatsch, M., Kies, M., Gordon, S. and Alvord, E., The encephalitogenic activity of myelin isolated by ultracentrifugation, J. Exp. Med. 115 (1962) 777-788.

19. Luft, J.H., Improvements in epoxyresin embedding methods, J. Biophys. Biochem. Cytol. 9 (1961) 409-419.

20. Mehl, E. and Wolfgram, E., Myelin types with different protein components in same species, J. Neurochem. 16 (1969) 1091-1097.
21. Palo, J., Savolainen, H. and Haltia, M., Proteins of peripheral nerve myelin in diabetic neuropathy, J. neurol. Sci. (1972) 193-199.
22. Reisfeld, R.A., Lewis, U.J. and Williams, D.E., Disk electrophoresis of basic peptides on polyacrylamide gels, Nature 195 (1962) 281-283.
23. Shapiro, A.L., Vinuela, E. and Maizel, J.V., Molecular weight estimation of polypeptide chain by electrophoresis in SDS polyacrylamide gel, Biochem. Biophys. Res. Comm. 28 (1967) 815-820.
24. Singer, S.J. and Nicolson, G.L., The fluid mosaic model of the structure of cell membranes, Science 175 (1972) 720-730.
25. Singh, H. and Spritz, N., Polypeptide components of myelin from rat peripheral nerve, Biochim. Biophys. Acta 351 (1974) 379-386.
26. Spritz, N., Singh, H. and Geyer, B., Myelin from human peripheral nerves, J. Clin. Invest. 52 (1973) 520-523.
27. Uyemura, K., Kato-Yamanaka, T. and Kitamura, K., Distribution and optical activity of the basic protein in bovine peripheral nerve myelin, J. Neurochem. 29 (1977) 61-68.
28. Uyemura, K., Kitamura, K., Ogawa, Y. and Matsuyama, H., Studies on the antigenic protein to induce experimental allergic neuritis, in The Aetiology and Pathogenesis of the Demyelinating Disease (H. Shiraki, T. Yonezawa and Y. Kuroiwa, eds.) (1976) Japan Science Press, pp. 181-192.
29. Uyemura, K., Kitamura, K. and Suzuki, M., Distribution and developmental changes of membrane glycoproteins in peripheral nerve myelin, Abstr., 6th Int. Meet. Int. Soc. Neurochem. Copenhagen (1977).
30. Uyemura, K., Tobari, C. and Hirano, S., Purification and properties of basic proteins in pig spinal cord and peripheral nerve, Biochim. Biophys. Acta 214 (1970) 190-197.
31. Uyemura, K., Tobari, C., Hirano, S. and Tsukada, Y., Comparative studies on the myelin proteins of bovine peripheral nerve and spinal cord, J. Neurochem. 19 (1972) 2607-2614.
32. Vacher-Lepretre, M., Nicot, C., Alfsen, A., Jolles, J. and Jolles, P., Study of the apoprotein of Folch-Pi bovine proteolipid, Biochim. Biophys. Acta 420 (1976) 323-331.
33. Waksman, B.H. and Adams, R.D., Allergic neuritis: An experimental disease of rabbits induced by the injection of peripheral nervous tissue and adjuvants, J. Exp. Med. 103 (1955) 213-235.
34. Wood, J.G. and Dawson, R.M.C., A major myelin glycoprotein of sciatic nerve, J. Neurochem. 21 (1973) 717-719.

PROTEIN HETEROGENEITY IN RAT CNS MYELIN SUBFRACTIONS

T.V. Waehneldt

Max-Planck-Institut für experimentelle Medizin,
  Forschungsstelle Neurochemie
3400 Göttingen, G.F.R.

SUMMARY

Microsomal fraction-free myelin from forebrain and spinal cord of young and mature rats, when subjected to hypo-osmotic shock and slow speed centrifugation, yielded a myelin pellet and a supernatant fraction (SN 4). Fraction SN 4 consisted of small vesicular profiles in which the major myelin proteins were reduced whereas high molecular weight material such as Wolfgram protein, myelin-associated glycoprotein and CNP were substantially increased over myelin. A close correlation of the SN 4 fraction to the myelin-like fraction of Davison and coworkers was suggested.

The myelin pellets were subfractioned on zonal sucrose gradients to yield bell-shaped particle distributions. Besides shifts in densities of the maxima between myelin of young and mature forebrain and spinal cord, a decrease was observed from the light to the heavy gradient end in basic proteins, and an increase in Wolfgram protein and other high molecular weight proteins. Proteolipid protein took an intermediate position. Light fractions from adult spinal cord displayed CNP activities below those of the total homogenate. This result, together with the very high CNP activities in fraction SN 4 casts some doubt on CNP being a marker for compact myelin; rather it appears that CNP is a marker for the process of myelin formation.

INTRODUCTION

Soon after methods were developed for the solubilization and fractionation of membrane proteins and applied to the analysis of CNS myelin (19, 34) it was evident that the proteins of myelin

not only included the classical myelin components basic protein and
proteolipid protein (21) but also other proteins of lower and higher
molecular weight. Among these were the small basic protein in
rodents (15), a DM-20 (3) or intermediate protein (23), a group of
high molecular weight proteins, commonly called "Wolfgram proteins"
(38), and a myelin-associated glycoprotein (27). In this protein
context, there appears to be enough evidence for at least two enzyme activities to be labelled as myelin-specific (12-14).

The protein compositional heterogeneity of myelin proved to be
still more complex in that certain changes occur during ontogeny
(11, 23, 39, 40) and that myelin can be subfractionated by density
gradient centrifugation into lighter and heavier subfractions (1,
5-7, 11, 16, 20, 40). Moreover, there exist membrane fractions
which might be of early or immature myelin origin (2, 4, 5, 23, 30,
36).

In this paper it is shown how numerous myelin subfractions from
the CNS of one species (rat) can be separated and analyzed for
morphology, protein composition, and marker enzyme distribution.
A hypothetical scheme is presented which attempts to unify the experimental data.

EXPERIMENTAL

Wistar rats were used in all experiments. Myelin fraction (My)
and fraction SN 1 and SN 4 were prepared as shown in Fig. 1 and as
outlined previously (37). Continuous density gradient centrifugations were carried out with a zonal rotor, using either a linear
0.32-1.0 M sucrose gradient (Fig. 3, My) or a linear 0.32-1.6 M
sucrose gradient (Fig. 6; SN 1; SN 4) (Matthieu and Waehneldt,
submitted). Enzyme assays, electron microscopy (37) and gel electrophoresis (35) were described earlier.

RESULTS

Characterization of fraction SN 1, SN 4 and My. The electron
microscopic examination of fractions SN 1, SN 4 and My (Fig. 2)
showed that SN 1 consisted of small single-membrane vesicles some
of which were flattened out. In fraction SN 4, too, small vesicular
structures were prevailing; most of these had only a few layers,
in contrast to the myelin fraction with its large and multilayered
rounded shapes. The morphological differences among the three
fractions were also reflected in the gel protein profiles (Fig. 2):
My consisted largely of a limited number of typical low molecular
weight proteins and SN 1 mostly of numerous high molecular weight
proteins, whereas fraction SN 4 held an intermediate position with,
however, a pronounced Wolfgram protein band.

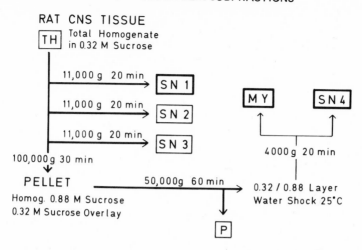

Fig. 1. Preparation of the microsomal fractions SN 1, SN 2 and SN 3 and of the fractions My and SN 4. After threefold washing under isotonic conditions, removing large amounts of microsomal material, the myelin is floated up and thereafter subjected to hypo-osmotic conditions. This yields the myelin pellet (My) and the myelin-related supernatant fraction SN 4.

The Wolfgram protein band, together with high 2',3'-cyclic nucleotide 3'-phosphohydrolase (CNP) specific activity (Table 1) and elevated proportions of the myelin-associated glycoprotein, was found characteristic for fraction SN 4 (36, 37).

Enzyme data are given in Table 1 for CNP, regarded as a positive myelin marker (13, 14), and for acetylcholinesterase, regarded as a marker for neuronal plasma and endoplasmic reticular membranes (see 32 for references). While in the total homogenate the CNP value of forebrain was only half that of spinal cord the AChE values showed opposite trends, reflecting the larger amount of myelin deposited in spinal cord. The same was found for fraction SN 1, however with a pronounced enrichment in AChE. The AChE values for My from both regions were low, pointing to high purity of the preparations, while fraction SN 4 maintained intermediate values indicating some non-myelinic contamination. Despite these AChE values fraction SN 4 showed very high CNP specific activities in forebrain when compared to My, much less so in spinal cord.

Zonal centrifugation. Further fractionation was carried out on linear sucrose gradients (Fig.3), showing the bell-shaped dispersion of myelin particles from adult rat forebrain as an example. Individual fractions were symmetrically pooled to yield the five subfractions Li, LiM, M, MH, H.

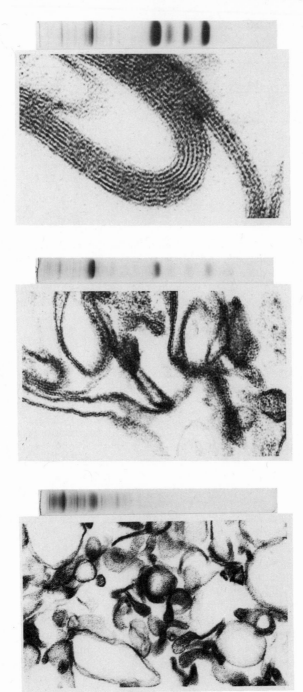

Fig. 2. Electron microscopical examination and gel protein analysis of fractions SN 1, SN 4, and My. SDS electrophoresis on 12% gels, Coomassie blue staining. The anode is at the bottom.

Table 1. CNP and AChE specific activities of the total homogenates (TH) and subcellular fractions of forebrain and spinal cord from adult rats.

	TH	SN 1	My	SN 4
CNP Forebrain	250±12	227±26	1116±167	3138±422
Spinal cord	516±70	569±109	698±126	927±167
AChE Forebrain	7.72±0.77	14.81±1.55	0.74±0.23	3.49±1.04
Spinal cord	4.25±0.60	7.49±1.13	0.85±0.10	1.75±0.17

Values are expressed as µmole hydrolyzed . mg protein^{-1} . h^{-1} and are means of 3 determinations each of three separate experiments ± SEM.

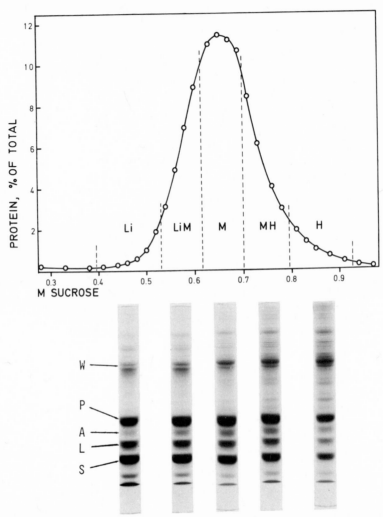

Fig. 3. Distribution of myelin from adult rat forebrain (expressed as per cent protein of the total) on a linear zonal sucrose gradient. Individual samples were pooled so that five symmetrically pooled subfractions were obtained. Li, light; LiM, light-medium; M, medium; MH, medium-heavy; H, heavy. Below are representative gels of these 5 subfractions. The anode is at the bottom. S, small basic protein; L, large basic protein; A, DM-20 protein (3, 23); P, proteolipid protein; W, Wolfgram protein.

The peak position in adult rat forebrain myelin centered near
0.67 M sucrose, whereas that from young rats had a lower density
(0.58 M sucrose); in spinal cord myelin the peak position remained
near 0.58 M sucrose throughout development (Waehneldt, submitted).
In the lower half of Fig. 3 actual gels from the 5 subfractions
are shown, while in Fig. 4 the dye binding capacities of individual
myelin proteins from forebrain and from spinal cord are found. The
scans of the two basic proteins were combined, as were the hydrophobic proteolipid and DM-20 proteins. From the light (Li) to the
heavy (H) fraction the basic proteins decreased in both regions,
with higher values at the light end in spinal cord. Generally higher
values were found for the Wolfgram protein in forebrain, increasing
from the light to the heavy end, while the hydrophobic proteins
maintained an intermediate position reaching the highest values in
the medium fraction of forebrain and in the heavy fractions in
spinal cord. This result is at variance with those of others who
found largely constant proportions for the proteolipid protein
throughout the density range examined (16, 40).

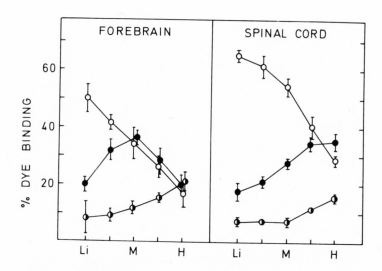

Fig. 4. Protein distribution in myelin subfractions from adult
rat forebrain and spinal cord. Expressed as per cent Coomassie
blue binding capacity. Means are shown from 3 gels each, run in
3 separate experiments ± SEM. - O, S + L (for abbreviations see
Fig. 3); ●, P + A; ◑, W. Residual proteins, largely of high
molecular weight, form the difference to 100%.

The ratio S/L is displayed in Fig. 5 and also that of the sum of the two hydrophobic proteins over the sum of the two hydrophilic basic proteins, P + A/S + L. S/L decreases from the light to the heavy side of the zonal gradients, with generally higher values for spinal cord myelin subfractions. No such marked differences were observed between the two regions in the case of ratio P + A/S + L. In forebrain and in spinal cord averages of respectively 0.90 and 0.65 were found. The decrease in caudal direction is in agreement with earlier results (31, 39).

AChE analyses of the zonal subfractions (Table 2) showed that contamination with non-myelin material was rather low in both regions, slightly increasing toward the heavy side. Increases were also found for CNP; the values for all forebrain myelin subfractions were substantially above those of the total homogenate whereas in spinal cord the light fractions had values below that of the corresponding total homogenate.

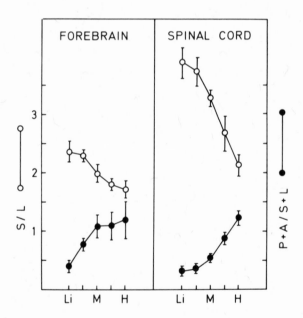

Fig. 5. Illustration of the changes in the S/L and P + A/S + L ratios in adult rat forebrain and spinal cord myelin subfractions.

Fig. 7. Specific activities of rat forebrain subfractions obtained by zonal distribution (see Figs. 3 and 6). O, SN 1; ●, SN 4; +, My. Expressed as μmole substrate hydrolyzed . mg protein^{-1} . h^{-1}. Despite substantial overlap upon zonal centrifugation (Fig. 6) and certain similarities in electrophoretic profiles (Fig. 2) the subfractions from SN 1 and SN 4 show drastic differences in enzyme distribution.

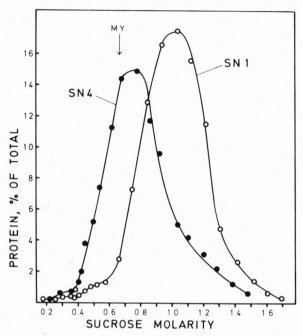

Fig. 6. Comparison of the particle dispersion on linear zonal gradients of fractions SN 1 and SN 4 from adult rat forebrain. Expressed as per cent protein of the total. "My" plus arrow in- dicates the peak position of the parent myelin (Figs. 1 and 3) which would form a rather narrow band on this wider ranging ab- scissa. Substantial overlap is noticeable.

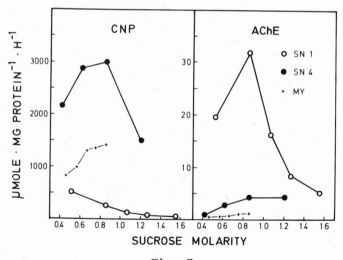

Fig. 7

Table 2. CNP and AChE specific activities of the subfractions obtained by zonal centrifugation of myelin from forebrain and spinal cord of adult rats.

	TH+	Li	LiM	M	MH	H
CNP Forebrain	250	824	997	1307	1375	1405
Spinal cord	516	360	288	481	820	1202
AChE Forebrain	7.72	0.50	0.55	0.73	1.04	1.03
Spinal cord	4.25	0.53	0.49	0.60	0.95	1.46

+The total homogenate (TH) is listed for comparison.
Figures represent the means of 3 determinations each of three separate experiments and are expressed as μmole hydrolyzed $\cdot$ mg protein$^{-1} \cdot$ h^{-1}.

When subjecting fractions SN 1 and SN 4 from adult forebrain to zonal centrifugation on a wide range density gradient (Fig. 6) fairly symmetrical distributions were obtained, the maxima being at 0.73 M and 1.0 M sucrose for SN 4 and SN 1, respectively. It is worth noting that a sizable portion of fraction SN 4 had densities higher than 0.88 M sucrose although it was derived from a fraction which banded on this density prior to hypo-osmotic treatment. There is substantial overlap between the profiles of SN 4 and SN 1; nevertheless, the enzyme analysis of the four (SN 4) and five (SN 1) subfractions showed entirely opposite trends (Fig. 7). While the CNP activities of SN 4 were high (ranging from 1,500 to 3,000 μmoles hydrolyzed) the values for SN 1 were only 500 in the lightest subfraction and decreasing rapidly toward minimal values at the heavy end. Myelin subfractions showed intermediate CNP values. On the other hand, the figures for AChE showed opposite trends: SN 4 subfractions were low, increasing slightly toward the heavy end of the gradient, while SN 1 reached its highest value of 32 μmoles hydrolyzed in a subfraction which has maximal density overlap with the SN 4 subfraction of highest CNP specific activity.

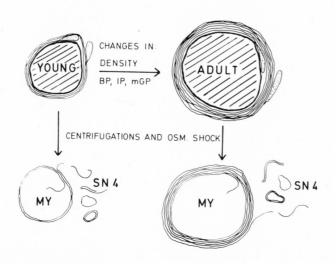

Fig. 8.   Relatively large amounts of fraction SN 4 are obtained from myelin of young animals (36, 37). With maturational increase in axon diameter and in number of lamellae the density of the myelin changes (see text) and also the ratios of the two basic proteins (39), of the two intermediate (23) or DM-20 proteins (3, 10) and of the myelin associated glycoproteins (17, 28).

DISCUSSION

When myelin is washed free from microsomal material avoiding
hypo-osmotic conditions, a fraction (SN 4) can thereafter be liberated by osmotic shock which remains in the supernatant of a slow
speed centrifugation (Fig. 1). Fraction SN 4 consists of small-
sized vesicles of nearly microsomal dimensions; however it has
some compaction of membranes similar to the layers in typical
myelin. Thus, the low density and the large size of multilayered
myelin has been used as a "handle" to preserve hypo-osmotically
labile portions of the myelin superstructure (probably tongue and
loop regions and some shavings of lamellae) (Fig. 8) which upon
immediate hypo-osmotic treatment (24) would have been lost in microsomal washings.

Fraction SN 4 is of interest in that it represents a fraction
which is directly related to myelin but which differs from myelin
in its protein composition: the typical low molecular weight myelin
proteins (<24,000 D) are reduced, while the high molecular weight
proteins such as Wolfgram protein, myelin-associated glycoprotein
and CNP are increased (36, 37). Moreover, recent observations point
to higher specific activities of carbonic anhydrase (M.B. Lees and
V. Sapirstein, personal communication), sulphotransferase and
galactosyltransferase (L.L. Sarlieve and N.M. Neskovic, personal
communication) in SN 4 as compared to the parent myelin. Therefore, SN 4 can be regarded as a compositional extreme in the wide
spectrum of myelin or myelin-related fractions which has been obtained to date. Myelinic fractions of similar high CNP specific
activity have also been recently described by others (18, 33).

Subjecting large sized myelin to continuous density gradient
centrifugation (Fig. 3) results in a symmetrical curve. Similar
observations have been made by Adams and Fox (1) who also noted
an increase in density of the peak position with   ontogeny. This
bell-shaped particle dispersion offers a simple explanation for
the varying yields of myelin which have been obtained by arbitrarily placing discontinuities of sucrose molarities (7, 11, 40; see
also 29).

The size of the myelin particles from forebrain and spinal cord
remains fairly constant throughout the density range (Waehneldt,
submitted); however, the proportion of the myelin proteins varies
substantially from the light to the heavy fractions. In general,
the typical myelin proteins are prevailing near the light end of
the gradient, pointing to later developmental stages (see also
7-9). This is underlined by a higher S/L ratio, which is a sensitive indicator for myelin maturation (39). Therefore, the
lightest subfractions of spinal cord myelin represent the most
mature stages, in that they have very high S/L ratios, low P +
A/S + L ratios, low percentages of high molecular weight proteins,
and low AChE and CNP specific activities, more pronounced than the
corresponding forebrain fraction. The CNP values are below that

of the total homogenate which casts some doubt on CNP being a marker
for mature myelin; rather it appears that this enzyme of unknown
function could serve as an excellent indicator for the membraneous
stages leading to mature myelin.

As yet neither myelin totally devoid of all high molecular
weight proteins has been prepared nor has a fraction been isolated
which lacks the typical myelin proteins but instead has still higher
proportions of Wolfgram protein, myelin-associated glycoprotein,
CNP, and possibly other proteins. Nevertheless, these two protein
compositions can be regarded as conceptual extremes and are as such
tentatively labelled SN 4-type and myelin-type (Fig. 9). By combining the results on the disposition of proteins in the multilayered myelin structure (25, 26) with the data of this paper it

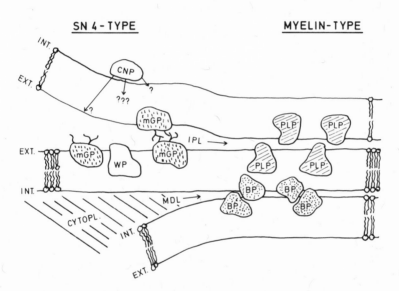

Fig. 9. Hypothetical scheme of the change from the single membrane
SN 4-type extreme to the fully compacted myelin-type superstructure.
Any transitional stage can be visualized resulting in a compositional continuum of particles. Int., cytoplasmic, and Ext., extracellular side of the membrane; MDL, major dense line; IPL, interperiod line; mGP, myelin-associated glycoprotein; WP, Wolfgram
protein; PLP, proteolipid protein; BP, basic protein; CNP, cyclic
nucleotide phosphohydrolase. The membrane disposition of these
myelin proteins follows the results of Poduslo and Braun (25) and
Poduslo et al. (26). The location of CNP is not known; however,
the ease with which this enzyme is activated by non-ionic detergents
makes a hydrophobic site deep within the lipid bilayer rather unlikely.

appears that a transition occurs from single oligodendroglial
membranes to fused membranes by replacing the high molecular weight
proteins with the typical low molecular weight myelin proteins.
It is possible that the proteins of the SN 4-type membrane, which
represents an example of an "oligodendroglia-derived membrane" (29),
serve specific tasks: Wolfgram protein, to function as a backbone
protein to be replaced by proteolipid protein and DM-20 protein;
CNP, to be involved in phosphorus metabolism of newly inserted
basic protein which in the altered state fuses the cytoplasmic
sides by dimerization (22); myelin-associated glycoprotein, to
help align the external sides of the membranes, not necessarily to
fuse them (17). Whether such a dilution of the high molecular
weight proteins occurs in specific cytoplasm-containing locations
(paranodal loops, inner and outer tongues, clefts) or more ubiqui-
tously (mesaxonal formations) remains an open question. It could
well be that this transition is a gradual one and that certain
molar threshold quantities of low molecular weight myelin proteins
are required to initiate and propagate the fusion of lamellae in
a 2-dimensional "zipper-like" mode.

Acknowledgements. The author wishes to thank Prof. V. Neuhoff
and Dr. J.-M. Matthieu for discussion and Dr. R. Sammeck for electron micrographs. Supported by a grant from the Deutsche Forschungsgemeinschaft (SFB 33).

REFERENCES

1. Adams, D.H. and Fox, M.E., The homogeneity and protein composition of rat brain myelin, Brain Res. 14 (1969) 647-661.
2. Agrawal, H.C., Banik, N.L., Bone, S., Davison, A.N., Mitchell,
   R.F. and Spohn, M., The identity of myelin-like fraction
   isolated from developing brain, Biochem. J. 120 (1970) 635-
   642.
3. Agrawal, H.C., Burton, R.M., Fishman, M.A., Mitchell, R.F.
   and Prensky, A.L., Partial characterization of a new myelin
   protein component, J. Neurochem. 19 (1972) 2083-2089.
4. Agrawal, H.C., Trotter, J.L., Mitchell, R.F. and Burton, R.M.,
   Criteria for identifying a myelin-like fraction from developing
   brain, Biochem. J. 136 (1973) 1117-1119.
5. Agrawal, H.C., Trotter, J.L., Burton, R.M. and Mitchell, R.,
   Metabolic studies on myelin: evidence for a precursor role of
   a myelin subfraction, Biochem. J. 140 (1974) 99-109.
6. Autilio, L.A., Norton, W.T. and Terry, R.D., The preparation
   and some properties of purified myelin from the central nervous
   system, J. Neurochem. 11 (1964) 17-22.
7. Benjamins, J.A., Miller, K. and McKhann, G.M., Myelin subfractions in developing rat brain: characterization and sulphatide metabolism, J. Neurochem. 20 (1973) 1589-1603.

8. Benjamins, J.A., Miller, S.L. and Morell, P., Metabolic relationships between myelin subfractions: entry of galacto-lipids and phospholipids, J. Neurochem. 27 (1976) 565-570.

9. Benjamins, J.A., Gray, M. and Morell, P., Metabolic relation-ships between myelin subfractions: entry of proteins, J. Neurochem. 27 (1976) 571-575.

10. Cammer, W. and Norton, W.T., Disc gel electrophoresis of myelin proteins: new observations on development of the inter-mediate proteins (DM-20), Brain Res. 109 (1976) 643-648.

11. Fujimoto, K., Roots, B.I., Burton, R.M. and Agrawal, H.C., Morphological and biochemical characterization of light and heavy myelin isolated from developing rat brain, Biochim. Biophys. Acta 426 (1976) 659-668.

12. Igarashi, M. and Suzuki, K., Solubilization and characteriza-tion of the rat brain cholesterol ester hydrolase localized in the myelin sheath, J. Neurochem. 28 (1977) 729-738.

13. Kurihara, T. and Tsukada, Y., The regional and subcellular distribution of 2',3'-cyclic nucleotide 3'-phosphohydrolase in the central nervous system, J. Neurochem. 14 (1967) 1167-1174.

14. Kurihara, T. and Tsukada, Y., 2',3'-cyclic nucleotide 3'-phosphohydrolase in the developing chick brain and spinal cord, J. Neurochem. 15 (1968) 827-832.

15. Martenson, R.E., Deibler, G.E. and Kies, M.W., The occurrence of two myelin basic proteins in the central nervous system of rodents in the suborders Myomorpha and Sciuromorpha, J. Neuro-chem. 18 (1971) 2427-2433.

16. Matthieu, J.-M., Quarles, R.H., Brady, R.O. and Webster, H. deF., Variations of proteins, enzyme markers and gangliosides in myelin subfractions, Biochim. Biophys. Acta 329 (1973) 305-317.

17. Matthieu, J.-M., Brady, R.O. and Quarles, R.H., Change in a myelin-associated glycoprotein in rat brain during development: metabolic aspects, Brain Res. 86 (1975) 55-65.

18. McIntyre, R.J., Quarles, R.H., Webster, H. deF. and Brady, R.O., Isolation and characterization of myelin-related mem-branes, Trans. Am. Soc. Neurochem. 8 (1977) 159.

19. Mehl, E. and Wolfgram, F., Myelin types with different protein components in the same species, J. Neurochem. 16 (1969) 1091-1097.

20. Mehl, E., Separation and characterization of myelin proteins, Adv. Exp. Med. Biol. 32 (1972) 157-170.

21. Mokrasch, L.C., Biophysical chemistry and dynamics of myelin, in Myelin (L.C. Mokrasch, R.S. Bear and F.O. Schmitt, eds.) Neurosciences Res. Progr. Bull. 9 (1971) 452-506.

22. Moore, W.J., Smith, R. and Chapman, B.E., Conformation and function of myelin basic proteins, Trans. Am. Soc. Neurochem. 8 (1977) 67.

23. Morell, P., Greenfield, S., Costantino-Ceccarini, E. and Wis-niewski, H., Changes in the protein composition of mouse brain

myelin during development, J. Neurochem.19 (1972) 2545-2554.

24. Norton, W.T. and Poduslo, S.E., Myelination in rat brain:
method of myelin isolation, J. Neurochem. 21 (1973) 749-758.

25. Poduslo, J.F. and Braun, P., Topographical arrangement of
membrane proteins in the intact myelin sheath, J. biol. Chem.
250 (1975) 1099-1105.

26. Poduslo, J.F., Quarles, R.H. and Brady, R.O., External labeling of galactose in surface membrane glycoproteins of the intact myelin sheath, J. biol. Chem. 251 (1976) 153-158.

27. Quarles, R.H., Everly, J.L. and Brady, R.O., Evidence for the
close association of a glycoprotein with myelin in rat brain,
J. Neurochem. 21 (1973) 1177-1191.

28. Quarles, R.H., Everly, J.L. and Brady, R.O., Myelin-associated
glycoprotein: a developmental change, Brain Res. 58 (1973)
506-509.

29. Quarles, R.H., The biochemical and morphological heterogeneity
of myelin and myelin-related membranes, in Biochemistry of
Brain (S. Kumar, ed.) Pergamon Press Ltd., in press.

30. Sabri, M.I., Tremblay, C., Banik, N.L., Scott, T., Gohil, K.
and Davison, A.N., Biochemical and morphological changes in
the subcellular fractions during myelination of rat brain,
Biochem. Soc. Trans. (London) 3 (1975) 275-276.

31. Smith, M.E. and Sedgewick, L.M., Studies of the mechanism of
demyelination. Regional differences in myelin stability in
vitro, J. Neurochem. 24 (1975) 763-770.

32. Storm-Mathisen, J., Localization of transmitter candidates
in the brain: the hippocampal formation as a model, Prog. Neuro-
biol.8 (1977) 119-181.

33. Toews, A.D., Horrocks, L.A. and King, J.S., Simultaneous isolation of purified microsomal and myelin fractions from rat spinal
cord, J. Neurochem. 27 (1976) 25-31.

34. Waehneldt, T.V. and Mandel, P., Proteins of rat brain myelin.
Extraction with sodium dodecylsulphate and electrophoresis on
analytical and preparative scale, FEBS Lett. 9 (1970) 209-212.

35. Waehneldt, T.V. and Neuhoff, V., Membrane proteins of rat brain:
compositional changes during postnatal development, J. Neurochem. 23 (1974) 71-77.

36. Waehneldt, T.V., Ontogenetic study of a myelin-derived fraction
with 2', 3'-cyclic nucleotide 3'-phosphohydrolase activity
higher than that of myelin, Biochem. J. 151 (1975) 435-437.

37. Waehneldt, T.V., Matthieu, J.-M. and Neuhoff, V., Characterization of a myelin-related fraction (SN 4) isolated from rat
forebrain at two developmental stages, Brain Res., in press.

38. Wolfgram, F., A new proteolipid fraction of the nervous system.
I. Isolation and amino acid analysis, J. Neurochem. 13 (1966)
461-470.

39. Zgorzalewicz, B., Neuhoff, V. and Waehneldt, T.V., Rat myelin
proteins. Compositional changes in various regions of the
nervous system during ontogenetic development, Neurobiology 4
(1974) 265-276.

40. Zimmermann, A.W., Quarles, R.H., Webster, H. deF., Matthieu,
     J.-M. and Brady, R.O., Characterization and protein analysis
     of myelin subfractions in rat brain: developmental and regional
     comparison, J. Neurochem. 25 (1975) 749-757.

THE PREPARATION AND ANALYSIS OF MYELIN FROM SMALL QUANTITIES OF

CENTRAL NERVOUS TISSUE: REGIONAL STUDIES OF THE QUAKING MOUSE

G.E. Fagg, T.V. Waehneldt and V. Neuhoff

Max-Planck-Institut für Experimentelle Medizin,
  Forschungsstelle Neurochemie
3400 Göttingen, G.F.R.

SUMMARY

Myelin of considerable purity may be isolated from small
(minimum 1 mg wet weight) samples of central nervous tissue, using
a 4-step centrifugation procedure. The separation of myelin proteins by micro-linear gradient polyacrylamide gel electrophoresis
yields similar results to those obtained by macro-scale (homogeneous) gel systems. These techniques have been employed for a
preliminary study of the regional composition of myelin fractions
from the Quaking mouse.

INTRODUCTION

This communication describes methods for the isolation and
protein analysis of myelin from small (minimum 1 mg wet weight)
samples of central nervous tissue. A survey of the literature
revealed several potential investigations which would be facilitated by such methodology. Myelination in the central nervous
system (CNS), for example, has commonly been studied biochemically
using myelin isolated from the whole brains of developing animals,
although it is well documented that the onset of this process
shows marked regional variation. Similarly, biochemical studies
of the dysmyelinating Quaking mouse (19) have generally involved
total brain fractionation, whilst morphological investigations
indicate the existence of a gradient in the myelin deficit throughout the mutant CNS (5, 25).
    The procedures to be described are rapid, and are particularly
suitable for investigations employing small animals, or for

135

situations when little tissue is available. A myelin fraction of
considerable purity may be isolated and analysed with high resolution using micro-gradient gel electrophoresis (17). The use of the
techniques is illustrated with a preliminary study of the protein
composition of myelin fractions prepared from six different regions
of Quaking mice.

EXPERIMENTAL

The isolation of myelin from small tissue samples. Samples
of brain and spinal cord tissue from young (30-day-old) and adult
Wistar rats ot either sex (Winkelmann, Borchen, G.F.R.) were used
for the development of the small-scale myelin isolation method.
The final procedure adopted for the preparation of a myelin fraction
of high purity (as determined by SDS gel electrophoresis) is described below. All operations were performed at $0-4^{\circ}C$, and centrifugations were carried out in an Omega II ultracentrifuge (Heraeus-
Christ) using a 6x5 ml swinging-bucket rotor.
Tissue samples were weighed on a torsion balance and homogenised in 0.9 M sucrose (Merck) in either 0.6 ml or 5 ml cellulose
nitrate ultracentrifuge tubes (Beckman), using 8-10 strokes
(750 r.p.m.) of a loosely-fitting Teflon pestle. A 5% (w/v)
homogenate was prepared from samples of wet weight greater than 10
mg, and smaller pieces of tissue were homogenised in 0.2 ml of
sucrose solution. The homogenate was overlayered with 0.32 M
sucrose, and tubes were centrifuged at 100,000 g_{av} for 60 min.
The interfacial material (crude myelin) was collected with
a syringe, transferred to a second cellulose nitrate tube, diluted
5-fold with water and centrifuged at 2400 g_{av} for 20 min. The
cloudy supernatant was discarded, the pellet was re-suspended in
water by hand-homogenisation, and the slow-speed centrifugation repeated. This process of osmotic shock and differential centrifugation was carried out once more (discarding all supernatants),
and the final myelin pellet was then frozen at $-20^{\circ}C$ until further
analysis.
For comparison, myelin was prepared from adult rat forebrains
using a macro-scale procedure (22) designed to give a highly pure,
microsome-free fraction (21).
The isolation of a myelin fraction from different regions of
the CNS of Quaking mice. Male Quaking and littermate control mice
(5 of each) were obtained from the C.S.E.A.L., Orleans, France,
and were killed by decapitation at 40 days of age. The entire brain
and spinal cord was rapidly removed from each animal and dissected
into optic nerves, spinal cord, brain stem (medulla and pons),
cerebellum, diencephalon (mesencephalon and thalamic nuclei) and
telencephalon (remainder of forebrain, minus the rhinencephalon).
Tissue pieces were weighed ($\pm$ 1 mg) and frozen ($-20^{\circ}C$) until myelin
isolation (1-5 days later).
A crude myelin fraction was prepared from each tissue sample
as described above (Quaking and control samples were processed in

parallel). In order to obtain a reasonable yield of myelin and related membranes, however, the subsequent slow-speed differential centrifugation steps were omitted, since morphological studies have shown that myelin sheaths are thin and poorly compacted in the CNS of the Quaking mouse (18, 25). Instead, the crude material was diluted with water and centrifuged at 150,000 g_{av} for 20 min. The supernatant was discarded, and the process of water washing repeated.

Micro-gel electrophoresis. The protein composition of all myelin fractions was determined by SDS polyacrylamide gel electrophoresis using the linear gradient gels described by Rüchel et al. (17). Gels of approximately 1-30% (w/v) acrylamide concentration were cast in 10 μl capillaries, and electrophoresis was performed (about 30 min running time at a constant 70 V) using the 0.35 M Tris-sulphate pH 8.4/0.05 M Tris glycine pH 8.4 discontinuous buffer system. The electrophoresis buffer contained 0.1% SDS. Bromophenol red was used as the tracking dye.

Myelin fractions were hand-homogenised in 0.14 M Tris-sulphate pH 8.4 containing 1% SDS and 10% sucrose, to give a protein concentration of 0.5 - 1.0 mg/ml. After centrifugation at 30,000 g_{av} for 20 min, the supernatant was used for electrophoresis.

Gels were stained (10 min) in 0.25% (w/v) Coomassie Brilliant Blue-R250 in 46% (v/v) methanol containing 7.5% (v/v) acetic acid. Scanning was performed at 515 nm, using a micro-cuvette attachment (Schütt, Göttingen) for a Zeiss (ZK4) gel scanner. The area under each protein peak was determined using a pen recorder with incorporated integrator (Servogor, RE 544). There was a linear relationship between the mean peak area of each of the major myelin proteins - Wolfgram proteins (WP), proteolipid protein (PLP), DM-20 protein (1), large (LBP) and small basic (SBP) proteins - and the amount of protein applied to triplicate gels, over the range of 0.2 - 1.5 μg total myelin protein. Above this level, overloading of the gels was apparent, and staining became non-linear, notably in the cases of the basic proteins.

For comparison, purified myelin was also fractionated on 12% (w/v) polyacrylamide gels (macro-scale) as described by Waehneldt and Neuhoff (23), but stained with Coomassie Blue according to Allison et al. (3).

Protein estimation. The protein content of solubilised myelin fractions was estimated using the method of Lowry et al. (9), with bovine serum albumin as standard.

RESULTS

The separation of myelin proteins by micro-gradient gel electrophoresis. Myelin isolated from adult rat forebrains (macro-scale procedure) was fractionated into 5 major bands and several minor bands by both micro- and macro-gel electrophoresis (Fig. 1). The overall protein patterns obtained were similar to those described by other authors (1, 2, 20, 26). The two components of the DM-20

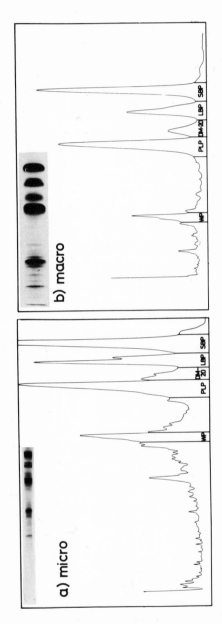

c) Quantitative evaluation of myelin fractionation by micro- and macro-gel electrophoresis

	WP	PLP	DM-20	LBP	SBP	Residual proteins
Micro-scale :	9.5(5.3)	17.0(3.5)	5.5(2.5)	10.2(2.9)	17.7(3.3)	40.1(1.7)
Macro-scale:	8.7(3.9)	28.6(5.8)	6.7(3.9)	13.3(4.3)	26.5(6.6)	16.2(24.8)

Fig. 1. SDS electrophoresis of adult rat forebrain myelin using (a) micro-gradient (1-30%) and (b) macro(12%)-polyacrylamide gels. The protein composition of this fraction (expressed as percentages of the total dye bound) is also shown (c). Values are means (coefficients of variation) of 5 observations.

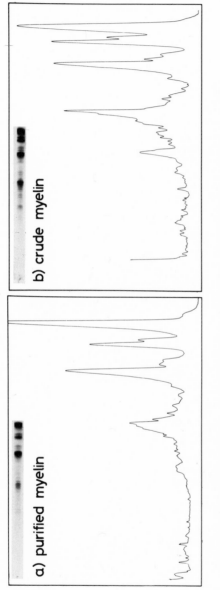

a) purified myelin

b) crude myelin

c) Protein composition of myelin fractions isolated from small tissue samples

	WP	PLP	DM-20	LBP	SBP	Residual proteins
Purified myelin:	10.1	17.1	5.0	11.7	22.5	33.7
Crude myelin :	11.4	13.0	4.4	11.9	16.6	42.8

Fig. 2. Micro-SDS gradient gel electrophoresis of (a) purified and (b) crude myelin fractions prepared from aliquots (equivalent to 20 mg wet weight tissue) of a homogenate of adult rat fore-brain (see Experimental section). Values for the protein composition of these fractions (percentages of the total dye bound) are means of data from 3 separate experiments.

protein (4, 6, 11), previously only consistently resolved in 15%
acrylamide gels (4), and of LBP (3, 8, 27) were more clearly separated by electrophoresis in micro-gradient gels, than in the macro-
scale (homogeneous) system employed (Fig. 1). Furthermore, scans
of micro-gels indicated the presence of a distinct shoulder on the
high molecular weight side of PLP, an observation also noted by
several other investigators (4, 12, 15). The Wolfgram protein
complex was generally visible as two major components (6, 14, 24).
One disadvantage of this system was that the DM-20 protein doublet
was not always well separated from PLP, although, as will be shown
below, this did not preclude reproducible determinations of these
proteins.

Comparison of the relative proportions of the major myelin
proteins separated by electrophoresis either on micro-gradient
gels or on macro-scale homogeneous (12%) gels showed that there
were essentially no differences between the two techniques, although
a high level (40%) of "residual proteins" was apparent when using
the former method (Fig. 1c). This may result from 1) the greater
resolution of higher molecular weight material in micro-gradient
gels and, to a smaller extent, 2) the presence of a low level of
background staining near the gel tops. This staining was demonstrated both in gels which had not been subjected to electrophoresis, and also in those which had been electrophoresed normally
after loading with only sample buffer (no protein) and tracking
dye. Nevertheless, separation on the micro-scale was highly reproducible, as evidenced by coefficients of variation of less than
4% for all myelin proteins except the Wolfgram protein complex
(Fig. 1c).

The protein composition of myelin isolated from small tissue
samples. Using the isolation procedure described, myelin fractions
have been prepared from samples of central nervous tissue as small
as 1 mg wet weight. Analyses of these fractions have so far been
restricted to protein composition, since the protein profile of
myelin, as determined by SDS polyacrylamide gel electrophoresis,
is clearly distinguishable from that of other (microsomal, mitochondrial, synaptosomal and "myelin-like") subcellular fractions
(2), and therefore provides a useful indicator of the presence
and purity of this material (13).

A comparison of micro- and macro-scale myelin isolation
procedures was achieved by using aliquots (equivalent to 20 mg
wet weight) of a homogenate (5% w/v; 0.9 M sucrose) of whole
adult rat forebrain for the micro-preparation. The protein composition of the resultant myelin fraction was qualitatively (Fig.
2a) and quantitatively (Fig. 2c) similar to that of myelin isolated
using the macro-scale technique (Fig. 1), with a slightly lower
proportion of "residual proteins" in the micro-preparation. Thus,
myelin isolated by this simple small-scale method appears to be of
high purity.

It was found that re-cycling (2-8 times) the myelin through
the isolation procedure did not alter the protein composition of
the resultant fraction, although the low-speed differential

centrifugation step, which was designed to reduce microsomal contamination, did remove predominantly high molecular weight material
from the crude myelin (Fig. 2).

<u>The protein composition of myelin isolated from different
regions of the CNS of Quaking mice.</u> The mean ($\pm$ SEM) body weight
(12.6$\pm$0.8 g) and brain weight (383$\pm$8 mg - not including spinal cord)
of Quaking mice were slightly less (P < 0.05; Student's t-test) than
those of controls (17.8$\pm$0.8 g and 424$\pm$14 mg, respectively). The
yield of crude myelin from the various CNS regions ranged from
1.2$\pm$0.1 µg protein/mg wet weight tissue (telencephalon) to 6.1$\pm$0.6
µg protein/mg tissue (spinal cord) in Quaking animals, and from
4.5$\pm$0.1 µg protein/mg tissue (telencephalon) to 22.1$\pm$0.8 µg
protein/mg tissue (spinal cord) in controls. The protein contents
of myelin fractions from Quaking mice were significantly different
(P < 0.05) from those of controls in all regions examined.

The composition of all myelin fractions was examined by micro-
gel electrophoresis, and the contents of SBP, LBP, DM-20 and PLP
were estimated (based on Coomassie Blue staining). All material
of electrophoretic mobility lower than that of PLP was designated
high molecular weight (HMW), whilst the band migrating ahead of
SBP (generally more prominent in the fractions from Quaking mice
- see also ref. 10) was labelled low molecular weight (LMW).
No attempt was made to quantitate WP, since it was difficult to
define this material in the Quaking myelin fractions, which contained a high percentage of HMW proteins. Experiments in which
solubilised myelin fractions from Quaking and controls were mixed
and electrophoresed, confirmed that the bands labelled SBP, LBP,
DM-20 and PLP in Quaking gels co-migrated with those similarly
labelled in controls.

Fig. 3 shows that, in all regions analysed, the proportions
of SBP and LBP were significantly lower in fractions from Quaking
than in those from control mice. With the exception of optic
nerve fractions, a similar pattern was observed for PLP. The
DM-20 protein was present in the spinal cord myelin fraction from
Quaking animals at essentially a control value, but at progressively lower levels in fractions from more rostral CNS areas (Quaking
optic nerve fractions, like those from spinal cord, contained
control levels of DM-20). Expressed as a percentage of the control
levels, a caudo-rostral gradient was also apparent, but less marked,
for the contents of SBP, LBP and PLP in fractions from Quaking
animals.

                              DISCUSSION

A combination of small-scale centrifugation and micro-gradient
polyacrylamide gel electrophoresis (17) techniques has been used
for the isolation and protein analysis of myelin fractions from
small samples of central nervous tissue. These procedures have
been subsequently utilised for a preliminary study of the protein

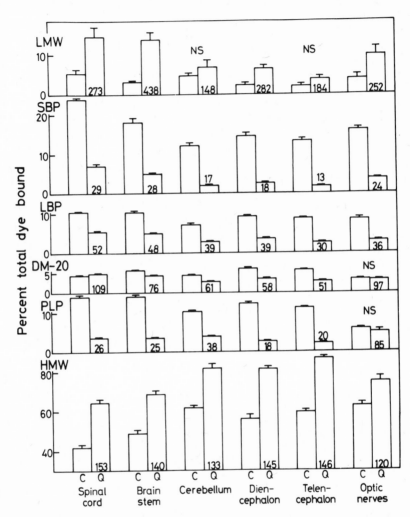

Fig. 3. The protein composition (expressed as percentages of the total dye bound to micro-gradient gels) of myelin fractions isolated from various CNS regions of 40-day-old Quaking (Q) and control (C) mice. Values are means and SEM's (bars) of data from 5 experiments. Numbers within the histogram express the Quaking value as a percentage of the control. NS=P ⊳0.05 (Student's t-test), for comparisons (within regions) of Quaking and control protein contents. For all other comparisons, P⊲ 0.05.

composition of a myelin fraction prepared from different regions of the CNS of the myelin-deficient Quaking mouse.

Theoretical considerations suggest that pore-gradient gel electrophoresis will be advantageous for the resolution of multi-component systems since, at least transiently during an electrophoretic run, any component pair will be separated under optimal conditions (16). Indeed, in the present study, myelin preparations were fractionated with a high resolution by micro-gradient gel electrophoresis, although the four major low molecular weight proteins were not as cleanly separated as by electrophoresis on homogeneous (12%; macro-scale) gels. However, employing the gradient gel system, which allowed a greater degree of resolution over a wider molecular weight range, it was demonstrated that the composition of myelin was more complex than the apparently simple picture obtained by homogeneous gel electrophoresis. Resolution of the two components of DM-20 and LBP, and of the high molecular weight shoulder of PLP (see Results section for details) has not been previously reported in a single gel electrophoresis system. Furthermore, the reproducibility of separation by micro-gel electrophoresis was at least equal to that achieved with the macro-scale system.

In addition to their separation qualities, the micro-gradient gels possess several advantages. Firstly, gels may be stored for long periods of time, thereby eliminating the need to prepare them regularly prior to use. Secondly, only small amounts of material (0.5 - 1.0 μg total myelin protein) are required for a single electrophoresis run. Finally, but perhaps most importantly, the time for electrophoresis (30 min), staining (10 min) and destaining is considerably less than that needed for macro-scale systems.

The small-scale myelin isolation procedure, which is a modification of the "rapid" method described by Agrawal et al. (1), yielded a myelin fraction of similar purity (as determined by SDS gel electrophoresis) to that prepared by a standard macro-scale technique (22). Four steps only are involved, with a total centrifugation time of 120 min, in contrast to the 9 steps and nearly 4 hours required for the macro-procedure.

Preliminary experiments using the myelin-deficient Quaking mouse have confirmed the results of previous studies, which showed that myelin from whole mutant brains contains reduced levels of proteolipid and basic proteins (6, 7). It is interesting that the deficit of myelin proteins is greater in myelin fractions from more rostral regions (with the exception of the optic nerves) of the Quaking neuraxis, since morphological studies indicate that such a gradient also exists with regard to the degree of myelination in these animals (5, 25). One mechanism by which this may occur is that myelination may be arrested (25) at different stages of its development throughout the mutant CNS. If this is so, further studies of the regional composition of myelin fractions isolated from the Quaking mouse may yield valuable information about the temporal sequence of events during early myelinogenesis.

Acknowledgements. It is a pleasure to thank Dr J.D. Lane for many valuable discussions, and Mr J. Malotka for his skillful technical assistance. G.E.F. acknowledges with gratitude the receipt of a post-doctoral fellowship from the Royal Society (Great Britain). This work was supported in part by a grant from the Deutsche Forschungsgemeinschaft (SFB 33).

REFERENCES

1. Agrawal, H.C., Burton, R.M., Fishman, M.A., Mitchell, R.F. and Prensky, A.L., Partial characterisation of a new myelin component, J. Neurochem. 19 (1972) 2083-2089.

2. Agrawal, H.C., Trotter, J.L., Mitchell, R.F. and Burton, R.M., Criteria for identifying a myelin-like fraction from developing brain, Biochem. J. 136 (1973) 1117-1119.

3. Allison, J.H., Agrawal, H.C. and Moore, B.W., Effect of N,N, N',N'-tetramethylethylenediamine on the migration of proteins in SDS polyacrylamide gels, Anal. Biochem. 58 (1974) 592-601.

4. Cammer, W. and Norton, W.T., Disc gel electrophoresis of myelin proteins: new observations on development of the inter- mediate proteins (DM-20), Brain Res. 109 (1976) 643-648.

5. Friedrich, V.L., The myelin deficit in Quaking mice, Brain Res. 82 (1974) 168-172.

6. Greenfield, S., Norton, W.T. and Morell, P., Quaking mouse: isolation and characterisation of myelin protein, J. Neurochem. 18 (1971) 2119-2128.

7. Gregson, N.A. and Oxberry, J.M., The composition of myelin from the mutant mouse "Quaking", J. Neurochem. 19 (1972) 1065-1071.

8. Kelly, P.T. and Luttges, M.W., Mouse brain protein composition during postnatal development: an electrophoretic study, J. Neurochem. 27 (1976) 1163-1172.

9. Lowry, O.H., Rosebrough, N.J., Farr, L.A. and Randall, R.J., Protein measurement with the Folin phenol reagent, J. biol. Chem. 193 (1951) 265-275.

10. Matthieu, J-M., Brady, R.O. and Quarles, R.H., Anomalies of myelin-associated glycoproteins in Quaking mice, J. Neurochem. 22 (1974) 291-296.

11. Morell, P., Greenfield, S., Costantino-Ceccarini, E. and Wis- niewski, H., Changes in the protein composition of mouse brain myelin during development, J. Neurochem. 19 (1972) 2545-2554.

12. Morell, P., Lipkind, R. and Greenfield, S., Protein composition of myelin from brain and spinal cord of several species, Brain Res. 58 (1973) 510-514.

13. Norton, W.T., Recent developments in the investigation of purified myelin, Adv. exp. Med. Biol. 13 (1971) 327-337.

14. Nussbaum, J.L., Delaunoy, J.P. and Mandel, P., Some immuno-chemical characteristics of W1 and W2 Wolfgram proteins isolated from rat brain myelin, J. Neurochem. 28 (1977) 183-191.

15. Poduslo, J.F., Everly, J.L. and Quarles, R.H., A low molecular weight glycoprotein associated with isolated myelin: distinction from myelin proteolipid protein, J. Neurochem. 28 (1977) 977-986.

16. Rodbard, D., Kapadia, G. and Chrambach, A., Pore gradient electrophoresis, Anal. Biochem. 40 (1971) 135-157.

17. Rüchel, R., Mesecke, S., Wolfrum, D-I. and Neuhoff, V., Micro-electrophoresis in continuous-polyacrylamide-gradient gels, II, Hoppe-Seylers Z. Physiol. Chem. 355 (1974) 997-1020.

18. Samorajski, T., Friede, R.L. and Reimer, P.R., Hypomyelination in the Quaking mouse, J. Neuropath. exp. Neurol. 29 (1970) 507-523.

19. Sidman, R.L., Dickie, M.M. and Appel, S.H., Mutant mice (Quaking and Jimpy) with deficient myelination in the central nervous system, Science 144 (1964) 309-311.

20. Waehneldt, T.V., Ontogenetic study of a myelin-derived fraction with 2',3'-cyclic nucleotide 3'-phosphohydrolase activity higher than that of myelin, Biochem. J. 151 (1975) 435-437.

21. Waehneldt, T.V. and Mandel, P., Isolation of rat brain myelin, monitored by polyacrylamide gel electrophoresis of dodecyl sulphate-extracted proteins, Brain Res. 40 (1972) 419-436.

22. Waehneldt, T.V., Matthieu, J.-M. and Neuhoff, V., Characterisation of a myelin-related fraction (SN4) isolated from rat forebrain at two developmental stages, Brain Res., in press.

23. Waehneldt, T.V. and Neuhoff, V., Membrane proteins of rat brain: compositional changes during postnatal development, J. Neurochem. 23 (1974) 71-77.

24. Wiggins, R.C., Joffe, S., Davison, D. and Del Valle, U., Characterisation of Wolfgram proteolipid protein of bovine white matter and fractionation of molecular weight heterogeneity, J. Neurochem. 22 (1974) 171-175.

25. Wisniewski, H. and Morell, P., Quaking mouse: ultrastructural evidence for arrest of myelinogenesis, Brain Res. 29 (1971) 63-73.

26. Zgorzalewicz, B., Neuhoff, V. and Waehneldt, T.V., Rat myelin proteins: compositional changes in various regions of the nervous system during ontogenetic development, Neurobiology 4 (1974) 265-276.

27. Zimmerman, A.W., Quarles, R.H., Webster, H.de F., Matthieu, J.-M. and Brady, R.O., Characterisation and protein analysis of myelin subfractions in rat brain: developmental and regional comparisons, J. Neurochem. 25 (1975) 749-757.

STUDIES ON THE ACTION OF MYELIN BASIC PROTEIN (MBP) IN RAT BRAIN

C.G. Honegger, W. Bucher and H.P. von Hahn

Abteilung Neurochemie, Neurologische-Universitäts-
 klinik
Basel, Switzerland [+]

SUMMARY

The specificity of I^{125}-MBP uptake and subcellular distribution on a discontinuous sucrose density gradient, compared to those of histone H 4 and cytochrome c, showed a high affinity of MBP for mitochondria and heavy synaptosomes, and of histone H 4 for lighter synaptosomes. One heavier synaptosomal subpopulation was almost equally labelled by both proteins. Cytochrome c showed only a low uptake into particular material. Receptor interaction studies of MBP with H^3-labelled 5-hydroxytryptamine and naloxone gave negative results.

INTRODUCTION

The main interest in MBP up to now has been in its antigenic properties in inducing experimental allergic encephalomyelitis (EAE). Since this protein is present in relatively high concentrations in myelin (3.2×10^{-6} moles/g myelin, or about 60 mg per g) and has a significant turnover rate (rate constant k = 2.8×10^{-7}, giving 0.9×10^{-12} moles/sec) (18), its general physiological properties in the central nervous system, other than that as a structural myelin membrane protein, are of considerable interest. The question of the level of free MBP in the brain is not yet settled. Westall (18) speculated that, according to the calculated turnover rate, free MBP could reach a level of 1.2×10^{-8} moles/g myelin. There is also some indication that this level could be much higher in

---

[+] Address for correspondence: Dr. C.G. Honegger, Abteilung Neurochemie, Neurologische Klinik, Socinstrasse 55, CH-4051 Basel, Switzerland.

demyelinating diseases. Cohen et al. (5) found a 10 to 100 fold
increase in MBP over the normal 0-2 ng/ml in the cerebrospinal
fluid of MS patients in an acute stage. If one considers the rapid
endogenous breakdown of MBP by proteinases, then the local level
of this protein must be temporarily quite high. Another interesting aspect of MBP is that it could be the source of a number of
peptides which are physiologically active in the brain.

We have been particularly interested in the electrophysiological action of MBP on neurones. Thus we found that the injection
of 2-4 μl of 1x10^{-4}M MBP into the rat spinal cord in situ produced
marked inhibition of ventral root responses (10). In cerebellar
tissue cultures, 5x10^{-8} to 5x10^{-6}M MBP inhibited the spontaneous
activity of Purkinje cells. Several antagonists to known neurotransmitters such as haloperidol, propanolol, phenoxybenzamine and
bicuculline failed to block this action (10).

In recent experiments, the physiological action of MBP was
tested by unilateral injection (1 μl of 1.2x10^{-3}M MBP) into the
substantia nigra of rats, where various neurotransmitters such as
GABA, dopamine, 5-hydroxytryptamine, acetylcholine and substance
P are active. MBP was about 10 times as active in inducing contra-
versive turning as substance P at the same molar concentration,
while cytochrome c (another basic protein of similar molecular
weight) was inactive. Since substance P has excitatory activity,
a similar action may be postulated for MBP (Olpe and Honegger, in
preparation). This possibility has been corroborated in the isolated spinal cord preparation, where 10^{-4}M MBP has a depolarizing
effect qualitatively similar to that of 10^{-3}M glutamate. The
ventral root response to MBP is of slower onset but longer duration
(Isler and Honegger, in preparation). These experiments suggest
that either MBP acts directly or indirectly as an excitatory substance, or it interacts with a biochemical or biophysical process
vital for normal bioelectrical activity.

In order to elucidate the action of MBP we undertook biochemical studies on its uptake and release in rat cortex and liver
slices. We found that in brain I^{125}-labelled MBP is accumulated
preferentially by a subpopulation of heavy mitochondria and a subpopulation of very heavy synaptosomes (1, 2). The T/M ratio of
MBP is relatively small compared with those of actively transported low molecular weight substances. MBP levels are dependent
on concentration and show distinct compartment differences. In
liver the uptake into mitochondria resulting in high relative
specific labelling is typical. It is not yet known whether the
compartment differences are caused by transport mechanisms or
binding to negative charges (1, 2). MBP at concentrations above
10^{-5}M slightly inhibited the uptake of H^3-5-hydroxytryptamine and
H^3-noradrenaline into rat cortex slices, whereas the K$^+$-stimulated
release of noradrenaline, 5-hydroxytryptamine and GABA was not affected (11).

Since the electrophysiological results obtained with different
test systems indicated that MBP interferes with neuronal activity

in a way which is not yet clearly understood, we decided to extend our studies in two directions: 1) In order to define precisely the specificity of unusual subcellular distribution of MBP after uptake into cortex slices, we compared it with those of two other basic proteins of similar molecular weight. 2) Since our biochemical results indicate that the neurochemical site of action of MBP is not pre-synaptic, we must now consider its possible interaction with various postsynaptic neurotransmitter receptor sites. We report here on first results with the 5-hydroxytryptamine and endogenous opiate receptors.

EXPERIMENTAL

Materials. Cytochrome c was obtained from Serva A.G., Heidelberg. Histone H 4 was kindly provided by Dr. E.W. Johns (Chester Beatty Research Institute, London). Bovine myelin basic protein (MBP) was prepared from fresh spinal cord using a slight modification of the standard method (6, 7). H^3-5-hydroxytryptamine (H^3-5HT), 26.6 Ci/mmole, and H^3-Naloxone, 19.9 Ci/mmole, were obtained from New England Nuclear, cold Naloxone from Endo Laboratories, Inc., Garden City, N.Y., cold 5-hydroxytryptamine (5-HT) from Serva A.G., Heidelberg. TRIZMA^R-7.4 and 7.7 buffers from Sigma Chemical Co., St. Louis. I^{125}-labelled proteins were prepared with NaI^{125} by a modification (9) of the original procedure of Greenwood et al. (8) and stored at -20°C.

Uptake and subcellular distribution of I^{125}-labelled proteins. We followed the method of Honegger et al. (12), using adult male SIV Ivanovas rats (200-300 g). 100 mg cortex slices (0.225x0.225 x1.0 mm) were preincubated for 5 min at 25°C in 1.9 ml Krebs-Henseleit medium. The I^{125}-labelled proteins were then added to give a final concentration of $1x10^{-7}$M, and incubation continued for 10 min at 25°C. After washing with 5 ml cold medium the slices were homogenized in 0.9 ml 0.32 M sucrose, and the homogenate was centrifuged for 10 min at 600 g to sediment the nuclei. 0.5 ml of the nuclei-free supernatant was layered on a 10-step discontinous sucrose density gradient (for details see ref. 12) and centrifuged for 90 min at 60,000 g_{av}. Thirty-three fractions were collected for scintillation counting. Protein was determined by absorption at 280 nm.

Binding to 5HT-receptor. Whole rat brain was homogenized in 40 vol. (per fresh weight) cold 50 mM TRIZMA-7.7 with a Polytron Pt-10 homogenizer (setting 7) for 30 sec. After 10 min centrifugation at 48,000 g the supernatant was discarded, the pellet resuspended in the same volume of TRIZMA-7.7 for 30 sec with the Polytron homogenizer, and again sedimented for 10 min at 48,000 g. The second pellet was homogenized for 30 sec in 60 vol. of cold 50 mM TRIZMA-7.7 containing 10^{-5}M ascorbic acid and 10^{-6}M pargyline. This final suspension was pre-incubated for 10 min at 37°C, and stored in ice until used. To measure the interaction of MBP with 5-HT-receptor 750 μl pre-incubated homogenate were added to 250 μl 10^{-8}M H^3-5HT (final concentration 2×10^{-9}M), and 250 μl MBP solution (final concentrations 10^{-9} to 10^{-5}M). For total binding, MBP was replaced by TRIZMA-7.7 (with 10^{-5} ascorbic acid), and for unspecific binding by cold 5HT (10^{-5}M final concentration). The filtration method of Pert and Snyder (14) was used for the assays. The reaction mixtures were incubated for 60 min at room temperature with shaking, and the reaction terminated by filtration, and washing with 5 ml cold TRIZMA-7.7. The filters were sucked dry and added to 10 ml cold Instagel in counting vials. After shaking overnight at room temperature and precooling they were counted in a Packard Tricarb scintillation counter. Specific 5HT binding was calculated as the difference between total and unspecific binding, and the effect of MBP was expressed in percentage of the specific binding.

Binding to opiate (naloxone) receptor. Whole rat brain was homogenized for 30 sec in 50 mM TRIZMA-7.7 buffer with the Polytron homogenizer. The pellet obtained after 10 min centrifugation at 48,000 g was rehomogenized in the same way in 30 vol. TRIZMA-7.7 and this second homogenate incubated for 30 min at 37°C with shaking. A second pellet was obtained by 10 min centrifugation at 48,000 g, which was homogenized for 30 sec in 100 vol. (per fresh weight) TRIZMA-7.4 with the Polytron homogenizer. The incubation mixtures contained 900 μl of this final homogenate, 50 μl 2×10^{-8}M H^3-Naloxone (in TRIZMA-7.4) (final concentration 10^{-9}M), and 50 μl MBP solutions (in TRIZMA-7.4) giving final concentrations of 10^{-9} to 10^{-5}M. The effect of 0.1 M NaCl was determined by adding 50 μl 2 M NaCl in TRIZMA-7.4 when required. For total binding MBP was replaced by TRIZMA-7.4 and for unspecific binding by 10^{-5}M Naloxone in TRIZMA-7.4 (final concentration). After 40 min incubation with shaking at room temperature the reaction was terminated by filtration and washing with 5 ml cold TRIZMA-7.4. The filters were sucked dry and added to 10 ml Instagel in counting vials for liquid scintillation counting after shaking overnight at room temperature and pre-cooling. The effect of MBP was calculated as described for the 5HT-receptor. In 4 of the 8 naloxone experiments the membranes were isolated by centrifugation as described by Closse and Hauser (4).

RESULTS

Uptake and subcellular distribution of 10^{-7}M I^{125}-labelled basic proteins in rat cortex slices. The three basic proteins MBP (M.W. 18,300), histone H 4 (M.W. 11,300) and cytochrome c (M.W. 13,000) are transported at different rates into rat cortex slices. As the tissue/medium ratios after 10 min incubation at 25°C show (Table 1), there is no accumulation of cytochrome c (T/M = 0.64). The small amount of radioactive label found in the slices is probably accounted for by diffusion into the extracellular space during swelling and by binding to negative charges.

Table 1. Tissue/Medium ratios (c.p.m. per g tissue/c.p.m. per ml medium) for the uptake of $10^{-7}M/I^{125}$-labelled MBP, cytochrome c and histone H 4 into rat cortex slices (10 min incubation at 25°C).

	N	T/M ratio
MBP	10	1.13+0.12
Cytochrome c	10	0.64+0.05
Histone H 4	4	1.61+0.23

With both MBP and histone H 4 (arginine-rich histone, formely F2al) the T/M ratios are greater than 1.0, indicating at least some active accumulation into the tissue. The comparison of the T/M ratios in Table 1 shows that not all basic proteins of similar size are transported in the same way into cortex:there is clearly a certain amount of specificity in the mechanisms involved.

After subcellular fractionation of the homogenized nuclei-free cortex slices on a ten-step discontinuous sucrose density gradient, the three I^{125}-labelled proteins show distinctly different distribution patterns. This is particularly the case for MBP and histone H 4 (Fig. 1). When the distribution is calculated on a protein basis as "Relative Specific Labelling" (RSL = percent c.p.m. per percent protein in each gradient fraction) it is apparent that MBP is strongly accumulated by the two mitochondrial subpopulations (at 1.4 and 1.3 M sucrose) and by the two heavier of our 4 synaptosomal subpopulations (at 1.2 and 1.1 M sucrose) (Fig. 2). In contrast, neither histone H 4 nor cytochrome c are found in high concentrations (RSL above 1.0) in the mitochondria. Histone H 4 is most actively accumulated by all 4 synaptosomal subpopulations (at 1.2, 1.1, 1.0 and 0.9 M sucrose). Cytochrome c is most actively bound to the lightest material (0.6 and 0.3 M sucrose), the highest RSL-values being found in the top of the gradient where the sample had been applied. It should be noted that while the three lighter synaptosomal subpopulations (at 1.1, 1.0 and 0.9 M sucrose) show relatively little contamination, the "very heavy synaptosomes" sedimenting to the 1.2 M-sucrose step have not yet been clearly identified by electron microscopy, and probably contain a mixed population of synaptosomes and mitochondria. In the myelin-step of our gradient (0.8 M sucrose, fractions 26-29) only histone H 4 has RSL values significantly above 1.0, MBP is clearly not bound here, and there is only a weakly defined shoulder for cytochrome c, perhaps caused by strong contamination from the heavily labelled material in the supernatant fractions (0.6 M sucrose, fractions 30-33).

Receptor binding studies: displacement of H^3-labelled 5-hydr-
oxytryptamine and naloxone by MBP. The possibility that MBP has a
post-synaptic site of action was studied by receptor experiments
using the 5-hydroxytryptamine and opiate (naloxone) receptors.
These particular receptors were chosen because of the suggestion
that MBP has structural similarity with the 5-hydroxytryptamine
receptor (3), and because the so-called "endogenous opiates", the
endorphins and enkephalins, are peptides. Under our experimental
conditions, 5-hydroxytryptamine (5HT) had an ED_{50} of 1.5×10^{-8}M,
and naloxone of 2.7×10^{-9}M both with and without 0.1 M NaCl.

The displacement curve for 2×10^{-9}M H^3-5HT is shown in Fig. 3.
Up to 10^{-6}M MBP the specific binding of H^3-5HT is increased by
approximately 10%. When the MBP concentration is further raised
to 10^{-5}M, inhibition is observed. The 50% inhibitory concentration
(IC_{50}) is approximately 8×10^{-6}M MBP.

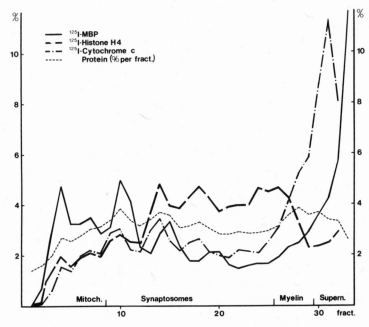

Fig.1. Subcellular distribution of 10^{-7}M I^{125}-labelled MBP, histone
H 4 and cytochrome c on a 10-step discontinuous sucrose density
gradient, after 10 min uptake at 25°C into rat cortex slices, homogenization and removal of the cell nuclei by centrifugation. Percent
c.p.m. per fraction (total c.p.m. recovered from the gradient =
100%). Protein in percent of total recovered. ————— = MBP
(N=10); —— —— = Histone H 4 (N=4); ——·—— = Cytochrome c (N=10);
-------- = Protein.

The displacement curves for 1×10^{-9}M H^3-naloxone in the presence and in the absence of 0.1 M NaCl are shown in Fig. 4. The presence of NaCl increases the IC_{50} by at least one order of magnitude, from about 2×10^{-6}M to about 2×10^{-5}M. This type of behaviour has been described as characteristic of opiate agonists (15). In all experiments with 5-HT displacement the filtration method, as described in the Experimental section, was used. For the naloxone experiments, centrifugation and filtration methods gave identical results, which have therefore been pooled in Fig. 4.

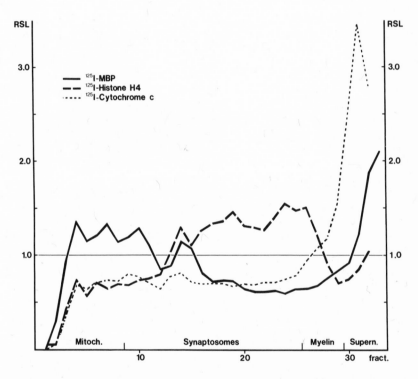

Fig. 2. Relative Specific Labelling (RSL) in percent c.p.m. per percent protein in each fraction for the subcellular distribution of MBP, histone H 4 and cytochrome c as shown in Fig. 1. Values for RSL above 1.0 indicate fractions with proportionately high labelling, pointing to specific accumulation of the labelled substance. ——————— = MBP; —— —— = Histone H 4; ---------- = Cytochrome c.

DISCUSSION

The distribution of relative specific labelling (RSL) values (Fig. 2) for our three basic proteins indicates that while MBP and histone H 4 are actively taken up into particle populations on our gradient, cytochrome c is not. The selectivity of mitochondria for MBP is as striking as that of the lighter synaptosomes for histone H 4. It should be noted that one of the heavier synaptosomal subpopulations accumulates MBP and H 4 almost equally. Our earlier results on the uptake of MBP into certain types of synaptosomes (1) were taken to indicate that its mode of action could be presynaptic interference with an inhibitory neurotransmitter. Our latest biochemical results have not supported such a mechanism (11) for the transmitters tested.

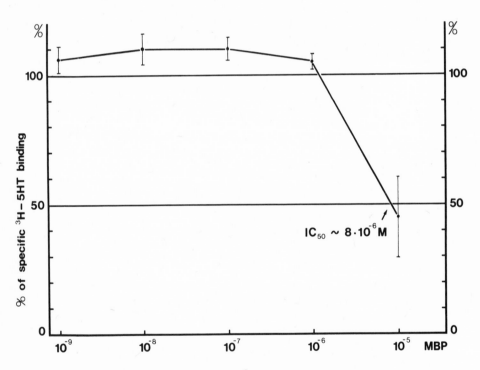

Fig. 3. Displacement of 2×10^{-9}M H^3-5-hydroxytryptamine by increasing concentrations of MBP from the 5-hydroxytryptamine receptor. The ordinate gives percent of specific H^3-5HT binding. IC_{50} = Concentration of MBP giving 50% inhibition of 5HT binding. Averages of 5 experiments, $\pm$ SD.

In this connection the studies of McIlwain (13) and Schwarz (16, 17) are of interest. They found that some basic proteins render cerebral tissue unresponsive to electrical excitation. They concluded that the observed changes in excitability were due to an interference with the re-establishment of membrane potentials, resulting from a hindering of particular ion movement. This action was antagonized by acidic substances such as gangliosides (13). The inhibitory effect was associated with the ATP system involved in active cation transport. These studies on the cellular energetics of basic proteins revealed a marked stimulation of mitochondrial respiration and ATPase, and an inhibition of ADP-ATP exchange (16, 17).

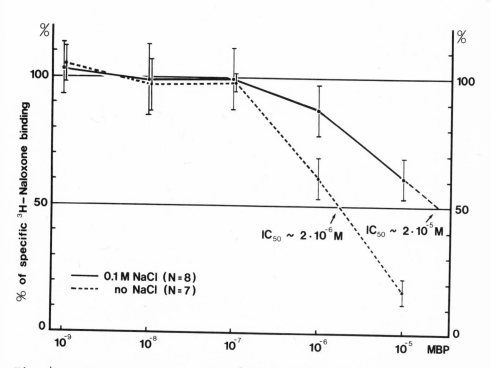

Fig. 4. Displacement of 10^{-9}M H^3-naloxone by increasing concentrations of MBP from the opiate receptor in the presence and absence of 0.1 M NaCl. The ordinate gives percent of specific H^3-naloxone binding. IC_{50} = Concentration of MBP giving 50% inhibition of naloxone binding. Averages of 8 experiments with NaCl and 7 without NaCl, $\pm$ SD. —————— = With 0.1 M Nacl; -------- = No NaCl.

The possible post-synaptic action of MBP induced us to study its interaction with receptors. Our results show that there is indeed an interaction with the opiate receptor and with that for 5-HT. This, however, only occurs at very high concentrations, 100-1000 times the ED_{50} of these two substances. Carnegie (3) has suggested that MBP possesses a binding site for 5HT. Our results show that MBP is taken up into particulate structures, including certain synaptosomes (Fig. 1 and 2). Our receptor studies indicate that Carnegie's suggestion might be correct, since an increased binding of 5HT (average 10%) occurs in the range of 10^{-9} to 10^{-6}M MBP. However, this result must be substantiated by direct saturation binding studies, which are now in progress. If this interpretation of the results proves right, then the possibility must be considered that MBP competes for 5-HT with the natural receptor. There are clearly also other possibilities for a direct or indirect action of MBP. This enquiry is also worth pursuing because an elucidation of the mechanism of action of MBP may have a bearing on various human pathological conditions.

Acknowledgments. We would like to thank Dr. D. Hauser for assistance in methodology problems, and Dr. E.W. Johns for a gift of histone H 4. Mrs. L. Krepelka and Mrs. M. Häusler gave skillful technical assistance. This work was supported by the Swiss Multiple Sclerosis Society.

REFERENCES

1. Bucher, W. and Honegger, C.G., Uptake and subcellular distribution of I^{125}-myelin basic protein (MBP) in rat cortex slices (Abstract), Experientia 32 (1976) 766.
2. Bucher, W. and Honegger, C.G., Uptake and release of I^{125}-myelin basic protein (MBP) in rat cortex and liver slices, 6th Meeting of the ISN, Copenhagen, August 1977, p. 118.
3. Carnegie, P.R., Properties, structure and possible neuro-receptor role of the encephalitogenic protein of human brain, Nature, London 229 (1971) 25.
4. Closse, A. and Hauser, D., Dihydroergotamine binding to rat brain membranes, Life Sciences 19 (1976) 1851-1854.
5. Cohen, S.R., Herndon, R.M. and McKhann, G.M., Radioimmunoassay of myelin basic protein as an index of demyelination, New Engl. J. Med. 295 (1976) 1455-1457.
6. Deibler, G.E., Martenson, R.E. and Kies, M.W., Large scale preparation of myelin basic protein from central nervous tissue of several mammalian species, Prepar. Biochem. 2 (1972) 139-165.
7. Dunkley, P.R. and Carnegie, P.R., Isolation of myelin basic proteins, Research Methods in Neurochemistry 2 (1974) 219-246.
8. Greenwood, F.C., Hunter, W.M. and Glover, J.S., The preparation of ^{131}I-labelled human growth hormone of high specific radioactivity, Biochem. J. 89 (1963) 114-123.

9. Hendry, I.A., Stoeckel, K., Thoenen, H. and Iversen, L.L.,
    The retrograde axonal transport of nerve growth factor, Brain
    Research 68 (1974) 103-121.
10. Honegger, C.G., Gähwiler, B.H. and Isler, H., The effect of
    myelin basic protein (MBP) on the bioelectric activity of
    spinal cord and cerebellar neurones, Neuroscience Letters 4
    (1977) 303-307.
11. Honegger, C.G., Krepelka, L.M., Steiner, M. and von Hahn, H.P.,
    The effect of bovine myelin basic protein on uptake and release
    of H^3-labelled 5-hydroxytryptamine, L-noradrenaline and γ-
    aminobutyric acid in rat cortex slices, Experientia 33 (1977)
    294-296.
12. Honegger, C.G., Krepelka, L.M., Steinmann, V. and von Hahn,
    H.P., Distribution of ^3H- and ^{14}C-labelled potential neuro-
    transmitters on a discontinuous density gradient after uptake
    into rat cerebral cortex slices, Europ. Neurol. 12 (1974)
    236-252.
13. McIlwain, H., Chemical exploration of the brain, Elsevier,
    Amsterdam (1963).
14. Pert, C.B. and Snyder, S.H., Properties of opiate-receptor
    binding in rat brain, Proc. Nat. Acad. Sci. USA 70 (1973)
    2243-2247.
15. Pert, C.B. and Snyder, S.H., Opiate receptor binding of agonists
    and antagonists affected differentially by sodium, Molec.
    Pharmacol. 10 (1974) 868-879.
16. Schwarz, A., The effects of histones and other polycations on
    cellular energetics. I. Mitochondrial oxidative phosphoryla-
    tion, J. biol. Chem. 240 (1965) 939-943.
17. Schwarz, A., The effects of histones and other polycations
    on cellular energetics. II. Adenosine triphosphatase and
    adenosine diphosphate-adenosine triphosphate exchange reactions
    of mitochondria, J. biol. Chem. 240 (1965) 944-948.
18. Westall, F.C., Released myelin basic protein: the immunogenic
    factor?, Immunochemistry 11 (1974) 513-515.

IN VIVO INCORPORATION OF ^{32}P INTO MYELIN BASIC PROTEIN FROM

NORMAL AND QUAKING MICE[+]

Jean-Marie Matthieu and Adrien D. Kuffer

Laboratoire de Neurochimie, Service de Pédiatrie,
   Centre hospitalier universitaire vaudois
1011 Lausanne, Switzerland

SUMMARY

Myelin basic protein in normal mice is phosphorylated. Since
phosphorylation can decrease the net positive charge of the myelin
basic protein, this could affect molecular interactions between this
protein and other myelin components. In this study ^{32}P incorporation
into the small and large components of the myelin basic protein was
studied in immature and young adult mice and also in Quaking mutants
which have a severe myelin deficit. We found a short   half-life
of ^{32}P in myelin basic protein. The ^{32}P specific activity of myelin
basic protein was higher in immature and Quaking mice than in young
adult animals.
   Of the ^{32}P-labeled basic proteins of control and Quaking mice,
the small component had a slightly higher specific activity than the
large component. Although the small basic protein is quantitatively
decreased in Quaking mice, the ratio of specific activity of small
to large basic protein is similar in control and Quaking animals.
Since Quaking and immature mice have many uncompacted myelin
lamellae, these preliminary results suggest that phosphorylation
and dephosphorylation could be involved in compaction mechanisms.

INTRODUCTION

   Since 1973, we know that myelin basic protein (BP) can be
phosphorylated (7) and, subsequently, that phosphorylation takes
place only on serine and threonine residues (7, 27, 38). Martenson

[+]Supported by the Swiss National Science Foundation, grant 3.684-76
and the Swiss Multiple Sclerosis Society.

et al. (22) demonstrated that phosphorus was confined to the carboxy-terminal half of component 3 and Chou et al. (9) further found
that the phosphorus content of component 3 was fully accounted for
by phosphothreonine 97 and phosphoserine 164. Recently, a report
appeared indicating that basic amino acids like arginine and
histidine could also be phosphorylated in myelin basic protein (37).
In vivo, only BP is phosphorylated (27, 38) but when myelin is
incubated in vitro other proteins can be phosphorylated (28). This
could indicate that in vivo BP may be the only protein accessible
to the endogenous protein kinase which was reported to be present
in myelin (8, 27, 28, 38). Previous studies (27, 38) indicated a
rapid turnover of the basic protein phosphate and the presence of
a myelin—bound phosphatase could be demonstrated (21). Although
these reports suggest that BP phosphorylation and dephosphorylation
could play an important role during myelin formation and for the
maintenance of myelin, the function of phosphorylation is still
unknown.

Myelin deficient mutants (34) have been useful in investigating
myelin composition and the mechanisms involved in myelin formation.
One of these mutants, the Quaking mouse, presents compaction
anomalies of the myelin lamellae (3, 32, 39, 40, 41). Biochemists
have studied extensively anomalies involving lipids (2, 4, 5, 10,
12, 15, 18), myelin proteins (13, 16, 17, 23, 30) and glycoproteins
(23, 26). Brostoff et al.(6) suggested that the synthesis of BP
in Quaking mouse proceeds at a normal rate but the incorporation of
basic protein into myelin is deficient. This and another report
(12) could indicate a possible defect in the mechanism of final
myelin assembly. In a recent study we have shown that the anomalies
of myelin proteins and glycoproteins are not caused by contaminants
and that they are present in compact myelin as well as in membranes
which are transitional between the glial plasma membrane and the
myelin sheath (26).

We present now results of a work where we investigated the
incorporation of radioactive phosphate into BP of Quaking mice
and compared it with immature and young adult controls. Our preliminary study is compatible with the hypothesis that the degree
of phosphorylation could play a role in molecular interactions
between basic protein and other components of the myelin membrane.

EXPERIMENTAL

Animals and materials. Quaking mice and their littermates of
strain C57BL/6J-Qk were from our local breeding colony, originally
obtained from the Jackson Laboratory, Bar Harbor, Maine, U.S.A.
For time course studies, normal mice of the same C57BL strain were
obtained from Hoffman-La Roche Tierfarm, Fuellinsdorf, Switzerland.
In a typical experiment, the mice were injected, under slight ether
anesthesia, intracerebrally in two different sites 16 h before

sacrifice with 26 µCi/animal of [^{32}P]sodium phosphate (specific
activity $\geq$ 9.6 mCi/mg phosphorus) in 12 µl physiological saline.
For double label experiments, 15 µCi of L-[4,5-^{3}H]leucine (30 Ci/
nmol) and 26 µCi ^{32}P were injected together into the same animal.
Radioactive phosphate was obtained from Eidgenossisches Institut
für Reactorforschung, Wuerenlingen, Switzerland, and radioactive
leucine from New England Nuclear Corporation, Boston, Mass., U.S.A.

For in situ autolysis studies, the mice were sacrificed by
fracturing the cervical column. The control brains were rapidly
removed and frozen at -70°C. For the purpose of the study, some
animals were kept after death in sealed plastic containers at 19°C
for 24 h. After this period, the brains were removed and stored at
-70°C.

Brain homogenate and myelin isolation. With the exception of
the autolysis experiments, the brains were homogenized immediately
after sacrifice in 0.32 M sucrose and myelin was purified (29).
For autolysis experiments, the frozen tissue was thawed in chilled
0.32 M sucrose and otherwise processed as mentioned above. Aliquots
from brain homogenates and myelin suspension were taken for protein
(20) and radioactivity determination.

Solubilization of proteins and polyacrylamide gel electrophoresis. Myelin was partially delipidated with ether-ethanol
(3:2, v/v, ref. 16) and proteins were solubilized in sodium dodecyl
sulfate (SDS)-mercaptoethanol for gel electrophoresis (24).
Aliquots of 150 µg of protein were separated in the presence of SDS
on a 15% polyacrylamide gel and stained with 1% Fast Green (24).
For the quantitation of BP, pure myelin basic protein from rabbit
brain (11) was used as a standard. For each protein determination,
a standard curve was made with gels prepared, electrophoresed and
stained at the same time as the myelin protein samples. The Fast
Green stained gels were scanned on a Guilford spectrophotometer and
the proteins quantitated by cutting out the peaks and weighing.
The standard curve was linear from 1-15 µg of BP. Radioactive
labelled proteins were determined by cutting out the stained basic
protein bands from the gels and by solubilizing in 35% H_2O_2. The
radioactivity$_R$was counted on a liquid scintillation spectrometer
using Aquasol^R (New England Nuclear Corporation, Boston, Mass.,
U.S.A.) as scintillation solution and the results were corrected
for quenching and decay.

RESULTS

^{32}P incorporation into mouse brain, myelin and myelin basic
protein. A time course study in whole brain, myelin and the two
components of basic protein (Fig. 1) from normal young adults,
showed that the level of ^{32}P in whole brain did not change, whereas
in myelin the incorporation of ^{32}P reached a plateau after 1 h. In
the basic proteins, after some fluctuations during the first hour,

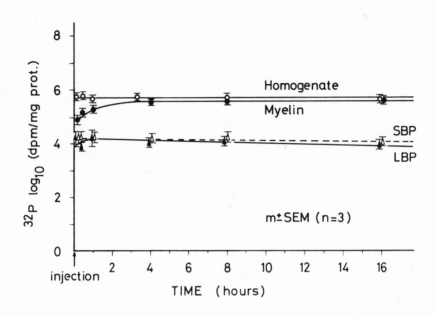

Fig. 1. <u>In vivo</u> incorporation of ^{32}P into mouse brain. Radioactivity was measured 10, 30, 60 min, 4, 8 and 16 h after intracerebral injection. Results are expressed in d.p.m. (disintegration
per minute) per mg of total protein for homogenate, per mg of myelin
protein for myelin and per mg of BP for the large, LBP, and small,
SBP, components of myelin basic protein. Mean $\pm$ standard error of
the mean (m $\pm$ SEM) from 3 separate experiments.

both components leveled off. The apparent half-life of ^{32}P in the
large basic protein (LBP) was 7.2 days while the half-life of the
small basic protein (SBP) was slightly longer, 8 days.
    The incorporation of ^{32}P into the whole homogenate did not
reveal significant differences between immature, young adult controls
and 25-day-old Quaking mutants (Table 1). In myelin, about 30 to
50% of the radioactivity was bound to lipids removed by the ether-
ethanol wash. The radioactivity was higher in the protein fraction
of myelin from Quaking and immature control mice than in young adult
controls (Table 1).
    <u>Effect of autolysis on myelin basic protein from normal 25-</u>
<u>day-old mice</u>. Myelin prepared from autolyzed brain (24 h at 19°C)
lost approximately 40% of basic protein. The specific ^{32}P –

Table 1. ^{32}P incorporation into whole brain and purified myelin.
The results represent the means $\pm$ SEM from 6 to 8 experiments.

| | | 10^{-5} d.p.m. mg protein^{-1} | |
| | | Control | Quaking |
	25 days	10 days	25 days
Homogenate	4.2$\pm$0.3	7.5$\pm$0.8	5.5$\pm$0.5
Myelin			
Protein fraction*	4.2$\pm$0.4	11.7$\pm$1.4	6.0$\pm$0.7
Lipid fraction**	2.4$\pm$0.3	10.4$\pm$1.0	4.6$\pm$0.6

*Protein fraction: myelin delipidated with ether-ethanol and
solubilized in SDS. **Lipid fraction: radioactivity extracted in
ether-ethanol.

Table 2. Effect of autolysis on ^{32}P basic protein. The results
represent the means $\pm$ SEM from 6 separate experiments. A, percent
of the dye binding capacity; B, 10^{-3} d.p.m. mg BP^{-1}. p, Student's
test significance; N.S., not significant.

		-70°C	$+19^{\circ}$C	p
LBP,	A	15.1$\pm$0.6	9.4$\pm$0.7	<0.05
	B	8.0$\pm$1.3	7.6$\pm$0.6	N.S.
SBP,	A	18.3$\pm$0.5	11.9$\pm$0.9	<0.001
	B	9.0$\pm$1.3	7.6$\pm$0.7	N.S.

radioactivity of the two myelin basic components did not change
significantly under these conditions (Table 2) suggesting that
phosphorus is not preferentially lost during in situ autolysis
but that the molecule is degrading in toto.

   Protein composition and phosphorylation of purified myelin.
The relative amount of the myelin proteins, expressed in percent
of the dye binding capacity after scanning of Fast Green stained
bands on polyacrylamide gels, is shown in Table 3. Quaking mice
differed from immature and same age controls by their very low
proteolipid protein content and by a decrease of the SBP component.
The high molecular weight proteins were relatively increased in
Quaking and also in immature control animals.

Table 3. Protein composition of purified myelin. Each individual
value represents the percent of the dye binding capacity (the mean
from two separate experiments). - HMW(-), high molecular weight
proteins without V and W bands; V, a high molecular weight band
migrating close to the W band; W, the major high molecular weight
protein, also called Wolfgram protein; PLP, proteolipid protein;
I, intermediate or DM-20 protein; LBP, large, and SBP, small
components of the myelin basic protein.

	Control (25 d.)	Control (10 d.)	Quaking (25 d.)
HMW(-)	19.8	28.3	30.7
V	4.8	6.7	6.7
W	7.6	5.7	7.1
PLP	18.9	11.0	4.4
I	7.2	7.2	8.2
LBP	15.9	17.4	16.8
SBP	17.8	16.4	12.7

The distribution of ^{32}P-radioactivity in myelin proteins
separated by gel electrophoresis (Fig. 2) showed in control and
Quaking animals that, in vivo, only the two basic protein components
incorporated ^{32}P. A large peak of radioactivity was measured in a
turbid band at the bottom of the gel; it represents lipids which
were not removed by ether-ethanol extraction (Fig. 2).

Determination of myelin basic protein, ^{32}P specific activity
and ^{32}P/^{3}H ratio. Determination of myelin basic protein using pure
BP as a standard confirmed our findings using the dye binding
capacity. In comparison to same age control, the Quaking mouse had
only 58% of the small basic protein, whereas the large component was
normal (Table 4). Very immature animals had also an important reduction of the SBP.

The ^{32}P specific activity in both components of the myelin
basic protein from Quaking and immature mice was significantly
higher than in normal young adults (Table 5). In both Quaking and
age-matched controls, the SBP component had a slightly higher
specific activity (55%) than the LBP component (45%). This trend
was also present, but to a lesser extent, in immature animals. The
ratios of ^{32}P specific activity between the small and large basic
protein were: 1.22, 1.27 and 1.11 for 25-day-old control and Quaking
mice, and 10-day-old mice, respectively.

The BP was labeled with two different precursors, radioactive
sodium phosphate and leucine, injected together into the animals.
The change in the ratio ^{32}P/^{3}H should allow comparisons between
phosphorylation and protein turnover. The ratio ^{32}P/^{3}H was lower
in both immature and Quaking mice than in 25-day-old controls
(Table 6). This fall of the ratio was observed while the ^{32}P
specific activity was high and reflects a simultaneous larger [^{3}H]
leucine incorporation.

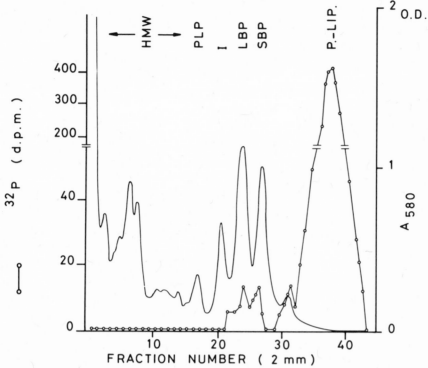

Fig. 2. ^{32}Phosphorus distribution (0———0) and densitometric scan of Fast Green stained proteins (solid line) in myelin of 25-day-old Quaking mice after separation on a 15% polyacrylamide gel. The ^{32}P labeled gel was cut into 1 mm slices and 2 mm fractions were counted. The gel contained 150 µg of ether-ethanol delipidated protein. HMW, high molecular weight proteins; PLP, proteolipid protein; I, intermediate protein; LBP, large, and SBP, small components of myelin basic protein; P-LIP, phospholipids.

Table 4. Myelin basic protein determination. The values represent the means ± SEM from 5 to 7 separate experiments.

	µg BP, mg total myelin protein^{-1}	
	LBP	SBP*
Control, 25 days	67.4± 3.5	87.7± 3.6^{A,B}
10 days	60.8±10.5	59.3±12.0^{B}
Quaking, 25 days	68.5± 5.4	50.5± 4.1^{A}

*p value between same letters: A < 0.01, B < 0.05 (Student's t-test).

Table 5. ^{32}P specific activity of myelin basic protein. The values represent the means ± SEM from 7 to 8 separate experiments.

	10^{-4} d.p.m. mg BP^{-1}	
	LBP*	SBP*
Control, 25 days	1.1±0.1^{A,B}	1.3±0.1^{C,D}
10 days	1.7±0.1^{A}	1.8±0.1^{C}
Quaking, 25 days	1.6±0.1^{B}	2.0±0.1^{D}

*Student's t-test values between same letters: $p < 0.01$; when not stated, not significant.

Table 6. Ratio ^{32}P/^{3}H-leucine incorporated into myelin basic protein. The values represent the means ± SEM from 3 separate experiments.

	LBP	SBP
Control, 25 days	0.53±0.18	0.71±0.13
10 days	0.13±0.02	0.45±0.10
Quaking, 25 days	0.35±0.06	0.25±0.10

DISCUSSION

Our results confirm that myelin from Quaking mice has a drastic decrease of proteolipid protein and to a lesser extent lower levels of the small component of the myelin basic protein (13, 16, 17, 23, 30). It was suggested recently that the synthesis of BP was normal but its incorporation into the membrane could be abnormal (6). Since phosphorylation will decrease the net positive charge of the BP, it could influence the interactions between myelin lamellae during sheath formation (21) or between this protein and the other myelin components. Therefore we were interested to study the radioactive phosphate incorporation into myelin proteins of the Quaking mutant. In normal mice only the two basic protein components were phosphorylated in vivo as reported previously (27, 38) and the specific activity of ^{32}P in myelin basic protein was not affected by in situ degradation. In Quaking mice the two basic protein components were also the only myelin proteins to incorporate radioactive phosphate. Contrary to the results of Miyamoto and Kakiuchi (27) we found that SBP had a slightly higher ^{32}P specific activity than LBP. Neither did we observe the rapid fall of ^{32}P radioactivity in brain homogenate, myelin and myelin basic protein reported by Miyamoto and Kakiuchi. Nevertheless, the half-life of ^{32}P measured in BP was short and is in agreement with the rapid turnover demonstrated by Steck and Appel (38). The rapid turnover rate of phosphate in BP is probably controlled by a myelin endogenous protein kinase (21, 27, 28, 38) and phosphatase (21, 27). This contrasts with the very slow turnover rates reported for myelin proteins (31, 33, 36). The evaluation of myelin protein turnover is difficult (19) since reutilization (14, 19, 31, 33) and membranous precursors of myelin (1) could influence the turnover and be responsible for the apparent metabolic stability of myelin.

Although SBP was quantitatively decreased in Quaking mice, the ratio of specific activity of small to large basic proteins was similar in control and Quaking animals. This indicates that the mechanism involved in the increased specific activity of Quaking basic proteins is the same for both basic proteins. The important difference found in this study was the higher ^{32}P specific activity measured in immature and particularly in Quaking BP. In vitro, also immature animals showed a higher phosphate incorporation than adult animals (38).

When ^{32}P and ^{3}H-leucine were incorporated simultaneously into BP the ratio between the two isotopes was lower in both basic protein components from Quaking and immature mice than in 25-day-old control animals. This decreased ratio occurred with high ^{32}P specific activities and indicates that the protein moiety has a very high turnover rate in immature and Quaking mice.

Our preliminary results which indicate a higher ^{32}P specific activity of BP in immature and Quaking mice which have many uncompacted myelin lamellae could be an indication that phosphorylation and dephosphorylation could be involved in compaction mechanisms. Studies to ascertain the activity in myelin of both protein kinase and phosphatase and to evaluate the turnover rate of basic protein phosphate of Quaking mice are presently in progress.

REFERENCES

1. Agrawal, H.C., in Fundamentals of Lipid Chemistry (R.M. Burton and C.E. Guerra, eds.) B-Science Publications, Wester Grooves, MO. (1974) pp. 511-531.

2. Baumann, N.A., Harpin, M.L. and Bourre, J.-M., Long chain fatty acid formation: key step in myelination studied in mutant mice, Nature 227 (1970) 960-961.

3. Berger, B., Quelques aspects ultrastructuraux de la substance blanche chez la souris Quaking, Brain Res. 25 (1971) 35-53.

4. Bourre, J.M., Daudu, O.L. and Baumann, N.A., Fatty acid biosynthesis in mice brain and kidney microsomes: comparison between Quaking mutant and control, J. Neurochem. 24 (1975) 1095-1097.

5. Bowen, D.M. and Radin, N.S., Hydrolase activities in brain of neurological mutants: cerebroside galactosidase, nitrophenyl galactoside hydrolase, nitrophenyl glucoside hydrolase and

sulfatase, J. Neurochem. 16 (1969) 457-460.

6. Brostoff, S.W., Greenfield, S. and Hogan, E.L., The differentiation of synthesis from incorporation of basic protein in Quaking mutant mouse myelin, Brain Res.120 (1977) 517-520.

7. Carnegie, P.R., Kemp, B.E., Dunkley, P.R. and Murray, A.W., Phosphorylation of myelin basic protein by an adenosine 3':5'-cyclic monophosphate-dependent protein kinase, Biochem. J. 135 (1973) 569-572.

8. Carnegie, P.R., Dunkley, P.R., Kemp, B.E. and Murray, A.W., Phosphorylation of selected serine and threonine residues in myelin basic protein by endogenous and exogenous protein kinases, Nature 249 (1974) 147-149.

9. Chou, F.C.-H., Chou, C.-H.J., Shapira, R. and Kibler, R.F., Basis of microheterogeneity of myelin basic protein, J. biol. Chem. 251 (1976) 2671-2679.

10. Costantino-Ceccarini, E. and Morell, P., Quaking mouse: in vitro studies of brain sphingolipid biosynthesis, Brain Res. 29 (1971) 75-84.

11. Deibler, G.E., Martenson, R.E.and Kies, M.W., Large scale preparation of myelin basic protein from central nervous tissue of several mammalian species, Prep. Biochem. 2 (1972) 139-165.

12. Deshmukh, D.S. and Bear, W.D., The distribution and biosynthesis of the myelin-galactolipids in the subcellular fractions of brains of Quaking and normal mice during development, J. Neurochem. 28 (1977) 987-993.

13. Druse, M.J. and Hogan, E.L., Composition of myelin proteins in murine genetic myelin dysgenesis: the Quaking mutant, Proc. Soc. Exp. Biol. Med. 145 (1974) 747-751.

14. Druse, M.J., Brady, R.O. and Quarles, R.H., Metabolism of a myelin-associated glycoprotein in developing rat brain, Brain Res. 76 (1974) 423-434.

15. Eto, Y. and Suzuki, K., Enzymes of cholesterol ester metabolism in the brain of mutant mice, Quaking and Jimpy, Exper. Neurol. 41 (1973) 222-226.

16. Greenfield, S., Norton, W.T. and Morell, P., Quaking mouse: isolation and characterization of myelin protein, J. Neurochem. 18 (1971) 2119-2128.

17. Gregson, N.A. and Oxberry, J.M., The composition of myelin from the mutant mouse "Quaking", J. Neurochem. 19 (1972) 1065-1071.

18. Hogan, E.L. and Joseph, K.C., Composition of cerebral lipids in murine leucodystrophy: the Quaking mutant, J. Neurochem. 17 (1970) 1209-1214.

19. Lajtha, A., Toth, J., Fujimoto, K. and Agrawal, H.C., Turnover of myelin proteins in mouse brain in vivo, Biochem. J. 164 (1977) 323-329.

20. Lowry, O.H., Rosebrough, N.J., Farr, A.L. and Randall, R.J., Protein measurement with the Folin phenol reagent, J. biol. Chem. 193 (1951) 265-275.

21. McNamara, J.O. and Appel, S.H., Myelin basic protein phosphatase in rat brain, J. Neurochem. 29 (1977) 27-35.

22. Martenson, R.E., Kramer, A.J. and Deibler, G.E., Micro-heterogeneity and phosphoaminoacids in the carboxy-terminal half of myelin basic protein, J. Neurochem. 26 (1976) 733-736.
23. Matthieu, J.-M., Brady, R.O. and Quarles, R.H., Anomalies of myelin associated glycoproteins in Quaking mice, J. Neurochem. 22 (1974) 291-296.
24. Matthieu, J.-M., Quarles, R.H., Poduslo, J.F. and Brady, R.O., ^{35}S sulfate incorporation into myelin glycoproteins. I. Central nervous system, Biochim. Biophys. Acta 392 (1975) 159-166.
25. Matthieu, J.-M., Koellreutter, B. and Joyet, M.-L., Changes in CNS myelin proteins and glycoproteins after in situ autolysis, Brain Res. Bull. 2 (1977) 15-21.
26. Matthieu, J.-M., Koellreutter, B., Joyet, M.-L. and Gautier, E., Protein and glycoprotein composition of Quaking myelin subfractions, Trans. Am. Soc. Neurochem. 8 (1977) 202.
27. Miyamoto, E. and Kakiuchi, S., In vitro and in vivo phospho-rylation of myelin basic protein by exogenous and endogenous adenosine 3':5'-monophosphate-dependent protein kinases in brain, J. biol. Chem. 249 (1974) 2769-2777.
28. Miyamoto, E., Phosphorylation of endogenous proteins in myelin of rat brain, J. Neurochem. 26 (1976) 573-577.
29. Norton, W.T. and Poduslo, S.E., Myelination in rat brain: method of myelin isolation, J. Neurochem. 21 (1973) 749-758.
30. Nussbaum, J.L. and Mandel, P., Brain proteolipids in neurolog-ical mutant mice, Brain Res. 61 (1973) 295-310.
31. Sabri, M.I., Bone, A.H. and Davison, A.N., Turnover of myelin and other structural proteins in the developing rat brain, Biochem. J. 142 (1974) 499-507.
32. Samorajski, T., Friede, R.L. and Reimer, P.R., Hypomyelination in the Quaking mouse, J. Neuropath. exp. Neurol., 29 (1970) 507-523.
33. Shapira, R., McKneally, S., Re, P.K. and Kibler, R.F., Turn-over of myelin basic protein in the mature rabbit, Trans. Am. Soc. Neurochem. 3 (1972) 120.
34. Sidman, R.L., Dickie, M.M. and Appel, S.H., Mutant mice (Quaking and Jimpy) with deficient myelination in the central nervous system, Science 144 (1964) 309-311.
35. Singh, H., Spritz, N. and Geyer, B., Studies of brain myelin in the "Quaking mouse", J. Lipid Res. 12 (1971) 473-480.
36. Smith, M.E., The turnover of myelin proteins, Neurobiology 2 (1972) 35-40.
37. Smith, L.S., Kern, C.W., Halpern, R.M. and Smith, R.A., Phosphorylation on basic amino acids in myelin basic protein, Biochem. Biophys. Res. Commun. 71 (1976) 459-465.
38. Steck, A.J. and Appel, S.H., Phosphorylation of myelin basic protein, J. biol. Chem. 249 (1974) 5416-5420.
39. Suzuki, K. and Zagoren, J.C., Quaking mouse: an ultrastructural study of the peripheral nerves, J. Neurocytol. 6 (1977) 71-84.

40. Watanabe, I. and Bingle, G., Dysmyelination in "Quaking" mouse.
     Electron microscopic study, J. Neuropath. exp. Neurol. 31
     (1972) 352-369.
41. Wisniewski, H. and Morell, P., Quaking mouse: ultrastructural
     evidence for arrest of myelinogenesis, Brain Res. 29 (1971)
     63-73.

ABNORMAL MYELIN MATURATION IN VITRO: THE ROLE OF CEREBROSIDES

Keith Bradbury

Department of Pathology, University of Leeds

Leeds LS2 9NL, England

SUMMARY

Myelinating neonatal rat cerebellar explants were maintained for up to 130 days in vitro. Myelin fractions were extracted from explants of different ages and purified by density gradient centrifugation. The three fractions obtained were termed "light myelin", "heavy myelin" and "membrane fraction" and were deficient in glycolipids compared to myelin fractions prepared from 15-day-old rat cerebellum. The culture myelin has an apparently normal ultrastructure but may not be as stable as myelin with a normal glycolipid composition.

INTRODUCTION

Organotypical myelinating explants have been studied for over 25 years since the first report of myelination in vitro (14) and their ultrastructure, physiology, and their pathology related to demyelinating disease, have been the subject of many studies. Two reviews (12, 13) have summarised much of the early work and culturing methods. In contrast the metabolism and biochemistry of the organ cultures have received little attention. Patterns of enzyme activity during explant development were the subject of two reports (3, 10) and some of the changes in substrate utilisation observed could be related to myelination.

The myelinating explant, lacking a functional vasculature, and deprived of the humoral and metabolic influences of the intact animal, offers unique opportunities for studying myelination. The present investigation was directed to the study of the biochemistry of myelin development in vitro.

171

EXPERIMENTAL

Cerebella of neonatal rats were cut into 8 parasagittal slices and placed on collagen-coated coverslips maintained at 36.5°C in roller tubes containing 1.25 ml of nutrient feed. The feed comprised 25% each of bovine serum ultrafiltrate, human ascitic fluid and chick embryo extract, 20% Simm´s balanced salt solution and 5% medium 199. Glucose was added to give a final concentration of 600 mg %. Explants were routinely transferred to Maximov chambers for light-microscope examination.

To prepare myelin fractions, homogenates of 200 or more explants in 0.32 M sucrose were overlaid on 1.0 ml of 0.70 M sucrose and centrifuged at 15,000 g for 30 min. A crude myelin layer was recovered and incubated in deionised water for 100 min at 4°C, followed by centrifugation at 45,000 g for 10 min and twice at 100,000 g for 10 min. The recovered pellet, termed partially purified myelin, was layered on a discontinuous gradient of 0.32 to 0.80 M sucrose and centrifuged for 1 h at 75,000 g. The three layers recovered were centrifuged twice in deionised water at 100,000 g for 15 min. Myelin fractions were similarly prepared from the cerebella of surviving littermates.

Lipids were extracted by the method of Folch et al. (7). Cholesterol was determined by the method of Rappaport and Eichhorn (16), glycolipids by GLC (4) and phospholipids by neutron activation. Myelin protein was determined by the method of Lowry (11). The activity of 2',3'-cyclic nucleosidemonophosphate phosphodiesterase (CNP) (EC 3.1.4.16) (9) and L-leucyl-2-naphtylamidase was examined in each layer.

RESULTS

Myelination of cerebellar explants commences at 7 DIV (days in vitro), on approximately the same postnatal day as cerebellar myelination commences in vitro. The refractility of the living myelin increases rapidly and the fibres are free of blebs or herniations (Fig. 1). By 28 DIV large myelin tracts are visible (Fig. 2), creating some foliar architecture typical of the developing cerebellum. The increase in the quantity and refractility of the living myelin observed under the light microscope can be related to the increasing yield of myelin on the centrifugation of homogenates from older explants.

The three layers recovered after centrifuging crude myelin on a discontinuous gradient were termed "light myelin", "heavy myelin" and "membrane fraction". At 7 DIV when the number of myelin sheaths is few, only a membrane fraction was recovered, which may indicate that this fraction is a precursor of the compact myelin. Under the electron microscope the heavy myelin, characterised by large aggregates of up to 20 lamellae, had the appearance of normal compact myelin. The light myelin was similar except that large aggregates were absent, and the membrane fraction comprised thin-walled vesicles usually bounded by a single electron-dense line. The layers prepared from the cerebella of littermates presented a comparable ultrastructural appearance to that of the culture myelin layers.

Cholesterol and total phospholipid values of the culture light and heavy myelin were similar (Table 1) and did not alter significantly between 14 and 60 DIV. In contrast, the membrane fraction contained relatively small amounts of cholesterol and phospholipid, and proportionately more protein than the light and heavy myelin. A membrane fraction prepared from 15 day old rat brain by Agrawal et al. (2) was similarly deficient in lipids.

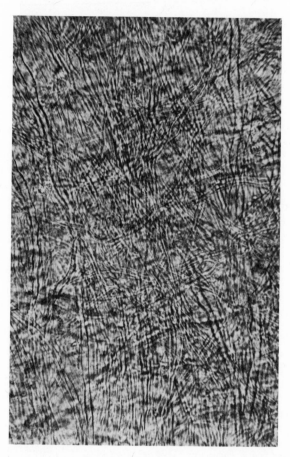

Fig. 1. Living rat cerebellar explant. 14 days in vitro. Myelinated axons cover the entire field in this central zone of the explant. Larger calibre axons probably originate in the dentate nucleus. The remaining axons are derived from Purkinje neurones. x 1000.

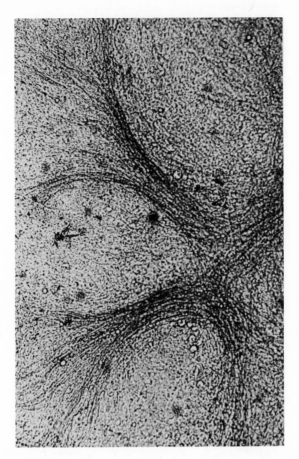

Fig. 2. Living rat cerebellar explant. 28 days in vitro. Visible
myelination is complete. Large tracts of myelinated axons emerge
from the centre of the explant (bottom). x 40.

        The major biochemical abnormality of the culture myelin lies
in the low levels of glycolipids in all fractions. Between 14 and
60 DIV the proportion of cerebroside and sulphatide in the light
and heavy culture myelin had effectively doubled but remained low.
The full extent of the glycolipid deficiency can be assessed by
comparing lipid molar ratios (Table 2). In the light and heavy
myelin of 15-day rat cerebellum the cholesterol:phospholipid:
galactolipid ratio is approximately 1:1:0.60 whereas the corresponding 14 DIV fractions have ratios closer to 1:1.50:0.05. It appears
that some of the glycolipid deficiency of young culture myelin is
balanced by an increase in phospholipid. By 60 DIV the proportion
of phospholipid in the light and heavy myelin fractions declines
as the glycolipids begin to increase, a trend which becomes more
evident in the 130 DIV preparations.

Table 1. Lipid composition of culture myelin. The results are expressed as μmol lipid/mg protein and the number of preparations of 200 or more myelinating cerebellar explants examined at each age is given in parentheses. - a = Light myelin; b = Heavy myelin; c = Membrane fraction.

Lipid	Days in vitro					
	14(3)			60(4)		
	a	b	c	a	b	c
Cholesterol	2.8±0.21	2.8±0.15	0.31±0.02	3.1±0.12	2.6±0.09	0.29±0.04
Total phospholipid	3.9±0.25	4.2±0.31	0.48±0.07	4.1±0.37	4.0±0.22	0.56±0.02
Cerebrosides and sulphatides	0.10±0.01	0.13±0.01	0.02±0.001	0.23±0.03	0.23±0.02	0.02±0.002

Table 2. Cholesterol:phospholipid:galactolipid ratios of culture myelin fractions. The number of preparations of 200 or more myelinating cerebellar explants examined at each age is given in parentheses.

Fraction	Days in vitro					15-day-rat cerebellum+
	7(3)	14(3)	21(3)	60(4)	130(2)	
Light myelin	-	1:1.37:0.04	1:1.46:0.04	1:1.33:0.07	1:1.11:0.29	1:1.10:0.59
Heavy myelin	-	1:1.49:0.05	1:1.62:0.05	1:1.54:0.09	1:1.40:0.31	1:1.23:0.55
Membrane fraction	1:1.14:0.03	1:1.55:0.05	1:1.70:0.05	1:1.89:0.07	1:1.56:0.04	1:1.36:0.08

+ Cerebellar myelin fractions derived from the surviving littermates of the animals used for explantation.

L-leucyl-2-naphtylamidase activity was highest in the light
myelin and membrane fraction of the culture myelin, and CNP levels
in the light myelin, heavy myelin and membrane fraction were
comparable to those reported for myelin in vivo (2).

DISCUSSION

The chemical composition of CNS myelin is known to change
during early development and these changes have been termed "myelin
maturation" (6).   Maturation is characterised by a relative increase
in glycolipids, particularly cerebrosides, in the brain of the
young rodent (8) and in man (5).   The exceedingly low glycolipid
levels of all the culture myelin fractions up to 60 DIV implies
that the cerebellar explants undergo early myelination without a
normal maturation process.   The only fractions previously prepared
from crude myelin which had a similar deficiency of glycolipids
were the myelin-like (1) and membrane fractions (2) from 15-day -
old rat brain where little or no cerebroside could be detected.
On the basis of isotope labelling experiments Agrawal et al. (2)
considered that the myelin-like and membrane fractions could be
precursors of myelin.   The light and heavy myelin fractions of
cerebellar explants have a high lipid/protein ratio - revealed
both by their buoyant densities and by chemical analysis - and
are similar in this respect to the light and heavy myelin prepared
from a range of mammals.   However, the light and heavy myelin
fractions of explants up to 60 DIV exhibit a lipid composition
similar to that of the corresponding membrane fraction and to
myelin-like and membrane fractions of rat whole-brain.   Between 60
and 130 DIV a relatively rapid increase of cerebrosides in the light
and heavy myelin fractions of the explants demonstrates that a significant accretion of glycolipid can take place in culture and may
indicate that in even older explants the myelin would assume a composition more like that in vivo.
A change in myelin composition could result from the deposition
of new membrane rich in glycolipids or the intersusception of
glycolipid molecules into the existing lamellae.   By 60 DIV myelin
lamellation in vitro is over and the glycolipids which accrue in
the culture myelin between 60 and 130 DIV are probably incorporated
into the existing lamellae.   The late incorporation of glycolipids
into the culture myelin is a particularly striking demonstration
that myelination is at least a two-stage process.   In the 15-day-
rat cerebellum (Table 2) the accretion of cerebroside in myelin is
already considerable, implying that any early cerebroside-deficient
myelin membrane formation in vivo is occurring pari passu with the
deposition of cerebroside.   In culture the two stages are out of
phase so that a glycolipid-deficient myelin can be laid down before
significant glycolipid deposition begins.   In spite of the glycolipid
deficiency the culture myelin has an apparently normal ultrastructure.   However, the stability of young culture myelin under

challenge may be impaired. Raine et al. (15) tested sera from
multiple sclerosis patients on myelinated mouse spinal cord explants
and noted that the characteristic demyelination which ensued was of
greater severity in the 21 DIV explants as compared with those of
42 DIV. If glycolipid incorporation into myelin was delayed in the
spinal cord explants, then the results obtained with demyelinating
sera might reflect the greater stability of the 42 DIV myelin with
a higher glycolipid content.

The cause of the delay in myelin maturation in vitro remains
elusive. The myelinating explant follows much of the normal
ontogenic development of the tissue. Cellular differentiation,
axon growth, synapse formation, bioelectric activity and myelination
in vitro are ample confirmation of this development (12). However, there are important differences between the cerebellar
explant and the cerebellum in vivo. One difference is the large
number of intermediate or undifferentiated glia which persist in
explants (12), and these cells together with the delayed myelin
maturation in vitro may both be symptoms of a failure of the ex-
planted cerebellum to sustain all aspects of development.

Acknowledgements. This work was supported by the North Humber-
side Branch of the Multiple Sclerosis Society of Great Britain and
Northern Ireland and by the Wolfson Foundation. The assistance
of Mrs Mary Firth and Mrs Patricia Hartley is gratefully acknowledged.

REFERENCES

1. Agrawal, H.C., Banik, N.L., Bone, A.H., Davison, A.N.,
    Mitchell, R.F. and Spohn, M., The identity of a myelin-like
    fraction isolated from developing brain, Biochem. J. 120
    (1970) 635-642.
2. Agrawal, H.C., Trotter, J.L, Burton, R.M. and Mitchell, R.F.,
    Metabolic studies on myelin. Evidence for a precursor role
    of a myelin subfraction, Biochem. J. 140 (1974) 99-109.
3. Aparicio, S.R., Bradbury, K., Bradbury, Margaret and Howard,
    L., Organ cultures of nervous tissues, in Organ culture in
    biomedical research. British Society for Cell Biology
    Symposium I (M. Balls and M.A. Monnickendam, eds.) Cambridge
    University Press, Cambridge (1976) pp. 309-354.
4. Carter, H.E. and Gaver, R.C., Improved reagent for trimethyl-
    silylation of sphingolipid bases, J. Lipid Res. 8 (1967)
    391-395.
5. Eng, L.F., Chao, F.-C., Gerstl, B. Pratt, D. and Tavaststjerna,
    M.G., The maturation of human white matter myelin. Fractiona-
    tion of the myelin membrane proteins, Biochemistry (Wash.) 7
    (1968) 4455-4465.
6. Eng, L.F. and Noble, E.P., The maturation of rat brain myelin,
    Lipids 3 (1968) 157-162.

7. Folch, J., Lees, M. and Sloane-Stanley, G.H., A simple method
    for the isolation and purification of total lipides from animal
    tissues, J. Biol. Chem. 226 (1957) 497-509.
8. Horrocks, L.A., Composition of mouse brain myelin during de-
    velopment, J. Neurochem. 15 (1968) 483-488.
9. Kurihara, T. and Tsukada, Y., The regional and subcellular
    distribution of 2',3'-cyclic nucleoside 3'-phosphohydrolase
    in the central nervous system, J. Neurochem. 14 (1967)1167-1174.
10. Lehrer, G.M., The tissue culture as a model for the biochemistry
    of brain development, in Progress in Brain Research, Vol. 40:
    Neurobiological aspects of maturation and aging (D.H. Ford,
    ed.) Elsevier, Amsterdam (1973) pp. 219-230.
11. Lowry, O.H., Rosebrough, N.J., Farr, A.L. and Randall, R.J.,
    Protein measurement with Folin phenol reagent, J. Biol. Chem.
    193 (1951) 265-275.
12. Lumsden, C.E., Nervous tissue in culture, in The structure
    and function of nervous tissue, Vol. I: Structure I. (G.H.
    Bourne, ed.) Academic Press, New York (1968) pp. 67-140.
13. Murray, Margaret R., Nervous tissue in vitro, in Cells and
    tissues in culture. Methods, Biology and Physiology, vol. 2
    (E.N. Willmer,ed.) Academic Press, London (1965) pp. 373-455.
14. Peterson, E.R., Production of myelin sheaths in vitro by
    embryonic spinal ganglion cells, Anat. Rec. 106 (1950) 232.
15. Raine, C.S., Hummelgard, A., Swanson, E. and Bornstein, M.B.,
    Multiple sclerosis: serum-induced demyelination in vitro. A
    light and electron microscopic study, J. Neurol. Sci. 20
    (1974) 127-148.
16. Rappaport, D.F. and Eichhorn, F., Valoracion clinica y mejoras
    al methodo Sidney Pearson y colaboradores para determinacion
    de cholesterol total, Revta med. Cordoba 43 (1955) 86-89.

RETARDATION OF BRAIN MYELINATION BY MALNOURISHMENT AND FEEDING

LOW PROTEIN IRRADIATED DIET IN RATS

Mohammad Habibulla and Hema Krishnan

Neurobiology Laboratory, School of Life Sciences,
  Jawaharlal Nehru University
New Delhi-110057, India

SUMMARY

The effect of feeding low protein diet, and the low protein irradiated diet on the deposition of myelin in the brains of rats over two generations showed that malnourishment lowered the CNP enzyme activity when compared to the normal (high protein) diet fed control rats during early postnatal period. Irradiated low protein diet, when fed within 21 days of irradiation (15 Krads Gamma radiation, 60_{Co} rays), produced still lower CNP enzyme activity. This also enhanced other effects of retarding the brain development, by lowering the protein and lipid contents of the brain during a period from the 4th to 25th day of postnatal development. This suggests the possibility that feeding irradiated low protein food to malnourished developing mammals could cause serious problems like mental retardation.

INTRODUCTION

Malnourishment affects the vulnerable period of growth of an organism. This is particularly so with the brain where the embryological process of development is rapid and extensive during gestation (15, 17) and early postnatal life (20, 23). An unbalanced diet not only has influence on the total proteins and glial cell specific proteins, but may also induce changes in the lipid content of the brain (3-5, 10). Myelination is very fast in rat during the later half of the suckling period (6, 10), and once nutritious food is deprived at this stage, the damage caused is irreparable. Much of the increase in the wet weight of the brain

is due to the increase in myelination (1, 2). Besides malnutrition being widely prevalent, in many developing countries irradiation is being resorted to as one of the means to prevent the in-
festation of stored grains by pests. For complete irradiation of
these pests, the recommended irradiation dose falls in the range
of 10 to 25 Krads (14). In many developing countries where most of
the pregnant women and growing children are deprived of nutritious
diet, irradiation of food may further cause deleterious effects on
the development of brain.

Hence, an attempt was made to follow the postnatal development
of brain by studying the changes occurring in the myelin marker
enzyme, 2', 3'-cyclic nucleotide-3'-phosphohydrolase (CNP enzyme)
in the Holtzman strain of rats after feeding irradiated protein
deficient diet. Changes in the protein and lipid content were also
followed.

EXPERIMENTAL

The Holtzman strain rats were bred in an animal house where the
temperature was maintained at $24\pm1^{\circ}C$. They were maintained on
different kinds of diets, A, B and C, for two generations. After
that the litters born from each group were decapitated starting 4
days after birth to 25th postnatal day at intervals of 4 days.
Each time 4 pups were sacrificed.

Diets. Diet A consisted of crude protein 24%, ether extract 4%,
crude fiber 4%, ash(max.) 8%, calcium 1%, phosphorus 0.6%, and
nitrogen extract 50% (metabolizable energy 3200 cal/kg).

Diet B consisted of 1 part of Diet A + 3 parts of powdered rice
(containing 6% protein) by weight.

Diet C consisted of Diet B irradiated with 15 Krads Gamma radiation (60_{Co} rays) at the rate of 90 rad/sec. This irradiated diet
was fed within 3 weeks of irradiation.

Homogenate preparation. Immediately after decapitation, the
entire brains were homogenized in cold 0.1 M Tris-HCl buffer (pH
7.4) in a motor driven homogenizer with a teflon pestle. A total
of 2 ml buffer was used for homogenizing each brain. The homogenate
was then stored at $-20^{\circ}C$ until required.

Protein estimation. The total soluble protein in 0.1 M Tris-HCl
buffer (pH 7.4) was estimated from an aliquot (0.5 ml) of the brain
homogenate (16) in each case.

Lipid estimation. The total lipids were extracted and estimated according to conventional methods (12). The chloroform
fraction from the Silica gel column contained the neutral lipids.
The neutral lipid was estimated gravimetrically after evaporating
chloroform with nitrogen in preweighed glass tubes.

CNP enzyme estimation. The method of Olafson et al.(19) and
Drummond et al.(8) method was preferred for CNP enzyme estimation,
after dialysing the sample in 0.1 M Tris-HCl buffer (pH 7.5) at 4°C

to free endogenous phosphate. The incubation mixture consisted of
0.1 ml homogenate added to a tube containing 50 μmoles of Tris
buffer (pH 7.5).   0.16 μmoles of deoxycholate solution was added
to liberate the membrane bound enzyme. To this was added 1 μmole
of 2',3'-cyclic AMP solution containing 6.25 mg/ml egg albumin
in Tris buffer (pH 7.5). The mixture was incubated at 30°C for
20 min in a shaking water bath. The reaction was terminated by
the addition of 1 ml 3% TCA. A known volume of this mixture was
used for the estimation of phosphorus (11). Two controls, one
with no enzyme and the other with no substrate were maintained.
The number of micromoles of phosphorus liberated was a measure of
CNP enzyme activity.

RESULTS

   Proteins. The effect of different diets on the soluble proteins
of the rat brain during early postnatal development is given in
Table 1. When compared with protein rich diet A, the protein deficient diet B appears to be instrumental in reducing the protein
content of the developing rat brain. The same diet B, when irradiated (diet C) and fed, still lowers the protein content of the
brain tissue. The effect that is brought about by malnourishment
appears to be further accentuated by irradiating diet B.

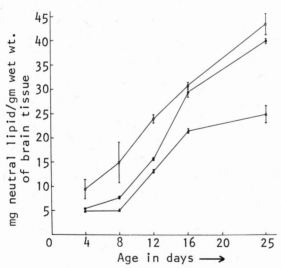

Fig. 1. Graph depicting the effect of feeding protein deficient
and irradiated protein deficient diet on the neutral lipid content
of the rat brain during development.
o———o protein rich diet, ●———● protein deficient diet,
△———△ irradiated protein deficient diet.

Table 1. Effect of different diets on the total soluble protein content (mg of total soluble protein/g wet weight of brain tissue) of the rat brain during postnatal development.

Age in days	Diet A (protein-rich)	Diet B (protein-deficient)	Diet C (irradiated protein-deficient)
4	72.8±0.8	47.0±0.7	46.1±0.6
8	101.9±1.0	91.9±1.2	78.1±1.7
12	137.5±1.3	120.2±1.3	110.6±4.6
16	153.6±2.2	141.0±0.6	136.2±0.5
20	163.9±2.2	155.7±0.5	135.6±1.5
25	175.6±1.7	164.5±2.0	143.4±1.3

Each value represents the mean of four readings ± SE.

Table 2. Effect of different diets on the total lipid content (mg of lipid/g wet weight of brain tissue) of the rat brain during postnatal development.

Age in days	Diet A (protein-rich)	Diet B (protein-deficient)	Diet C (irradiated protein-deficient)
4	52.5±1.8	30.0±1.0	21.2±1.2
8	91.2±4.3	72.5±4.0	65.0±1.6
12	100.0±0.8	91.2±1.8	85.0±4.4
16	185.0±9.8	158.7±4.2	158.7±1.6
20	220.0±9.1	220.0±3.6	172.5±4.1
25	295.0±2.2	272.0±4.1	202.5±5.3

Each value represents the mean of four readings ± SE.

Lipids. The effect of various diets on the lipid content of the rat brain during early postnatal development is shown in Table 2. Diet B brings about the depletion of lipid content in the brain when compared to the protein rich diet A. This effect is further amplified when the irradiated low protein diet C is fed to the rats. A similar picture appears when neutral lipids were estimated (Fig. 1).

CNP enzyme. Retardation of myelination is evident during the development of brain in the rats that were fed diet B and diet C. The myelin marker enzyme CNP is found to be effected by malnourishment. Irradiation of the malnourished diet C further accentuates this undesirable effect (Fig. 2).

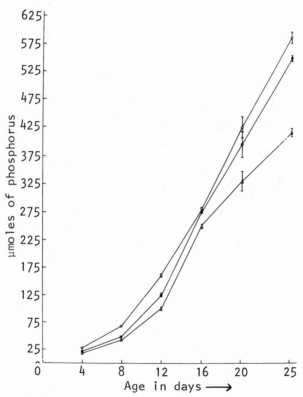

Fig. 2. Graph showing the effect of feeding protein deficient and irradiated protein deficient diet on the total activity of CNP (myelin marker) enzyme in the rat brain during development.
o————o protein rich diet,   •————• protein deficient diet,
Δ————Δ irradiated protein deficient diet.

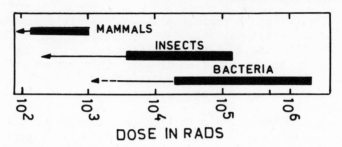

Fig. 3. Diagram to show the comparative sensitivity of different groups of organisms to single acute dose of Gamma radiation. Note that the bacteria and the insects are more resistant   than mammals.

DISCUSSION

The retardation in the early postnatal development of the brain of rat is evident from the profile of proteins, lipids and the marker enzyme studies. Development of the brain appears to be susceptible to even slight deficiency in the major items constituting a balanced diet (21). In the context of protein deficiency being a formidable problem facing many developing countries, nutritional status of the mother clearly effects the foetus (21, 24). Hence a pregnant woman deprived of proper nutrition would produce an offspring with improper development. Further, irradiation of such food can accentuate the effects of malnourishment.

Although the recommended irradiation dose is up to 25 Krads because of the high resistance of insects (14), as shown in Fig. 3, even 15 Krads markedly effect the myelin formation and the brain development, if fed within 3 weeks after irradiation.

CNP enzyme has been found to be a specific marker for myelin formation (13). The specific activity of the enzyme in the developing brain diminishes as a result of feeding protein deficient diet (18). The present study also showed that irradiation of low protein diet enhances the retarding effects.

It is possible that irradiation further lowers the protein content (7) of an already protein deficient diet. It is also possible that the vitamins are destroyed. Irradiation produces free radicals. These might initiate secondary reactions (7) which can cause the observed differences. It is known that the life of some of these radicals, or the chain reactions triggered by them, could last for more than 3 weeks. It is also to be noted that in the non-metabolizing systems like the stored grain, scavenging of the free radicles by enzymes like peroxidases is minimal.

Although the precise mechanism of action is not known, irradiated protein deficient diet further enhances the undesirable effects produced by the protein deficiency on the development of brain. It is of concern to note that feeding irradiated wheat also brings about chromosomal aberrations in the bone marrow cells of malnourished rats (22).

REFERENCES

1. Davison, A.N. and Dobbing, J., Myelination as a vulnerable period in brain development, Brit. Med. Bull. 22 (1966) 40-44.
2. Davison, A.N. and Dobbing, J., The developing brain, in Applied Neurochemistry (A.N. Davison and J. Dobbing, eds.), Blackwell, Oxford (1968) pp. 253-286.
3. Dickerson, J.W.T. and Dobbing, J., Proc. Roy. Soc. Med.166 (1967) 384.
4. Dickerson, J.W.T., Dobbing, J. and McCance, R.A., The effect of undernutrition on the development of brain and cord in pigs, Proc. Roy. Soc. Med. 166 (1967) 396-407.
5. Dobbing, J. and Widdowson, E.M., The effect of undernutrition and subsequent rehabilitation on myelination of rat brain as measured by its composition, Brain 88 (1965) 357-366.
6. Dobbing, J., The influence of early nutrition on the development and myelination of brain, Proc. Roy. Soc. B. 159 (1964) 503-509.
7. Dole, M., The radiation chemistry of macromolecules (1973).
8. Drummond, G.I., Eng, D.Y. and McIntosh, C.A., Ribonucleoside 2',3'-cyclic phosphate diesterase activity and cerebroside levels in vertebrate and invertebrate nerve, Brain Res. 28 (1971) 153-163.
9. Eng, L.F. and Noble, E.P., The maturation of rat brain myelin, Lipids 3 (1968) 157-162.
10. Fishman, M.A., Prensky, A.E. and Dodge, P.R., Low content of certebral lipids in infants suffering from malnutrition, Nature 221 (1969) 552-553.
11. Fiske, C.H. and Subbarow, Y., in Experimental Biochemistry (J.M. Clark, Jr., ed.) Freeman and Co., San Francisco (1962).
12. Folch, J., Lees, M. and Sloane-Stanley, G.H., A simple method for the isolation and purification of total lipid from animal tissue, J. Biol. Chem. 226 (1957) 497.
13. Himwich, W., Biochemistry of the Developing Brain, Vol. I Marcel Dekker Inc., New York (1973).
14. Hoedaya, M.S., Hutabarat, D., Sastradihadja, S.I. and Soetrisno, S., Radiation effects on four species of insects in stored rice and the use of radiation disinfestation in their control, in Radiation preservation of food, Proceedings of a symposium B-17, jointly organized by the IAEA and FAO (1972).
15. Jacobson, M., Effects of nutrition, hormones and metabolic factors on the development of the nervous system, in Developmental Neurobiology (1971).

16. Lowry, O.H., Rosebrough, M.J., Farr, A.L. and Randall, R.J.,
     Protein measurement with the Folin phenol reagent, J. Biol.
     Chem. 193 (1951) 265-275.
17. Mitchell, R.G., Nutritional influences in early life, Proc.
     Roy. Soc. Med. 59 (1966) 1013-1076.
18. Nakhasi, H.L., Toews, A.D. and Horrocks, L.A., Effects of
     postnatal protein-deficiency on the content and composition
     of myelin from brains of weanling rats, Brain Res. 83 (1975)
     176-179.
19. Olafson, R.W., Drummond, G.I. and Lee, J.F., Studies on 2',3'-
     cyclic-nucleotide-3'-phosphohydrolase from brain, Canad. J.
     Biochem. 47 (1969) 1961-1966.
20. Platt, B.S., Proteins in nutrition, Proc. Roy. Soc. London
     156 (1962) 337.
21. Sterman, M.B., McGinty, D.J. and Adinolfi, A.M., Nutrition
     deprivation and neural development, in Brain Development and
     Behaviour, Academic Press, New York and London (1971) pp. 354-
     381.
22. Vijaylaxmi and Sadasivan, G., Chromosomal aberrations in rats
     fed on irradiated wheat, Int. J. Radiat. Biol. 27 (1975) 135-
     142.
23. Winick, M., Malnutrition and brain development, J. Pediat. 74
     (1969) 667-679.
24. Zamenhof, S. and Marthens, E.V., Study of factors influencing
     prenatal brain development, Molec. Cell. Biochem. 4 (1974)
     157-168.

MYELINATION

Molecular Organization

THE MOLECULAR ARCHITECTURE OF MYELIN: IDENTIFICATION OF THE

EXTERNAL SURFACE MEMBRANE COMPONENTS

Joseph F. Poduslo

Neuroimmunology Branch, National Institute of Neurological
   and Communicative Disorders and Stroke,
   National Institutes of Health
Bethesda, Maryland 20014, U.S.A.

SUMMARY

Basic information concerning the molecular organization of the myelin membrane is an intrinsic requirement for understanding the neurochemical events leading to myelination, as well as the potential mechanism of demyelination that might exist at the molecular level for a variety of neurological diseases. The application of chemical, enzymatic, fluorescent, and immunological membrane probes has contributed significantly to this end, although the diverse structural complexity of the myelin sheath has permitted only a rudimentary understanding of its molecular organization. Nevertheless, compelling evidence is accumulating which suggests that components of myelin are asymmetrically distributed in the membrane. Such membrane asymmetry should not only provide important clues to the mechanisms of membrane assembly in the process of myelination, but should also serve as a paradigm for potential functional asymmetry of the individual components at the molecular level. One particularly useful membrane probe is galactose oxidase which has the capacity for identifying surface galactose residues in both glycoproteins and glycolipids on the external surface of the myelin sheath. The identification of these surface components on the myelin sheath is of primary importance since such components might be more readily susceptible to immunological damage or act as a viral receptor which ultimately might lead to demyelination.

INTRODUCTION

Evidence is rapidly accumulating which indicates that myelin
may not be the atypical membrane that it was once thought to be.
Myelin resembles other cellular membranes in many respects and,
in fact, may be structurally organized in a manner similar to the
fluid lipid - globular protein mosaic model described for other
biological membranes (21, 24, 25).

Such structural similarities for the myelin bilayer are pre-
dicated on a variety of more recent observations. In particular,
the investigations of Feinstein and Felsenfeld (6, 7) revealed
that the binding properties of the fluorescent probes 8-anilino-
1-naphthalenesulfonate (ANS) and 2-p-toluidinylnaphthalene-6-
sulfonate (TNS) to purified myelin were very similar to that of
other cellular membranes. The binding of these probes to isolated
myelin was compared with the binding to isolated basic protein and
to proteolipid protein, as well as with the binding of these proteins
incorporated into lipid vesicles. Significant differences were
revealed which were attributed as being characteristic of myelin
membrane proteins having a more integral (intrinsic) or peripheral
(extrinsic) location in the membrane as defined by the fluid mosaic
model (21). In addition, Williams and Cordes (26) could not exclude the possibility of translational fluidity of the lipid matrix
of isolated bovine myelin using natural abundance carbon-13 nuclear
magnetic resonance measurements. Moreover, the observations of
Curatolo et al.(4) indicate that the fluidity of the myelin membrane may be strongly influenced by intrinsic membrane proteins as
well as by both the phospholipid acyl chains and the presence of
cholesterol. Such a conclusion was based on x-ray diffraction
studies and differential scanning calorimetry of recombinants of
the myelin proteolipid apoprotein with dimyristoyllecithin. Similar
conclusions can be obtained from the investigations of Boggs et al.
(3) who studied recombinants of myelin proteolipid protein with
phosphatidylserine and dipalmitoylphosphatidylcholine. These observations, coupled with the high-resolution proton magnetic resonance spectra on sciatic nerve (5) allow the conclusion that myelin
indeed resembles other cellular membranes in that there are discrete
fluid hydrophobic regions.

An important aspect of the fluid mosaic model is the gross
organization of the proteins and lipids in the membrane. This
information is discernible only when the different membrane components are identified in the membrane. Such an identification
requires information concerning the distribution of these components in the membrane. Possible distributions for the different
components of myelin include:
A. Distribution across the bilayer.
B. Distribution along the membrane surface.
C. Distribution at each layer of a multilamellar structure.
D. Distribution at specialized membrane regions.

The topographical distribution of the different components across the bilayer could be asymmetrical in which each copy will have the same orientation in an all or none fashion. Examples of this asymmetrical distribution involve both proteins and carbohydrates with the carbohydrates complexed either as external glycoproteins or glycolipids. In addition, the distribution across the bilayer could be one of partial asymmetry in which certain components may be present on both sides of the membrane in different amounts. This distribution is not an all or none phenomenon and can be highly variable among different types of membranes. Examples of this partial asymmetry involve phospholipids where in the erythrocyte membrane, phosphatidylcholine and sphingomyelin are preferentially localized at the outer surface whereas most of the phosphatidyl-ethanolamine and all of the phosphatidy-serine are localized at the inner surface. Finally certain components could have a symmetrical distribution where they exist on both membrane surfaces in nearly equal amounts. Cholesterol appears to be an example of this symmetrical distribution (13, 14), although Fisher (8) has reported more cholesterol on the external surface of the erythrocyte membrane. Gottlieb (10) has also reported differences in the re-activity of cholesterol to cholesterol oxidase in the erythrocyte membrane with only the inner surface cholesterol being oxidized. It is apparent, therefore, that the application of a variety of chemical, enzymatic, fluorescent, and immunological membrane probes has contributed significantly to the understanding of the topo-graphical distribution of membrane components across the bilayer.

The distribution along a membrane surface could be uniform or more typically non-uniform for the different components. Exclusion or sequestration on the membrane surface could occur as a result of a wide variety of different associations, including protein-protein, protein-lipid, protein-carbohydrate, lipid-lipid, lipid-carbohydrate, carbohydrate-carbohydrate, protein-solid phase lipid, protein-liquid phase lipid, etc. Such associations could readily influence membrane fluidity. Interactions with extrinsic membrane proteins through ionic interactions and hydrogen bonding could affect the distribution on both membrane surfaces. Moreover, inner surface components could interact with cytoskeletal microfilaments, thick filaments, or microtubules. Such near neighbor relationships become an important consideration in evaluating functional roles for these different components.

The complex lamellar structure of the myelin sheath necessi-tates further definition of the possible distributions for the different membrane components. The maintenance of the topographical distribution across the bilayer for the different membrane com-ponents at each layer of the multilayered structure must be con-sidered. Similarly questions concerning maintenance of the inter-actions among the different membrane components at each layer must also be answered. Specifically, is there a contiguity in the distribution of the different membrane components at the external membrane surface with the intraperiod line of myelin? In addition,

is there a contiguity of distribution between the inner membrane
surface and the major dense line of myelin? Although such questions
concerning the uniform distribution of components throughout the
myelin sheath are difficult to answer experimentally, they should
be considered in any model of the myelin structure.

Another important area of consideration unique to the myelin
sheath is the specialized external surface regions which include:

A. Oligodendroglial - myelin transition region.
B. Outer belt region.
C. Outer surface of internode region.
D. Paranodal region (lateral belts).

Several of the regions indicated might be highly specialized such
that the surface components at one area might be quite different
from those at other regions. Furthermore, restrictive labeling of
the surface components at any of the specialized regions could occur
because of a diffusion restriction of the membrane probes. Consequently, immunocytochemical techniques studied electron microscopi-
cally as well as the correlation of myelin subfractions with specialized regions would be ways of evaluating the precise localization of
the surface components.

In recent investigations, I have been focusing on the identification of the external surface components on the intact myelin sheath
(17, 19). The identification of surface components is of primary
importance because of the potential recognition roles they may play
in the process of myelination or myelin maintenance. In addition,
such components may be more readily susceptible to immunological
damage or even act as specific receptors for viruses and thereby
initiate the process of demyelination.

Since carbohydrate containing lipids and proteins are likely
candidates for an external surface localization, it was rationalized
that a membrane probe with a high degree of specificity for carbohydrate residues should facilitate the identification of myelin surface constituents. Consequently, the enzymatic membrane probe,
galactose oxidase, was chosen for the covalent labeling of surface
membrane glycoproteins and glycolipids. This procedure has been
particularly useful for identifying a variety of carbohydrate-
bearing macromolecules on the surface of cell membranes (9, 22, 23).
In this chapter, I will summarize the results of recent investigations concerning the identification of the external surface components of the intact myelin sheath.

EXPERIMENTAL

Adult rat spinal cord preparations were used in all experiments. This preparation allows the investigation of structurally
intact myelin and obviates the ambiguities inherent in investigating
the external surface components of isolated myelin where the inner
and outer membrane surfaces can no longer be distinguished. The
incubation of the spinal cord preparations with galactose oxidase
and the subsequent reduction with tritiated sodium borohydride

were performed in specially designed chambers according to procedures
described previously (19). The reaction, as indicated in Fig. 1,
involves the oxidation of D-galactose and related carbohydrates at
the C-6 position by galactose oxidase to form D-galactohexodialdose.
This resulting aldehyde group can then be labeled by reduction back
to the primary hydroxyl group with the tritiated borohydride.
Because of the specificity of the reaction and the impermeant nature
of the enzyme, only those sugar residues accessible to the enzyme
will be labeled. Because of the possible penetration of the
tritiated sodium borohydride, appropriate controls for non-specific
reduction were included in all experiments.

The experimental protocol is summarized in Fig. 2. The radioactively labeled spinal cord preparation is homogenized, and myelin
is isolated according to the procedure of Norton and Poduslo (15).
The isolated myelin is then analyzed for radioactive label associated
with either the glycoproteins by SDS-polyacrylamide gel electrophoresis or with the glycolipids by thin-layer chromatography.
Further details concerning the methodology have been described
previously (17, 19). For those experiments involving the galactose
oxidase labeling of surface membrane glycoproteins, rats, after being
lightly anesthetized with ether, were injected intracisternally with
0.18 μmoles (10 μCi per rat) of $[1-{}^{14}C]$-L-fucose (New England Nuclear)
in 10 μl 0.85% (w/v) NaCl. The animals were sacrificed 18-22 hours
later, and the spinal cords removed and used for the surface labeling
of glycoproteins with galactose oxidase. The coincidence of tritium
label with that of $[{}^{14}C]$fucose used as an internal marker for the
glycoproteins on gel electrophoresis was indicative of an external
surface location.

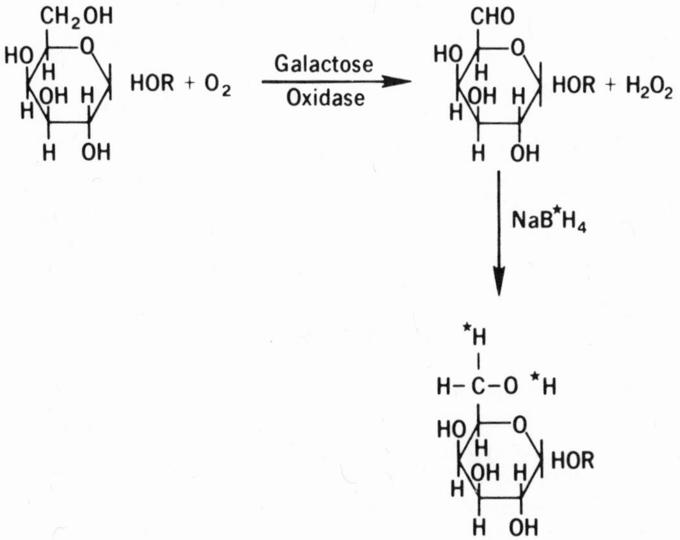

Fig. 1. The galactose oxidase reaction.

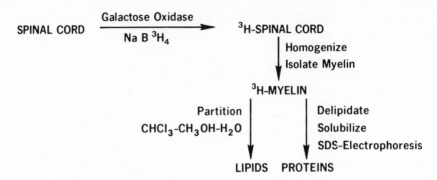

Fig. 2.   The experimental design.

RESULTS

    A typical densitometric scan at 555 nm of the Coomassie blue
stained myelin proteins on a 15% acrylamide separating gel with a
6% acrylamide spacer gel (sample numbers 1-3) from adult rat spinal
cord is illustrated in Fig. 3.   The major staining myelin protein
bands are identified, including the small and large basic protein,
the intermediate protein, proteolipid protein, and a major high
molecular weight protein, sometimes designated as the Wolfgram
protein.   A large number of high molecular weight proteins which
are not well separated in this electrophoretic system are observed.
    Also indicated in Fig. 3 is the radioactive profile of $[^{14}C]$
fucose associated with the spinal cord myelin glycoproteins after
electrophoresis.   Three major peaks of radioactive fucose, designated 1, 2, and 3, are observed as well as several smaller peaks.
This pattern is reproducible and similar to the fucose incorporation
observed in myelin isolated from brain.   The levels of fucose incorporation into spinal cord myelin as a result of the intracisternal injection, however, is usually less than that incorporated into whole brain myelin after intracerebral injection.   Peak
1 corresponds to the location of the major myelin glycoprotein,
whereas peak 3 is the glycoprotein which migrates in a similar
position as proteolipid protein on gel electrophoresis.   This glycoprotein (peak 3) has been shown to be distinctly different from
proteolipid protein (20).

Fig. 3.   Fucose incorporation into purified rat spinal cord myelin.
Top: densitometric scan at 555 nm of Coomassie blue stained proteins
after electrophoretic separation on a polyacrylamide gel; Bottom:
radioactive profile of $[^{14}C]$ fucose associated with the myelin
proteins   as the result of intracisternal injection 20 hours prior
to the death of the animal.

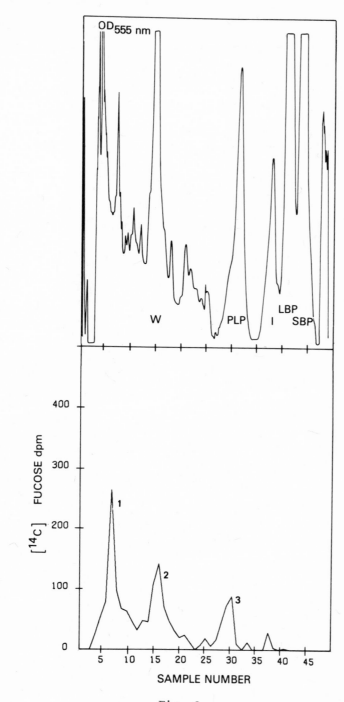

Fig. 3

A similar densitometric scan at 555 nm of the Coomassie blue stained proteins from myelin isolated from the adult rat spinal cord is illustrated in Fig. 4A. The dashed line and right-hand scale of Figures 4B and 4C indicate the profile of $[^{14}C]$fucose associated with myelin proteins isolated from two different rat spinal cord preparations after a 24 h incorporation. The fucose profile resembles that of Fig. 3, although there was little incorporation in the experiment shown in Fig. 4C. The absolute amount of fucose incorporation varies from experiment to experiment; however, difficulties inherent with intracisternal injections most likely account for these variations.

The results of treating the intact spinal cord with galactose oxidase followed by reduction with tritiated sodium borohydride are shown in Fig. 4B (left-hand scale, solid line). Fig. 4C indicates the levels of nonspecific reduction as a result of treatment of the spinal cord in the absence of galactose oxidase. The most striking observation is the high levels of nonspecific reduction in the proteolipid region of the gel. On other regions of the gel lower levels of reduction are also observed; however, there does appear to be an enhancement of label after treatment with galactose oxidase in certain areas of the gel. This observation is more apparent in Fig. 5 which shows the tritium incorporation by galactose oxidase after correcting for nonspecific reduction. The major myelin glycoprotein (peak 1) appears associated with a shoulder of tritium radioactivity in this gel system. By employing other gel systems which permit maximal separation of the high molecular weight proteins, it has been shown that this major glycoprotein is labeled by the oxidase reaction (19). The coincidence of the tritium radioactivity at peak 2 with that of radioactive fucose is also an indication of an accessible surface location for this glycoprotein. Furthermore, hydrolysis of the high molecular weight proteins and the subsequent identification of radioactive galactose has confirmed the specificity of the reaction for these glycoproteins. The enhancement of radioactive label in the proteolipid protein region of the gel (peak 3) as a result of galactose oxidase treatment has been observed in a variety of experiments.

Fig. 4. Internal and external surface labeling of glycoproteins of the intact rat spinal cord preparation. A: densitometric scan at 555 nm of the proteins from isolated myelin on a polyacrylamide gel stained with Coomassie blue; B: radioactivity associated with the proteins of myelin isolated from the intact spinal cord preparation as a result of reduction by tritiated sodium borohydride after treatment with galactose oxidase; C: radioactivity associated with the proteins as a result of reduction by borohydride in the absence of galactose oxidase. Internal labeling of glycoproteins with $[^{14}C]$fucose (----); external labeling of proteins with NaB^3H_4 (——).

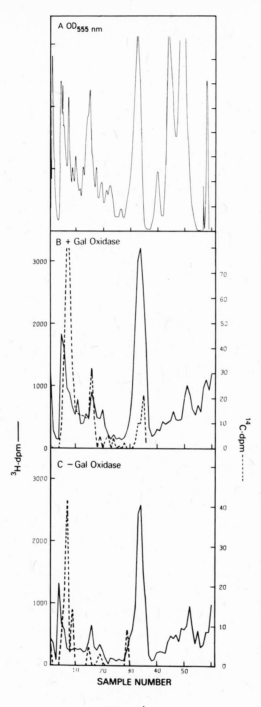

Fig. 4

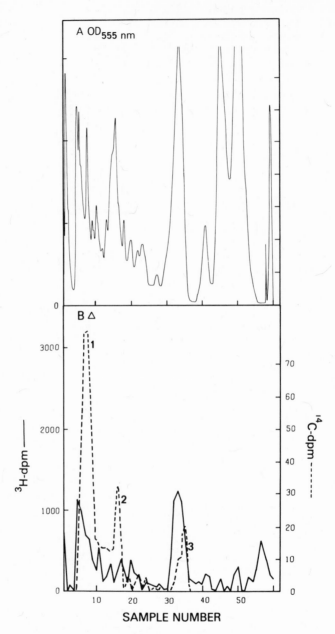

Fig. 5. Tritium incorporation by galactose oxidase into surface glycoproteins of the intact rat spinal cord preparation after correcting for nonspecific reduction.

This observation, therefore, strongly indicates that this fucose containing glycoprotein is also on the outer membrane surface. Further experiments, however, are necessary to distinguish the labeling of this glycoprotein by galactose oxidase from the non-specific reduction of the proteolipid protein.

All of the glycoproteins in isolated myelin from rat brain or spinal cord are quantitatively minor components. The major glyco-protein probably has a genuine association with the myelin or the oligodendroglial plasma membrane (20). The relationship of the other minor glycoproteins to myelin, however, has not been estab-lished. If these glycoproteins are true myelin associated compo-nents, they could have an external surface localization at any of the myelin specialized regions indicated above.

The use of galactose oxidase as a membrane probe for the intact myelin sheath has also provided interesting information concerning the distribution of the lower phase glycosphingolipids. Fig. 6 illustrates the radioactive pattern of a typical thin-layer chroma-togram of the lower phase lipids. The locations of the different myelin lipids are marked at the top of the figure. This identifi-cation of the myelin lipids was also correlated with known lipid standards. The levels of nonspecific reduction by tritiated sodium borohydride as a result of treatment of the intact spinal cord pre-paration in the absence of galactose oxidase are shown in the radio-active profile in Fig. 6A. The majority of the radioactive label was associated with the normal fatty acid galactocerebroside which accounted for 42-49% of the recovered counts. Only 4% of the radioactivity was observed at the hydroxy fatty acid galactocere-broside region, whereas sulfatide accounted for 12-14% of the radioactivity. Other smaller, undefined, radioactive peaks were also observed. A variety of experiments on different spinal cord preparations consistently produced this pattern of nonspecific re-duction.

Fig.6B illustrates the radioactive pattern after treatment of the intact spinal cord preparation with galactose oxidase followed by reduction with the borohydride. A 1.6-1.9 fold stimulation of tritium incorporation into the normal fatty acid galactocerebroside was consistently observed in a variety of separate experiments. In contrast to this enhancement of radioactivity is the absence of label associated with the hydroxy fatty acid galactocerebroside. Sulfatide also displayed a 1.4-2.0 fold stimulation of radioactive label. In addition, no label was observed associated with the monogalactosyl diglyceride (not shown) under the conditions of the experiments. These observations were consistently observed in a variety of chromatograms using different solvent systems. In addition, removal of the phospholipids by the $HgCl_2$ - saponification procedure of Abramson et al. (1) did not alter this labeling pat-tern. The specificity of the reaction for the normal fatty acid galactocerebroside has been confirmed by the identification of labeled galactose after hydrolysis of this isolated glycolipid (17).

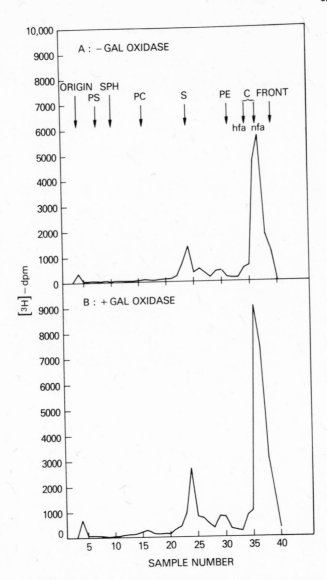

Fig. 6. Thin-layer chromatogram of lower phase lipids from rat spinal cord myelin. A: radioactive profile of the lower phase lipids as a result of non-specific reduction by NaB^3H_4 of the intact spinal cord preparation in the absence of galactose oxidase; B: radioactivity associated with the lipids after treatment of the spinal cord preparation with galactose oxidase followed by reduction. Solvent system: $CHCl_2/MeOH/H_2O$: 70/30/4, v/v/v; PS: phosphatidyl serine; SPH: sphingomyelin; PC: phosphatidylcholine; S: sulfatide; PE: phosphatidylethanolamine; C: cerebroside; hfa: 2-hydroxy fatty acid; nfa: non-hydroxy (normal) fatty acid.

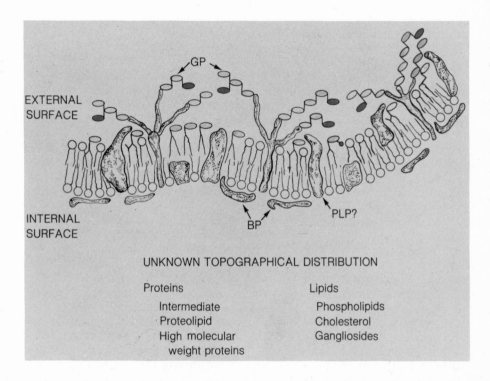

Fig. 7.   Fluid mosaic model of the myelin membrane.

DISCUSSION

The investigations summarized in this chapter have identified
several of the external surface components of the intact myelin
sheath. These results are illustrated in Fig. 7 and described in
terms of a fluid mosaic model for the myelin membrane. Arbitrarily
identified on the external membrane surface are glycoproteins,
which could include the major myelin glycoprotein (peak 1), a
second glycoprotein (peak 2), and a glycoprotein (peak 3) which
migrates with the proteolipid protein on gel electrophoresis.
Further information which would distinguish these glycoproteins
from one another in terms of their amino acid or carbohydrate composition is not available. There are, however, differences in the
molecular weights of these glycoproteins, their solubility in organic solvents, etc. (20).

Also illustrated on the external membrane surface are the
normal fatty acid galactocerebroside and sulfatide. The lack of
label associated with the hydroxy fatty acid galactocerebroside and
the monogalactosyl   diglyceride permits several possible interpretations (17). One of these interpretations is that the unlabeled
glycolipids are sterically inaccessible to galactose oxidase because
of masking by adjacent myelin components. This is illustrated in
Fig. 7; however, the low concentrations of the monogalactosyl
diglyceride in myelin (16) might be outside the levels of detecta-
bility using this labeling procedure.

Basic protein is illustrated in the model as an extrinsic protein associated with the cytoplasmic membrane surface. Such a conclusion is based on a variety of investigations, including the
utilization of the lactoperoxidase iodination technique (18), immunochemical techniques (12), and the use of chemical reagents (27).

The localization of the proteolipid protein is less clear.
The observation of a low molecular weight glycoprotein (peak 3)
which migrates with proteolipid protein on gel electrophoresis necessitates a re-evaluation of the lactoperoxidase iodination found
in this region of the acrylamide gel (18). A more likely candidate
for this labeling by the impermeant lactoperoxidase would be the
glycoprotein on the external surface. Furthermore, the negligible
binding of fluorescent probes to the proteolipid protein in myelin
and in lipid recombinants compared to the isolated protein suggests
a position more deeply embedded in the membrane (6, 7). In addition
the observations of Curatolo et al. (4) also imply a more inaccessible location for this protein. It is interesting to speculate
that the myelin proteolipid protein might be analogous to bacteriorhodopsin in the purple membrane from Halobacterium halobium. This
transmembrane protein apparently does not protrude significantly
above the lipid bilayer on either side of the membrane (1). The
extent of projection for these bacteriorhodopsin molecules, however, is uncertain (2).

Information about the localization of the other myelin proteins, including the remaining high molecular weight proteins and the intermediate protein, is not available. Several high molecular weight proteins were predominantly labeled by lactoperoxidase iodination (18); however, these proteins have not been further characterized. The proteins labeled by iodination do not include the major myelin glycoprotein as determined by the lack of coincidence of the [^{3}H]fucose labeled glycoprotein with the iodinated high molecular weight proteins (unpublished observations).

The phospholipid, cholesterol, and ganglioside localization within the myelin sheath also has not been determined. Further information concerning the topographical distribution of these other myelin components is therefore necessary. Near neighbor relationships should provide additional information concerning the functional roles for these different components. Questions concerning their distribution at each layer of the multilamellar structure will also have to be investigated. Finally, the diverse structural complexity of the myelin sheath necessitates a consideration of the different external surface regions. It is apparent, therefore, that our understanding of the molecular architecture of the myelin sheath is at a rudimentary level; however, the merging of biochemical, biophysical, and immunological techniques should significantly facilitate future investigations of the myelin membrane.

REFERENCES

1. Abramson, M.B., Norton, W.T. and Kutzman, R., Study of ionic structures in phospholipids by infrared spectra, J. Biol. Chem. 240 (1965) 2389-2395.
2. Blaurock, A.E. and King, G.I., Asymmetric structure of the purple membrane, Science 196 (1977) 1101-1104.
3. Boggs, J.M., Wood, D.D., Moscarello, M.A. and Papahadjopoulos, D., Lipid phase separation induced by a hydrophobic protein in phosphatidyserine-phosphatidylcholine vesicles, Biochemistry 16 (1977) 2325-2329.
4. Curatolo, W., Sakura, J.D., Small, D.M. and Shipley, G.G., Protein-lipid interactions: Recombinants of the proteolipid apoprotein of myelin with dimyristoyllecithin, Biochemistry 16 (1977) 2313-2319.
5. Dea, P., Chan, S.I. and Dea, F.J., High-resolution proton magnetic resonance spectra of a rabbit sciatic nerve, Science 175 (1972) 206-209.
6. Feinstein, M.B. and Felsenfeld, H., Reactions of fluorescent probes with normal and chemically modified myelin, Biochemistry 14 (1975) 3041-3048.
7. Feinstein, M.B. and Felsenfeld, H., Reactions of fluorescent probes with normal and chemically modified myelin basic protein and proteolipid. Comparisons with myelin, Biochemistry 14 (1975) 3049-3056.

8. Fisher, K.A., Analysis of membrane halves: Cholesterol, Proc. Nat. Acad. Sci. USA 73 (1976) 173-177.

9. Gahmberg, C.G. and Hakomori, S., External labelling of cell surface galactose and galactosamine in glycolipid and glycoprotein of human erythrocytes, J. Biol. Chem. 248 (1973) 4311-4317.

10. Gottlieb, M.H., The reactivity of human erythrocyte membrane cholesterol with a cholesterol oxidase, Biochim. Biophys.Acta 466 (1977) 422-428.

11. Henderson, R. and Unwin, P.N.T., Three-dimensional model of purple membrane obtained by electron microscopy, Nature 257 (1975) 28-32.

12. Herndon, R.M., Rauch, H.C. and Einstein, E.R., Immuno-electron microscopic localization of the encephalitogenic basic protein in myelin, Immunol. Comm. 2 (1973) 163-172.

13. Higgins, J.A., Florendo, N.T. and Barrnett, R.J., Localization of cholesterol in membranes of erythrocyte ghosts, J. Ultrastruct. Res. 42 (1973) 66-81.

14. Lenard, J. and Rothmun, J.E., Transbilayer distribution and movement of cholesterol and phospholipid in the membrane of influenza virus, Proc. Nat. Acad. Sci. USA 73 (1976) 391-395.

15. Norton, W.T. and Poduslo, S.E., Myelination in rat brain. Method of myelin isolation, J. Neurochem. 21 (1973) 749-757.

16. Pieringer, R.A., Deshmukh, D.S. and Flynn, T.J., The association of the galactosyl diglycerides of nerve tissue with myelination, Progress in Brain Res. 40 (1973) 397-405.

17. Poduslo, J.F., J. Biol. Chem.(1977), submitted for publication.

18. Poduslo, J.F. and Braun, P.E., Topographical arrangement of membrane proteins in the intact myelin sheath, J. Biol. Chem. 250 (1975) 1099-1105.

19. Poduslo, J.F., Quarles, R.H. and Brady, R.O., External labeling of galactose in surface membrane glycoproteins of the intact myelin sheath, J. Biol. Chem. 251 (1976) 153-158.

20. Poduslo, J.F., Everly, J.L. and Quarles, R.H., A low molecular weight glycoprotein associated with isolated myelin: Distinction from myelin proteolipid protein, J. Neurochem. 28 (1977) 977-986.

21. Singer, S.J. and Nicolson, G.L., The fluid mosaic model of the structure of cell membranes, Science 175 (1972) 720-731.

22. Steck, T.L., The organization of proteins in human erythrocyte membranes, in Membrane Research (C.F. Fox, ed.) Academic Press, New York (1972) pp. 71-93.

23. Steck, T.L. and Dawson, G., Topographical distribution of complex carbohydrates in the erythrocyte membrane, J. Biol. Chem. 249 (1974) 2135-2142.

24. Vanderkooi, G. and Green, D.E., Biological membrane structure, I. The protein crystal model for membranes, Proc. Nat. Acad. Sci. 66 (1970) 615-621.

25. Wallach, D.F.H. and Zahler, P.H., Protein conformations in cellular membranes, Proc. Nat. Acad. Sci. 56 (1966) 1552-1559.

26. Williams, E.C. and Cordes, E.H., Natural abundance carbon-13 nuclear magnetic resonance studies of bovine white matter and myelin, Biochemistry 15 (1976) 5792-5799.
27. Wood, D.D., Epand, R.M. and Moscarello, M.A., Localization of the basic protein and lipophilin in the myelin membrane with a non-penetrating reagent, Biochim. Biophys. Acta 467 (1977) 120-129.

CONFORMATION OF MYELIN BASIC PROTEIN AND ITS ROLE IN MYELIN FORMATION

B.E. Chapman, L.T. Littlemore and W.J. Moore

School of Chemistry, University of Sydney

N.S.W. 2006, Australia

SUMMARY

High resolution ^{13}C and ^{1}H NMR spectra of myelin basic protein over a range of pH and concentrations indicate that intramolecular folding of the polypeptide chain occurs in aqueous solution in the region of residues 85 to 116. At pH 4 in D_2O solution, the ^{13}C resonances due to nonprotonated carbons of phenylalanine and tryptophan are broadened and chemically shifted compared to the same resonances when the protein is dissolved in 6M guanidinium hydrochloride. These residues occur in the region of the polypeptide chain in which the intramolecular folding may occur. As the pH is raised and the positive charge on the protein reduced from 28 to 18, intermolecular aggregation occurs, which appears to involve these same folded regions. Data on T_1 (longitudinal relaxation times) of protons indicate also that amino-acid sidechains vary considerably in their motional freedoms. The concentration dependence of the proton NMR spectra provides further information on association of protein monomers.

The region of the protein involved in folding, polymerization and substrate specificities is conservative in various species and we can surmise that it may have a specialized role in protein-lipid interactions in the myelin membrane. We suggest that the protein forms dimers across the cytoplasmic apposition during the formation of myelin. Estimates of the repulsive energies of interaction between approaching membranes suggest that some special mechanism of this kind is required to overcome the repulsive forces due to breakdown of water structure and electrostatic interaction.

INTRODUCTION

The conformations of myelin basic protein (MBP) in aqueous and lipid media may provide evidence for its function in formation and breakdown of myelin. Many techniques have been used to study the conformation of myelin basic protein: viscosity, ultracentrifugation, low angle x-ray scattering, electron microscopy, light scattering and circular dichroism. These techniques yield information only about the gross conformational properties of the protein. They indicate that in aqueous solution MBP has an elongated structure without alpha-helical content, but that probably the polypeptide chain includes at least one bend to yield a hairpin conformation. In some nonaqueous solvents, the protein is partly or entirely alpha-helical. When the protein is mixed with lipids or detergents some alpha-helical conformation also occurs. Two groups have obtained proton nuclear magnetic resonance (NMR) data, which give evidence of marked aggregation of the protein to yield oligomeric species at pH above about 7.0 (1, 14), and our laboratory has published a preliminary account of some ^{13}C NMR studies (5).

With NMR spectroscopy it is often possible to obtain information about the conformation of a protein in the neighborhood of individual amino acid residues. Both the chemical shift and the line width of an NMR peak from an individual nucleus are sensitive to the chemical environment of the nucleus and the line width depends also on the dynamic mobility of the nucleus and its environs. Thus in principle it should be possible to obtain detailed conformational information about individual amino acid residues in a protein from its NMR spectrum. In practice as the chemical shifts of ^{1}H peaks cover a small range (approx. 10 ppm) and the widths of individual proton peaks tend to be large (5-30 Hz), a ^{1}H NMR spectrum usually consists of broad bands of overlapping resonances, making it difficult to resolve peaks from individual protons. A favorable aspect of ^{1}H NMR spectroscopy is that its high sensitivity allows dilute solutions of proteins to be used. ^{13}C NMR chemical shifts cover a much wider range (approx. 200 ppm) which leads to less overlapping of peaks than is obtained with ^{1}H NMR. Thus there is a greater probability that information on individual amino acid residues can be obtained from a ^{13}C NMR spectrum than from a ^{1}H NMR spectrum of the same protein. An unfavorable aspect of ^{13}C NMR spectroscopy is its low sensitivity compared with ^{1}H NMR (approx. 10^{-4} at the same molar concentration of protein). This aspect of ^{13}C NMR means that more scans of a spectrum must be averaged to improve the signal/noise ratio, with consequent increase in instrumental time, than are needed for a ^{1}H spectrum. More importantly, high concentrations of protein have to be used, typically 10^{-2} M vs. 10^{-3} M used in ^{1}H NMR, to obtain the signal/noise ratios needed for a usable ^{13}C NMR spectrum. These high concentrations may lead to intermolecular interactions, such as formation of oligomers, which would alter the NMR spectrum. The problem of separating intramolecular from intermolecular effects can be a difficult one.

The dynamic properties of nuclei in NMR experiments can also be studied more directly by measurements of the longitudinal (spin lattice) relaxation time T_1. This relaxation time is usually controlled by magnetic dipole interactions with neighboring nuclei and theoretical expressions are available such as the Solomon-Bloembergen equations (24) to relate T_1 to the correlation times of the internuclear motions.

EXPERIMENTAL

^{13}C NMR spectra at 22.625 MHz were obtained, using 15 ml sample tubes, on a Bruker HX-90 spectrometer by the Fourier transform method. Each spectrum was obtained by averaging approximately 40,000 transients at a 5,000 Hz spectral width, 1.5 s recycle time, 1 Hz digital broadening and 8,192 time domain addresses. A 7 µs (45°) pulse was used to excite the nuclei. Protons were decoupled from carbon nuclei using a Bruker broadband decoupler. Chemical shifts are reported as parts per million from Me_4Si. Dioxane (67.86 ppm downfield from Me_4Si) was used as the internal reference. The concentration of protein was 100 to 200 mg/ml. The ^{13}C spectra at 67.9 MHz were obtained on a Bruker HX-270 spectrometer at the National NMR Center, Canberra, Australia. 97,000 transients were averaged at 15,000 Hz spectral width with 2.5 s recycle time. Protons were decoupled as stated previously. The ^{1}H spectra were obtained at 270 MHz at Canberra, in 10 mm tubes, over a range of concentrations from 1 to 200 mg/ml and pH from 3.5 to 8.0.

Proton T_1 experiments were performed on a Bruker HX-90 spectrometer using the standard-τ-90 method with a recycle time of 5 s. The number of transients averaged varied from 50 to 500 depending on the protein concentration used.

Bovine protein was prepared by the method of Eylar (21), porcine protein was kindly provided by Eli Lilly & Co, Indianapolis. Purity of proteins was controlled by polyacrylamide gel-SDS-electrophoresis.

RESULTS AND DISCUSSION

A basic type of experiment consists in examining the spectrum of the protein in its native state and then re-examining the spectrum of the protein in the presence of a powerful denaturing agent. Solutions of 6M guanidinium hydrochloride have been shown to convert globular proteins to random coil conformations and also to destroy quaternary structure of the protein (after reduction of any S-S bonds).

Fig. 1 (from ref. 5) shows the spectra obtained in D_2O at pH 4 in both presence and absence of 6 M Gu.DCl. The protein has a

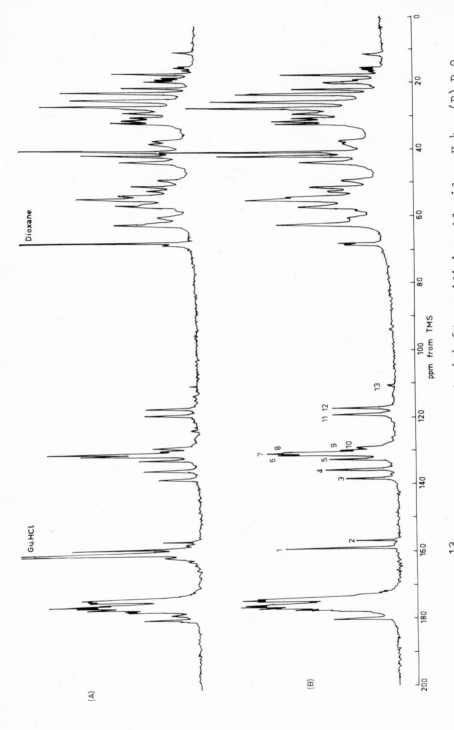

Fig. 1. 22.625 MHz ^{13}C NMR spectra of MBP in (A) 6M guanidinium chloride, pH 4, (B) D$_2$O, pH 3.9.

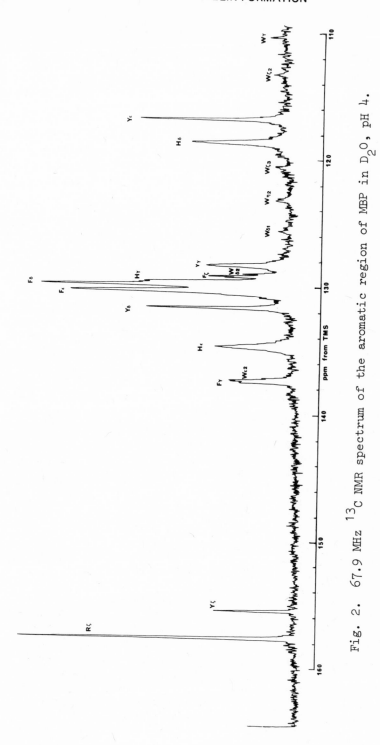

Fig. 2. 67.9 MHz ^{13}C NMR spectrum of the aromatic region of MBP in D_2O, pH 4.

net positive charge of 28 at this pH and is thought to exist predominantly as a monomer (14). Peaks fall into three main groups,
from carbonyl (165-180 ppm), aromatic (105-145 ppm) and aliphatic
(10-70 ppm) carbon atoms.

The ^{13}C NMR spectrum of MBP in D_2O shows mainly the sharp
peaks characteristic of a random-coil conformation, with a number
of broader peaks. This type of spectrum is consistent with the
occurrence in the protein of some regions which have tertiary or
quaternary structure and others which are capable of unstructured
motion as in a random coil. These broadened peaks sharpen when the
protein is placed in the denaturant 6M Gu.DCl as is consistent with
the protein being completely in a monomeric random-coil conformation
in this medium.

Peaks in the aromatic region can be identified as (1) the Cδ
of arginine (2) the Cδ of tyrosine (3) the Cγ of phenylalanine (4)
the Cεl of histidine (5) the Cδ of tyrosine (6) the Cε of phenylalanine (7) the Cδ of phenylalanine (8) the Cγ of histidine (9)
the Cδ of phenylalanine (10) the Cγ of tyrosine (11) the Cδ2 of
histidine (12) the Cε of tyrosine and (13) the Cγ of the sole
tryptophan residue.

The aliphatic region has not been completely assigned. Some
peaks of interest are the isoleucine δ and ε methyl carbons at 11.7
and 16.2 ppm, the valine methyl carbons at 16.9 and 19.3 ppm, and
the leucine methyls at 20.4 and 23.6 ppm. In going from D_2O to
6 M Gu.DCl the peaks that sharpen are those mentioned above in the
aliphatic region and those arising from phenylalanine residues and
the sole tryptophan residue, indicating that some of these residues
are involved in regions of restricted mobility in the protein.
Other peaks in the aliphatic region of the spectrum that sharpen
on going from D_2O to 6 M Gu.DCl are at 60, 55, 53 and 23 ppm. These
are composite peaks from a number of amino acid residues. If
residues that contribute in only one of these peaks are eliminated
we are left with valine, leucine, isoleucine and proline residues.

The sharpening of certain peaks in the ^{13}C spectrum at pH 4 in
6 M Gu.DCl as compared with D_2O could be due to (a) unfolding of a
structured region in the protein, (b) breaking of dimers or higher
oligomers, or a combination of both processes. As the pH is raised,
and charge on the protein decreases, aggregation increases. From
an examination of a ^{13}C NMR spectrum of MBP obtained at pH 7 (Fig.
2 of ref. 5) it appeared that the peaks that broadened most on
aggregation were those that were already broad in the spectrum obtained at pH 4. This relation could indicate either that the
protein is aggregating through structured regions of the polypeptide
chain or that this pH dependent aggregation is merely an extension
of concentration dependent aggregation already present at pH 4.

To differentiate between the two mechanisms giving rise to
broadened peaks it is necessary to study the protein at low concentration where aggregation would be eliminated or minimized.
As there are problems associated with obtaining sufficient

signal/noise ratio in ^{13}C NMR using low protein concentrations, a study was made of the ^1H NMR spectra of MBP.

Measurements of aggregation of protein from ^1H NMR. The aggregation of myelin basic protein is being studied as a function of pH using 270 MHz ^1H NMR spectroscopy and a technique first applied by Chan et al. (22) to aggregation of histone IV. Series of spectra taken at increasing total protein concentrations at a given pH show an absolute deficit in integrated peak intensities which may be attributed to the formation of aggregated species, the NMR peaks of which have linewidths of at least several hundred hertz. The amount of aggregate detected in this way increases with increasing pH; however, from the criterion of absolute intensity, a small amount of aggregate is present even at pH = 3.7 at concentrations in excess of 5%. Examples of these measurements of aggregation are given in Table 1.

Table 1. Formation of large MBP aggregates, monitored by the loss in intensity of the upfield methyl peak in 270 MHz ^1H NMR spectra.

Total protein concentration (w/w)	pD	% loss of intensity of ^1H NMR peak
0.2%	7.5	5.0
0.5%	7.5	17.0
1.0%	7.5	26.0
5.0%	7.5	42.0
10.0%	3.7	4.0

A separate phenomenon observed is a general decrease in linewidth of observed peaks with decreasing concentration. These results indicate that the natural linewidth of monomeric MBP proton peaks is considerably less than those previously reported (14).

Although further data are required for quantitative analysis of the spectra, it appears that formation of dimers of MBP is associated with broadening of spectral lines, whereas formation of larger aggregates is linked to losses in absolute intensity. Thus our tentative interpretation of the concentration dependence of the myelin basic protein data differs in detail from that of Chan et al. (22) for histone IV.

Further evidence for dimerisation comes from a study of the proton relaxation rates of the phenylalanine and methyl residues of the proteins as a function of concentration (6). Residues in freely mobile regions of the protein will have relatively long relaxation times as compared to those in restricted regions. If the same type of residue exists in both environments, biphasic behavior will be observed in the relaxation-time experiment. Biphasic behavior was observed for both phenyl and methyl peaks at concentrations of 1 to 20% protein, indicating that more than one relaxing species is present in both peaks. For the methyl peaks the fastest relaxing species has a relaxation time (T_1) of approximately 0.2 s. This T_1 was constant through the concentration range. For the phenyl peak the relaxation time of the fastest relaxing species varied from 0.48 s for a 1% solution to 0.35 s for a 20% solution, showing a slight effect of increased concentration in decreasing the mobility of some of the phenylalanine residues.

Chemical shifts in ^{13}C spectra. The NMR results support but do not yet prove the concept that MBP in D_2O contains regions of the polypeptide chain that have some tertiary structure and that aggregation of the protein at high pH is through these structured portions of the molecule. It is difficult, however, quantitatively to separate effects in the ^{13}C spectra that are caused by dimerisation from those caused by possible structure.

Further evidence for a structured region in the protein is shown in Fig. 2. This is a ^{13}C NMR spectrum of the aromatic region obtained at 67.9 MHz. There is a splitting of the phenylalanine γ and δ peaks due to resonances from individual phenylalanine side-chains with slightly different chemical shifts. This splitting indicates that the phenylalanine residues occupy different environments, which would not be expected if the protein existed as a random coil. This effect on the phenylalanine spectrum is similar to that shown by Jardetsky for parvalbumin (19) in which some phenylalanine residues occupy internal positions in a structured protein.

From an analysis of the amino acid sequence, the region from residues 85 to 118 in MBP comprises a large proportion of the amino acid residues that give broadened peaks. Residues 84-118 have a constant amino acid sequence in all species reported to date and this region is the locus of several chemical specificities of the protein. Figure 3 shows a graph of sequence variation for human, bovine, monkey and small MBP from rat, using the sequence numbering for human MBP. There are constant regions from 17-39, 85-118 and 157-170.

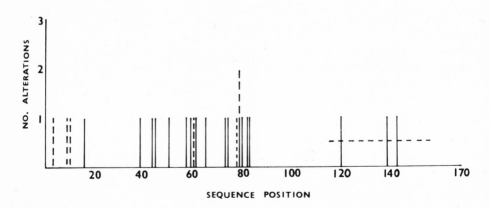

Fig. 3. Variation in MBP sequence from different species. Solid lines substitutions. Dashed lines insertions or deletions.

The sequence of three proline residues at 99-101 was suggested by Brostoff and Eylar (3) as the site of a hairpin fold. Theoretical calculations (17) indicate a deep minimum of potential energy at $\psi_1 = \psi_2 = 165°$ for the proline C^{α}-C bonds. If the suggested fold extended to the phenylalanines at 89-90 it would provide an explanation of the chemical splitting shown in Fig. 2.

Formation of Myelin

When we contemplate the 19 net positive charges on MBP at pH 7 and the array of negatively charged phospholipids on the surfaces of membrane bilayers, it would seem reasonable to believe that the role of MBP is to neutralise these negative surface charges. With their electrostatic repulsions largely eliminated, opposed membranes could approach each other to form a close packed lamellar sheath. Certainly there are enough net positive charges on MBP to perform such a function. We can calculate that MBP spread over one surface of a myelin bilayer membrane would provide 4×10^{13} positive charges/cm². This figure can be compared with the estimate of $\sigma = 5 \times 10^{13}$ charges/cm² as an upper limit for the surface density of net negative charge on the lipid components (17). Thus MBP appears to be designed with almost stoichiometric efficiency to produce an electrically neutral membrane surface. If negative charges on the membrane are uniformly distributed there would be 1 charge per 200 Å². From the X-ray data MBP has a radius of gyration of 46 Å and axial ratio 5; thus at pH 7, its average charge density is ~ 1 charge per 200 Å².

The predicted electrostatic repulsions are greatly lowered by the formation of an electric double layer due to counterions at the membrane surfaces. If the ionic concentration in the cytoplasm is taken to be 150 mM (of 1:1 electrolyte, presumably mostly KCl) the corresponding thickness of the double layer (Debye length) would be

$$\kappa^{-1} = (\varepsilon kT/8\pi ne^2 z^2)^{1/2} = 8.1 \times 10^{-8} \text{ cm.}$$

The dielectric constant ε was taken to be the value for bulk water.

The electrostatic repulsion between the double layers can be calculated from the theory of Verwey and Overbeek (25). We use the theoretical expressions derived by Gregory (8) for the case in which the surface charges on the membranes remain constant as the intermembrane spacing d is varied. The energy of interaction V is

$$V = \frac{2nkT}{\kappa} \left[2\bar{y} \ln \left(\frac{B + \bar{y} \cosh (\kappa d/s)}{1 + y} \right) \right.$$

$$\left. - \ln(\bar{y}^2 + \cosh d + B\sinh \kappa d) + xd \right].$$

Here n is the ionic concentration, $\bar{y} = ze\psi/kT$ where ψ is the potential at the surface, and

$$B = \left[1 + \bar{y}^2 \operatorname{csch}^2 \left(\frac{\kappa d}{2} \right) \right]^{1/2}$$

The surface potential is related to the surface charge density by

$$\sinh (\bar{y}/2) = \sigma(2\pi/n\epsilon kT)^{1/2}.$$

The computed electrostatic repulsion energies are plotted in Fig. 4 for $\sigma = 5 \times 10^{13}$ cm^{-2}. These calculations do not take into account the discrete nature of the distribution of membrane charge, which would be expected to reduce the electric field in the double layer by about 25% (18).

The calculated electrostatic repulsion energies are quite large, even though reduced by the shielding effect of the double layer. At $d = 10^{-7}$ cm, for example, and for a surface site of area 2×10^{-14} cm^2, $V/kT = 1.93..$

These electrostatic effects are not the only source of repulsions between approaching bilayers. Even between neutral membranes powerful repulsive forces arise as a result of changes in the structure of the intervening water layer as the membranes begin to approach each other closely (13). In lecithin bilayers these forces were measured experimentally by LeNeveu et al. (12) by an ingenious technique of osmotic compression. Marcelja and Radic (16) have outlined the theory of this repulsive interaction. Israelach-vili and Adams (9) found further evidence for these forces in direct measurements of forces between mica plates. We shall call these forces due to change in water structure, chaotropic forces. By integration of the experimental force – distance relation for lecithin bilayers we obtained the repulsive energy vs. distance curve included in Fig. 4. We see that at distances below 10^{-7} cm the chaotropic repulsion exceeds the electrostatic repulsion.

The van der Waals attractive forces between neutral membranes balance the repulsive forces at a separation of about 2.7 nm. At 2.0 nm, for our model myelin membrane, the electrostatic repulsion, chaotropic repulsion, and van der Waals attraction energies would be estimated to be 17×10^{-2}, 5×10^{-2} and -3×10^{-2} erg/cm^2, respectively. The van der Waals attractive energy was estimated by the method of Nir and Anderson (20).

It is evident that membrane fusion of phospholipid bilayer membranes, with or without net surface negative charges, will be energetically most unfavorable. Some other factor must be added to the model in order to permit closer approaches of the double membranes. We do not have any high resolution X-ray analyses of CNS myelin but the experiments indicate that the spacings between the unit membranes are all very close (10).

Neutron diffraction data are as yet available only for sciatic nerve myelin (11). These data suggest that the intracellular cleft is about 3 nm wide and the extracellular cleft about 4 nm. A considerable concentration of protein is detected in this aqueous region between the bilayers, a volume fraction of 0.09 to 0.14.

The process of myelin formation. Myelin basic protein may serve two functions in the formation of myelin: (1) It will largely neutralize the net negative charges on the inside of the oligo-dendroglial membrane; (2) It will introduce hydrophobic (oily)

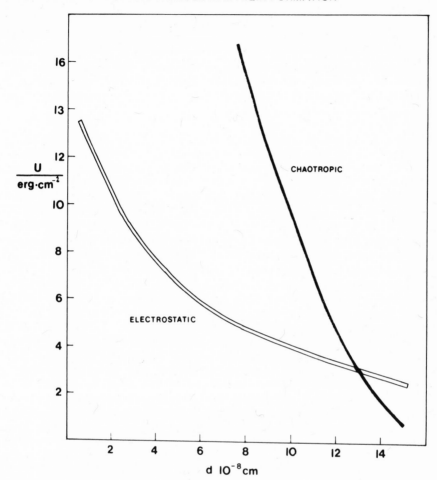

Fig. 4. Calculated repulsive energies between planar membranes with surface charge density, $\sigma = 5 \times 10^{13} cm^{-2}$, showing the electrostatic part and the chaotropic part (due to breakdown of water structure).

patches into a highly polar membrane surface. These hydrophobic patches will greatly reduce the chaotropic forces of repulsion between membranes, and may indeed actually associate across the cleft through strong hydrophobic interactions (2, 23).

The association of myelin basic protein that has been observed in the NMR studies and by other methods therefore becomes relevant for the structural role of MBP in myelin.

There is increasingly good evidence that MBP resides predominantly at the intracellular surfaces of the myelin membranes. The ionic gradients across the glial cell membrane would lead to a high electric field gradient, with the outside of the membrane being positive with respect to the inside. The actual potential difference $\Delta\phi$ across the membrane differs from the p.d. ΔV between the extracellular and intracellular fluids because of the surface double layer (4). For a protein with 19 positive charges a p.d. of 50 mV across the membrane corresponds to a free energy difference of 91 kJ/mol. Thus once MBP is attached to the inner side of the membrane a flip-flop migration to the outside will be unlikely.

It may be noted that Van Deenen et al. (15) suggested that "The basic protein is the organizer molecule and the initiator of the spiral winding of the myelin around the axon". They believed, however, that MBP was localized at the intraperiod lines in myelin and that MBP did not occur in the oligo-cell membranes.

We can distinguish two distinct processes in the winding of the myelin sheath, (1) the condensation of a pair of plasma membranes from the oligodendroglial cell, which after suitable modification become a unit of the myelin structure, and (2) the coiling of these double membranes about the axon. This coiling process is quite independent of the condensation process. Coiling takes place by a spiral motion of the myelin sheath, in which the doublets move relative to one another at the extracellular spacing. The leading nose of the myelin sheath rotates about the axon. Essentially it must be driven by the new myelin being spun off by the oligodendroglial cell. We do not know whether it is driven by diffusion or by plastic flow, but renewal of an already formed sheath was shown by Dawson and Gould (7) to be a diffusion process, and the rate of diffusive flow would also be adequate for growth.

A serious problem for any autoimmune mechanism of demyelination that directly involves MBP is the relative inaccessibility of this protein in the cell interior. Although various ad hoc ways to overcome this difficulty may be suggested, they suffer from various degrees of implausibility. It has seemed necessary to invoke a viral agent to accomplish the release of the MBP in the first place, and persistence of the same agent to bring MBP into contact with the sensitized T cells. We can, however, suggest a physical mechanism to bring MBP to the extracellular surface. When a nerve cell fires, the high electric field across its membrane is reversed for about a millisecond. Although the oligodendroglial cell is not itself electrically excitable, the part of the myelin sheath in the neighborhood of the node of Ranvier will experience large changes in electric field whenever the action potential occurs at the node. Thus transmembrane "flip-flops" of MBP molecules may sometimes occur in the myelin adjacent to the nodes.

Acknowledgements. Mr Lee Klososzczyk, electronics engineer, has devoted much skillful work to the installation and operation of the NMR laboratory. We have had help and advice from Dr Ross Smith in many aspects of the research. The work was supported by the National Health and Medical Research Council of Australia.

REFERENCES

1. Block, R.E., Brady, A.H. and Joffe, S., Conformation and aggregation of bovine myelin proteins, Biochem. Biophys. Res. Comm. 54 (1973) 1595-1602.

2. Braun, P.E., Molecular architecture of myelin, in Myelin (P. Morell, ed.) Plenum Press, New York (1977) pp. 91-116.

3. Brostoff, S.W. and Eylar, E.H., Localization of methylated arginine in A1 protein from myelin, Proc. Nat. Acad. Sci.(USA) 68 (1971) 765-772.

4. Chandler, W.K., Hodgkin, A.L. and Meves, H., The effect of changing the internal solution on sodium inactivation and related phenomena in giant axons, J. Physiol. 180 (1965) 821-836.

5. Chapman, B.E. and Moore, W.J., Conformation of myelin basic protein in aqueous solution from nuclear magnetic resonance spectroscopy, Biochem. Biophys. Res. Comm. 73 (1976) 758-765.

6. Chapman, B.E. and Moore, W.J., ^{13}C and ^{1}H/NMR studies on the conformation of myelin basic protein, in preparation.

7. Gould, R.M. and Dawson, R.M.C., Incorporation of newly formed lecithin into peripheral nerve myelin, J. Cell. Biol. 68 (1976) 480-496.

8. Gregory, J., Interaction of unequal double layers at constant charge, J. Colloid Interface Sci. 51 (1975) 44-51.

9. Israelachvili, J.N. and Adams, G.E., Direct measurement of long range forces between two mica surfaces in aqueous KNO_3 solutions, Nature (Lond.) 262 (1976) 774-776.

10. Kirschner, D.A. and Caspar, D.L.D., Diffraction studies of molecular organization in myelin, in Myelin (P. Morell, ed.) Plenum Press, New York (1977) pp. 51-89.

11. Kirschner, D.A., Caspar, D.L.D., Schoenborn, B.P. and Nunes, A.C., Neutron diffraction studies of nerve myelin, in Neutron Diffraction for the Analysis of Biological Structures (B.P. Schoenborn, ed.) Brookhaven Symposia in Biology No. 28 (1975) pp. 68-76.

12. LeNeveu, D.M., Rand, R.P. and Parsegian, V.A., Measurement of forces between lecithin bilayers, Nature (Lond.) 259 (1976) 601-603.

13. LeNeveu, D.M., Rand, R.P., Parsegian, V.A. and Gingell, D., Measurement and modification of forces between lecithin bilayers, Biophys. J. 18 (1977) 209-230.

14. Liebes, L.F., Zand, R. and Phillips, W.D., Solution behavior, circular dichroism and 220 MHz PMR studies of the bovine myelin basic protein, Biochim. Biophys. Acta 405 (1975) 27-39.

15. London, Y., Demel, R.A., van Kessel, W.S.M.G., Vossenberg, F. G.A. and van Deenen, L.L.M., The protection of A1 myelin basic protein against the action of proteolytic enzymes after interaction of the protein with lipids at the air-water interface, Biochim. Biophys. Acta 311 (1973) 520-530.

16. Marčelja, S. and Radić, N., Repulsion of interfaces due to boundary water, Chem. Phys. Letters 42 (1976) 129-130.

17. Moore, W.J., Contribution of phospholipids to the surface charge of neuronal membranes, in Function and Metabolism of Phospholipids in Central and Peripheral Nervous System (G. Porcellati, L. Amaducci and C. Galli, eds.) Plenum Press, New York (1976) pp. 21-24.

18. Nelson, A.P. and McQuarrie, D.A., The effect of discrete charges on the electrical properties of a membrane, J. Theor. Biol. 55 (1975) 13-27.

19. Nelson, D.J., Opella, S.J. and Jardetzky, O., ^{13}C nuclear magnetic resonance study of molecular motions and conformational transitions in muscle calcium binding parvalbumins, Biochemistry 15 (1976) 5552-5559.

20. Nir, S. and Andersen, M., van der Waals interactions between cell surfaces, J. Membrane Biol. 31 (1977) 1-18.

21. Oshiro, Y. and Eylar, E.H., Allergic encephalomyelitis: Preparation of the encephalitogenic basic protein from bovine brain, Arch. Biochem. Biophys. 138 (1970) 392-396.

22. Pekary, A.E., Hsueh-Jei, L., Chan, S.I., Chen-Jung, H. and Wagner, T.E., Nuclear magnetic resonance studies of histone IV solution conformation, Biochemistry 14 (1975) 1177-1184.

23. Smith, R., Noncovalent cross-linking of lipid bilayers by myelin basic protein. A possible role in myelin formation, Biochim. Biophys. Acta , in press.

24. Solomon, I., Relaxation processes in a system of two spins, Phys. Rev. 99 (1955) 559-565.

25. Verwey, E.J.W. and Overbeek, J.T.G., Theory of the Stability of Lyophobic Colloids, Elsevier, Amsterdam (1948).

CROSS-LINKING OF LIPID BILAYERS BY CENTRAL NERVOUS SYSTEM MYELIN

BASIC PROTEIN: AGGREGATION OF FREE AND VESICLE-BOUND PROTEIN

Ross Smith

School of Chemistry, University of Sydney

Sydney, Australia 2006

SUMMARY

Central nervous system myelin basic protein binds to the zwitterionic lipid, egg diacylphosphatidylcholine, over a wide range of pH and ionic strength. Lipid vesicles containing the protein have been observed to increase in size and to aggregate. The size increase is most marked at very low ionic strengths whereas aggregation is evident at ionic strengths from 0.001 to 0.35. The pH and ionic-strength dependence of this aggregation closely follows that of the self-association of the protein, suggesting that vesicle association is mediated by binding between polypeptides attached to different vesicles. Basic protein is monomeric at low pH but above pH 6 self-associates yielding primarily small oligomers (probably dimers) and minor amounts of higher species. It is envisaged that each protein molecule possesses two distinct binding sites, one capable of association with lipid bilayers and the second with another protein molecule.

Basic protein is found predominantly on the intracellular surface of the myelin membrane. Given the ability of the protein to act as a bridge between lipid bilayer vesicles in vitro it is proposed that it may perform a similar function in vivo, serving to cross-link the inner surfaces of the oligodendroglial cell membrane. This protein function could lead to formation of the long cellular processes which encircle the nerve cell axon and could assist in stabilizing the highly ordered myelin structure which results.

Abbreviations used: PC - phosphatidylcholine; PS - phosphatidyl-serine.

INTRODUCTION

Myelin basic protein has long been envisaged as being an extrinsic membrane protein held at the lipid bilayer by ionic attraction, serving primarily to neutralize the charge on the lipids and to thus allow close juxtaposition of membranes.

Some recent observations however challenge this concept. Demel et al. (2), by examining the expansion of lipid monolayers by basic protein, observed a dependence on lipid alkyl chain length indicative of some hydrophobic interaction. Similar conclusions have been reached from thermal and permeability studies of lipid vesicles containing this protein (6). In our laboratory we have shown that protein interaction with deoxycholate, an anionic surfactant, and a negatively charged lipid, diacylphosphatidylserine (PS), induces formation of a small proportion of helical secondary structure in the protein which in water is without detectable α- or β-structure. Neither this structural change nor protein binding to these amphiphiles is significantly affected by variation in ionic strength or pH (11,and M.A. Keniry, B.J. McDonald and R. Smith, unpublished). We have also found that the protein attaches to vesicles of the zwitterionic lipid, diacylphosphatidylcholine (PC), and it has previously been shown to bind lysophosphatidylcholine (1), in both cases undergoing a conformational change similar to that caused by the negatively charged amphiphiles. Thus, it seems that despite its high proportion of polar residues basic protein is capable of binding hydrophobically to lipid bilayers and other amphiphiles. More direct, but preliminary, evidence for such an intrusion into the hydrophobic region of PS bilayers has recently been obtained using ^{13}C natural-abundance NMR spectroscopy (M.A. Keniry and R. Smith, unpublished).

In the course of the above-mentioned studies of interaction with PS and PC we observed that basic protein dramatically increased the light scattering of solutions of PC vesicles. This apparent aggregation of PC was remarkable in that it occurred under conditions where the lipid-protein complexes carried a large net positive charge and hence could be expected to be kept well-dispersed by intervesicular electrostatic repulsion. Subsequent examination of this phenomenon has suggested a possible role for basic protein in central nervous system myelin and has led to a more detailed study of the aggregation of the protein at near-neutral pH.

EXPERIMENTAL

Human and bovine myelin basic proteins were isolated by acidification of a chloroform-methanol extract of fresh white matter: the preparation followed the method of Oshiro and Eylar (5). The small basic protein from rat was kindly supplied by Dr. P.R. Carnegie, Biochemistry Department, University of Melbourne, Australia. The

purity of the proteins was determined to be better than 99% by
electrophoresis at pH 4.3 (9) or at pH 7.2 in sodium dodecyl sulphate solution (15).

Egg L - α - diacylphosphatidylcholine (Sigma Chemical Co.,
St. Louis, U.S.A.) was verified to be homogeneous by thin-layer
chromatography. For some experiments this lipid was subjected to
further purification by preparative chromatography. Vesicles of this
lipid were prepared by sonication in a bath-type sonicator at 4°C
under nitrogen.

Light scattering was measured as the absorbance at 450 nm.
Scattering from solutions of protein and lipid alone was also
measured to enable deduction of the light-scattering caused by the
protein-lipid complex alone.

PC binding to vesicles was estimated by determination of protein concentrations in solution before and after sedimentation of
the lipid-protein complexes at approximately 90,000 x g for 2 h at
room temperature. Under these conditions no phospholipid remained
in the supernatant.

Electron micrographs were obtained on a Phillips 300 electron
microscope at 60 kV using a pH 8.5 solution of 2% ammonium molybdate
as the negative stain.

Sedimentation velocity and equilibrium experiments were carried
out in a Beckman Model E ultracentrifuge equipped with interference
and schlieren optics. Determinations of the sedimentation co-
efficient were made using a double-sector synthetic-boundary cell.

RESULTS

Experiments with purified PC showed that small amounts of basic
protein are bound almost quantitatively (Fig. 1). The amount bound
is pH dependent and varies a little from one vesicle preparation
to another; in the pH range 7.5-9 it is about 0.15 g protein/g
lipid.

In an attempt to determine the nature of the forces leading to
complex formation the pH and ionic-strength dependence of binding
was examined. Above pH 7 protein binding is insensitive to pH
variation; below this value less is bound (Table 1). It appears
unlikely that this reduction in binding is caused by increased
electrostatic repulsion between protein molecules as the association
is not significantly ionic-strength dependent (Table 2). At the
higher protein concentrations used for these binding measurements
there is some precipitation: this has been allowed for in calculating the amounts bound to the vesicles.

Above pH 6 attachment of protein to PC vesicles also causes a
large increase in the light scattering from the solution. Electron
microscopy reveals that at low ionic strength there is a 10-30 -fold
increase in vesicle size (12). In solutions containing more than
0.07 M sodium chloride far smaller increases in vesicle size are

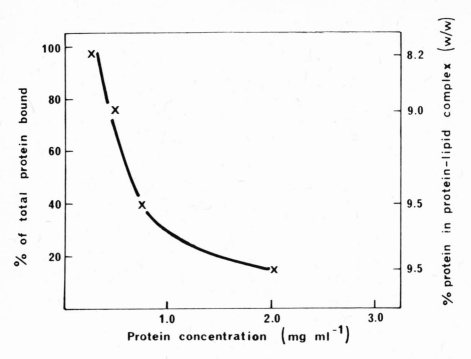

Fig. 1. Binding of human basic protein to PC vesicles at pH 8.9 in 0.10 M tris buffer. The PC concentration. was 2.88 mg.cm^{-3}.

Table 1. Effect of pH on binding of basic protein to PC vesicles. - The PC concentration was 3.64 mg/cm^3 in 0.02 M buffer containing 0.27 M sodium chloride (at pH 6.40 and 8.75) or in 0.005 M buffer (pH 5.52).

pH	Protein bound g/g lipid
5.52	0.028±0.003
6.40	0.025±0.004
8.75	0.110±0.006

Table 2. Effect of ionic strength on binding of basic protein to
PC vesicles. - The PC concentration was 3.64 mg/cm^3 in 0.02 M
buffer (pH 5.59 and 8.60) or in 0.005 M buffer (pH 5.52 and 8.67).

pH	Sodium chloride concentration (M)	Protein bound g/g lipid
5.52	0	0.028±0.003
5.59	0.27	0.032±0.003
8.67	0	0.181±0.007
8.60	0.27	0.150±0.006

observed: Fig. 2 shows the change induced by addition of human
basic protein to a solution of PC vesicles. At all ionic strengths
studied there was also a concomitant aggregation of protein-lipid
complexes (Fig. 2b). It was found that the negative stain used for
electron microscopy does not increase the light scattering of these
samples and hence it is unlikely that the observed aggregation is
an artifact introduced by the specimen preparation method adopted
for electron microscopy. This conclusion is confirmed by light
scattering studies described below.

Light scattering by PC solutions (as measured by absorbance
at 450 nm) increases as more protein is bound to the vesicles (Fig.
3). Further addition of protein beyond the level where the vesicles
are saturated with protein causes only minor scattering increases
which are attributable to precipitation of some protein.

Above an ionic strength of 0.07 light scattering increases as
salt is added to the lipid-protein complexes: this change is reversible and is presumably caused by increased aggregation (Fig. 4).

Turbidity changes caused by aggregation and by vesicle growth
are distinguished by study of the pH-dependence of scattering. In
solutions containing basic protein, PC, and 0.13 M sodium chloride,
only minor scattering increases are observed between pH 5 and pH
6, but there is a sharp rise between pH 6 and pH 9 (Fig. 5). On
reversal of this titration the scattering falls in a pattern parallel to the previous increase, but even below pH 5 it does not return
to the initial value at this pH.

It is known that reduction of PC vesicle size is achieved only
with difficulty (14)whereas disaggregation of the enlarged vesicles
should be relatively fast. The electron microscopic and scattering
studies are therefore consistent with minor vesicle growth and
aggregation as the pH is increased, with disaggregation only occurring when the pH is subsequently lowered.

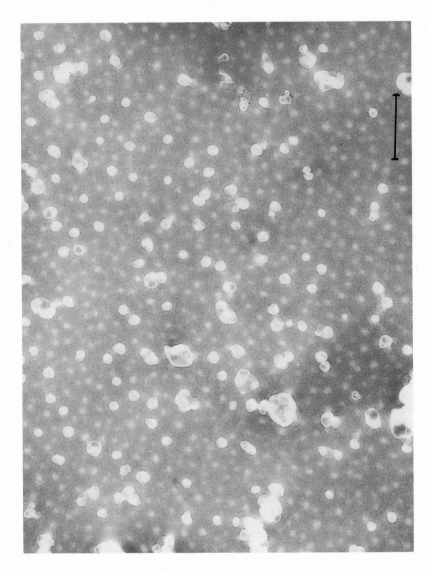

Fig. 2a

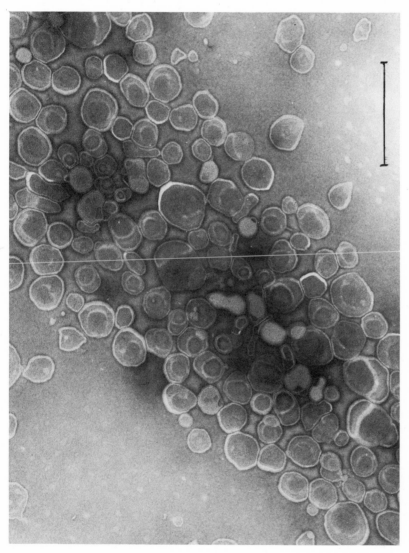

Fig. 2b. Representative electron micrographs obtained by negative staining with ammonium molybdate. Samples were taken from a solution containing (a) 7.6 mg·cm^{-3} PC at pH 8.9 in 0.002 M tris buffer, and (b) the same solution containing additionally 1.8 mg·cm^{-3} human basic protein. In both micrographs the bar in the lower right corner represents 250 nm.

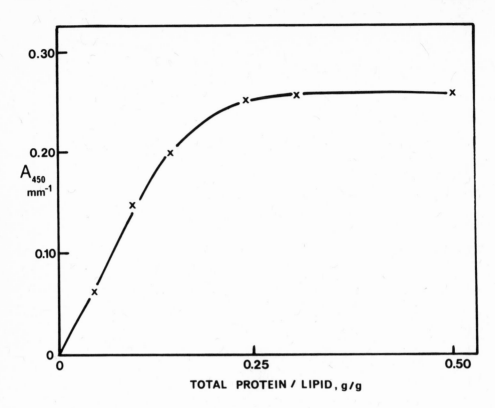

Fig. 3.   Changes in light scattering by a solution of PC vesicles
as basic protein is added. The PC concentration was 3.13 mg.cm^{-3}
in 0.10 M tris buffer at pH 8.9. Scattering caused by unbound
protein has been subtracted.

The small basic protein from rat myelin at pH 9.0 in 0.14 M
tris buffer caused similar aggregation to that induced by the human
protein. At a PC concentration of 2.4 mg.cm^{-3}, 0.47 mg.cm^{-3} human
protein raised the absorbance at 450 nm by 0.38 (mm^{-1}) above the
vesicle solution alone; the rat protein caused an increase of 0.49
at a concentration of 0.55 mg.cm^{-3}.

The demonstration that basic protein could cause vesicle
aggregation under conditions where the lipid-protein complexes
carry a large positive charge has led us to examine the self-association of the protein in more detail. As described by Liebes et al.
(4), the onset of aggregation is evident in light scattering
studies near pH 7. Fig. 6 shows that the scattering rises gradually
until just above pH 10, where it increases sharply. In the pH range
6-10 addition of 0.3 M sodium chloride causes a small but reproducible increase in scattering at a protein concentration of 2-3 mg.
cm^{-3}; at higher protein concentrations this difference is more

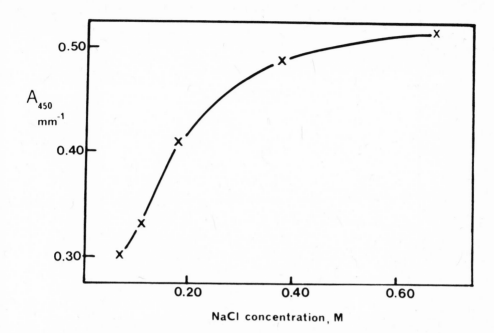

Fig. 4. Effect of ionic strength on the light scattering of PC-basic protein vesicles. The PC concentration was 2.88 mg.cm^{-3} and the protein concentration 0.44 mg.cm^{-3} in 0.001 M tris buffer, pH 8.9. Scattering from PC vesicles alone is negligible under these conditions: the curve has been corrected for scattering from unbound protein.

marked. Above pH 10 the trend reverses with a far larger turbidity in salt-free solutions. The isoelectric point of basic protein is close to 10 (10) and the precipitation at this pH is probably caused by the fluctuating charge attraction (13); this electrostatic attraction is lessened at high ionic strength. In the range pH 7-9 the protein carries a net positive charge of about 20 and the self-association exhibits an altered dependence on ionic strength, and must be caused by quite different forces.

Sedimentation equilibrium experiments yield unambiguously the weight-average molecular weight or, with auxiliary information, the association constants for oligomerization for a self-associating molecule. In such experiments the initial protein concentration is near 0.4 mg.cm^{-3}: at this concentration at pH 4.8 and 4°C bovine basic protein exhibits the expected molecular weight of 18,500, but at pH 6.8 the protein appears slightly heterogeneous with a molecular weight near 26,000. These changes indicate limited self-association at the latter pH.

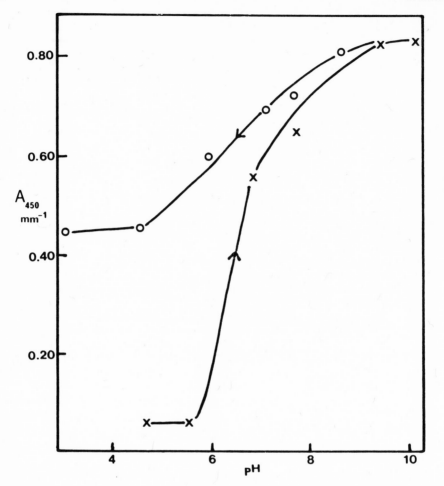

Fig. 5. Effect of pH on the turbidity of PC-basic protein vesicles.
The PC concentration was 4.0 mg.cm^{-3} and the basic protein concentration 1.93 mg.cm^{-3} in 0.4 M NaCl. Solutions were titrated
with small volumes of 2 M NaOH or HCl. Scattering due to unbound
protein has been subtracted.

     At higher concentrations at neutral pH solutions of both human
and bovine protein are turbid, showing the presence of large aggregates. However, at 5-7 mg.cm^{-3} only a minor amount of the protein
precipitates; the remainder is present as small aggregates.
Although sedimentation velocity experiments allow study of these
more concentrated solutions interpretation of the data is more
complex. At pH 7.4 in 0.30 M sodium chloride the sedimentation
co-efficient $(S_{20,w})$ of the bovine protein remaining in solution
rises from 1.20S below 1.0 mg.cm^{-3} to 1.45S at 8-10 mg.cm^{-3}. This

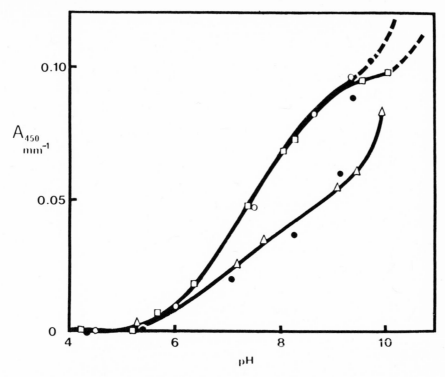

Fig. 6. Light scattering by human basic protein as a function of pH. Basic protein concentrations were 2.35 mg.cm^{-3} (□ , 0) and 2.06 mg.cm^{-3} (△ , ●) in water (o , ●) and in 0.3 M NaCl (□, △). The volume of base added during the titration was negligible.

change in the weight-average sedimentation co-efficient is also consistent with formation of dimers or small oligomers. Further experiments are being undertaken to delineate more fully the nature of this protein-protein interaction.

Some of our preparations of bovine basic protein (but not our single preparation of the human protein) have shown evidence of proteolysis when left several hours at room temperature at pH 7.4. The sedimentation velocity experiments appear unaffected by this: there was no change in the apparent sedimentation constant during the course of these experiments, which were performed at 20°C.

DISCUSSION

We have demonstrated interaction of basic protein with zwitter-ionic PC bilayer vesicles at salt concentrations up to 0.3 M, providing additional evidence that this protein can interact with lipid molecules through other than ionic bonds. But it is not this interaction _per se_ which is at present the focus of our attention. PC was chosen as the lipid for these aggregation studies because it is zwitterionic, and consequently the lipid-protein complexes are expected to be always positively charged, obviating the possibility of protein binding inducing vesicle aggregation by charge neutralization. A more specific intervesicular attraction is therefore implicated in this aggregation.

A close parallel may be drawn between the aggregation of the protein alone and of the lipid-protein complex. Light scattering from preformed pure PC vesicles is almost invariant from pH 5 to 10 whereas scattering from solutions of protein or of protein-containing vesicles increases above pH 6; the similarity of these changes is evident in Figs. 5 and 6. In solutions containing more than 0.07 M sodium chloride, where there is no large increase in vesicle size on protein addition, the scattering from the PC complexes becomes more intense as the salt concentration is increased (Fig. 4). Salt also lowers the solubility of the isolated protein. From this correlation it is inferred that the same associative forces are probably operative in both systems, vesicular aggregation being mediated by intermolecular contacts between protein molecules attached to different vesicles.

No detailed studies of the self-association of basic protein have been reported. In the pH range 6-9 this association occurs despite the large charge carried by each polypeptide chain: it is clearly distinguished from the isoelectric precipitation near pH 10 by its intensification on addition of salt. The rise in turbidity observed above pH 6 in solutions containing up to a few mg.cm^{-3}, observed also by Liebes _et al_. (4), appears to be caused by precipitation of only a small fraction of the protein. Sedimentation experiments at 5 mg.cm^{-3} in pH 7.4 buffer have revealed that the protein is present primarily as monomer and small oligomers (possibly dimers). Further sedimentation analyses are being pursued in our laboratory. Dimerization of histone IV, which is considered on the basis of sequence homology to be closely related to myelin basic protein, has also been postulated from recent NMR experiments (7).

Some progress has been made toward defining the polypeptide segments which are involved in protein-lipid and protein-protein binding. The small basic protein from rat myelin differs from the bovine and human proteins principally in that it has an internal deletion of residues 118 to 157. As it can still effect vesicular aggregation it is unlikely that either the lipid- or protein-protein binding sites are contained within the 118-157 segment of the human and bovine proteins. Digestion with intracellular proteinase, cathepsin D, is being employed in our laboratory to obtain peptides containing residues 1 to 43, 44 to 89, and 90 to 170. The self-association and lipid-binding properties of these segments will also be examined in an attempt to establish more closely which regions of the protein contain the two binding sites. Other attempts to define the amino-acids participating in protein oligomerization, using ^{1}H and ^{13}NMR spectroscopy are being made in the laboratory of Professor W.J. Moore (see this volume).

The above vesicle and protein aggregation studies have suggested a possible role for basic protein in myelin. Each protein molecule is envisaged as possessing two distinct sites one of which can interact with the hydrophobic region of lipid bilayers (this may be assisted by some electrostatic attraction if the lipids are anionic), the second is capable of binding to other protein molecules.

Recent chemical labelling experiments have shown that basic protein is confined to the intracellular surface of the myelin membrane (8). At this site the protein should be able to bring about the same non-covalent cross-linking observed *in vitro* with PC vesicles and by such bridging maintain the intracellular surfaces at the close separation observed in X-ray diffraction studies of myelin (16). Certainly it is expected that some specific attraction between the cytoplasmic membrane surfaces of the oligodendroglial cell is necessary, as has been suggested by Geren for peripheral nervous system myelin (3), to bring about fusion of these surfaces and form the long process which encircles the nerve cell axon. Myelin basic protein may fill this role, providing a molecular trigger for the sequence of events leading to myelinogenesis and serving to stabilize the highly ordered membrane array that is formed.

Acknowledgements. Thanks are extended to Drs. L.A. Littlemore and B.E. Chapman, Mr M.A. Keniry and Mr B.J. McDonald, and Professor W.J. Moore for stimulating discussions. This work was supported by the Australian Research Grants Committee.

REFERENCES

1. Anthony, J.S. and Moscarello, M.A., A conformation induced in the basic encephalitogen by lipids, Biochim. Biophys. Acta 243 (1971) 429-433.
2. Demel, R.A., London, Y., van Kessel, W.S.M.G., Vossenberg, F.G.A. and Van Deenen, L.L.M., The specific interaction of myelin basic protein with lipids at the air-water interface, Biochim. Biophys. Acta 311 (1973) 507-519.
3. Geren, B.B., The formation from the Schwann cell surface of myelin in the peripheral nerves of chick embryos, Exp. Cell. Res. 7 (1954) 558-562.
4. Liebes, L.F., Zand, R. and Phillips, W.D., Solution behaviour, circular dichroism and 220 MHz PMR studies of the bovine myelin basic protein, Biochim. Biophys. Acta 405 (1975) 27-39.
5. Oshiro, Y. and Eylar, E.H., Allergic encephalomyelitis: A comparison of the encephalitogenic A1 protein from human and

bovine brain, <u>Arch. Biochem. Biophys.</u> 138 (1970) 606-613.

6. Papahadjopoulos, D., Moscarello, M., Eylar, E.H. and Isac, T., Effects of proteins on thermotropic phase transitions of phospholipid membranes, <u>Biochim. Biophys. Acta</u> 401 (1975) 317-335.

7. Pekary, A.E., Li, H.-J., Chan, S.I., Hsu, C.-J. and Wagner, T.E., Nuclear magnetic resonance studies of histone IV solution conformation, <u>Biochemistry</u> 14 (1975) 1177-1184.

8. Poduslo, J.F. and Braun, P.E., Topographical arrangement of membrane proteins in the intact myelin sheath, <u>J. Biol. Chem.</u> 250 (1975) 1099-1105.

9. Reisfeld, R.A., Lewis, U.J. and Williams, D.E., Disk electrophoresis of basic proteins and peptides on polyacrylamide gels, <u>Nature</u> 195 (1962) 281-283.

10. Schäfer, R. and Franklin, R.M., Resistance of the basic membrane proteins of myelin and bacteriophage PM2 to proteolytic enzymes, <u>FEBS Letters</u> 58 (1975) 265-268.

11. Smith, R., The secondary structure of myelin basic protein extracted by deoxycholate, <u>Biochim. Biophys. Acta</u> 491 (1977) 581-590.

12. Smith, R., Non-covalent cross-linking of lipid bilayers by myelin basic protein: a possible role in myelin formation, <u>Biochim. Biophys. Acta</u>, in press.

13. Tanford, C., <u>Physical Chemistry of Macromolecules</u>, Wiley, New York (1961) pp. 231-233.

14. Tanford, C., <u>The Hydrophobic Effect</u>, Wiley, New York (1973) pp. 100-101.

15. Weber, K. and Osborn, M., The reliability of molecular weight determinations by dodecylsulphate-polyacrylamide gel electrophoresis, <u>J. Biol. Chem.</u> 244 (1969) 4406-4412.

16. Worthington, C.R., X-ray diffraction studies on biological membranes, <u>Current Topics in Bioenergetics</u> 5 (1973) 1-39.

MOLECULAR ORGANISATION IN CENTRAL NERVE MYELIN

A.J. Crang and M.G. Rumsby

Department of Biology, University of York

Heslington, York, YO1 5DD, U.K.

SUMMARY

Pertinent data from the literature and in press is summarised and used to construct a model for the molecular arrangement of lipid and protein in the lamellae of compact central nerve myelin. For the lipid phase of myelin the available data is best interpreted in terms of a bilayer arrangement while physical studies suggest that the lipids are in an intermediate fluid state maintained by the presence of cholesterol and water in the system. Lipids will interact to maintain this condition. The proteins of myelin differ in their membrane locations. The high molecular weight proteins are considered to be intrinsic components with at least part of their polypeptide chains in the lipid phase. The proteolipid protein is also intrinsic and may be completely buried in the lipid phase. The basic protein of myelin is an extrinsic component and must be localised at the surface of the lipid phase at either the external or cytoplasmic face of the lamellae. Present results suggest an elusive location at the cytoplasmic apposition region. The lipid-interacting properties of the basic protein are segregated on the polypeptide chain of the molecule and this may be important for the possible role of the basic protein in bridging adjacent lamellae at the cytoplasmic apposition. It is speculated that association of the proteolipid protein with the basic protein in a 1:1 molar ratio would form an effective lipid-complexing nucleus in the lipid rich myelin lamellae but experimental data to support this idea is lacking at present.

INTRODUCTION

In a recent review on structural organisation in central nerve myelin (36) an attempt has been made to summarise the relevant data on the way in which lipids and proteins are arranged in this membrane system. This communication presents some of the major points on myelin structure which now allows us to see how the individual constituents of the myelin sheath are distributed and arranged in the lamellae. An appreciation of the molecular structure of the myelin sheath is essential if we are to understand how the membrane system is degraded in both experimental and pathological demyelinating states. It should be stressed that in this report we are referring to myelin in central nerve tissue.

Myelin can be isolated in good yield and purity and thus we have a clear knowledge of the main constituents of the membrane system. Compact myelin has a unique lipid to protein ratio compared with other membranes (14) being very rich in lipid. This lipid to protein ratio of about 3:1 on a dry weight basis has led to myelin being termed a "simple" or "minimal" membrane. Myelin is, however, typical of other membrane structures in that its main constituents are lipid and protein and that its composition is designed specifically to fit its role in situ. The lipid-rich nature of compact myelin is fully in keeping with the role of the lamellae in providing insulation around the axon (15). It is our view that the way in which lipid and protein molecules interact and are organised in the myelin sheath will follow the principles now established for biological membranes in general. Our interpretation of myelin structure is based on such principles and the individual lipid and protein components of the membrane can now be considered from a structural point of view.

The chemistry of compact myelin in the central nervous system of several animal species has been well documented (e.g. 25, 26, 36). The precise information on the nature and proportions of the different constituents of myelin has facilitated a consideration of organisation in the membrane.

The lipids of myelin account for the main part of the membrane on a dry weight basis. The major lipid classes are amphipathic in nature and are cholesterol, phospholipids and glycolipids which occur in an approximately 1.25:1:0.6 molar ratio for animal species such as man, ox, guinea-pig and rat. The molar proportions of cholesterol to other amphipathic lipids are in a ratio of about 1:1.25. Cholesterol is thus not complexed with phospholipid and glycolipid completely in a 1:1 molar ratio. The high proportions of cerebroside and phosphatidyl ethanolamine are notable in the myelin sheath. It is also important to note, in a structural context, that the sphingolipids in myelin (sphingomyelin, cerebroside and cerebroside sulphate) contain high proportions of saturated and monoenoic fatty acids which have C24 chain lengths. Such long-chain acyl groups result in the sphingolipids, especially the glycosphingolipids, having considerably higher endothermic phase transitions than the glycerol-based phospholipids as reviewed by Rumsby and Crang (36).

EXPERIMENTAL STUDIES

An evaluation of the structural form of lipid in myelin has come from the application of two main techniques, X-ray diffraction and electron microscopy. X-ray diffraction analyses, which have the great advantage that they can be applied to myelin in situ in fresh nerve tissue, have provided data on myelin (Fig. 1) which can best be interpreted in terms of a bilayer arrangement for lipid in the lamellae, as reviewed by Rumsby and Crang (36). It has to be appreciated, however, that the technique produces an averaged result and the possibility that small regions of the lipid phase adopt other structural forms cannot be excluded. The bilayer interpretation is supported by the evidence from electron microscopy, notably the freeze-fracture method (e.g. 38) where the lamellar structure of the lipid-rich myelin is preserved. Alternative structural arrangements for lipid, such as the hexagonal phase are preserved through the freeze-fracture technique and produce different images from the lamellar system (e.g. 28). The best data for the structural form of lipid in myelin lamellae would seem to be principally in the bilayer arrangement. In central nerve myelin the width of the lipid phase (Fig. 1) is some 47 Å, one bilayer being separated from its adjacent bilayer at the cytoplasmic and extracellular appositions by a channel of some 30 Å and 31 Å respectively. Such channels may be water-filled with much of this water being highly structured.

Within the lipid phase in compact myelin individual classes of lipids will be arranged to suit the requirements of the membrane system in terms of gel or liquid-crystalline nature, interactions with proteins and in the maintenance of the multilamellar nature of the compact myelin where membrane surfaces approach at the external and cytoplasmic apposition sites.

There are no firm data for the arrangement of lipid classes within the two halves of the lipid bilayer but some pointers are available which may be relevant. Remembering that compact myelin is in continuity with the plasma membrane of the oligodendrocyte and with reference to the red cell plasma membrane some asymmetry of lipid components in the bilayer might be expected. By extrapolation from the red cell membrane phosphatidyl choline and sphingomyelin, the zwitterionic phospholipids, could be predominantly located on the external surface of the bilayer while we can place the acidic lipids phosphatidyl serine, phosphatidyl inositol and cerebroside sulphate on the cytoplasmic surface of the bilayer where they would be able to interact through ionic forces with the basic protein which has a favoured location at this apposition.

Studies investigating the action of small covalently-reacting probe molecules with isolated myelin suggest that some phosphatidyl ethanolamine is availabe at the external surface (6, 7, 37). Different probes yield different amounts of phosphatidyl ethanolamine exposed but the figure may be as high as 50% located at the external half of the bilayer. Experiments on the location of cerebroside in myelin are also in progress. Póduslo (33) has noted that cerebrosides become labelled in studies with galactose oxidase on an intact dorsal root preparation. Isolated myelin preparations with lamellae swollen apart in hypotonic media at the external apposition have cerebroside exposed to reaction with galactose oxidase and periodate (21). It is thus possible that this major

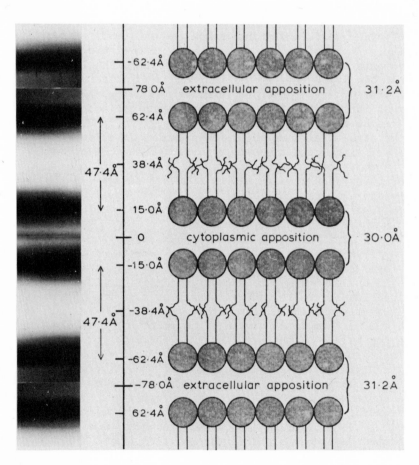

Fig. 1. Diagrammatic representation of the electron density profile of central nerve myelin as revealed by X-ray diffraction (left) and its interpretation in terms of a lipid bilayer model (right).

myelin lipid is partially located on both the external and cytoplasmic faces of the bilayer.

The role of cholesterol in animal cell plasma is seen in terms
of creating an intermediate liquid-crystalline environment in the
centre of the lipid phase. In myelin cholesterol may well perform
a similar function for the importance of this sterol and water in
maintaining a liquid-crystalline state in the lipid phase has been
demonstrated by Ladbrooke et al. (19). The observation that
hydrated myelin does not show an endothermic phase transition on
heating is taken to indicate that the lipid phase is in an intermediate fluid state which will provide for lateral mobility of
lipid and protein components in the plane of the membrane. It
should be noted, however, that cholesterol does not occur in high
enough concentration to associate with all other lipid on a 1:1
molar basis. The possibility that some phospholipid is removed
from the bulk phase by interaction with protein and thus does not
contribute to the phase transition may bring the cholesterol to
other lipid ratio to nearer to a figure of 1:1. Suggestions that
cholesterol may be asymmetrically distributed in the lipid bilayer
do not yet seem to have been substantiated.

The proteins of myelin have received wide investigation. Two
protein species comprise some 80% of the total myelin protein. The
properties of these proteins are summarised in Table 1. The minor
protein components which can be detected in central nerve myelin
preparations are, in our view, derived at least in part by a
dilution of normal proteins located in the plasma membrane of the
oligodendrocyte. Such proteins are most probably intrinsic in
nature and are embedded in the lipid phase requiring detergents
for their activation or extraction. Such proteins will be asymmetrically distributed in the lipid phase depending on their
function in the membrane system.

The proteolipid protein of myelin also has the properties of
an intrinsic protein component. Myelin has to be solubilised with
detergents or solvents to release this protein component. Certain
probe studies (reviewed in 36) suggest that a part of the proteolipid protein may be exposed at the external surface of the membrane in compact myelin. Taking the molecular weight of this
protein in central nerve myelin as 23,500 daltons (27) calculations
show that as a sphere the proteolipid protein would have a diameter
of about 38 Å (36). This size would allow the proteolipid protein
to occupy the lipid phase almost completely with a slight exposure
at the external surface (34). Proteolipid protein in this position
would be exposed by cleavage of the bilayer along the central
hydrocarbon phase in freeze-fracture studies and there is some
dispute about whether particles can be seen in the fracture plane
of myelin lamellae. In our view it is unlikely that the proteolipid
protein will be identifiable by such techniques as the small size
of the protein (38 Å) puts it on the limits of resolution for the
freeze-fracture technique (reviewed in 36). Aggregation of

Table 1. Summary of physical properties of myelin protein components. The numbers in parentheses refer to the corresponding publications in the reference list.

Protein component	Mol. wt.	Molecular size	Class (13)	Lipid interactions in model systems
Basic protein	18,400[+] (9)	Prolate ellipsoid 150x15 Å[++++] (8)	Extrinsic	Phosphatidyl serine, cerebroside, sulphate (23), triphosphoinositide (29)
Proteolipid apoprotein	23,500[++] (27)	Sphere 38 Å[++++]	Intrinsic	Cholesterol, phosphatidylcholine, cerebroside (1)
High molecular weight components	⩾50,000 (35)		Intrinsic	

[+]Bovine myelin basic protein; [++]Human myelin proteolipid apoprotein; [+++]Isolated myelin basic protein; [++++]Calculated diameter for spherical PLP, MW 23,500, partial specific volume, 0.725 cm^3G^{-1}.

proteolipid protein molecules during such a process would substantially increase the size of such a component making it more
easily identified.

The properties of the basic protein of myelin have been
frequently reviewed in detail (e.g. 3). The basic protein resembles
an extrinsic protein more closely. It can be recovered from myelin
without the use of detergents or solvents to break the lipid phase.
The basic protein is not labelled in various probe studies (e.g.
12, 34) and this is taken to be the best evidence to date that the
protein is located at the cytoplasmic apposition face in myelin
(Fig. 2). This apposition site shows a marked tendency to remain
closed under conditions when the lamellae have separated wide apart
at the external apposition region (11, 24). An indication of the
way in which lipid-interacting groups on the basic protein are
structured has been gained. Thus the N-terminal part of the
polypeptide chain favours interaction with lipid through hydrophobic
associations (22, 23). Ionic interactions with lipid occur along
the C-terminal portion of the chain (17). This distribution of
groups on the basic protein may be vital in the maintenance of the
cytoplasmic apposition region in compact myelin. We do not think
it likely that the basic protein has a dual location in compact
myelin at both the external and the cytoplasmic surfaces because
of the different mechanisms within the cell for synthesising
proteins for intracellular and extracellular use.

Fine detail about the exact molecular shape of the proteolipid
protein in myelin is lacking. In organic solvents the protein has
a high helical content and this is lost when the protein is transferred to an aqueous phase. Thus the proteolipid protein has considerable conformational flexibility. The high non-polar amino
acid content of the proteolipid protein is in keeping with the
intrinsic character of this molecule in the membrane.

Much more information is available about the basic protein
especially in isolated form. This protein is considered in aqueous
solution to have a random coil conformation as little evidence for
α-helical or β-structure can be detected (e.g. 20). The basic
protein has an open yet ordered structure in which tyrosine and
tryptophan species are largely exposed to the solvent (17). It has
been proposed that the protein adopts the form of a prolate
ellipsoid with approximate dimensions of 150x15 Å in aqueous
solution (8). A β-bend in the molecule is compatible with and is
necessary to explain the axial ratio of 10:1. The possibility that
the triproline sequence in the polypeptide chain could provide such
a bend in the molecule has been discussed (2). More recently
physical chemical studies on the isolated basic protein have indicated that intramolecular folding of the polypeptide chain occurs
in the region of residues 85-116 which are invariant for several
animal species (4). In relation to the structure of the protein
in situ in myelin it is of interest to note that in organic solvents the α-helical content of the protein is increased (e.g. 20)

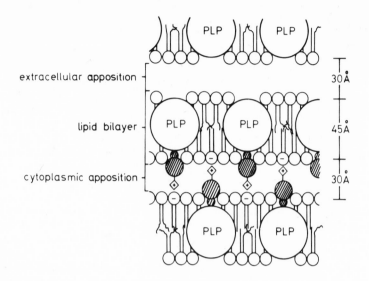

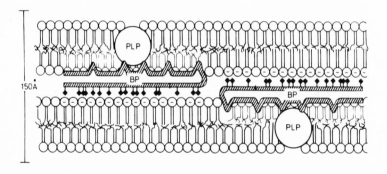

Fig. 2. (Upper) Cross-section through the proposed proteolipid
protein - basic protein subunits in compact myelin. The proteolipid protein is essentially buried within the bilayer but is
slightly exposed at the extracellular surface. The basic protein
interacts both hydrophobically and ionically between adjacent
cytoplasmic surfaces in compact myelin. (Lower) Longitudinal
section through compact myelin lamellae incorporating the basic
protein in the folded conformation as discussed in the text. This
view indicates the proposed hydrophobic penetration of the lipid
bilayer by the "amino-half" of the basic protein and the ionic
interactions across the cytoplasmic apposition by the basic residues
on the "carboxyl-half" of the molecule. Basic amino acid residues
indicated as ◆. (Reproduced from 36 with permission).

while interaction of the protein with acidic lipids on anionic detergents such as sodium dodecyl sulphate also leads to changes in the structure of the protein molecule.

Differences in the respective lipid affinities of the proteo-lipid protein and the basic protein have been well documented (e.g. 36) and are summarised in Table 1. The basic protein shows a clear preference for interaction with acidic lipid species such as phosphatidyl serine, phosphatidyl inositol and cerebroside sulphate while the proteolipid protein interacts equally well with charged and uncharged species including cholesterol. Thermal techniques have provided some understanding of how the two pro-teins influence the properties of a bulk lipid phase but it should be emphasised that the effects are observed at protein to lipid ratios which are much higher than occur normally in myelin. Inter-action of the basic protein with an acidic lipid phase causes a reduction in the temperature of the phase transition indicating an increased fluidity in the system due to partial "penetration" of protein into the acyl chain region of the lipid phase (30). No interaction with uncharged lipid species was observed. The proteolipid protein, on the other hand, on interaction with a phosphatidyl choline bulk phase causes a decrease in the enthalpy of the transition which is interpreted as indicating that lipid is bound to protein and is thus removed from the bulk lipid phase contributing to the phase transition (31). It is possible from such work to calculate that some 15 phospholipid molecules bind to each protein monomer.

Having summarised the properties of the lipid and protein components of myelin it is now possible to attempt to locate the components in the membrane system. A model showing the result is included (Fig. 2). Lipid is shown in a bilayer arrangement through-out.

As an intrinsic protein the proteolipid protein can be located within the lipid phase where its calculated diameter of 38 Å means that it will almost span the bilayer. Labelling studies suggest that the proteolipid may have some partial exposure at the external surface of the lipid phase and this feature is incorporated into the model shown in Fig. 2. The basic protein is an extrinsic component and as such could be located at either the external or the cytoplasmic apposition surface. As stated above a dual location for this protein is not favoured and, in our view, a localisation at the cytoplasmic apposition region is indicated from the probe-labelling studies of Poduslo and colleagues (12, 34). At this apposition the exclusive location of the basic protein would result in a 27% coverage of the surface of a lipid phase (calculations in 36). It should be appreciated that the opposing lipid surface will also have a 27% coverage of basic protein and thus some 54% of the total cytoplasmic apposition surface area will be occupied by the basic protein. The fluid nature of the bulk lipid phase in myelin (19) will allow ionic interactions between acidic lipid and basic protein to be maximised. High molecular weight proteins and glycoproteins in myelin as intrinsic protein species will, presumably, be located in the lipid phase at both the external and cytoplasmic faces depending on their function in situ. Glycoproteins may be located at the external appositions in the multilamellar structure of myelin.

The structuring of lipid-interacting groups along the polypeptide chain of the basic protein makes this molecule particularly suitable for a role in bridging between the two opposing lipid faces at the cytoplasmic apposition and the differing natures of the lipid interactions involved on the protein – ionic and hydrophobic – may account for the stability of this apposition region to swelling, etc. Thus a possible role for the basic protein in compact myelin may be to bring together opposing lipid faces and yet to maintain a discrete separation between them. The structure and lipid-interacting properties of the protein are compatible with such a role.

In a speculative vein we have noted (36) that in central nerve myelin the basic protein and the proteolipid protein occur in about equimolar proportions. The two proteins have distinctly different lipid-binding properties and interaction of the two proteins on a 1:1 molar basis in the membrane, probably through hydrophobic bonding, would produce a protein nucleus for binding and stabilising lipid in the membrane. Such a complex is shown in Fig. 3 though basic protein and proteolipid protein are also shown in weak association in Fig. 2. It can be calculated that with the basic protein having dimensions of 150x15 Å and the proteolipid protein of diameter 38 Å such a nucleus would have dimensions of 150x38x45 Å, the last figure being the depth of the lipid bilayer. The complete lipid-protein subunit would occupy about 80% of the myelin bilayer the distance between each unit being about 15 Å. Such spaces will be occupied by other protein components or by lipid which shows little or no affinity for either major protein species. The presence of such subunits in compact myelin may be vital for introducing long-range order and stability into this lipid-rich system.

DISCUSSION

Several questions remain to be answered about the lipids which occur in compact myelin. For example we are not yet in a position to explain the high concentration of cerebroside in myelin and to define a role for this lipid class in the membrane system. Is it the galactose moiety of this lipid class which is required to provide a non-charged headgroup which can react well with water through hydrogen bonding or are cerebrosides present because such sphingolipids provide long chain fatty acyl groups to the membrane? A possible clue to the role of such lipids in myelin can be seen in the recent report of Pascher (32) who notes that sphingolipids

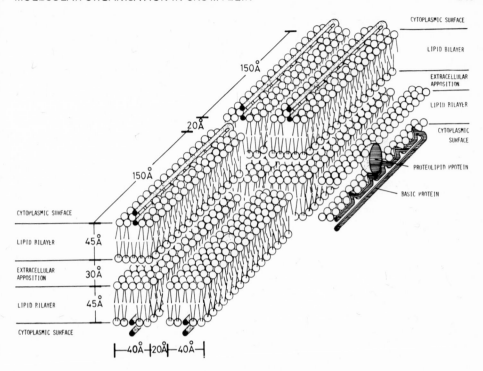

Fig. 3.   Cross-sectional perspective view of the proposed proteolipid protein-basic protein subunits in compact myelin to show the
arrangement of the component lipid molecules and the possible
packing arrangement of the subunits.

can act as hydrogen bond donors as well as acceptors while glycerol-
based lipids with ester bonds can only act as hydrogen bond
acceptors. The ability of such molecules to form lateral hydrogen
bonds within the membrane layer thus increasing membrane stability
and reducing permeability would be of relevance to the function of
the lipid-rich myelin system in its function in situ. Another
question which remains unanswered to date concerns the role of
plasmalogens in the membrane and why so much of the ethanolamine-
containing lipids are plasmalogenic in form. Such questions will,
no doubt, be answered as interest in the role of individual lipid
types in various membrane systems is persued.
     The way in which cholesterol is distributed in myelin is not
clear but we do know that this sterol has a vital function, with
water, in maintaining an intermediate fluid state in myelin. In
the membrane it is not known whether cholesterol associates

preferentially with lipids which contain more unsaturated fatty
acids (18). Such an effect could produce a non-random distribution
of cholesterol in the lipid phase. Although the molar ratio of
cholesterol to other amphipathic lipids is about 1 to about 1.3
some lipids may be removed from the bulk phase as boundary lipids
around intrinsic protein components in the membrane. Thus the true
cholesterol to other lipid ratio may be nearer the 1 to 1 situation
which is optimal for the interaction of the sterol with amphipathic
lipids. In any case the results of Clowes et al. (5) have shown
that the high transition temperature of the cerebrosides can be
reduced markedly by interaction with other amphipathic lipids such
as phosphatidyl choline up to a 1:1 molar ratio. It would seem,
however, that previous models for the arrangement of cholesterol
and phospholipid (10, 39) in a 1:1 molar association in myelin must
be reappraised now in terms of phospholipid structure, acyl chain
fluidity and the manner of cholesterol interaction.

Acknowledgements. We are grateful to The Multiple Sclerosis
Society of Great Britain and Ireland, The Wellcome Trust and the
Science Research Council for supporting our work over the years.

REFERENCES

1. Braun, P.E. and Radin, N.S., Interactions of lipids with a
    membrane structural protein from myelin, Biochem. 8 (1969)
    4310-4313.
2. Brostoff, S. and Eylar, E.H., Localisation of methylated
    arginine in the A1 protein from myelin, Proc. Natl. Acad. Sci.
    U.S. 68 (1971) 765-769.
3. Carnegie, P.R. and Dunkley, P.R., Basic proteins of central and
    peripheral nervous system myelin, in: Advances in Neurochemistry
    (B.W. Agranoff and M.H. Aprison, eds.) Vol. 1, Plenum Press,
    New York (1975) pp. 95-126.
4. Chapman, B.E. and Moore, W.J., Conformation of the myelin basic
    protein in aqueous solution from nuclear magnetic resonance
    spectroscopy, Biochem. Biophys. Res. Comm. 73 (1976) 758-766.
5. Clowes, A.W., Cherry, R.J. and Chapman, D., Physical properties
    of lecithin-cerebroside films, Biochim. Biophys. Acta 249
    (1971) 301-307.
6. Crang, A.J., Grainger, J.M. and Rumsby, M.G., Covalent probe
    investigations with central nerve myelin, in: Myelination
    and Demyelination, Recent Chemical Advances, Satellite
    Symposium of the ISN, Helsinki, August 1977.
7. Crang, A.J. and Rumsby, M.G., The labelling of lipid and
    protein components in isolated central nervous system myelin
    with dansyl chloride, Biochem. Soc. Trans. 5 (1977) 110-112.
8. Epand, R.M., Moscarello, M.A., Zierenberg, B. and Vail, W.J.,
    The folded conformation of the encephalitogenic protein of the
    human brain, Biochem. 13 (1974) 1264-1267.

9. Eylar, E.H., Amino acid sequence of the basic protein of the myelin membrane, Proc. Natl. Acad. Sci. U.S. 67 (1970) 1425-1431.

10. Finean, J.B., Phospholipid-cholesterol complex in the structure of myelin, Experientia 9 (1953) 17.

11. Finean, J.B. and Burge, R.E., The determination of the Fourier transform of the myelin layer from a study of swelling phenomena, J. Mol. Biol. 1 (1963)

12. Golds, E.E. and Braun, P.E., Organisation of membrane proteins in the intact myelin sheath, J. Biol. Chem. (1976) 4729-4735.

13. Green, D.E., Membrane proteins, Science 174 (1971) 863-867.

14. Guidotti, G., Membrane proteins, Ann. Rev. Biochem. 41 (1972) 731-752.

15. Henn, F.A. and Thompson, T.E., Properties of lipid bilayer membranes separating two aqueous phases: composition studies J. Mol. Biol. 31 (1968) 227-235.

16. Jones, A.J.S. and Rumsby, M.G., Intrinsic fluorescence properties of the myelin basic protein, J. Neurochem. 25 (1975) 565-572.

17. Jones, A.J.S. and Rumsby, M.G., Localisation of sites for ionic interaction with lipid in the C-terminal third of the bovine myelin basic protein, Biochem. J. (1977) in press.

18. de Kruyff, B., VanDijek, P.W.M., Demel, R.A., Schnijff, A., Brants, F. and van Deenen, L.L.M., Non-randon distribution of cholesterol in phosphatidyl choline bilayers, Biochim. Biophys. Acta 350 (1974) 1-7.

19. Ladbrooke, B.D., Jenkinson, T.J., Kamat, V.B. and Chapman, D., Physical studies on myelin, Biochim. Biophys. Acta 164 (1968) 101-109.

20. Liebes, L.F., Zand, R. and Phillips, W.D., Solution behaviour, circular dichroism and 220 MHz PMR studies on the bovine myelin basic protein, Biochim. Biophys. Acta (1975) 27-39.

21. Linington, C. and Rumsby, M.G., On the accessibility and localisation of cerebrosides in central nervous system myelin, in: Myelination and Demyelination, Recent Chemical Advances, Satellite symposium of the ISN, Helsinki, August 1977.

22. London, Y., Demel, R.A., Beurts van Kessel, W.S.M., Vossenberg, F.G.A. and van Deenen, L.L.M., The protection of A1 myelin basic protein against the action of proteolytic enzymes after interaction of the protein with lipids at the air-water interface, Biochim. Biophys. Acta 311 (1973) 520-530.

23. London, Y. and Vossenberg, F.G.A., Specific interaction of central nervous system myelin basic protein with lipids, Biochim. Biophys. Acta 307 (1973) 478-490.

24. McIntosh, T.J. and Robertson, J.D., Observations on the effect of hypotonic solutions on the myelin sheath in the central nervous system, J. Mol. Biol. 100 (1975) 213-217.

25. Mokrasch, L.C., Bear, R.S. and Schmitt, F.O., Myelin, Neurosciences Research Bulletin 9 (1971) 440-598.

26. Norton, W.T., Myelin: Structure and biochemistry, in: The
     Nervous System (D.B. Tower, ed.) Vol. 1, Raven Press, New
     York (1975) pp. 467-481.
27. Nussbaum, J.L., Rouayrenc, J.L., Mandel, P., Jolles, J. and
     Jolles, P., Isolation and terminal sequence determination of
     the major rat brain myelin proteolipid P7 apoprotein,
     Biochem. Biophys. Res. Comm. 57 (1974) 1240-1247.
28. Olive, J., Cryo-ultramicrotomy and freeze-etching of lipid-
     water phases, in: Freeze Etching Techniques and Applications
     (E.L. Benedetti and P. Favard, eds.) S.F.M.E., Paris (1973)
     pp. 187-198.
29. Palmer, F. and Dawson, R.M.C., The isolation and properties
     of experimental allergic encephalitogenic protein, Biochem.
     J. 111 (1969) 629-636.
30. Papahadjopoulos, D., Moscarello, M., Eylar, E.H. and Isac, T.,
     Effects of proteins on thermotropic phase transitions of
     phospholipid membranes, Biochim. Biophys. Acta 401 (1975)
     317-335.
31. Papahadjopoulos, D., Vail, W.J. and Moscarello, M., Interaction
     of a purified hydrophobic protein from myelin with phospholipid
     membranes, J. Membrane Biol. 22 (1975) 143-164.
32. Pascher, J. Molecular arrangements in sphingolipids: Conforma-
     tion and hydrogen bonding of ceramide and their implication in
     membrane stability and permeability, Biochim. Biophys. Acta
     455 (1976) 431-451.
33. Poduslo, J.F., Distribution of galactose residues in surface
     membrane glycoproteins and glycolipids of the intact myelin
     sheath, Fifth ISN Conference, Barcelona (1975) Abstract No.
     319.
34. Poduslo, J.F. and Braun, P.E., Topographical arrangement of
     membrane proteins in the intact myelin sheath, J. Biol. Chem.
     250 (1975) 1099-1105.
35. Reynolds, J.A. and Green, H.O., Polypeptide chains from porcine
     cerebral myelin, J. Biol. Chem. 248 (1973) 1207-1210.
36. Rumsby, M.G. and Crang, A.J., The myelin sheath - a structural
     examination, in: Cell Surface Reviews (G. Poste and G.L.
     Nicholson, eds.) Vol. 4, North Holland, New York (1977) in
     press.
37. Rumsby, M.G. and Grainger, J.M., Reaction of the covalently-
     binding probes trinitrobenzene sulphonic acid and dinitro-
     fluorobenzene with isolated myelin sheath preparations,
     Biochem. Soc. Trans. 5 (1977) in press.
38. daSilva, P.P. and Miller, R.G., Membrane particles on fracture
     faces of frozen myelin, Proc. Natl. Acad. Sci. U.S. 72 (1975)
     404-406.
39. Vandenheuvel, F.A., Biological structure at the molecular level
     with stereomodel projections, J. Am. Oil Chem. Soc. 40 (1963)
     455-472.

COVALENT PROBE INVESTIGATIONS WITH ISOLATED CENTRAL NERVE MYELIN

PREPARATIONS

A.J. Crang, Jacqueline Grainger and M.G. Rumsby

Department of Biology, University of York

Heslington, York, YO1 5DD, U.K.

SUMMARY

The interaction of the covalently reacting probes dansyl chloride, fluorodinitrobenzene and trinitrobenzene sulphonic acid with isolated central nerve myelin sheath preparations has been studied. The three probes interact preferentially with accessible amino groups on lipid and protein in the membrane. With isolated myelin some 13% of the total phosphatidyl ethanolamine is labelled with dansyl chloride while the figure is 66% with fluorodinitro benzene and 47% with trinitrobenzene sulphonic acid. Lower levels of phosphatidyl serine are labelled. Phosphatidyl ethanolamine seems to be more accessible to probes in the myelin sheath than is phosphatidyl serine perhaps because the ethanolamine-containing lipid class is localised partially at the external apposition surfaces of the membrane which are most accessible to the probes. The serine phospholipids may not react so well because they are preferentially distributed at the cytoplasmic surface of the system. Analysis of protein labelling patterns after reaction of intact myelin with dansyl chloride indicates that the high molecular weight proteins and the proteolipid protein is accessible to the probe while the basic protein is not, even though this latter component is readily labelled with dansyl chloride in purified form. It is suggested that the inability of the basic protein to react with myelin is perhaps due to the fact that it is occluded from inter- action with the probe at the cytoplasmic apposition surfaces of the lamellae.

INTRODUCTION

The use of covalently-reacting probe molecules in the study
of the surface architecture of membranes has yielded significant
data on the asymmetric organisation of lipid and protein components
in a variety of membrane systems (10). Carraway (1) and Hubbard
and Cohn (5) have comprehensively reviewed the use of probe molecules
in such work.

This approach can be applied to the myelin sheath to elucidate
details of the surface structure of the lamellar system in health,
during development and in disease. Already Poduslo and colleagues
(4, 8, 9) have used probe methods with lactoperoxidase, galactose
oxidase and pyridoxal phosphate applying them to the intact dorsal
column from the spinal cord. Labelling of proteins, glycoproteins
and glycolipids has been described under a variety of reaction
conditions. This system, however, may not be fully representative
of compact myelin and may bear more relation to a membrane structure
which is intermediate in composition between the oligodendroglial
cell plasma membrane and compact myelin. In another approach Wood
et al. (13) have labelled isolated human myelin with tritiated
4,4'-diisothiocyano-2,2'-ditritio stilbene disulphonic acid (DIDS)
to examine the disposition of proteins in the membrane. In this
work lyophilised resuspended myelin samples were used for labelling
and we have already (11) referred to the problems which may occur
when myelin samples are dehydrated. In our view freshly isolated
myelin should be used for labelling studies. Only then can the
rearrangements of lipid and protein which may occur in the membrane
due to the removal of water be overcome.

We are studying the interaction of dansyl chloride (DC),
fluorodinitrobenzene (FDNB) and trinitrobenzene sulphonic acid
(TNBS) with isolated central nerve myelin preparations. In such
samples we consider that a uniform surface of the membrane system,
the external surface, is presented to the probe. During treatment
of myelin in hypotonic media separation of the lamellae only occurs
at the external apposition (the intraperiod dense line of electron
micrographs) while the cytoplasmic apposition remains closely
opposed (3, 6, 7). Some initial findings on the interaction of
these three covalently-binding probes with isolated myelin have been
described previously (2, 12) and are continued in this report. Some
details of the interaction of the probes with amino group-containing
phospholipids in purified form are included for such studies yield
important data on how the probes react with lipids free of constraint
in the membrane situation.

EXPERIMENTAL

The probes. The three probes in use all react covalently with
available amino groups on lipid and protein under the correct
conditions while other groups such as -OH and -SH may react. The

REAGENT	CLASS	REACTIVE GROUPS	REACTION CONDITIONS
Dansyl chloride m.w. 270 7 x 12 A 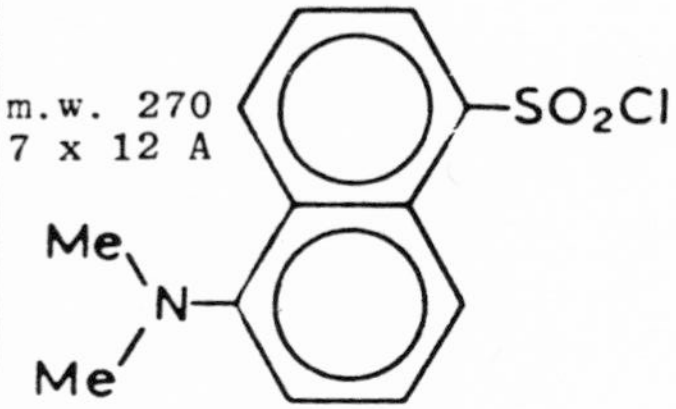	Permeant	$-NH_2$ $-OH$ $-SH$	10mM Tris/HCl or 10mM bicarbonate buffer, pH 8.3. Dansyl chloride introduced as 10% (w/v) solution in acetone. Final acetone concentration in reaction buffer does not exceed 2.5% (v/v). Reaction followed up to 16 hours.
Fluorodinitrobenzene 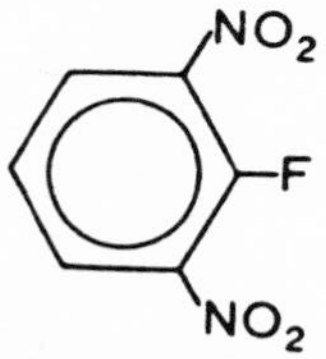 m.w. 186 7 x 10 A	Permeant	$-NH_2$ $-OH$ $-SH$	120mM sodium bicarbonate/40mM sodium chloride buffer, pH 8.3. FDNB introduced as water-immiscible liquid. Reaction followed up to 24 hours.
Trinitrobenzene sulphonic acid 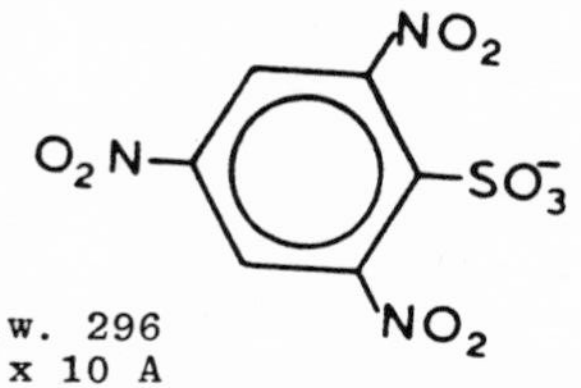 m.w. 296 9 x 10 A	Impermeant	$-NH_2$	120mM sodium bicarbonate/40mM sodium chloride buffer, pH 8.3. TNBS introduced as solid, water soluble. Reaction followed up to 24 hours.

Fig. 1. Summary of properties and reaction conditions of covalent probes used to label myelin.

structure, size, some properties and the reaction conditions for the three probes are summarised in Fig. 1. It is vital to be certain of the permeant or impermeant nature of the probes used in this approach to membrane structure. The available evidence suggests that dansyl chloride and FDNB are permeant to lipid layers while TNBS, reacting in bicarbonate buffer at pH 8.3, is impermeant. The use of probes with different permeability characteristics is important for it increases the data on the accessibility of amino groups at the surfaces of the multilamellar membrane system. It is probable, however, that the penetrability of a small probe molecule through a lipid layer has to be worked out for the specific membrane system under investigation.

For myelin lipids the three probes should chiefly report on the disposition of phosphatidyl ethanolamine (PE) and phosphatidyl serine (PS) in the membrane. Probe-lipid complexes can be separated from unlabelled lipid by thin-layer chromatography as the R_f properties of the labelled compound differ from the pure lipid component. Further the probes possess different characteristic features. Dansyl-lipids can be detected by their fluorescence while DNB- and TNB-lipids are yellow. The reaction conditions for the probes are summarised in Fig. 1 and the general methodology for interaction with myelin is set out in Table 1. It is essential that reaction of the probe is terminated before the myelin is disrupted with solvent or detergent for analysis for artifactual post-disruption labelling could occur. We avoid this possibility as shown in Table 1 by the use of repeated centrifugation to separate probe-labelled membrane from free unreacted probe when reactions are terminated.

RESULTS AND DISCUSSION

Reaction of the probes with pure lipid systems. The reaction of dansyl chloride, FDNB and TNBS with amino group-containing phospholipids in pure and mixed lipid dispersions has been studied to give information on the accessibility of amino groups on these lipids under controlled conditions. It provides data on the way in which headgroup accessibility is influenced by the presence of adjacent lipid molecules of similar and different form. This is important for an understanding of how the probes react with PE and PS in the myelin membrane.

The reaction of dansyl chloride with phosphatidyl ethanolamine in mixed PE/sphingomyelin dispersions at pH 9 and 17°C is shown in Fig. 2. Within about 100 minutes some 80% of the available PE reacts to give the dansyl-PE product and this represents the limit of the reaction. The reaction of PS and PE dispersions with FDNB and TNBS at pH 8.3 and 20°C is shown in Fig. 3. With PS the permeant FDNB labels over 60% of the available lipid amino groups in six hours and nearly 100% in 22 hours. On the other hand TNBS reacts to a more limited extent some 30% of the lipid complexing in six hours

Table 1. Reaction scheme showing the interaction of covalent probes
with isolated myelin preparations and for the termination of the
reaction and removal of unreacted probe prior to membrane disruption.

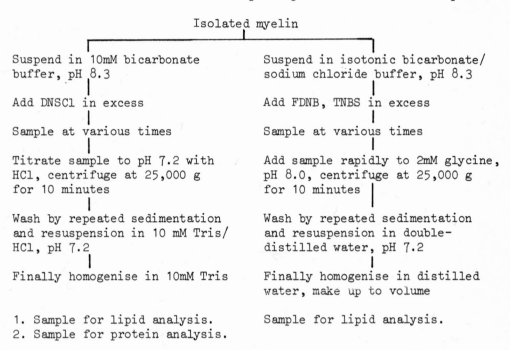

Isolated myelin

Suspend in 10mM bicarbonate buffer, pH 8.3	Suspend in isotonic bicarbonate/ sodium chloride buffer, pH 8.3
Add DNSCl in excess	Add FDNB, TNBS in excess
Sample at various times	Sample at various times
Titrate sample to pH 7.2 with HCl, centrifuge at 25,000 g for 10 minutes	Add sample rapidly to 2mM glycine, pH 8.0, centrifuge at 25,000 g for 10 minutes
Wash by repeated sedimentation and resuspension in 10 mM Tris/ HCl, pH 7.2	Wash by repeated sedimentation and resuspension in double- distilled water, pH 7.2
Finally homogenise in 10mM Tris	Finally homogenise in distilled water, make up to volume
1. Sample for lipid analysis. 2. Sample for protein analysis.	Sample for lipid analysis.

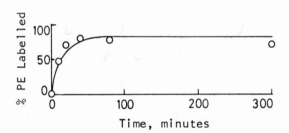

Time, minutes

Fig. 2. Reaction of phosphatidyl ethanolamine in phosphatidyl
ethanolamine/sphingomyelin dispersions with dansyl chloride. PE/
sphingomyelin dispersions were prepared in 10mM Tris/40mM sodium
chloride, pH 9.0, by sonication at 17°C for 20 minutes. Large
aggregates in the suspension were removed by centrifugation at
150,000 g for 60 minutes. Samples were taken at intervals and the
labelling reaction was stopped by titrating the buffer to pH 7.2
with 1N HCl. Lipid extracts were prepared by a Folch wash of the
reaction buffer.

and this increasing to about 45% overnight. With PE both probes
show very similar reaction effects complexing with some 60% of the
lipid in six hours and this increasing only very little more overnight.

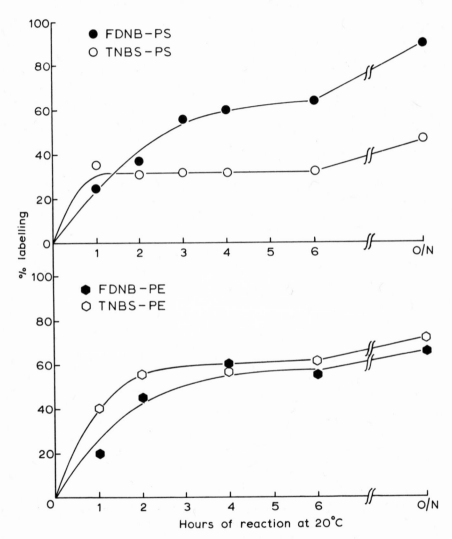

Fig. 3. Reaction of PE and PS dispersions with FDNB and TNBS.
Lipid dispersions were prepared in bicarbonate buffer by sonication
for 60 min at 18°C as described elsewhere (12). Probe concentration
was 2mM and the reaction was in the dark. At specific time intervals
aliquots of the reaction were removed and added to acid to terminate
the reaction. Lipids were recovered in a Folch wash system. Free
and probe-bound PE and PS were separated by thin-layer chromatography
and were quantitated by phosphate analysis.

These results of the probes with pure lipid systems are of interest for they tend to suggest for the dansyl chloride that some 20% of the PE in the mixed system (Fig. 2) is unavailable for reaction. The exact form of the mixed lipid dispersion is not clear, _i.e._ it may be multilamellar unsealed fragments or uni-lamellar or multilamellar sealed vesicles. The fact that some PE does not react with the probe suggests shielding of amino groups by adjacent lipid molecules, rather than that the probe cannot penetrate to some of the lipid. With pure PE dispersions which are thought to be in the form of unsealed multilamellar fragments, some 40% of the lipid does not react and must be shielded from interaction with the small probe molecules. It is probable that the mixture of PE with other amphipathic lipids increases the reactivity of individual PE molecules by dispersing them in the mixed lipid phase. With pure phosphatidyl serine liposomes the results (Fig. 3) suggest that TNBS is impermeable and can only react with amino groups on the outer surfaces of the vesicles. FDNB, on the other hand, by reacting with over 60% of the lipid molecules would seem able to penetrate the vesicles and react with headgroups on the inside of the liposomes. PE and PS headgroups in lipid dispersions thus show different reactivities to FDNB and TNBS. Further the permeability of FDNB through PE layers may be questionable.

Reaction of probes with lipids in isolated myelin samples. When purified myelin samples are reacted with dansyl chloride some 13% of the total PE becomes labelled (Fig. 4) even with long time exposures to the probe. Although dansyl-PS can be detected by fluorescence it was not detected by phosphorus assay. This puts the extent of PS labelling by dansyl chloride at less than 6% of the total PS available. The reaction of FDNB and TNBS with PE and PS in myelin is shown in Figs. 5 and 6. Considerably more labelling of lipids is detected with these probes than has been noted for dansyl chloride. Some 47% of the available PE is labelled

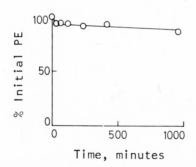

Fig. 4. Reaction profile for the labelling of PE in isolated myelin samples by dansyl chloride. 3.25 mg dansyl chloride was added as a 13% (w/v) solution in acetone to 90 mg myelin in 10 ml bicarbonate buffer. Reaction monitored at 20°C. Samples were taken and washed free of unreacted reagent as described in Table 1.

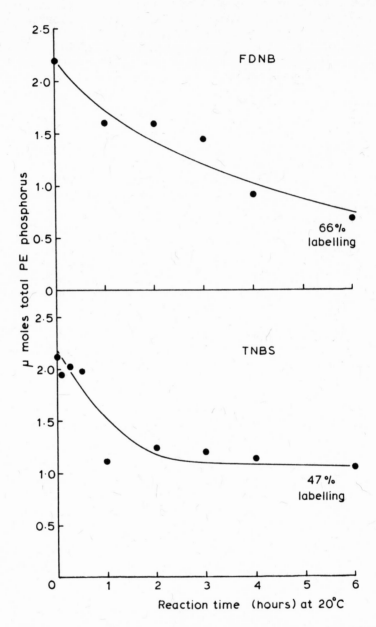

Fig. 5. Reaction of PE in isolated myelin samples with FDNB and TNBS. Fresh myelin (44 mg) in 100 ml bicarbonate/saline buffer (12) was made 2mM with respect to probe and then treated as shown in Table 1.

by the impermeant TNBS and this figure seems to represent a maximum.
With FDNB, however, the figure for PE labelling is 66% and this
level seems to be increasing with time, perhaps as the FDNB penetrates through the lipid phase of the membrane system. Both probes
label some 20 to 25% of the available PS in a six-hour-period the
reaction again tending to plateau out with TNBS but to continue with
FDNB.

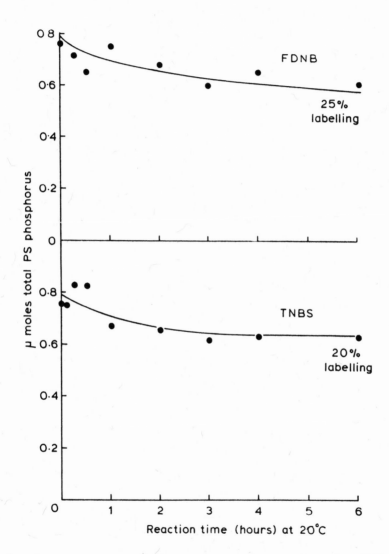

Fig. 6. Reaction of PS in isolated myelin samples with FDNB and
TNBS. Fresh myelin (44 mg) in 100 ml bicarbonate/saline buffer
(12) was made 2mM with respect to probe and treated as shown in
Table 1.

These results on the interaction of small probes with isolated
myelin samples provide some differences in interpretation in relation
to the accessibility and disposition of PE and PS in the system but
this will become easier when we have clarified how each probe penetrates into the isolated membrane system in which many of the fragments retain their multilamellar nature. The results do, however,
show that, in contrast to the pure lipid situation, PE labels more
readily than does PS with all three probes used and that even with
a supposedly impermeable probe like TNBS some 40 to 50% of the
available PE is labelled. As we consider that the preparation has
the external face of the membrane exposed to the medium it is
tempting to infer that a substantial proportion of the myelin PE is
localised at this surface. However, the reason why dansyl chloride
labels only some 13% of the PE while the other probes label much
increased levels is not understood at present. The way in which
the probes are presented to the membrane, dansyl chloride being
added in acetone solution (Fig. 1) may influence reactivity with the
membrane system. Again, FDNB and TNBS show a greater reaction with
PS in myelin than does dansyl chloride and this observation also
needs further investigation. It is tempting to speculate that the
lower level of PS labelling compared with PE indicates that the
bulk of this lipid is occluded from reaction with the probes by
localisation at the cytoplasmic apposition surface in the membrane.
We have yet to determine whether the probes can displace lipids
such as PS from reaction with proteins in a membrane so that an
artifactually high level of labelling is registered. Experiments
with model systems should clarify this point.

Interaction of probes with proteins in isolated myelin samples.
Thus far only the interaction of dansyl chloride with isolated
myelin samples has been studied in some depth (2) although it is
clear that the total proteins of myelin do acquire some label when
FDNB or TNBS are used. Such samples have yet to be analysed. With
dansyl chloride the evidence would tend to suggest that the high
molecular weight proteins and the proteolipid protein of myelin
react with dansyl chloride in the isolated membrane preparation
while the basic protein is not accessible. When dansyl chloride-
labelled myelin is solubilised in sodium dodecyl sulphate and
separated by gel filtration chromatography on a Sephadex G-200
column the elution profile shown in Fig. 7 is obtained. As described
previously (2) the resolution of the dansyl-fluorescence elution
profile from this system was facilitated by the different emission

---

Fig. 7. Separation of protein and phospholipid from myelin after
reaction of the intact preparation with dansyl chloride. Myelin,
after exposure to probe for 2 h at 4°C, was washed by repeated
centrifugation. The washed myelin was solubilised in a 7-fold
weight excess of sodium dodecyl sulphate. Myelin proteins were
separated on a calibrated Sephadex G-200 column eluted with 0.2%
SDS in 10mM Tris/HCl buffer pH 7.2 in 40mM NaCl. Fractions were
assayed for protein, phospholipid and for dansyl fluorescence.

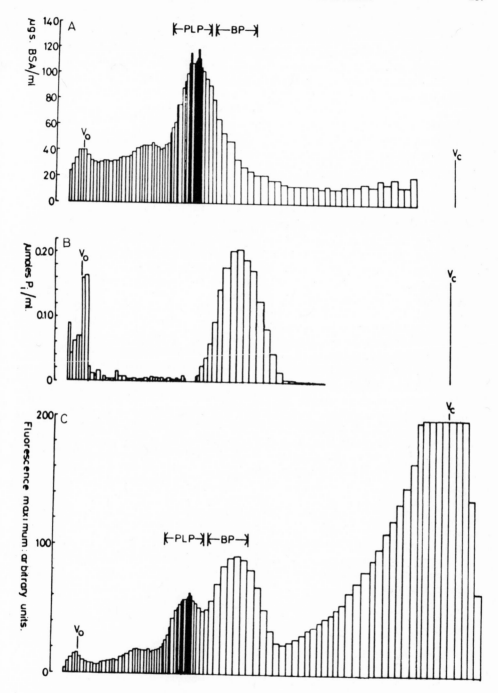

Fig. 7

characteristics of the dansyl-protein and the dansyl-lipid con-
jugates. The data indicate that dansyl chloride gives a significant labelling of the high molecular weight proteins and of the
proteolipid protein. The basic protein, however, does not become
labelled even though the molecule will in purified form out of the
membrane (P.R. Dunkley, personal communication).

This labelling result with the proteins is consistent with the
findings of Poduslo and colleagues (4, 8, 9). High molecular
weight and proteolipid proteins of myelin are exposed to probes
while the basic protein is not. Similarly Wood et al. (13)
have noted that with lyophilised resuspended myelin labelled with
DIDS the specific activity of the proteolipid protein is some ten
times greater than that of the basic protein even though the basic
protein labelled to a much greater extent than the proteolipid
protein in isolated form. Our results would tend to suggest that
high molecular weight proteins and the proteolipid protein are
accessible to probe at the external surface of the myelin preparation
and that the basic protein is occluded from interaction. The most
likely explanation for this is that the basic protein is situated
at the cytoplasmic apposition region of the membrane where it is
not accessible to the probes and where its amino groups may be
shielded by interaction with acidic lipids such as phosphatidyl
serine and phosphatidyl inositol and cerebroside sulphate.

Conclusions. It is felt that the results gained thus far with
these methods warrant further investigation and study as a means of
investigating ultrastructure in the myelin sheath. The preliminary
findings can be fitted into a model for myelin in which the basic
protein is localised at the cytoplasmic apposition (the main dense
line in electron micrographs) of the multilamellar membrane system
while the other main protein, the proteolipid protein and the high
molecular weight components are mainly localised at the external
apposition surface. The data would also suggest that PE and PS are
asymmetrically distributed in the lamellae with a substantial
proportion of the PE being localised on the external surface of the
system and the PS perhaps being preferentially located at the cytoplasmic surface. These findings and others have been discussed in
terms of myelin ultrastructure elsewhere in this book.

Acknowledgements. We thank The Wellcome Trust, the Science
Research Council and The Multiple Sclerosis Society of Britain for
supporting our work.

REFERENCES

1. Carraway, K.L., Covalent labelling of membranes, Biochim.
    Biophys. Acta 415 (1975) 379-410.
2. Crang, A.J. and Rumsby, M.G., The labelling of lipid and protein
    components in isolated central nervous system myelin with dansyl
    chloride, Biochem. Soc. Trans. 5 (1977) 110-112.
3. Finean, J.B. and Burge, R.E., The determination of the Fourier
    transform of the myelin layer from a study of swelling

phenomena, <u>J. Mol. Biol</u>. 1 (1963) 672-682.

4. Golds, E.E. and Braun, P.E., Organisation of membrane proteins in the intact myelin sheath, <u>J. Biol. Chem</u>. 251 (1976) 4729-4735.

5. Hubbard, A.L. and Cohn, Z.A., Specific labels for cell surfaces, in <u>Biochemical Analysis of Membranes</u> (A.H. Maddy, ed.) Chapman & Hall, London (1976) pp. 427-501.

6. Linington, C. and Rumsby, M.G., On the accessibility and localisation of cerebrosides in central nervous system myelin, in <u>Myelination and Demyelination, Recent Chemical Advances,</u> Satellite symposium of the ISN, Helsinki, August 1977.

7. McIntosh, T.J. and Robertson, J.D., Observations on the effect of hypotonic solutions on the myelin sheath in the central nervous system, <u>J. Mol. Biol</u>. 100 (1976) 213-217.

8. Poduslo, J.F. and Braun, P.E., Topographical arrangement of membrane proteins in the intact myelin sheath, <u>J. Biol. Chem.</u> 250 (1975) 1099-1105.

9. Poduslo, J.F., Quarles, R.H. and Brady, R.O., External labelling of galactose in surface membrane glycoproteins of the intact myelin sheath, <u>J. Biol. Chem</u>. 251 (1976) 153-158.

10. Rothman, J.E. and Lenard, J., Membrane asymmetry, <u>Science</u> 195 (1977) 743-753.

11. Rumsby, M.G. and Crang, A.J., The myelin sheath - a structural examination, <u>Cell Surface Reviews</u>, in press.

12. Rumsby, M.G. and Grainger, J.M., Reaction of the covalently-binding probes trinitrobenzene sulphonic acid and fluoro-dinitrobenzene with isolated myelin sheath preparations, <u>Biochem. Soc. Trans</u>, in press.

13. Wood, D.D., Epand, R.M. and Moscarello, M.A., Localisation of the basic protein and lipophilin in the myelin membrane with a non-penetrating reagent, <u>Biochim. Biophys. Acta</u> 467 (1977) 120-129.

ON THE ACCESSIBILITY AND LOCALISATION OF CEREBROSIDES IN CENTRAL

NERVOUS SYSTEM MYELIN

Christopher Linington and Martin G. Rumsby

Department of Biology, University of York

Heslington, York, YO1 5DD, U.K.

SUMMARY

Cerebrosides are concentrated in the myelin sheath where they account for about 20% of the total lipid of the membrane. The present paper is concerned with the role and localisation of these glycolipids in the myelin lamellae. Isolated central nerve myelin preparations have been treated with two probes to investigate cerebroside accessibility in the membrane. The action of galactose oxidase on the galactose headgroups of cerebrosides is followed and quantitated by recovery of the modified glycolipid and resolution of either the 6-aldehydo sugar or galactose remaining by gas-liquid chromatography. With isolated myelin preparations only some 40-50% of the cerebroside galactose is attacked by galactose oxidase at $20°C$. With periodate at $20°C$ over 90% of the galactose headgroups are oxidised in 3 h while the figure is 50-55% over the same time period at $4°C$ rising to 85% after 22 h. With multilamellar liposomes of mixed myelin lipids only some 20-25% of the available cerebroside is oxidised at $4°C$, the reaction being complete in 2 h. The results are discussed in relation to the disposition of cerebroside in the myelin lamellae. A major location on the external face of the membrane system (intraperiod dense line) is favoured. A role for cerebroside in myelin in terms of increasing the stability and resistance of the lipid phase to ion movement is suggested.

INTRODUCTION

One of the main characteristics of the myelin sheath in central nerve tissue is the high content of cerebroside which is

located in the membrane system. Cerebrosides and cerebroside
sulphate account for some 20% of the total lipid of the myelin
sheath from a variety of animal species. In no other natural
membrane system is this glycolipid class present in such high
levels. Yet we know little about the role of cerebrosides in
myelin and why such lipids are concentrated in the membrane. Our
studies on cerebrosides in myelin are directed to answering two
main questions which concern the role of cerebrosides as structural
components of compact myelin and how cerebrosides are localised in
the lipid phase of the membrane. Some preliminary results and
thoughts are presented in this communication.

Cerebrosides in myelin are characterised by a galactose headgroup and long chain saturated and monoenoic fatty acids some of
which contain an additional hydroxyl group at the 2-position of the
acyl chain. Cerebrosides are amphipathic lipids like the phospholipids of myelin but, unlike lipids such as phosphatidyl ethanolamine and phosphatidyl serine, cerebrosides carry no charge on the
headgroup. Yet these glycolipids form bilayer structures in an
aqueous phase (1) for the headgroup interacts with water by
hydrogen bonding.

The presence of long chain fatty acids in cerebrosides gives
the lipid a high phase transition temperature which is around $70^{o}C$
for cerebrosides in the hydrated state (7). The position of the
transition can be reduced by interaction of cerebroside with
cholesterol (10) or with phospholipids such as phosphatidyl choline
(3). The properties of cerebrosides in relation to their function
in the myelin sheath have been reviewed by Rumsby and Crang (14).

EXPERIMENTAL STUDIES

In the work described here in preliminary form we have examined
the way in which cerebrosides can be attacked in purified central
nerve myelin sheath preparations. Thus the accessibility of
cerebrosides in the membrane is being explored. To undertake this
aspect of the project two probes have been used which differ widely
in size. Thus the action of galactose oxidase (55,000 daltons)
is compared with that of sodium periodate, a small permeant probe
molecule. Both probes attack the galactose headgroup of cerebrosides. These two probes are being used with isolated myelin preparations in this report. Subsequently we shall go on and react
the probes with myelin in situ thus isolating the myelin for
analysis.

An important appreciation in this work with isolated myelin is
the view that a uniform face of the membrane, the external apposition
surface, is presented to the medium and thus to the probe during
labelling studies. Finean and Burge (4) and McIntosh and Robertson
(9) have shown that when myelin is treated with hypotonic media
the lamellae swell apart and separate only at the external apposition
region. The cytoplasmic apposition remains tightly opposed. During

the purification of myelin we see that splitting of lamellae occurs
exclusively at the external apposition (Fig. 1) to provide a uniform
labelling surface.

    Treatment with galactose oxidase. Poduslo et al. (13) have
studied the reaction of galactose oxidase with an intact dorsal
root preparation. Labelling of glycoproteins has been noted. Some
labelling of cerebrosides has also been reported (12). This has
been confirmed in the present work as is shown in Table 1 where
tritiated sodium borohydride reduction of oxidised galactose headgroups on cerebrosides has been employed to detect enzyme action.
It is difficult to obtain any quantitative estimate of the levels
of cerebroside attacked using this approach. However, the results
do show that radioactivity appears in cerebrosides indicating exposure of the galactose headgroup to the enzyme.

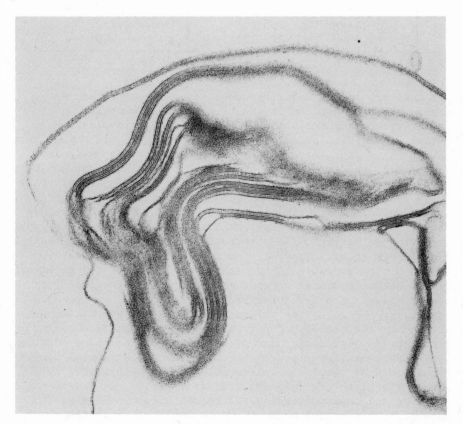

Fig. 1. Bovine brain myelin isolated by the method of Rumsby et al.
(15). Fixed with 3% glutaraldehyde and osmium tetroxide, then
stained with uranyl acetate and lead citrate. x 70,000.

Table 1.   Incorporation of tritium into the cerebrosides of isolated
bovine myelin by reduction with tritiated $NaBH_4$ after treatment with
galactose oxidase. - 75 mg of myelin (dry wt.) was incubated with
900 units of galactose oxidase and 3,000 units of catalase in 10 ml
of 0.1 M phosphate buffer, pH 7.2, at $25^\circ C$. At appropriate intervals
1.0 ml aliquots were removed and incubated with 5 mCi of tritiated
$NaBH_4$ for 5 min at $0^\circ C$, the lipids were then extracted by standard
techniques. The cerebrosides were isolated by thin-layer chromatography on silica gel H plates run in chloroform:methanol (185:15,
v/v) and were then scraped off the plates and counted.

Time (min)	D.p.m. per cerebroside spot		Specific incorporation of H^3 into cerebrosides (d.p.m./mg total lipid)
	Control	Experimental	
0	53,540	53,939	0
30	42,530	46,948	3,192
90	39,218	55,633	11,253
300	48,459	109,337	45,229

We have previously described how the action of galactose
oxidase on cerebrosides can be quantitated using a method which
does not involve radioactivity but which, rather, involves the
estimation of modified galactose residues by gas-liquid chromatography (GLC) (8). Thus, after galactose oxidase action on isolated
myelin samples, the cerebroside component of the lipid extract is
isolated and the unmodified galactose and the 6-aldehydo galactose
(produced by the action of the enzyme) are isolated and analysed
in derivative form. Quantitation of peaks resolved on GLC can be
effected with a suitable internal standard. In Fig. 2 a time course
experiment of galactose oxidase activity on isolated bovine central
nerve myelin is shown. The reaction was at $20^\circ C$ and shows that
after some 5 h of exposure to the enzyme about 50% of the galactose
headgroups become modified through enzyme action. The reaction
seems to plateau out after three hours.

Following the galactose oxidase reaction this way has been
complicated by the variety of derivative peaks produced during
splitting of the glycosidic bond of the cerebrosides and production
of forms for chromatography. It occurred to us that a much simpler
technique would be simply to follow galactose disappearance by GLC
using cholesterol as the internal standard. This idea has been
investigated and seems promising. A result is shown in Fig. 2.
The data from this method seem to agree very well with the other
route in which oxidised galactose moieties are examined. Again the
results show that galactose oxidase attacks some of the membrane
cerebroside and that some 45% of cerebroside headgroups become
modified in 5 h exposure to the enzyme at $20^\circ C$. Some 45-50% of the
myelin cerebroside is thus accessible to this enzyme.

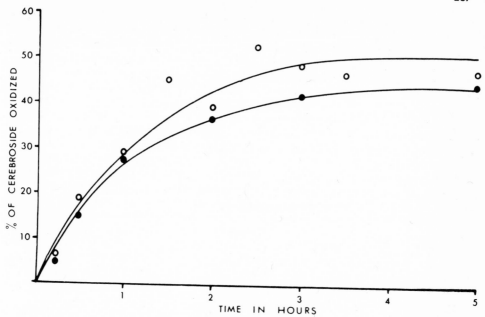

Fig. 2. The reaction of galactose oxidase with the cerebrosides of isolated bovine myelin. - Bovine myelin, isolated by the method of Rumsby et al. (15) was suspended in 10 mM phosphate buffer, pH 7.4, to give a final concentration of 5 mg (dry wt.) per ml. Galactose oxidase and catalase were added to give final concentrations of 300 and 500 units/ml, respectively, and the reaction mixture was then incubated at 20°C. At appropriate intervals aliquots were removed and the lipids extracted by standard procedures; the level of oxidation of the cerebroside headgroup was estimated by two procedures: (1) The total cerebrosides were isolated by thin-layer chromatography and their methyl galactosides prepared and purified, prior to analysis by GLC as their trimethylsilyl esters. The level of oxidation is calculated from the ratio of the oxidised to unoxidised galactosides relative to mannitol as an internal standard (8). (2) The total lipid is subjected to methanolysis and the total methanolysate analysed by GLC, the reaction can then be followed by measuring the loss of galactose relative to the cholesterol content of the lipid extract.

This approach has now been used on several different myelin preparations, all isolated from bovine central nerve tissue, with good agreement showing that some 36-50% of the cerebroside is attacked by the galactose oxidase. The enzyme can thus penetrate

to cerebroside in the isolated myelin sample. It should be stressed
that the reaction is carried out with myelin in hypotonic phosphate
buffer, 10 mM and pH 7.4, so that lamellae will be swollen apart at
the external apposition layer. The approach has now to be applied
to myelin from other sources and to myelin in situ followed by
purification of the membrane system.

Treatment with sodium periodate. When isolated myelin samples
are reacted with a molar excess of sodium periodate in 10 mM
phosphate buffer, pH 7.4, with the reaction in the dark at either
4°C or 20°C there is a rapid degradation of galactose headgroups
on cerebroside (Fig. 3). At 20°C some 90% of the cerebroside is
oxidised within 3 h while at 4°C this figure is about 50-55%. With
longer exposure times virtually all the galactose located on
cerebroside in myelin is attacked.

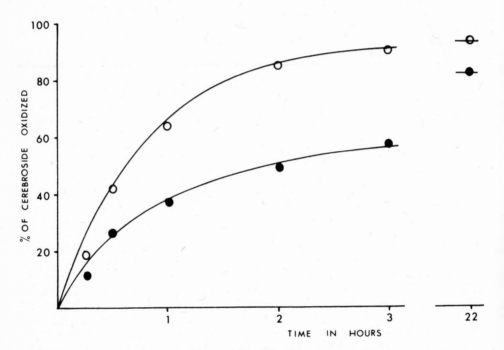

Fig. 3. Oxidation of the cerebrosides in isolated myelin by sodium
periodate. - Isolated bovine myelin was suspended in 10 mM phosphate
buffer, pH 7.4, and incubated in the dark with sodium periodate.
The concentration of periodate was adjusted to give a 10-fold molar
excess of periodate to cerebroside and the incubations carried out
at 4°C and 20°C.

Lipids were isolated by standard procedures and then separated
by thin-layer chromatography on Silica gel H plates in chloroform:
methanol (185:15, v/v). Cholesterol was used as an internal standard
and was estimated colorimetrically by the method of Sackett (16),
cerebrosides were estimated from their galactose content by the
phenol-sulphuric acid method.

Table 2. Oxidation of cerebrosides in sonicated liposomes made from total myelin lipids at 4°C, by sodium periodate. Results for two experiments, A and B, are shown. - An aliquot of total myelin lipids was dried down under nitrogen, 10 mM phosphate buffer, pH 7.4, was then added to the dried lipid and the resulting suspension sonicated at 15°C under a stream of nitrogen, for 2 h. The sonicated dispersion was then centrifuged to remove any large lipid aggregates and metal particles derived from the sonicator head. The final lipid concentration was from 9.0 to 12.0 mg/ml. Sodium periodate was added from a fresh 0.1 M solution to give a 10-fold molar excess of periodate to cerebroside, the reaction mixture was then incubated at 4°C in the dark with shaking. Aliquots were removed and the lipid separated by thin-layer chromatography in chloroform:methanol (185:15, v/v). Cerebroside galactose was estimated colorimetrically by the phenol-sulphuric acid method, cholesterol by the method of Sackett (16) and phosphate by Bartlett's method.

Time (min)	% of cerebrosides oxidised	
	A	B
0	0	0
15	5	-
30	7	6
60	16	19
120	18	26
180	19	17
overnight	15	23

The reactions with periodate are biphasic in character exhibiting a fast initial reaction in which at 20°C some 50-60% of cerebroside galactose is attacked. The second phase of the reaction is slower.

In experiments with several different myelin preparations from bovine brain tissue exposure to periodate at 20°C resulted in some 90% of the cerebroside galactose being degraded while at 0°C over the same 3-hour period this figure was between 45-54%.

This work with periodate was extended by looking at the action of the probe on multilamellar liposomes produced with mixed myelin lipids. Total lipids were extracted from isolated myelin by standard procedures. An aliquot of the total lipid was dried under nitrogen and liposomes produced by the addition of phosphate buffer followed by sonication under nitrogen at constant temperature (15°C). Periodate was then added in molar excess and the reaction monitored at 4°C, in the dark. The results are shown in Table 2 and indicate that only a limited proportion of the total cerebroside present is attacked at 4°C, the figures for two separate experiments being up to a maximum of about 20-25% of the total glycolipid present. Reaction was complete within about 2 h unlike the situation with myelin.

DISCUSSION

These preliminary studies clearly indicate that cerebrosides in isolated myelin preparations are accessible to probes and it is relevant therefore to go a step further and consider what the results may mean in terms of the structural disposition of cerebrosides in the lipid phase of the myelin sheath. The two probes used are vastly different in molecular size although they both attack the galactose headgroup of the glycolipid. Further, periodate is believed to be permeant to lipid membranes (6) while this seems not to be true of galactose oxidase which will therefore have a preference for reaction with easily-available cerebroside molecules.

The action of galactose oxidase on isolated myelin is to bring about the oxidation of some 50% of the total cerebroside of the preparation. This result can be interpreted in several ways. The most obvious possibility - bearing in mind that the reaction was carried out in hypotonic solution in which lamellae will have separated at the external apposition - is that the enzyme can penetrate freely to such sites and that cerebroside at that face of the lamellae is oxidised. This would indicate that at least half of the myelin cerebroside is located at the external apposition face of the membrane. It does not answer the question of the asymmetric distribution of the glycolipid for it is not possible yet to tell whether galactose oxidase attacks all galactose headgroups on adjacent cerebroside molecules. It should be noted that in the lipid phase of myelin cerebroside molecules are most probably not arranged in some form of lateral phase separation and are to be located interacting with other lipid species in the membrane to reduce the high phase transition of the lipid class. Studies with galactose oxidase on liposomes containing cerebrosides will also help answer this problem.

Another possibility is that in fact all the cerebroside, or the main bulk of the lipid, is located at the external apposition face of the lamellae and that this is all oxidised by the action of the enzyme. In this interpretation the galactose oxidase is considered unlikely to penetrate even swollen channels between myelin lamellae due to the structuring of water between adjacent bilayers at such sites. For sciatic nerve Blaurock (2) has indicated that separation of lamellae at the external apposition is about 9.5 nm for water and about 21.0 nm for 0.24 M sucrose. The width of the normal channel at the external apposition is wider in peripheral nerve myelin than in central nerve myelin as reviewed by Rumsby and Crang (14). It is thus quite probable that even in hypotonic conditions galactose oxidase does not penetrate into multilamellar fragments of myelin. The action of the enzyme is thus concentrated at the

surface of the myelin particles and the 50% degradation of cerebroside galactose must arise from a near complete oxidation of galactose
at the exposed external apposition face followed by dilution from
unattacked cerebroside from lamellae within the myelin fragment.
This interpretation is favoured at present and would indicate
that the bulk of the glycolipid is localised at the external face
of the lamellae in compact myelin. This possibility is in keeping
with the findings of Gregson (5) who in electrophoretic studies on
isolated myelin fragments has noted the presence of non-ionogenic
patches on the surface of the membrane particles.

The small oxidising agent, sodium periodate, at 20°C shows a
very rapid attack on cerebroside galactose in isolated myelin preparations so that virtually all the galactose headgroups are oxidised
within three hours. At 4°C the reaction is slower some 50% of the
cerebroside galactose being attacked over the same time period but
on increased exposure again nearly all the galactose headgroups
are being oxidised.

The results with liposomes composed of mixed myelin lipids
treated with periodate at 4°C are of interest in that they would
tend to suggest that in this system periodate does not penetrate
the lipid lamellae at the low temperature. Thus only cerebrosides
in the outer surface of the liposomes are attacked. This finding
has implications for the action of periodate on the isolated myelin
preparations at 4°C and an interpretation of the reaction can be
given in such terms. Periodate attacks surface cerebroside molecules very rapidly (50% oxidation in three hours). Subsequently
a slower oxidation of inner cerebroside occurs as periodate penetrates along the external apposition channels, the probe being
unable to cross the lipid phase at the low temperature conditions.
Such a result is in good agreement with the galactose oxidase data
and again tends to suggest that cerebroside may be asymmetrically
concentrated on the external apposition faces of the lipid phase
in compact myelin.

Until recently we have been unable to provide an answer to
explain why cerebrosides are concentrated in myelin and there is
still no firm data on this point or on why the sugar headgroup of
this glycolipid is galactose rather than glucose. A recent study
on molecular arrangements in sphingolipids by Pascher (11) does,
however, allow us to speculate on a possible function for cerebrosides and other sphingolipids in myelin. The conformation of
ceramides has been studied and it has been noted that such molecules
(and thus cerebrosides also) can function as hydrogen bond donors
as well as hydrogen bond acceptors. It should be noted that
glycerol-based phospholipids containing ester-linked fatty acids
can only function as hydrogen bond acceptors. Pascher speculates
that sphingolipids may thus be able to form lateral hydrogen bonds
within the membrane layer. This would increase the stability of
the membrane as well as decreasing the permeability of the system.
Such features would be of special significance in a lipid-rich
system such as myelin.

The other possible feature that cerebrosides contribute to myelin is that the galactose headgroup would have a considerable influence in structuring water molecules in its vicinity through hydrogen bonding while at the same time such molecules, unlike sphingomyelin, carry no charged groups in the polar moiety of the molecule. This feature may also be important for the overall structure of compact myelin where lamellae oppose at the external and cytoplasmic apposition regions. It is of interest that the tentative results presented in this report tend to locate cerebrosides predominantly at the external apposition where the features of the molecule discussed above fit in with the swelling and separation characteristics of this apposition site.

Acknowledgement. The Science Research Council is thanked for supporting this work (a research studentship to C.L.).

REFERENCES

1. Abrahamsson, S., Pascher, I., Larsson, K. and Karlsson, K.A., Molecular arrangements in glycosphingolipids, Chem. Phys. Lipids 8(1972) 152-179.

2. Blaurock, A.E., Structure of the nerve myelin membrane: proof of the low resolution profile, J. Mol. Biol.56 (1971) 35-52.

3. Clowes, A.W., Cherry, R.J. and Chapman, D., Physical properties of lecithin-cerebroside films, Biochim. Biophys. Acta 249 (1971) 301-307.

4. Finean, J.B. and Burge, R.E., The determination of the Fourier transform of the myelin layer from a study of swelling phenomena, J. Mol. Biol. 1 (1963) 672-682.

5. Gregson, N.A., Personal communication (1977).

6. Hubbard, A.L. and Cohn, Z.A., Specific labels for cell surfaces, in Biochemical Analysis of Membranes (A.H. Maddy, ed.) Chapman & Hall, London (1976) pp. 427-501.

7. Ladbrooke, B.D., Jenkinson, T.J., Kamat, V.B. and Chapman, D., Physical studies of myelin, Biochim. Biophys. Acta 164 (1968) 101-109.

8. Linington, C. and Rumsby, M.G., Localisation of cerebroside in central nervous system myelin lamellae: An initial approach, Biochem. Soc. Trans. 5 (1977) 196-198.

9. McIntosh, T.J. and Robertson, J.D., Observations on the effect of hypotonic solutions on the myelin sheath in the central nervous system, J. Mol. Biol. 100 (1976) 213-217.

10. Oldfield, E. and Chapman, D., Molecular dynamics of cerebroside-cholesterol and sphingomyelin-cholesterol interactions: Implications for myelin membrane structure. FEBS Letts. 21 (1972) 303-306.

11. Pascher, I., Molecular arrangements in sphingolipids: Conformation and hydrogen bonding of ceramide and their implication in membrane stability and permeability, Biochim. Biophys. Acta 455 (1976) 431-451.

12. Poduslo, J.F., Distribution of galactose residues in surface membrane glycoproteins and glycolipids of the intact myelin sheath, Abstract No. 319, Fifth ISN Conference, Barcelona (1975).

13. Poduslo, J.F., Quarles, R.H. and Brady, R.O., External labelling of galactose in surface membrane glycoproteins of the intact myelin sheath, J. Biol. Chem. 251 (1976) 153-158.

14. Rumsby, M.G. and Crang, A.J., The myelin sheath - a structural examination, Cell Surface Reviews 4 (1977) in press.

15. Rumsby, M.G., Riekkinen, P.J. and Arstila, A.V., A critical evaluation of myelin purification: Non-specific esterase activity associated with central nerve myelin preparations, Brain Res. 24 (1970) 495-516.

16. Sackett, D., Estimation of cholesterol, J. Biol. Chem. 64 (1925) 203.

DEMYELINATION

Experimental Demyelination

AUTOIMMUNITY IN MULTIPLE SCLEROSIS: DO WE HAVE AN EXPERIMENTAL

MODEL?

Marian W. Kies

Section on Myelin Chemistry, Laboratory of Cerebral
    Metabolism, National Institute of Mental Health
Bethesda, Maryland 20014, U.S.A.

SUMMARY

Experimental autoimmunity of the CNS has been well characterized - the antigen has been identified, effector cell specificity
has been defined, and the relationship between cellular sensitization and antibody production has been partially clarified. In the
guinea pig, experimental allergic encephalomyelitis (EAE) is induced by one injection of myelin basic protein in complete Freund's
adjuvant (BP/CFA). If BP/CFA is preceded by repeated injections
of basic protein in incomplete Freund's adjuvant(BP/IFA), EAE is
not induced; the guinea pigs survive and ultimately produce antibody. Induction and prevention of EAE as well as antibody induction by this schedule are dependent on the presence of the intact
encephalitogenic (T-cell) site in the polypeptide used for sensitization and preimmunization. In contrast, B-cell sites (those
peptide sequences which bind antibody) are independent of the T-
cell site. At least 5 specific antigenic regions (B-cell sites)
have been demonstrated in the BP molecule. High mycobacteria levels
bypass the specificity requirement of helper T-cells but cannot bypass the specificity requirement of effector T-cells. In spite of
the sophisticated immunologic techniques available, our knowledge
of humoral and cellular sensitivity in multiple sclerosis (MS)
patients is very limited. The experimental demonstration of an
analogy between EAE and MS is weak: a) Demonstration of BP-
sensitized cells or BP-specific antibodies in peripheral blood of
MS patients has not been successful. b) Anti-myelin serum factors
reported to be associated with both disease states (experimental
autoimmunity and MS) are clearly not identical. Nevertheless,
successful treatment of EAE in animals by BP/IFA injections has

encouraged consideration of clinical trials to test the therapeutic
value of BP injections in MS patients. If successful, the question
will be answered: if unsuccessful, the dilemma still remains.

INTRODUCTION

Author´s note:
The following letter, received during the preparation of the
manuscript on autoimmunity in multiple sclerosis (MS), was used
as an introduction to the oral presentation in Helsinki. I believe
it is also appropriate to include the letter and my answer in the
final publication:

"Dear Dr. Kies:
"I am very much interested in your work in research for a cure
for multiple sclerosis and am very much a victim of the disease.
Now twenty-one and one half years old, I have had MS since I was
nineteen. I am walking again but I want to run, I want to be able
to do what you can do. Of late, I type my letters because I can
barely write. I am fighting.
"I already generously support the NMSS. I did not allow the
"specificity" or "specialty" of your study to discourage me from
contacting you because your progress is mine. Your job, Dr. Kies,
since you have chosen to accept it, is to save me. What are you
doing about it? I really do want "it" to be cured during my life-
time. What am I to expect? "Learning to live with it", is a
platitude that means nothing to anyone but the victim.
"You´ll be hearing from me again. You have no right to forget
me. My life is too important for you not to make the most cease-
less and diligent efforts at your job. I speak for myself but I
represent too many. You owe me. Best Wishes."

"Dear _____:
"Your letter came just as I was preparing a paper on the topic
"Autoimmunity in Multiple Sclerosis." The question I asked was
"Do we have an experimental model?" Your questions (What are you
doing about it? and What am I to expect?) were helpful to me as I
planned what I would say. They suggested two more questions --
Is the concept of autoimmunity a valid one? If so, how does the
concept help us to understand MS; i.e.-- What can we expect?
"In answer to your first question, we are studying the cause,
prevention, and treatment of a disease induced in laboratory
animals with a protein isolated from white matter, or myelin. The
disease is called experimental allergic encephalomyelitis (EAE).
Because the protein is a normal brain constituent EAE is presumably caused by an autoimmune reaction. For a long time EAE was
considered to be the experimental model for MS, but as our knowledge of the experimental disease grew we became less certain of

the bridge between the two. For example, the evidence that MS
patients are sensitized to this protein has not been substantiated.
Why then do we continue to study this protein and the disease it
causes? First, because it is the only brain constituent ever found
that induces an immunologic disease which affects the brain and
spinal cord and secondly, because only with a well-defined experimental situation can we hope to understand the complex reactions
which must be involved in autoimmunity. Animals can be bred to be
either resistant or susceptible to EAE and thus we can study the
effect of their genetic backgrounds on disease. Information can
be obtained from large groups of experimental animals and this is
more valuable to us at the present stage of our study than information from one or two patients.

"And finally, there is still the possibility that our failure
to detect any connection between this protein and MS is caused by
our lack of knowledge rather than the fact that it is the wrong
antigen or that autoimmunity is not a factor in MS.

"I think we have a good experimental model for autoimmunity
and I believe that an autoimmune reaction is somehow involved in
the cause of MS. Whether we are studying the "right" antigen is
the question we have not been able to resolve. Whether it is the
"right" one or not, we hope that the development of techniques for
interfering with the experimental disease will eventually help us
to develop safe and effective techniques for the control of MS.

"I cannot predict what you can expect from our studies. I
can only say that your letter provided an incentive for me to work
even harder to attain our goal of understanding the underlying
mechanisms of autoimmune damage to the nervous system. For your
sake and for the others you have mentioned, I hope we are successful."

In 1957 Witebsky proposed four postulates which he considered
to be basic to the proof that a human disease is caused by an autoimmune reaction (29):

1) Circulating antibodies should be demonstrable in patients
(antibodies to the target organ).

2) The antigen against which the antibodies are directed should
be isolated and defined.

3) It should be possible to induce these antibodies experimentally in animals.

4) Animals in which antibodies had been induced should develop
lesions closely resembling those found in the human disease.

Witebsky visualized specific antibodies as playing an important
role in autoimmunity partly because immunology up to that time had
been a science of serology rather than cellular reactivity and
partly because his major interest had been in autoimmune thyroiditis
in which antibodies play an important role. Research on EAE and
its possible relationship to MS developed in a transitional period
in immunology when interest was shifting from the production of

circulating antibodies to the induction of sensitized cells. For
this reason, the postulates need to be modified to include cellular
phenomena as well as antigen-antibody reactions:

1) Demonstration of circulating antibodies and/or sensitized
cells.

2) Isolation of specific antigen.

3) Induction of antibodies and/or sensitized cells in experimental animals.

4) Concurrent induction of lesions resembling those of the
human disease.

The proof that EAE is an experimental autoimmune disease of
the central nervous system (CNS) has been reviewed many times
(1, 15, 28). In the context of Witebsky's postulates, the experimental disease resembles MS except for the first postulate -
that circulating antibodies (and/or sensitized cells) be demonstrated in patients. This remains the missing link in our chain of
evidence that MS is an autoimmune disease. Although there are many
reports that sensitization to myelin basic protein can be demonstrated in patients' cells, the evidence is weak that the reactions
are specific either to myelin basic protein (BP) or to the disease.

Even without the evidence required by the first postulate, the
possibility that MS is indeed caused by an autoimmune reaction
justifies our continued study of EAE. At present, it is the only
experimental disease linked to an autoimmune reaction in the CNS.
The antigen has been identified (17), localized in the target organ
(18) and well characterized (5, 11). Postulates 3) and 4) have
been satisfied by demonstrating that BP can be used for the induction
of disease which correlates well with the appearance of delayed
hypersensitivity to BP (23). Lesions and clinical signs resemble
those observed in MS patients. Most important is the fact that the
lesions are induced in normal recipients by transfer of lymphocytes
from BP-sensitized donors (9, 13).

What do we need to know about EAE as an autoimmune disease;
and how can we best use our knowledge of EAE to assist us in
understanding MS? If MS is a disease of autoimmunity, regardless
of the nature of the initiating event, it should be possible to
control the disease by interfering with the continued production
of sensitized cells. Attempts have been made to achieve this result by massive immunosuppression, but the potential harm of such
a drastic procedure is almost as great as that of the disease itself. Suppression of specific cells would be much safer and
probably more effective. For this reason I believe the greatest
benefit to be gained from a study of the experimental disease is
an understanding of the mechanisms by which specifically sensitized
cells are induced and suppressed. To this end we have carried out
many in vivo studies and are currently involved in a study of the
reactivity of BP-sensitized cells in vitro.

EXPERIMENTAL STUDIES AND DISCUSSION

Specifically, we have investigated procedures for interfering with the course of disease by various injection schedules of BP. It is well known that the induction of EAE in guinea pigs requires both BP and complete Freund´s adjuvant (CFA); BP in incomplete Freund´s adjuvant (IFA) is nonencephalitogenic, even if large amounts of antigen are injected repeatedly. But such injections can be used prior to <u>induction</u> to confer <u>protection</u>; after induction but before disease onset to confer <u>suppression</u>; and after disease onset to provide effective <u>treatment</u> (2).

Until recently we made no attempt to define the cell populations which were involved in the mechanisms of disease induction and intervention. We are not even sure that the same mechanism applies to each type of intervention. In the context of current theories of cellular immunology, however, we can postulate that injection of BP in CFA induces effector T-cells whereas injection of BP in IFA induces an opposing phenomenon (suppressor T-cells?). The role of effector T-cells in disease induction in rats is well documented (14, 22), but the role of suppressor T-cells is still somewhat in doubt. Such cells have been reported in EAE-resistant states in both rats (26) and mice (3), but we have so far been unsuccessful in demonstrating suppressor cells in guinea pigs.

I spoke earlier of the importance of designing a procedure which would not only be safe but effective as well. As far as we can tell BP in IFA is completely nonencephalitogenic in guinea pigs. Whether similar injections would be harmless in humans is still open to the question, but I think one must understand the animal model first before one can answer this question.

It seems to me that the most important task is to determine the optimum conditions for interrupting the processes involved in lesion formation. In order to induce tolerance, suppressor cells, or a permanent state of resistance (whatever one chooses to call it), the antigen of choice is the one which is most effective. In EAE that antigen is BP or an encephalitogenic fragment of BP. Other investigators have reported that certain nonencephalitogenic antigens are capable of preventing EAE. These include HNB-modified BP (24), a peptic fragment of BP (25), synthetic polymers of natural amino acids (27) and a spinal cord protein unrelated to BP (21).

Our search for a nonencephalitogenic fragment of BP that would be effective in preventing induction of EAE has convinced us that the specificity of protection is the same as that of induction - i.e., nonencephalitogenic fragments do not exert a protective effect (10). The results on which this conclusion is based are shown in Table 1. As additional evidence that our conclusions regarding the specific immunologic requirements of protection have even wider significance, I cite the data we have obtained with some of the other proposed "anti-encephalitogenic" materials (Table 2).

Table 1. Prevention of EAE with fragments of BP. Relationship between encephalitogenic activity and the ability to prevent disease.

Induction			Prevention	
Sensitization (Fragment in CFA)	Disease index[+] 5.4	27.0	Preimmunization[++] (Fragment in IFA)	Disease index (After BP in CFA)
	(nmoles)			
1-19	0	0	1-19	7.5±0.3
1-36	0	0	1-36	8.7±0.6
1-42	0	2.4±1.1	1-42	8.7±0.4
116-169	0	0.2±0.2	116-169	7.7±0.5
37-88	0	0	37-88	6.2±1.4
1-115[+++]	0	7.1±1.0	1-115	4.7±0.7
	0.27	27.0		
1-169 (BP)	8.0±0.2	7.8±0.6	1-169 (BP)	0.2±0.1
89-169	7.2±0.5	8.1±0.6	89-169	0.5±0.2
111-169	7.6±1.4	Not tested	111-169	1.5±0.5

[+]Disease severity based on combined clinical and histologic data; 0-10 (maximum disease).
[++]Guinea pigs were injected 10 times with 5.4 nmoles BP or fragment over a 3-week period. One week after the last IFA injection, they were injected with 5.4 nmoles BP + 0.1 mg mycobacteria.
[+++]Contamination of this peptide by uncleaved BP is suggested by its encephalitogenic activity at 27 nmoles.

Because of these results we feel that efforts expended in the search for a potentially safe procedure to treat patients would be better spent examining ways and means of enhancing the efficacy of the encephalitogenic protein itself rather than searching for new nonencephalitogenic compounds.

There are several variables which have to be taken into account in studying specific intervention of an immunologic reaction. By animal experimentation we can analyze these variables and attempt to judge whether they will be critical in patient studies. This is perhaps one of the strongest arguments for continuing our study of EAE.

One of the variables is the strength of sensitization. It is obvious that the greater the disease reaction, the more difficult it will be to overcome. A simple illustration is given in Table 3.

Table 2. Prevention of EAE - comparison of BP with nonencephalitogenic peptides.

Pretreatment[+]	Clinical No. positive/total	Survival No. survived/total	Disease index
GPBP (10 x 0.1 mg/IFA)	0/15	15/15	0.2±0.1
Cop I "	5/5	5/5	7.2±0.5
SCP (9 x 0.1 mg/IFA)	5/5	0/5	8.4±0.4
" (4 x 0.1 mg/IFA)	5/5	0/5	8.4±0.5
HNB-BP (10 x 0.1 mg/IFA)	10/10	2/10	7.4±0.7

+All groups challenged with 0.1 mg BP/0.1 mg mycobacteria.
Cop I supplied by Dr. Michael Sela; SCP, spinal cord protein supplied by Dr. Catherine MacPherson; HNB-BP, prepared in our laboratory by the formic acid procedure (6).

Table 3. Protection vs. challenge.

Challenge[+] mg		Clinical signs No. positive/total	Survival No. survivors/total	Disease index
BP	Mycobacteria			
0.1	0.1	0/15	15/15	0.2
0.5	0.5	3/5	4/5	3.7
0.5	2.5	8/9	9/9	4.3
Cord[++]	Mycobacteria			
5	0.1	10/10	6/10	8.0
50	2.5	5/5	0/5	9.0

↑ Increasing "strength" of challenge

→ Increasing effectiveness of protection

+All challenges were 100% effective in unprotected guinea pigs; all groups were preimmunized as in Table 1.
++5 and 50 mg cord ≅ 0.05 and 05. mg BP.

Table 4.   Duration of protection.[+]

Time interval[++] days	Clinical No. positive/ total	Survival No. survivors/ total	Disease index
7	0/15	15/15	0.2
46	0/5	5/5	0
95	0/5	5/5	0.6
180	3/4	3/4	4.0
240	2/2	1/2	9.0

[+]Pretreatment = 10 x 0.1 mg BP in IFA (3/wk x 3 wks).
[++]Length of time between end of pretreatment and challenge (0.1 mg BP/0.1 mg mycobacteria).

Coates et al.(7) also have studied the problem of balance between protection and challenge. They used a much weaker challenge than those illustrated in Table 3 and thus were able to demonstrate protection with less antigen in IFA.

Another variable is the duration of protection. This factor is of considerable importance in planning a treatment schedule for patients. In guinea pigs 3-5 months may elapse before the effectiveness of protection is lost (Table 4). Not only is it important to know how long the protection will last but also why it lasts as long as it does. Bernard et al. (4) have addressed themselves to this question and have reported results which agree in general with our observations. Their experimental design was complicated by the fact that they used repeated challenges and thus introduced an additional variable – the effect of a prior injection of CFA on disease induction. Preinjection of the latter also protects guinea pigs against EAE (16, 20), and we believe its effects cannot be ignored in such a study.

Although the experiments I have discussed pertain to protection we are keenly aware of the fact that experiments based on suppression and treatment of EAE are even more important when one considers the problems of control of MS. An early attempt to treat EAE in guinea pigs by injections of BP in saline after disease onset was only partially successful (12). Signs of disease were temporarily abolished, but guinea pigs treated with BP eventually succumbed to EAE. However, it was encouraging that lesions in treated animals were less severe than in control animals given saline injections alone. Later studies by other investigators in which rats (19) and monkeys (12) were treated with BP appeared to be more successful. By using IFA as the vehicle for the injected BP, we were able to treat guinea pigs with EAE successfully even after an excessive challenge (Table 5) (8). More importantly, we were able to show that lymphocytes from treated donors were unable to transfer EAE to normal recipients (9). This suggested that the

Table 5.   Successful treatment of EAE in guinea pigs (8, 9).

A) Effect of BP injections on recovery after active sensitization.		
Sensitization	Treatment	Success of treatment (No. recovered/No.treated)
0.5 mg BP + 2.5 mg mycobacteria "	BP in IFA IFA	16/17 0/12

B) Influence of donor treatment[+] on effectiveness of adoptive transfer			
	EAE in recipients		
No. of BP injections (Donors[++])	No. positive No. recipients	Time of onset (day after cell transfer)	Lesions No.positive No.tested
0	10/10	7.9$\pm$0.5	10/10
1[+++]	3/3	7, 7, 12	3/3
2	1/2	13, -	1/2
3	0/2	-	1/2
4	0/1	-	0/1

[+]Injections of BP in IFA were begun 24 h after onset of clinical signs. [++]Donors were sensitized as in A). [+++]After 2 injections of BP, cell donors showed definite signs of recovery.

beneficial effect of treatment had to be on the cells rather than on the CNS. What we hope to determine by in vitro studies is whether this was achieved by a direct action of BP on the sensitized cells themselves or by the stimulation of some opposing mechanism (possibly by suppressor cell induction).

In conclusion, I want to emphasize my belief that basic research on an experimental autoimmune disease is not only justifiable but extremely useful in providing a rationale for studies on multiple sclerosis. Even though our studies have not provided evidence that MS is an autoimmune disease, I believe that a clear understanding of autoimmunity and the knowledge of how to control it in the animal model will provide greater insight into the human disease. At the present time the best model available for such studies is experimental allergic encephalomyelitis.

Acknowledgements. I am grateful to my colleagues, Drs. B.F. Driscoll, R.E. Martenson, and E.C. Alvord, Jr., Mrs. G.E. Deibler, Mrs. M.L. Bacon and Mr. J.D. Stream for their help in the experiments described above.

Shortly after my return from Helsinki I was saddened by news of the death of Dr. Harry Weaver, one of the most dedicated

exponents of research on multiple sclerosis in the United States.
Officially, Dr. Weaver's contribution was made through his position
as Research Consultant for the National Multiple Sclerosis Society.
Unofficially, he contributed immeasurably to MS research through
discussion, criticism, advice and encouragement. In recognition
of the many helpful discussions I have had with him on the validity
of EAE as a model for MS, I would like to dedicate this chapter to
Dr. Weaver.

REFERENCES

1. Alvord, E.C., Jr., Acute disseminated encephalomyelitis and
    "allergic" neuro-encephalopathies, in Handbook of Clinical
    Neurology (P.J. Vinken and G.W. Bruyn, eds.) North-Holland
    Publishing Co.,Amsterdam (1970) pp. 500-571.
2. Alvord, E.C., Jr., Shaw, C.-M., Hrugy, S. and Kies, M.W.,
    Encephalitogen-induced inhibition of experimental allergic
    encephalomyelitis: prevention, suppression and therapy,
    Ann. N. Y. Acad. Sci. 122 (1965) 333-345.
3. Bernard, C.C.A., Suppressor T cells prevent experimental auto-
    immune encephalomyelitis in mice, Clin. Exp. Immunol. 29 (1977)
    100-109.
4. Bernard, C.C.A., MacKay, I.R., Whittingham, S. and Brous, P.,
    Durability of immune protection against experimental autoimmune
    encephalomyelitis, Cell. Immunol. 22 (1976) 297-310.
5. Carnegie, P.R., Amino acid sequence of the encephalitogenic
    basic protein from human myelin, Biochem. J. 123 (1971) 57-
    67.
6. Chao, L.-P. and Einstein, E.R., Localization of the active
    site through chemical modification of the encephalitogenic
    protein, J. Biol. Chem. 245 (1970) 6397-6403.
7. Coates, A., MacKay, I.R. and Crawford, M., Immune protection
    against experimental autoimmune encephalomyelitis: optimal
    conditions and analysis of mechanism, Cell. Immunol. 12 (1974)
    370-381.
8. Driscoll, B.F., Kies, M.W. and Alvord, E.C., Jr., Successful
    treatment of experimental allergic encephalomyelitis (EAE) in
    guinea pigs with homologous myelin basic protein, J. Immunol.
    112 (1974) 392-397.
9. Driscoll, B.F., Kies, M.W. and Alvord, E.C., Jr., Adoptive
    transfer of experimental allergic encephalomyelitis (EAE):
    prevention of successful transfer by treatment of donors
    with myelin basic protein, J. Immunol. 114 (1975) 291-292.
10. Driscoll, B.F., Kies, M.W. and Alvord, E.C., Jr., Protection
    against experimental allergic encephalomyelitis with peptides
    derived from myelin basic protein: presence of intact en-
    cephalitogenic site is essential, J. Immunol. 117 (1976) 110-
    114.

11. Eylar, E.H., Brostoff, S., Hashim, G., Caccam, J. and Burnett, P., Basic A1 protein of the myelin membrane. The complete amino acid sequence, J. Biol. Chem. 246 (1971) 5770-5784.

12. Eylar, E.H., Jackson, J., Rothenberg, B. and Brostoff, S.W., Suppression of the immune response: reversal of the disease state with antigen in allergic encephalomyelitis, Nature 236 (1972) 74-76.

13. Falk, G.A., Kies, M.W. and Alvord, E.C., Jr., Delayed hypersensitivity to myelin basic protein in the passive transfer of experimental allergic encephalomyelitis, J. Immunol. 101 (1968) 638-644.

14. Gonatas, N.K. and Howard, J.C., Inhibition of experimental allergic encephalomyelitis in rats severely depleted of T cells, Science 186 (1974) 839-841.

15. Kies, M.W., Experimental allergic encephalomyelitis, in Biology of Brain Dysfunction (G.E. Gaull, ed.) Plenum Press, New York (1973) pp. 185-224.

16. Kies, M.W. and Alvord, E.C., Jr., Prevention of allergic encephalomyelitis by prior injection of adjuvants, Nature 182 (1958) 1106.

17. Kies, M.W. and Alvord, E.C., Jr., Encephalitogenic activity in guinea pigs of water-soluble protein fractions of nervous tissue, in"Allergic" Encephalomyelitis (M.W. Kies and E.C. Alvord, Jr., eds.) Charles C. Thomas, Springfield, Ill. (1959) pp. 293-299.

18. Laatsch, R.H., Kies, M.W., Gordon, S. and Alvord, E.C., Jr., The encephalitogenic activity of myelin isolated by ultracentrifugation, J. Exp. Med. 115 (1962) 777-788.

19. Levine, S., Sowinski, R. and Kies, M.W., Treatment of experimental allergic encephalomyelitis with encephalitogenic basic proteins, Proc. Soc. Exp. Biol. Med. 139 (1972) 506-510.

20. Lisak, R.P. and Kies, M.W., Mycobacterial suppression of delayed hypersensitivity in experimental allergic encephalomyelitis, Proc. Soc. Exp. Biol. Med. 128 (1968) 214-218.

21. MacPherson, C.F.C. and Yo, S.-L., Studies on brain antigens. VI. Prevention of experimental allergic encephalomyelitis by a water-soluble spinal cord protein,β_1-SCP, J. Immunol. 110 (1973) 1371-1375.

22. Ortiz -Ortiz, L. and Weigle, W.O., Cellular events in the induction of experimental allergic encephalomyelitis in rats, J. Exp. Med. 144 (1976) 604-616.

23. Shaw, C.-M., Alvord, E.C., Jr., Kaku, J. and Kies, M.W., Correlation of experimental allergic encephalomyelitis with delayed-type skin sensitivity to specific homologous encephalitogen, Ann. N.Y. Acad. Sci. 122 (1965) 318-331.

24. Swanborg, R.H., Antigen-induced inhibition of experimental allergic encephalomyelitis. I. Inhibition in guinea pigs injected with non-encephalitogenic modified myelin basic protein, J. Immunol. 109 (1972) 540-546.

25. Swanborg, R.H., Antigen-induced inhibition of experimental allergic encephalomyelitis. III. Localization of an inhibitory site distinct from the major encephalitogenic determinant of myelin basic protein, J. Immunol. 114 (1975) 191-194.

26. Swierkosz, J.E. and Swanborg, R.H., Suppressor cell control of unresponsiveness to experimental allergic encephalomyelitis J. Immunol. 115 (1975) 631-633.

27. Teitelbaum, D., Meshorer, A., Hirshfield, T.,Arnon, R. and Sela, M., Suppression of experimental allergic encephalomyelitis by a synthetic polypeptide, Eur. J. Immunol. 1 (1971) 242-248.

28. Whipple, H.E., ed., Research in Demyelinating Diseases, Ann. N. Y. Acad. Sci. 122 (1965) 1-570.

29. Witebsky, E., The status of organ specificity, in "Allergic" Encephalomyelitis (M.W. Kies and E.C. Alvord, eds.) Charles C. Thomas, Springfield, Ill. (1959) pp. 321-347.

MOLECULAR BASES FOR THE DIFFERENCE IN THE POTENCY OF MYELIN

BASIC PROTEIN FROM DIFFERENT SPECIES IN LEWIS RATS

George A. Hashim

Department of Surgery and Microbiology, St. Luke's
  Hospital Center, and Columbia University
421 West 113th Street, New York, NY 10025, U.S.A.

SUMMARY

    The results of this study define the chemical bases for the
difference in the encephalitogenic potency reported for the bovine
and guinea pig myelin basic proteins. Studies with synthetic
peptides showed that the sequence of peptide S53, H-Ser-Gln-Arg-
Ser-Gln-Asp-Glu-Asn-OH, which is native to the guinea pig basic
protein, is the minimum amino acid sequence necessary for inducing
EAE in Lewis rats. The results of this study further showed that
specific sequence modifications rendered the native bovine sequence highly encephalitogenic.

INTRODUCTION

    Experimental allergic encephalomyelitis (EAE) is a cell-
mediated immune disease of the central nervous system induced in
animals by the myelin basic protein from several species including
man (1,2,5,11,19,21,25,28,29). The EAE-inducing potency of the
basic protein (BP) and the severity of disease in Lewis rats depend
upon the species from which the basic protein was derived (7,20-23,
28). The purpose of this presentation is to describe the minimum
amino acid sequence necessary for inducing EAE and define the molecular bases for the difference in the encephalitogenic potency
of myelin basic proteins from different species in Lewis rats.

EXPERIMENTAL

Preparation of antigens. The myelin basic protein was isolated from fresh frozen bovine and guinea pig spinal cords by
established procedures (11). All peptides were synthesized in the
laboratory by the general procedure of Merrifield (24) using Boc-
glycine-resin ester. The synthetic peptides were cleaved from the
resin and the side chains deprotected by treatment with hydrogen
fluoride at 0°C for 1 hour. The peptide was extracted with tri-
fluoroacetic acid, neutralized and chromatographed on a Sephadex
G10 column which was equilibrated and eluted with 0.1 M acetic
acid. Other details of the procedure were described previously
(16). Further purification of peptides was accomplished by preparative high voltage electrophoresis (14).

The EAE assay. Male Lewis rats (Microbiological Associates,
Walkersville, Md.) weighing 250-300 grams were used throughout this
study. They were housed in individual wire cages and provided with
food and water ad libitum. Saline solutions of antigens were emulsified with an equal volume of complete Freund's adjuvant and 0.1
ml emulsion containing the desired antigen concentration in addition
to 100 µg M. butyricum was injected in one hind foot pad. Challenged rats were weighed and inspected daily for clinical signs of
EAE. They were terminated between day 20 and 26 following challenge. The brain and spinal cord tissues were isolated for histology.

RESULTS AND DISCUSSION

The encephalitogenicity of myelin basic protein from bovine,
guinea pig and rat CNS-tissues has been demonstrated in several
laboratories, and in Table 1 we have assembled some of the published results (12,13,20,23). Regardless of the method of determining the incidence of EAE and the amount of adjuvant administered, it is clear that the basic protein from guinea pig CNS
myelin is a potent encephalitogen in Lewis rats compared to its
bovine or rat counterpart. Based on the development of hind leg
paralysis (HLP), the incidence of EAE was the same in rats challenged with either 1 µg guinea pig or 50 µg bovine basic protein.
Increasing the challenge dose to 100 µg bovine basic protein did
not increase the incidence of HLP. In contrast, the incidence of
HLP was 100% when each of 6 to 8 rats was challenged with either
10 or 50 µg guinea pig basic protein.

Differences in the encephalitogenic potency of the intact
basic proteins were also demonstrated by the administration of
fragments derived from the respective proteins (7,20,23). These
fragments may be defined by residues 44 to 89 of the bovine basic
protein sequence (9). The results of these studies,assembled in
Table 2, clearly demonstrate that fragment 44 to 89, like its
parent guinea pig basic protein, is the most potent encephalitogen

Table 1.   Encephalitogenic activity of intact guinea pig, rat and bovine basic proteins in Lewis rats.

Dose µg	Incidence of EAE		
	Guinea pig BP	Bovine BP	Rat S-BP
45	5/5	5/5	5/5
4.5	5/5	0/5	1/5
0.45	5/5	0/5	0/5
230		4/5	
46		3/5	
9		0/5	
0.36	4/5		
0.07	0/5		
100		1/6	
50	8/8	1/6	
10	6/6	1/6	
1	1/5		

The data presented in this table were assembled from the published results of McFarlin et al.(20), Martenson et al. (23), Hashim (12) and Hashim et al.(13).

compared to similar fragments derived from either rat or bovine basic proteins. The incidence of EAE increased from 20 to 100% (1/5 to 5/5) when the 0.1 µg doses were increased to 1.0 or 10 µg of guinea pig fragment 44 to 89. Similarly, 10 µg (but not 1 µg) of fragment 44 to 89 from rat basic protein was required to induce EAE in 100% (5/5) of the challenged animals. In contrast, fragment 44 to 89 from bovine basic protein was inactive at 10 and 52 µg levels (23), but at doses of 105 µg, the bovine fragment was mildly encephalitogenic (13,20). The addition of the N-terminal six amino acid residues to bovine fragment 44 to 89 rendered the resulting fragment 38 to 89 encephalitogenic at 50 µg but not at 10 µg doses (23).

Recent studies have demonstrated that the entire length of fragment 44 to 89 is not necessary for activity and that the en-cephalitogenic determinant for Lewis rats may be defined by a smaller portion of fragment 44 to 89. Selective enzymatic cleavage of this fragment released the C-terminal 19 amino acid residues, which retained the encephalitogenic activity of the parent fragment (5). Further cleavage of the C-terminal six residues rendered the resulting two peptides inactive (Table 3).

Table 2. Encephalitogenic activity of fragments from bovine, guinea pig and rat basic proteins in Lewis rats.

Fragment	Dose µg	Incidence of EAE		
		From guinea pig BP	From bovine BP	From rat BP
44–89	105		mild	
44–89	10	5/5	0/5	5/5
44–89	1	5/5	0/5	1/5
44–89	0.1	1/5		
44–89	4.2			6/6
44–89	52		0/5	
44–89	10		0/5	
38–89	50		5/5	
38–89	10		0/5	
44–89	0.08	5/5		
44–89	0.02	0/5		
38–89	0.08	4/5		
38–89	0.02	0/5		

The data presented in this table were assembled from the published results of McFarlin et al.(20), Chou et al.(6) and Martenson et al. (23).

Simultaneous studies from our laboratory have shown (12) that the encephalitogenic determinant for Lewis rats is located in the region defined by residues 68 to 84 of the bovine basic protein. The sequence of residues 68 to 84, H-Gly-Ser-Leu-Pro-Gln-Lys-Ala-Gln-Gly-His-Arg-Pro-Gln-Asp-Glu-Asn-OH, was synthesized by the Merrifiéd solidphase method (24) and purified by high voltage and paper chromatography as previously described (12,14,16). Similar to its parent bovine basic protein, the sequence of residues 68 to 84 (designated peptide S8) was shown to be mildly encephalitogenic, demonstrating that the C-terminal Pro-Val-Val-His-Phe-OH of the enzymatically derived fragment 69 to 89 (Table 3) was not necessary for encephalitogenicity. Deletion of Gly-His from peptide S8 gave rise to synthetic peptide S49 and rendered the resulting peptide S49 highly encephalitogenic (30). Compared to rats challenged with guinea pig myelin BP, histological scores were higher in rats challenged with peptide S49. The histological severity decreased when the challenging dose was reduced from 25 to 0.5 µg(13). This 50-fold dose reduction resulted in an approximately 4 to 6-fold decrease in histological severity. The severity of EAE in rats challenged with peptide S8 was milder even at doses 200 times higher

than those of peptide S49. Doses of 28 µg peptide S8 failed to
induce histological evidence of EAE. Similarly, rats challenged
with the adjuvant alone failed to develop any signs of EAE.

The minimum sequence requirement for encephalitogenicity in
Lewis rats was then investigated. In a series of shorter synthetic
peptides overlapping the sequence of peptide S49, we were able to
show (13) that the N-terminal sequence H-Gly-Ser-Leu-Pro-Gln-Lys--
was not essential for encephalitogenic activity of this determinant,
since deletion of Gly-Ser-Leu, Gly-Ser-Leu-Pro, or Gly-Ser-Leu-Pro-
Gln-Lys, as in peptides S52, S51 and S50 did not alter the encephalitogenic potency of the resulting peptides (Table 4). In
fact, full encephalitogenic activity of peptide S49 was retained
in the C-terminal eight amino acid residues found in peptide S50.
Deletion of additional residues from peptide S50 rendered the
resulting peptide S20a biologically inactive. Previous studies
have shown that enzymatic (10,15) or chemical modification (8,27)
of the intact basic protein and substitution (17,30) or deletion
(16,18) of residues from disease inducing determinants renders them
nonencephalitogenic. The encephalitogenic activity of peptide S49
and its shorter overlapping sequences of peptides S52, S51 and S50
provides the first documented evidence for the generation of encephalitogenic sequences that are native neither to the sequences
of the human and bovine CNS myelin basic proteins (4,9), to the
partially reported sequences of fragment 44 to 89 from rabbit,
guinea pig or monkey basic proteins (26),nor to the natural sequence of P1 protein of sciatic nerve myelin (3).

The question arose as to what is the native sequence of the
guinea pig basic protein that might account for its encephalitogenic
potency in Lewis rats. Comparison of the sequence of peptide S50
to the corresponding region of guinea pig basic protein revealed
the presence of an eight amino acid sequence (residues 74 to 84)
similar but not identical to the sequence of peptide S50. The
sequence from the guinea pig protein, H-Ser-Gln-Arg-Ser-Gln-Asp-
Glu-Asn-OH (designated peptide S53 in Table 4), was synthesized
(13). Compared to peptide S50, the sequence of peptide S53 has a
natural Gly-His deletion and Ser substitutions for Ala and Pro,
residues no. 75 and 80, respectively. At the lower doses tested
(0.5 µg or 5 nmoles), peptide S53 was as encephalitogenic as
peptide S50 (Table 4). It is of interest to note that the sequence
of peptide S53 is the shortest encephalitogenic determinant described for the basic protein.

Our studies with synthetic peptides show the presence of
encephalitogenic determinants in both bovine and guinea pig myelin
basic proteins. Both of these determinants have been chemically
synthesized and shown to differ in encephalitogenic potency similar
to their respective parent proteins. The potent encephalitogenic
determinant from the guinea pig protein, H-Ser-Gln-Arg-Ser-Gln-Asp-
Glu-Asn-OH, lacks the Gly-His sequence found naturally in the
corresponding region of the bovine basic protein.

Table 3. Encephalitogenic activity of guinea pig basic protein and its peptide fragments.

Generated peptide	Guinea pig myelin basic protein	EAE incidence
44–89	Fragment $\xrightarrow{\text{pepsin}}$ 44–89 $\xrightarrow{\text{chymotrypsin}}$	3/3
44–68	44 50 60 H-Phe-Gly-Ser-Asp-Arg-Ala-Ala-Pro-Lys-Arg-Gly-Ser-Gly-Lys-Asp-Ser-His-His- 55 65 68 Ala-Ala-Arg-Thr-Thr-His-Tyr-OH	0/4
69–89	69 75 85 H-Gly-Ser-Leu-Pro-Gln-Lys-Ser-Gln-(-)-(-)-Arg-Ser-Gln-Asp-Glu-Asn-Pro-Val- 89 Val-His-Phe-OH <u>and</u> 80 citraconic anhydride (modify lysine) $\xrightarrow{\text{trypsin}}$ 81	3/3
69–81	69 75 H-Gly-Ser-Leu-Pro-Gln-Lys-Ser-Gln-(-)-(-)-Arg-Ser-Gln-OH	0/4
82–89	82 89 H-Asp-Gly-Asn-Pro-Val-Val-His-Phe-OH <u>and</u>	0/4

The amino acid sequences of basic protein fragments were reproduced to correspond to the known sequence of the bovine basic protein (9). Methods for generating the above listed peptides, doses used for challenge and the EAE incidence were reported by Chou et al. (6).

Table 4. Encephalitogenic potency of synthetic peptide antigens in Lewis rats.

Challenging antigen	Amino acid sequence	EAE potency
	69 70 75 80 84	
Peptide S8	H-Gly-Ser-Leu-Pro-Gln-Lys-Ala-Gln-Gly-His-Arg-Pro-Gln-Asp-Glu-Asn-OH	+
Peptide S49	H-Gly-Ser-Leu-Pro-Gln-Lys-Ala-Gln-(-)-(-)-Arg-Pro-Gln-Asp-Glu-Asn-OH	++++
Peptide S52	H-Pro-Gln-Lys-Ala-Gln-(-)-(-)-Arg-Pro-Gln-Asp-Glu-Asn-OH	++++
Peptide S51	H-Gln-Lys-Ala-Gln-(-)-(-)-Arg-Pro-Gln-Asp-Glu-Asn-OH	++++
Peptide S50	H-Ala-Gln-(-)-(-)-Arg-Pro-Gln-Asp-Glu-Asn-OH	++++
Peptide S20a	H-Arg-Pro-Gln-Asp-Glu-(-)-OH	-
Peptide S53	H-Ser-Gln-(-)-(-)-Arg-Ser-Gln-Asp-Glu-Asn-OH	++++
Guinea pig BP		++++
Bovine BP		+

The listed peptides were synthesized in the laboratory. The amino acid residue numbers correspond to the bovine myelin basic protein (9). Partial amino acid sequence of the guinea pig basic protein is known (26). The EAE potency of listed antigens is compared to a challenging dose of 10 µg of guinea pig basic protein.

Table 5. Encephalitogenic activity of fragments from bovine and guinea pig basic proteins in Lewis rats.

Residue number	Amino acid sequence	Incidence of clinical EAE
	1 30 37 38 43	
1-89	N-Ac-Ala-(2-29)-Arg-His-Arg-Asp-Thr-Gly-Ile-Leu-Asp-Ser-Leu-Gly-Arg-Phe-(44-89)-OH	4/5
1-43	N-Ac-Ala-(2-29)-Arg-His-Arg-Asp-Thr-Gly-Ile-Leu-Asp-Ser-Leu-Gly-Arg-Phe-OH	5/5
1-37	N-Ac-Ala-(2-29)-Arg-His-Arg-Asp-Thr-Gly-Ile-Leu-OH	0/5
38-89	H-Asp-Ser-Leu-Gly-Arg-Phe-(44-89)-OH	5/5
44-89	H-(44-89)-OH	0/5
38-43 Conclusion:	H-Asp-Ser-Leu-Gly-Arg-Phe-OH	
	90 94 109 114	
90-170	H-Phe-Lys-Asn-Ile-Val-(95-108)-Leu-Ser-Leu-Ser-Arg-Phe-(115-170)-OH	3/5
90-153	H-Phe-Lys-Asn-Ile-Val-(95-108)-Leu-Ser-Leu-Ser-Arg-Phe-(115-153)-OH	1/5
111-170	H-Leu-Ser-Arg-Phe-(115-170)-OH	0/5
109-114 Conclusion:	H-Leu-Leu-Ser-Arg-Phe-OH	

The aminco acid sequences of basic protein fragments were reproduced to correspond to the known sequence of the bovine basic protein (9). Methods for generating some of the listed fragments doses used for challenge and the incidence of clinical EAE, were reported by Martenson et al. (23).

Studies with overlapping peptides suggested the presence of two mutually exclusive encephalitogenic determinants found in separate regions of both bovine and guinea pig basic proteins (23). The data presented in Table 5 provide a summary of reported findings (23) in addition to relevant amino acid sequences of overlapping peptides used. Comparison of the encephalitogenic activities of peptide fragments derived from the pepsin digest of myelin basic proteins revealed that the sequence of residues 1-37 was non-encephalitogenic compared to the overlapping sequence of residues 1 to 43 or the parent fragment 1 to 89. Similarly, the overlapping sequence of residues 38 to 89 was encephalitogenic compared to the shorter sequence of residues 44 to 89. The difference between encephalitogenic and non-encephalitogenic fragments is the presence of residues 38 to 43 at the C- and N-terminal ends of encephalitogenic fragments 1 to 43 and 38 to 89, respectively. The authors concluded that the sequence of residues 38 to 43 H-Asp-Ser-Leu-Arg-Phe-OH, "constitutes an encephalitogenic determinant" for Lewis rats.

The second encephalitogenic determinant was not as clearly defined as the first. The encephalitogenic activity of the second half of the basic protein molecule (residues 90 to 170) was localized in a shorter fragment made up of residues 90 to 153 but not in fragment 111 to 170 demonstrating that additional residues N-terminal to Leu (residue no. 111) are essential components of this determinant. Because of the difference in the encephalitogenic activities of fragments 90 to 153 and 111 to 170 and the sequence similarities to the first determinant, the authors concluded that the sequence of residues 109 to 114, Leu-Ser-Leu-Ser-Arg-Phe, might be the second encephalitogenic determinant for Lewis rats.

The amino acid sequences of the two proposed non-overlapping determinants were synthesized in our laboratory and their encephalitogenic activity could not be demostrated in Lewis rats. The data presented in Table 6 show that neither peptide S46, residues 38 to 43, nor peptide S47, residues 109 to 114, induced clinical or histological signs of EAE. It is not clear, however, whether the failure of peptides S46 and S47 to induce EAE is related to the absence of essential residues from the N-, C- or both ends of the synthetic sequences. In the intact basic protein, the C-terminal Phe of peptide S46 is followed by another Phe, residue no. 44. This Phe-Phe linkage is repeated twice in the sequence of the basic protein molecule (9). Synthetic peptide S45 (residues no. 85 to 93) with a Phe-Phe linkage was non-encephalitogenic in Lewis rats (Table 6). Deletion of His, residue no. 87, as in peptide S44, did not alter the non-encephalitogenic activity of this peptide. Similarly, the C-terminal Phe of peptide S47 is followed by Ser-Trp-Gly-Ala-Glu-Gly-Gln-Lys, residues 115 to 122. The sequence of this region, shown in peptide S3, is known to induce EAE in guinea pigs (16); however, the administration of peptide S3 or the encephalitogenic determinant for rabbits, peptide S24, failed to induce EAE in Lewis rats.

   An alternative explanation for the encephalitogenic activity
of basic protein fragments may be that other encephalitogenic
determinants are present as contaminants in the enzymatically prepared fragments from both bovine and guinea pig basic proteins.
Based upon equimolar doses, the encephalitogenic activity of bovine
and guinea pig basic proteins was accounted for by the activity
found for their respective fragments 38 to 89 (23). The encephalitogenic determinants in these fragments have been defined by
synthetic peptide S8 (bovine sequence) (12) and synthetic peptide
S53 (guinea pig sequence) (13). Although the presence of additional
determinants in regions of the basic protein molecule other than
fragment 38 to 89 has not been ruled out, our results strongly
suggest the presence of a single encephalitogenic determinant for
Lewis rats.

Table 6. Encephalitogenic activity of synthetic peptides in Lewis
rats.

Peptide	Amino acid sequence	EAE incidence
S46	38 43 H-Asp-Ser-Leu-Gly-Arg-Phe-OH 44 48 Phe-Gly-Ser-Asp-Arg-	0/4
S45 S46	85 93 H-Pro-Val-Val-His-Phe-Phe-Lys-Asn-Ile-OH H-Gly-Pro-Val-Val-(-)-Phe-Phe-Lys-Asn-Ile-OH	0/6 0/6
S47	109 114 H-Leu-Ser-Leu-Ser-Arg-Phe-OH 115 118 Ser-Trp-Gly-Ala	0/4
S3	114 122 H-Phe-Ser-Trp-Gly-Ala-Glu-Gly-Gln-Lys-OH	0/5
S24	65 74 H-Thr-Thr-His-Tyr-Gly-Ser-Leu-Pro-Gln-Lys-OH	0/5

Groups of Lewis rats were challenged with either of the above listed
peptides emulsified with complete Freund's adjuvant. Each rat was
injected in one hind foot pad with 0.1 ml emulsion containing 50
µg of peptide and 100 µg M. butyricum. All rats were terminated
between day 20 and 26 following challenge. The brain and spinal
cord were isolated for histology.

Acknowledgements. I am grateful to Drs. Hugh Fitzpatrick and Richard D. Sharpe for their advice and support; to Evelyn Carvalho, Chingmei Yu and Marvin Ellis for their technical assistance. This work was supported by NINCDS grant no. 5 R01 NS 12316-03; The National Multiple Sclerosis Society grant no. RG 1063-A-3 and a grant from The Margaret T. Biddle Foundation.

REFERENCES

1. Alvord, E.C. Jr., Etiology and pathogenesis of experimental allergic encephalomyelitis, in The Central Nervous System (O.T. Bailey and D.E. Smith, eds.), The Williams and Wilkins Co., Baltimore (1968) pp. 52-70.

2. Alvord, E.C. Jr., Acute disseminated encephalomyelitis and allergic neuroencephalopathies, in Handbook of Clinical Neurology Vol. 9 (P.J. Vinken and G.W. Bruyn, eds.) North-Holland Publishing Co., Amsterdam (1970) pp. 500-571.

3. Brostoff, S.W. and Eylar, E.H., The proposed amino acid sequence of the P1 protein of rabbit sciatic nerve myelin, Arch. Biochem. Biophys. 153 (1972) 590-598.

4. Carnegie, P., Properties, structure and possible neuroreceptor role of the encephalitogenic protein of human brain, Nature 229 (1971) 25-28.

5. Caspary, E.A. and Field, E.J., An encephalitogenic protein of human origin: some chemical and biological properties, Ann. N. Y. Acad. Sci. 122 (1965) 182-198.

6. Chou, J. C-H., Chou, F. C-H., Kowalski, T.J., Shapira, R. and Kibler, R.F., The major site of guinea pig myelin basic protein encephalitogenic in Lewis rats, J. Neurochem. 28 (1977) 115-119.

7. Dunkley, P.R., Coates, A.S. and Carnegie, P., Encephalitogenic activity of peptides from the smaller basic protein of rat myelin, J. Immunol. 110 (1973) 1699-1701.

8. Einstein, E.R., Chao, L.P., Csejtey, J., Kibler, R. and Shapira, R., Species specificity in response to tryptophan modified encephalitogen, Immunochemistry 9 (1972) 73-84.

9. Eylar, E.H., Brostoff, S., Hashim, G.A., Caccam, J. and Burnett, P., Basic A1 protein of the myelin membrane. The complete amino acid sequence, J. Biol. Chem. 246 (1971) 5770-5784.

10. Eylar, E.H. and Hashim, G.A., Allergic encephalomyelitis: cleavage of the C-tryptophyl bond in the encephalitogenic basic protein from bovine myelin, Arch. Biochem. Biophys. 131 (1969) 215-222.

11. Eylar, E.H., Salk, J., Beveridge, G.C. and Brown, L.V., Experimental allergic encephalomyelitis: an encephalitogenic basic protein from bovine myelin, Arch. Biochem. Biophys. (1969) 132: 34-48.

12. Hashim, G.A., Experimental allergic encephalomyelitis in Lewis rats: chemical synthesis of disease-inducing determinant, Science 196 (1977) 1219-1221.

13. Hashim, G.A., Carvalho, E.F. and Sharpe, R.D., Definition and synthesis of the essential amino acid sequence for experimental allergic encephalomyelitis in Lewis rats, J. Biol. Chem. (1977), submitted for publication.

14. Hashim, G.A. and Eylar, E.H., Allergic encephalomyelitis: isolation and characterization of encephalitogenic peptides from the basic protein of bovine spinal cord, Arch. Biochem. Biophys. 129 (1969) 645-654.

15. Hashim, G.A. and Schilling, F.J., Prevention of experimental allergic encephalomyelitis by nonencephalitogenic basic peptides, Arch. Biochem. Biophys. 156 (1973) 287-297.

16. Hashim, G.A. and Sharpe, R.D., Experimental allergic encephalomyelitis:the structural specificity of determinants for delayed hypersensitivity, Immunochemistry 11 (1974) 633-640.

17. Hashim, G.A. and Sharpe, R.D., Non-encephalitogenic synthetic analogues of the determinant for allergic encephalomyelitis in guinea pigs, Nature 255 (1975) 484-485.

18. Hashim, G.A., Sharpe, R.D., Carvalho, E.F. and Stevens, L.E., Suppression and reversal of experimental allergic encephalomyelitis in guinea pigs with a non-encephalitogenic analogue of the tryptophan region of the myelin basic protein, J. Immunol. 116 (1976) 126-130.

19. Kies, M.W. and Alvord, E.C. Jr (eds.), Encephalitogenic activity in guinea pigs of water soluble protein fractions of nervous tissue, in Allergic Encephalomyelitis, Charles C. Thomas Co., Springfield, Ill. (1959) pp. 293-299.

20. McFarlin, D.E., Blank, S.S., Kibler, R.F., McKneally, S. and Shapira, R., Experimental allergic encephalomyelitis in the rat: response to encephalitogenic proteins and peptides, Science 179 (1973) 478-480.

21. Martenson, R.E., Deibler, G.E., Kies, M.W. and Levine, S., Myelin basic protein of mammalian and submammalian vertebrates: encephalitogenic activities in guinea pigs and rats, J. Immunol. 109 (1972) 262-270.

22. Martenson, R.E., Deibler, G.E., Kramer, A.J. and Levine, S., Comparative studies of guinea pig and bovine myelin basic proteins. Partial characterization of chemically derived fragments and their encephalitogenic activities in Lewis rats, J. Neurochem. 24 (1975) 173-182.

23. Martenson, R.E., Levine, S. and Sowinski, R., The location of regions in guinea pig and bovine myelin basic proteins which induce experimental allergic encephalomyelitis in Lewis rats, J. Immunol. 114 (1975) 592-596.

24. Merrifield, R.B., Solidphase peptide synthesis. III. An improved synthesis of bradykinin, Biochemistry 3 (1964) 1385-1390.

25. Nakao, A., Davis, W.J. and Einstein, E.R., Basic protein from the acidic extract of bovine spinal cord. I. Isolation and characterization, Biochim. Biophys. Acta 130 (1966) 163-170.
26. Shapira, R., McKneally, S., Chou, F. C-H., and Kibler, R.F., Encephalitogenic fragment for myelin basic protein. Amino acid sequence of bovine, rabbit, guinea pig, monkey and human fragments, J. Biol. Chem. 246 (1971) 4630-4640.
27. Swanborg, R.H., Immunological response to altered encephalitogenic protein in guinea pigas, J. Immunol. 102 (1969) 381-388.
28. Swanborg, R.H. and Amesse, L.S., Experimental allergic encephalomyelitis: species variability of the encephalitogenic determinant, J. Immunol. 107 (1971) 281-283.
29. Waksman, B.H., Experimental allergic encephalomyelitis and the "auto-allergic" diseases, Int. Arch. Allergy Suppl. 14 (1959) 1-87.
30. Westall, F.C., Robinson, A.R., Caccam, J., Jackson, J. and Eylar, E.H., Essential chemical requirements for induction of allergic encephalomyelitis, Nature 229 (1971) 22-24.

COMPARISON OF THE RAT AND MOUSE ENCEPHALITOGENIC DETERMINANTS

K.T. Burgess, C.C.A. Bernard[+] and P.R. Carnegie

Russell Grimwade School of Biochemistry and
   Walter and Eliza Hall Institute,
   University of Melbourne
Parkville, 3052, Australia

Because of extensive knowledge of the regulation of the immune
response in the mouse it is an excellent animal for studying models
of human autoimmune disease. However, most strains of mice are
resistant to the induction of experimental autoimmune encephalomyelitis (EAE). The SJL/J and SJL/J/BALB/c hybrids are susceptible
to mouse spinal cord, mouse myelin basic protein and a peptide
corresponding to the region between amino acid residues 45 and 89
in other myelin proteins (2). However, even with this strain, relatively large doses of encephalitogen are necessary and the use
of pertussis vaccine as an additional adjuvant is essential (1).

The amino acid sequence of an encephalitogenic peptide from a
peptic digest of mouse myelin basic protein was determined (3).
This peptide was identical in amino acid sequence to the mid-region
of the rat protein (5) except for the insertion of the dipeptide
His-Gly in the C-terminal half of the peptide (Table 1).

Table 1 compares the encephalitogenic activity and amino acid
sequence of part of the myelin basic protein from four species.
Several groups (4, 7, 8) have recently concluded that the major
encephalitogenic determinant for the rat is contained within this
region of the protein. Because the only difference between the rat
and mouse peptic peptides was the deletion of the His-Gly sequence
and because the rat protein appeared to be less active in the mouse
it seems likely that the region between amino acid residues 75 and
87 is the encephalitogenic determinant for the mouse. The lack of

------

[+]Present address: Roche Institute for Immunology, Basel, Switzerland.

Table 1. Encephalitogenic activity and amino acid sequence of mid-region of myelin basic protein.

Protein	Activity in SJL/J mice	Amino acid sequence - residues 75-87*
Mouse	+++	75 87 Gln-Lys-Ser-Gln-His-Gly-Arg-Thr-Gln-Asp-Glu-Asn-Pro
Rat	++	Gln-Lys-Ser-Gln-(-)-(-)-Arg-Thr-Gln-Asp-Glu-Asn-Pro
Human	Not active	Gln-Lys-Ser-(-)-His-Gly-Arg-Thr-Gln-Asp-Gln-Asp-Pro
Bovine	++**	Gln-Lys-Ala-Gln-Gly-His-Arg-Pro-Gln-Asp-Glu-Asn-Pro

* Residue numbers and sequence for rat, human and bovine myelin basic proteins from (5, Fig.3); (-) indicates deletion.
** Data from Ref. 9.

activity of the human protein could be related to the deletion of glutamine-78. Synthetic peptides are being prepared in an effort to delineate the amino acid sequence of the mouse encephalitogen as has been done for the rat (6, 8).

Acknowledgements. Supported by the Australian Research Grants Committee, the Canadian Multiple Sclerosis Society (C.C.A.B.) and in part by the National Multiple Sclerosis Society (Grant No. 887-B-3).

REFERENCES

1. Bernard, C.C.A., Experimental autoimmune encephalomyelitis in mice: Genetic control of susceptibility, J. Immunogenetics 3 (1976) 263-274.
2. Bernard, C.C.A. and Carnegie, P.R., Experimental autoimmune encephalomyelitis in mice: Immunologic response to mouse spinal cord and myelin basic proteins, J. Immunol. 114 (1975) 1537-1540.
3. Burgess, K.T., Bernard, C.C.A. and Carnegie, P.R., Experimental autoimmune encephalomyelitis in mice: Isolation, amino acid sequence and immunological activities of an encephalitogenic fragment from the smaller basic protein from mouse myelin: in preparation.
4. Chou, C.-H. J., Chou, F. C.-H., Kowalski, T.J., Shapira, R. and Kibler, R.F., The major site of guinea pig myelin basic protein encephalitogenic in Lewis rats, J. Neurochem. 28 (1977) 115-119.
5. Dunkley, P.R. and Carnegie, P.R., Amino acid sequence of the smaller basic protein from rat myelin, Biochem. J. 141 (1974) 243-255.
6. Hashim, G.A., Amino acid sequence requirement for induction of experimental allergic encephalomyelitis in Lewis rats: Abstracts of the ISN Satellite Symposium on "Myelination and Demyelination - Recent Chemical Advances", Helsinki, August, 1977, p. 23.
7. Martenson, R.E., Nomura, K., Levine, S. and Sowinski, R., Experimental allergic encephalomyelitis in the Lewis rat: Further delination of active sites in guinea pig and bovine myelin basic proteins, J. Immunol. 118 (1977) 1280-1285.
8. Westall, F.C., Thompson, M. and Lennon, V.A., Hyperacute autoimmune encephalomyelitis induced by a synthetic auto-antigen, Nature, in press.
9. Yasuda, T., Tsumita, T., Nagai, Y., Mitsusawa, E. and Ohtani, S., Experimental allergic encephalomyelitis (EAE) in mice: 1. Induction of EAE with mouse spinal cord homogenate and myelin basic protein, Jap. J. Exp. Med. 45 (1975) 423-427.

THE ACTION OF TRYPSIN ON CENTRAL AND PERIPHERAL NERVE MYELIN

E.H. Eylar and M.W. Roomi

Playfair Neuroscience Unit and Department of Biochemistry,
   University of Toronto
Toronto, Ontario, Canada

SUMMARY

In contrast to other studies, our results demonstrate that low concentration of trypsin degrades a high proportion of proteolipid from CNS myelin. The Wolfgram protein and BP are vulnerable and completely lost on trypsinolysis, perhaps accounting for some of the peptides retained by the myelin. In PNS myelin, the major PO protein, a hydrophobic glycoprotein, is readily degraded to a stable 18,000-19,000 molecular weight unit, referred to as TPO protein, still retaining the carbohydrate unit which probably exists as a nonasaccharide grouping. Production of the TPO glycoprotein results from cleavage of a lysinyl-methionine or arginyl-methionine linkage probably found approximately 80-100 residues from the NH_2-terminal isoleucine of the PO molecule. This linkage must be especially accessible to trypsin since the TPO protein is also generated in high yield when isolated PO protein is treated with trypsin in solution for 0.5 hours. Further incubation for 24 hours fully degrades the TPO protein to over 20 tryptic peptides, shown by peptide mapping, unlike the situation in myelin where the TPO unit is stable and resists further proteolysis.

The TPO unit is also produced when PO protein is treated with BrCN. The PO protein contains 3 methionine residues but presumably the methionine residue in the trypsin-sensitive region is crucial; cleavage leads to the same TPO unit minus NH_2-terminal methionine. Another methionine residue also exists in the TPO protein but it may be resistant to BrCN cleavage or else occupy a near-end position.

Abbreviations used: EAE - experimental allergic encephalomyelitis; EAN - experimental allergic neuritis; BP - myelin basic protein; PAGE - polyacrylamide gel electrophoresis; PLP - proteolipid protein.

Other proteins were also identified on PAGE of trypsinized PNS myelin: albumin, P2 protein, and PO protein. Albumin and P2 protein were identified in the acidic extract by reaction with specific antibody. The PO protein was isolated; it moved similarly to standard protein on SDS-PAGE and gave the appropriate amino acid analysis. However, it cannot be determined at this time whether a portion of these proteins remains because they are partially inaccessible to trypsin, or else are slightly attacked and thus represent early stages of trypsinolysis. The P2 protein of trypsinized myelin appears to migrate slightly faster than standard P2 protein on PAGE. Further work should clarify this point.

Amino acid analysis and sequence data show that the PO protein is particularly hydrophobic, very likely existing in PNS myelin as an amphipathic molecule which penetrates the bilayer but which has a hydrophilic portion exposed. It is this hydrophilic region that contains much lysine, particularly the crucial lysinyl-methionine linkage, that is so trypsin-sensitive. Determination of the amino acid sequence of terminal portions of the isolated PO and TPO proteins serves to firmly establish the PO protein as a unique entity probably exclusive to PNS myelin. It can be concluded that the study of trypsin activity toward PNS myelin has made possible a new understanding of how proteins are positioned in the membrane, and provided valuable insight into the PO protein.

INTRODUCTION

Proteolysis appears to be a crucial step in the final stages of the inflammatory process. In experimental demyelinating diseases such as EAE and EAN the myelin is directly attacked by macrophages (22, 39), and it is reasonable to assume that degradation of the myelin fragments within the macrophage must involve proteolysis by lysosomal enzymes. It was found in EAE that proteolytic activity occurs in CNS lesions in monkeys and rats, particulary cathepsins D, B1 and A, and neutral proteases being active (14, 32, 37). In multiple sclerosis, acid protease appears to increase (10, 33) at the edge of plaques with concomitant loss of BP.

Interestingly, although acid proteases such as capthesin D have been emphasized in the breakdown of myelin (10, 33) or BP (9), it was found (6) that protease activity was just as high at pH 8 using BP as substrate. Moreover, in rats with EAE, much higher proteolytic activity was found at both neutral and acidic pH (6). Although cathepsin D activity is responsible for proteolysis of BP during preparation at the acid extraction step (26), we found (13) that BP was degraded in situ when spinal cords were kept at room temperature, presumably at a neutral pH. From these data it appears that neutral proteases may play as important a role as acid proteases in breakdown of myelin proteins in normal and pathologic processes.

Because trypsin is one of the most specific proteolytic enzymes, we decided to investigate the action of this enzyme on CNS and PNS myelin. Although the action of trypsin toward myelin has been the subject of numerous studies, in no case have the proteolytic products been seriously investigated. Isolated CNS myelin or intact myelin (previously frozen) is susceptible to trypsin attack as shown in early studies (1, 20) by loss of myelin BP. Other studies (2, 31) have concluded that both BP and certain lipids are released from CNS myelin on trypsin treatment even when very high or low concentrations of trypsin are used. Dickinson et al. (8) found that trypsin affected CNS myelin by release of BP and that concomitantly, the interperiod line was replaced by a dense line position, but other studies using immunohistological procedures appear more reliable and position BP at the major period line in CNS myelin (17).

In PNS myelin from sciatic nerve, the action of trypsin is more complex, in some respect reflecting the complexity imposed by a greater number of protein components than in CNS myelin. Not only do the basic proteins appear to be lost, but the main protein component, the PO glycoprotein, appears to be degraded to a smaller unit still retained in the myelin membrane as shown by PAGE (18). One of the main objectives of this study was to answer this question.

Although all of the past studies on the effect of trypsin on myelin indicate that BP is accessible and degraded, a number of questions remain. Are there any peptide products of BP retained in the myelin membrane, perhaps protected from attack? We (12, 16) have shown that isolated myelin BP is extremely sensitive to trypsin proteolysis due primarily to its relatively open conformation: 28 tryptic peptides were in fact isolated,   sequenced and positioned on a peptide map during the course of the complete sequencing of BP (12). Thus we have in the BP molecule a highly sensitive indicator of trypsin accessibility to myelin substructure.

Other questions concerned with trypsin-myelin interactions relate to other proteins such as proteolipid of CNS myelin, and the PO glycoprotein of PNS myelin. Are they resistant to attack, and if not, what are the degradation products? There appears to be some differences in interpretation; Peterson (29) states that basic proteins are lost from PNS myelin followed by loss of major proteins whereas it is clear from the PAGE of Wood and Dawson (42) that the major protein might be degraded to a smaller unit which is not lost. Besides, PAGE alone is not adequate to determine whether basic proteins (BP and P2) survive proteolysis or not. It is difficult to interpret results using only PAGE techniques since a faster migrating band may be ascribed either to a small undegraded protein or a degradation product of a larger protein. For these reasons, it seemed necessary and instructive to isolate and identify the products from trypsin-degraded myelin. We have addressed ourselves to this problem in the twofold hope of discovering further facts about individual proteins and a more

definitive picture of where the proteins are positioned in the
myelin stucture. Additionally, a comparison of known proteolytic
activity on a standard myelin sample may indicate the most vulnerable points for proteolytic attack during nerve degeneration or
demyelinating diseases.

EXPERIMENTAL METHODS AND RESULTS

Trypsin on CNS myelin. It is reasonable to suppose that
examination of proteins remaining in trypsin-treated myelin may be
informative. London et al.(24) found that when BP was incorporated
into surface films of cerebroside sulfate, it was immune from trypsin attack over most of its NH_2-terminal region up to the hairpin
bend. In view of the great vulnerability of the BP molecule to
trypsinolysis (16), these data imply that the lipid-protein interactions involving BP may be pronounced and protective.

CNS myelin used for this study was prepared from rabbit brain
according to the method of Suzuki et al. (38) and finally purified
on a discontinuous sucrose gradient. The myelin was incubated with
a low concentration of trypsin, 0.025 mg/ml, for 0.5 hours under
conditions shown in Fig. 1. All of the proteins appear to be degraded to varying degrees, but the Wolfgram protein and BP are
completely lost. Although some proteolipid (PLP) still remains,
possibly indicative of its known resistance to proteolysis, much
of the PLP has been degraded. Interestingly, three new bands appear
representing peptides with a molecular weight near 10,000 or less
and must represent degradation products of one or more of the major
proteins. In order to determine the origin of the peptides

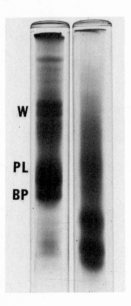

Fig. 1. The polyacrylamide gel electrophoresis pattern of normal (left) and
trypsinized (right) rabbit brain myelin
in SDS is shown as stained with Coomassie
blue. In untreated myelin, the basic
protein (BP), proteolipid (PL) and
Wolfgram (W) bands are clearly seen.
In the trypsinized myelin, peptide bands
migrating faster than BP are seen. For
both cases, 0.1 mg of ether-ethanol defatted myelin was used. For trypsinization, 20 mg of washed (or lyophilized)
myelin was incubated for 0.5 hours at
$25^{\circ}C$ in 3 ml of ammonium bicarbonate
buffer, 0.1 M, pH 8.0, containing 0.075 ml
of trypsin (1 mg/ml); final trypsin concentration is 0.025 mg/ml.

remaining in the myelin, studies are currently underway to isolate these peptides, and once purified, determine their amino acid composition and sequence and thereby their origin. Since the complete amino acid sequence of the BP is known (4, 12), peptides from this source can be easily identified. Peptides from PLP could be identified by the presence of half—cysteine, an amino acid absent from BP and Wolfgram protein. Moreover, some tryptic peptides have already been derived from PLP (proteolipid P7) and sequenced by Jolles et al. (19).

One of the most surprising findings of this study is that the PLP was substantially degraded by trypsin, even at the low level of enzyme used. Resistance to trypsin has long been cited as a characteristic of PLP and indeed, in the isolated state, it appears to be highly trypsin-resistant. In myelin, however, there are several variables to be considered. In a study of rat myelin by Wood et al.(44), only BP (large and small) was degraded, but an extremely low concentration of trypsin (0.001%) was used. When extremely high levels of trypsin were used on bovine myelin, chloroform-methanol soluble protein was greatly reduced (31). Classically, trypsin-resistant protein (TRPR) has been prepared from white matter after extensive trypsinolysis, and under such conditions, very likely some myelin remains inaccessible to the enzyme. It is not surprising therefore, that TRPR was found to be heterogeneous with PLP as the main component (23). Thus factors such as the state of the myelin, animal species, and trypsin concentration must be considered in interpreting these data.

It can be concluded from our results that PLP molecules in myelin are accessible to trypsin and are degraded. Other reports using modest concentrations of trypsin on CNS myelin also show some degradation of PLP (2). It is not too surprising that proteins of the myelin membrane are accessible to solvent and macromolecules. If the tissue had been frozen, as in our case, prior to isolation, then BP becomes reactive with immunoglobulin (17). Thus the myelin lamellae can be penetrated even at the minor period surface by macromolecules or other hydrophilic probes if modest disrupting procedures have been employed. In isolated myelin PLP is accessible and reactive with nonpenetrating membrane probes (40), and even in intact myelin, PLP will react with certain reagents (30). Thus PLP molecules are approachable in situ; their vulnerability to proteolysis while surprising, must be considered in light of studies (19, 23) showing that isolated PLP is attacked by trypsin in the presence of nonionic detergent. The detergent-treatment may promote trypsinization in two ways; by inducing a trypsinizable conformation, i.e. similar to that in situ, and by preventing peptide aggregation. Undoubtedly some PLP may be protected by the lamellar structure and thus digestion may not proceed completely.

The finding of proteolipid degradation by trypsin, and the retention of tryptic peptide fragments in the treated myelin are the major observations of this phase of the study. Whereas we found three peptides retained in the degraded myelin, it was reported (44) that no such products of BP degradation were observed. That study, however, does not rule out BP as the source of the peptides since an exceedingly mild trypsin concentration was used. Even the study of Norton <u>et al.</u> (27) using a very dilute macrophage extract, clearly produced degradation of BP from myelin with the concomitant appearance of peptide products. Identification of such degradation products could substantially assist our understanding of BP-lipid interactions within the myelin membrane, particularly if they involve the NH_2-terminal region of the BP molecule as found in model studies (24).

 <u>Trypsin on sciatic nerve myelin.</u> PNS myelin contrasts with CNS myelin in its more complex protein pattern on PAGE. At least nine protein bands, four of which are glycoproteins, can be routinely observed in sciatic nerve myelin from rabbit (Fig. 2), human or chicken sources (35). The major protein is the PO glycoprotein,

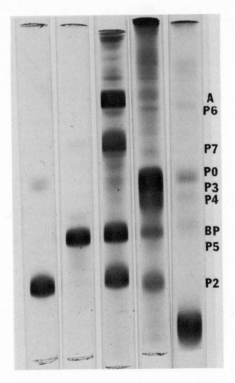

Fig. 2. SDS-PAGE of protein standards and whole defatted rabbit sciatic nerve myelin (from left to right): P2 protein; myelin BP; a mixture of P2, BP, ovalbumin and albumin; and myelin stained with Coomassie blue and PAS respectively. The amount of protein used was 0.020 mg except for defatted myelin where 0.1 and 0.3 mg was applied respectively.

molecular weight 28,000 (5). The BP, previously referred to as P1
protein, is also present as shown by isolation and comparison of the
amino acid sequence with BP from CNS myelin (4). Another major
protein is the P2 protein, molecular weight near 14,000 (18). The
BP and P2 proteins are basic proteins and comprise 13% and 7% respectively of rabbit sciatic nerve myelin proteins compared to 55%
for the PO protein (15). The other proteins are referred to as
P4, P5, P6, and P7 proteins, respectively. With the rabbit, human,
and chicken sciatic nerve myelin we routinely see four band staining
by the PAS method, the PO, P4, BP and P6 bands (35). The BP is
not a glycoprotein, but we have found that a glycoprotein does
migrate to that position and may be identical to the PASII glycoprotein isolated by Kitamura et al. (21). We also find routinely
that serum albumin binds to PNS myelin and thus is present as a
high molecular weight contaminant which can be isolated and identified (35).

The sciatic nerve myelin used for this study was prepared
initially by the method of Suzuki et al. (38) and then subjected
to discontinuous sucrose gradients (35). The middle band, 50% of
the total myelin, appeared highly purified based on electron
microscopy and the low level of enzymes from organelles. The
myelin from the gradient was washed in H$_2$O and lyophilized in some
cases.

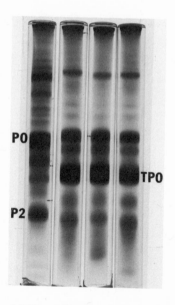

Fig. 3. SDS-PAGE of rabbit sciatic nerve myelin and trypsin-treated
myelin, from left to right: defatted myelin (0.1 mg); trypsin-
treated myelin (0.1 mg) incubated for 0.5, 3 and 24 hours respectively under conditions given in Fig. 1.

When frozen or lyophilized rabbit sciatic nerve myelin is treated with trypsin (0.025 mg/ml) for 0.5, 3 or 24 hours, the resulting protein pattern is nearly indistinguishable regardless of the time of incubation (Fig. 3). The most striking observation is the degradation of the PO protein and the appearance of a new band, referred to as TPO, near the BP band, confirming reports of Wood and Dawson (42) and Peterson (29). Since the TPO band is produced rapidly in high quantity, it is presumably derived from the PO protein, the major myelin protein.

Although the protein profile of the trypsinized myelin differs considerably from the untreated myelin, it is still quite complex. The band at the P2 protein position remains, although diminished, but it cannot be decided on the basis of the PAGE pattern alone whether it represents undegraded or possibly slightly degraded P2 protein or a breakdown product of some other protein. Several high molecular weight proteins are degraded and lost, but the albumin band remains prominent. Neither the PO nor P4 proteins are completely degraded; appreciable quantities remain even after 24 hours. The P5 band increases and as with CNS myelin, some peptide material appears which is smaller than the P2 protein. The differences between normal and trypsinized myelin are emphasized by the tracings shown in Fig. 4. The P2 band of the trypsinized myelin migrates faster than the normal P2 band (Fig. 4) and it is possible that the P2 protein has been partially degraded.

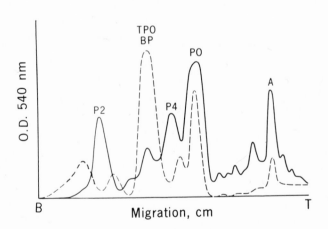

Fig. 4. Densitometric scan of rabbit sciatic nerve myelin (high PO peak) and trypsin-treated myelin incubated 0.5 hours under conditions given in Fig. 1.

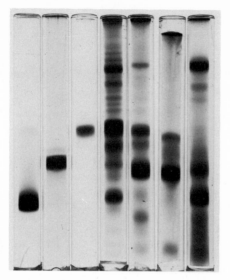

Fig. 5. SDS-PAGE (from left to right) of: (1) P2 protein; (2) BP; (3) PO protein; (4) defatted rabbit sciatic nerve myelin; (5) defatted trypsin-treated rabbit sciatic nerve myelin; (6) neutralized acid-insoluble residue; and (7) acid soluble proteins from trypsin-treated myelin. Except for standards, 0.1 mg of material was used.

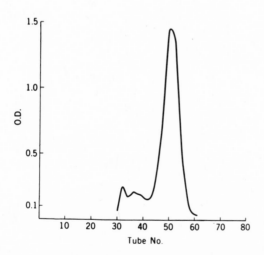

Fig. 6. Elution pattern (O.D. at 280 nm) of neutralized acid-insoluble trypsin-treated rabbit sciatic nerve myelin on an Agarose 0.5 m column, (8.3 x 2.7 cm) in 2% SDS-0.1 M phosphate buffer. Optical density at 280 nm is plotted against tube number (2.5 ml/ tube).

Isolation of TPO protein and other proteins. In order to determine the origin of the TPO band, we decided to attempt its isolation. When trypsinized PNS myelin is defatted with chloroform:
methanol and extracted at pH 2, approximately 15% of the protein is
extracted. As shown in Fig. 5, the acidic extract (gel 7) contains
material migrating at the P2 and albumin positions along with some
TPO and peptides as well. In the acidic residue (gel 6) TPO protein
predominates but some PO and P4 band material is also present.

In order to isolate the TPO protein, the pH 2-insoluble
material was chromatographed on a column of Agarose 0.5 m in 2%
SDS (Fig. 6). As shown by PAGE (Fig. 7), the TPO protein is concentrated in the latter part of the main peak. The small early
peak (gel 4) also contains TPO but in an aggregated state. When
the latter half of the main peak is rechromatographed under similar
conditions, the TPO protein can be obtained in a high degree of
purity as shown in Fig. 8. The TPO protein also contains carbohydrate as shown by the PAS reaction (gel 6). The isolation of TPO
protein by this procedure is much easier than isolation of PO protein, which can be accomplished in 2% SDS by the same procedure (21,
35), because potential contaminating proteins such as the P3 and P4
proteins are mainly destroyed by the trypsin treatment. Surviving
proteins, such as the P2 protein and albumin, are removed by acid
extraction. For these reasons, TPO protein can be prepared in a
37% yield compared to PO protein obtainable in a 7% yield (21).

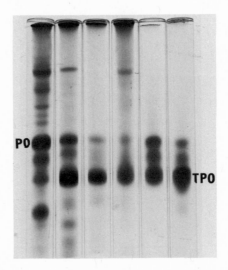

Fig. 7. SDS-PAGE of fractions obtained from chromatography of the
acid-insoluble residue from trypsinized PNS myelin as shown in Fig.
6 (left to right): (1) defatted rabbit sciatic nerve myelin; (2)
trypsin-treated sciatic nerve myelin; (3) acid-insoluble trypsin-
treated sciatic nerve myelin; (4) Tubes 30-40; (5) Tubes 42-50;
and (6) Tubes 51-58. Protein applied in each case is 0.1 mg.

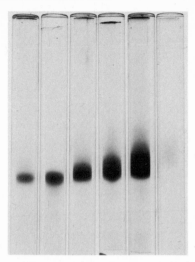

Fig. 8. SDS-PAGE of purified TPO protein. The amount applied is
(from left to right): 0.005 mg; 0.01 mg; 0.015 mg; 0.025 mg; 0.05
mg and 0.05 mg (PAS stained).

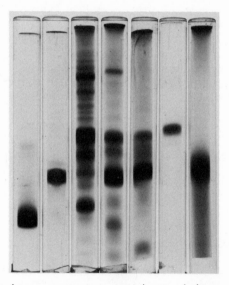

Fig. 9. SDS-PAGE (from left to right) of (1) P2 protein; (2) BP;
(3) defatted rabbit sciatic nerve myelin; (4) trypsin-treated
sciatic nerve myelin; (5) acid-insoluble trypsin-treated sciatic
nerve myelin; (6) PO protein isolated from trypsin-treated PNS
myelin; and (7) purified TPO protein.

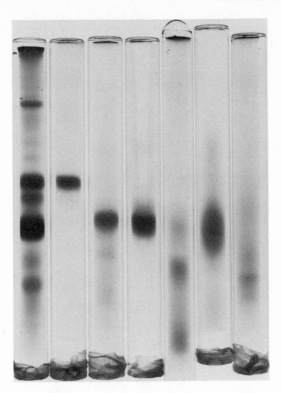

Fig. 10. SDS-PAGE (from left to right): (1) trypsin-treated
rabbit sciatic nerve myelin (conditions in Fig. 1); (2) PO protein;
(3) PO protein treated with BrCN; (4) TPO protein; (5) TPO protein,
treated with trypsin for 24 hours; (6) PO protein, treated with
trypsin for 0.5 hours; (7) PO protein, treated with trypsin for 24
hours. For BrCN treatment, a 100-fold excess of BrCN was used in
70% formic acid and incubated 2 days at 25°C. For trypsinization,
a 1:40 ratio of trypsin to protein was used under conditions given
in Fig. 1.

        Other proteins were also isolated from trypsinized PNS myelin.
From the acid extract, the P2 protein was isolated by procedures
described elsewhere (3). The P2 protein was convincingly demonstrated by amino acid analysis and immunodiffusion using goat antibody prepared against homogeneous rabbit P2 protein. Thus it
appears that the P2 protein in myelin is quite resistant to tryptic
digestion, unlike BP. It should be noted that trypsin will completely degrade P2 protein in solution (3, 5, 18). Whether small subtle
changes have occurred to the P2 protein during trypsinization of
myelin will be clarified by further study.

It was also possible to isolate PO protein from trypsinized myelin by chromatocraphy of the acidic residue on Agarose 0.5 m in 2% SDS as described elsewhere (35), in a manner similar to that of Kitamura et al. (21). The isolated PO protein showed a single band on PAGE (Fig. 9, gel 6), and gave the appropriate amino acid analysis (Table 1). Again, subtle changes not yet detected, may have occurred.

Degradation of isolated PO protein. One of the questions which arise is how trypsin acts on isolated PO protein compared to PO protein in situ. When PO protein is incubated for 0.5 hours under conditions identical to that used for PNS myelin, the major product is a 18,000-19,000 molecular weight unit which appears similar if not identical to TPO protein on SDS-PAGE (Fig. 10, gel 6). These results emphasize the vulnerability of a particular region of the PO molecule to trypsin attack. This result is identical to results obtained when PO protein is degraded in situ. In striking contrast to myelin, however, further incubation with trypsin (24 h) degrades the TPO unit to numerous peptides (Fig. 10, gel 7). Peptide mapping of the digested PO protein shows approximately 25-26 peptides, a figure somewhat less than the 35 expected peptides based on the number of lysine and arginine residues (Table 1). It is apparent however that trypsin can degrade the TPO protein to a high degree. This finding contrasts with TPO in myelin where the TPO unit is protected from further degradations by trypsin even after 24 hours. Treatment of the isolated TPO protein confirms this observation (gel 5). Peptide mapping of digested TPO protein shows 19-20 peptides that correspond precisely to peptides found on peptide mapping of the PO protein digested for 24 hours with trypsin. This result adds strong evidence that the TPO protein is derived from the PO protein.

BrCN treatment of PO protein also leads to a unit of same molecular weight as TPO protein (Fig. 10, gel 3). A reasonable interpretation of these data is that the BrCN treatment cleaves the PO molecular at a methionine residue occupying the trypsin-sensitive region. These results demonstrate that a crucial trypsin-sensitive region surrounding a methionine residue exists in PO protein; cleavage of the peptide linkage in this region either by trypsin or BrCN leads to formation of a 18,000-19,000 MW unit. This unit is protected in myelin but is further degraded by trypsin in solution.

Properties of the PO and TPO proteins. As shown by gel electrophoresis originally by Everly et al. (11) and Wood and Dawson (41), the PO protein reacts with the PAS reagent and thus is a glycoprotein (Fig. 2). Interestingly, the TPO unit is also a glycoprotein, having virtually the same monosaccharide analysis as the PO protein (Table 2). We have computed (34) that the carbohydrate of PO, and thus TPO, probably exists as a single nonasaccharide unit based on gas chromatography analysis of the trifluoroacetate derivatives of the methyl-glycosides. This carbohydrate unit is

not removed by the trypsin treatment of PO protein in intact myelin.
The carbohydrate unit comprises approximately 5.5% by weight of the
PO protein; mannose and N-acetylglycosamine predominate but N-acetyl-
galactosamine is absent.

The amino acid analysis of the PO and TPO proteins shows expected similarities (Table 1). Both are highly nonpolar and have
a small percentage of half-cysteine and methionine. Based on a
molecular weight of 28,000 there appears to be 3 methionine residues
in the PO protein. Thus treatment with BrCN could potentially lead
to four peptide products. The content of nonpolar residues is
high, and it is quite likely that the PO molecule is compact and
contains a high level of secondary structure. By comparison, the
TPO appears considerably more nonpolar than PO protein, having more
valine, leucine, phenylalanine etc. Interestingly, TPO contains
much less lysine; on a molar basis, 65% of the lysine is lost in
the conversion to the TPO protein. Furthermore, the TPO protein
has distinctly less polar and apolar amino acids and more nonpolar
amino acids than the PO protein.

Table 1. Amino acid composition of proteins derived from rabbit
sciatic nerve myelin.

AMINO ACID	Amino acid composition (moles %) PO	TPO
Lysine	9.0	4.0
Histidine	2.5	5.0
Arginine	7.0	5.6
Aspartic acid	9.0	6.6
Threonine	4.3	4.9
Serine	6.9	7.5
Glutamic acid	9.0	7.2
Proline	4.6	2.2
Glycine	10.0	8.0
Alanine	6.5	7.4
Half-cystine	1.6	1.5
Valine	8.9	11.9
Methionine	1.2	1.2
Isoleucine	4.4	6.0
Leucine	7.4	9.5
Tyrosine	4.4	4.7
Phenylalanine	3.9	6.8

Table 2. Carbohydrate composition of PO and TPO proteins from rabbit sciatic nerve myelin.

| Monosaccharide* | Weight %** | | Moles/mole protein |
	TPO	PO	
Galactose	11.0	9.2	1
Mannose	34.9	32.9	3
N-acetylglucosamine	29.3	26.8	2
Sialic acid	16.3	18.9	1
Fucose	8.5	12.1	1-2

*Determined as the TFA derivative of the O-methylglycoside.
**The total carbohydrate unit is 5.5% by weight of the PO protein (28,000 MW).

Table 3. Amino acid sequences of the NH_2-terminal regions.

	1		3		5	
PO Protein	NH_2 - Ile - Val - Val - Tyr - Thr - Asp
TPO Protein	NH_2 - Met - Leu - Leu - X - Leu - Leu
Proteolipid (Lipophilin)	NH_2 - Gly - Leu - Leu - Glu - Cys - Cys

| | 7 | | 9 | | 11 | | 13 |
| Pro - Gln - Val - Asn - Gly - Ala - Val |
| Gly - Ile - Ile - Val - Leu - X - Val |
| Ala - X - Cys - Leu - Val - Gly - Ala |

| | 15 | | | 17 | 19 |
| Gly - X - X - Val - Thr - Leu |
| Ala - Val - Leu - Val - Leu - Phe - Val |
| Pro - Phe - Ala - Ser - Leu - Val - Ala |

Thus it appears that trypsinization of the PO protein in myelin leads to a loss of a region with more polar and hydrophilic characteristics than the remaining TPO region.

In Table 3 the amino acid sequence of the NH_2-terminal regions of the PO and TPO proteins are compared with the PLP. There is no sequence homology with the PLP in this region thus establishing the PO protein as a unique myelin protein probably exclusive to the PNS. The NH_2-terminal residues of the PO and TPO proteins are isoleucine and methionine respectively. It is evident that the TPO sequence is the most hydrophobic of the three sequences shown.

DISCUSSION

Trypsin exhibits a definite action toward most of the CNS and PNS myelin proteins. With CNS myelin, all of the proteins are degraded to varying degrees; no trace of the original Wolfgram proteins and BP can be observed. In contrast, several proteins in PNS myelin partially resist proteolysis, such as the PO and P2 proteins, and most interestingly, the PO protein is degraded to a 18,000-19,000 molecular weight unit (TPO) which resists further proteolysis. One of the most immediate advantages of this phenomenon is that TPO protein can be isolated far more easier and in higher yield than PO protein itself.

In working with myelin a major problem exists in studying protein distribution and availability because myelin is not simply a bilayer but a multi-lamellar structure, and most proteins might theoretically not be accessible to reagents. When myelin is not previously frozen or disrupted prior to (or during) preparation, it appears to be nonpenetrable by macromolecules (17), and BP might resist tryptic attack if indeed it does occupy the cytoplasmic side (major period line) of the bilayer unit. In isolated myelin, however, where hypotonic solutions are used, BP becomes accessible to macromolecules such as immunoglobulin (17) and lactoperoxidase (30). In the present work highly purified myelin was derived from previously frozen sciatic nerve. Thus it is not surprising that trypsin exerts extensive attack on some of the myelin proteins. It is likely that these proteins become accessible because the myelin, when minimally disrupted, becomes penetrable by the solvent phase. Moreover, it is reasonable to assume that the proteins maintain their position in the isolated myelin and that accessibility to trypsin results from partial penetration of bilayers by solvent rather than some major reorientation of the proteins.

The loss of BP from both CNS and PNS myelin is not unexpected in view of its likely external localization due to its highly charged character. The BP molecule, however, probably penetrates the lipid layer at several positions (12, 24) but accessibility of one or two appropriate peptide linkages to trypsin could result in complete degradation, perhaps leading to some of the acid-soluble peptides observed on PAGE. The Wolfgram protein is also rapidly

removed and it is evident that much of the proteolipid also is
attacked. These results suggest that portions of each protein of
CNS myelin must be available at the surface, whether outer or cytoplasmic side, where some of its peptide bonds are hydrolyzed.

PNS myelin is more complex than CNS myelin; there are more
proteins with the PO protein predominating. As in CNS myelin, the
BP molecule appears readily attacked by trypsin since it was not
found in the acid extract. A search is planned for possible BP
peptide fragments remaining in the trypsinized myelin of CNS and
PNS myelin. With PO protein, however, the results are easiest to
interpret since it degrades to the TPO protein (MW 18,000-19,000).
Proof that the TPO protein is a degradation product of PO protein
comes from several sources: a) it is the major degradation product,
and PO protein is the major protein; b) its amino acid analysis is
similar to PO; c) its monosaccharide profile is nearly identical to
that in PO protein; d) the tryptic peptide maps show many overlapping peptides; e) a unit of the same size is obtained by treating PO protein in solution either with trypsin (0.5 hours) or with
BrCN; and f) the COOH-terminal residues are similar. All of these
data support the conclusion that the TPO glycoprotein is derived
from the PO protein.

In conversion of PO to TPO protein (Fig. 11) approximately
30% of the PO polypeptide chain is removed. The released peptide
was not isolated, but evidently must derive from the NH_2-terminal
end. If intact, it would have a molecular weight of 8,600-10,000
(80-100 amino acids) with NH_2-terminal isoleucine and COOH-terminal

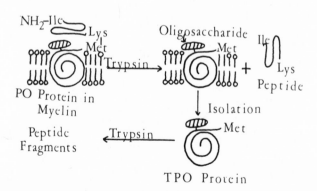

TPO Protein

Fig. 11. Trypsin activity of the PO protein. A conceptual view
of how the PO protein may be positioned as an amphipathic molecule
in the myelin membrane spanning the bilayer. Trypsin attacks the
exposed Lys-Met or Arg-Met linkage releasing a 80-100 residue
hydrophilic peptide. The remaining TPO glycoprotein is buried in
the membrane and immune to further tryptic attack; if isolated,
however, the TPO protein is vulnerable and broken down to peptides
by trypsin.

lysine or arginine. It is probably relatively rich in lysine, arginine, and hydrophilic residues as shown by comparison of amino acid analysis of PO and TPO proteins (Table 1). It can be concluded that most of the PO protein molecules in the myelin membrane have their NH_2-terminal region exposed to the polar phase where it is accessible to large molecules such as trypsin. The TPO product is likely submerged or deeply penetrating into the bilayer since it is resistant to further attack by trypsin even after 24 hours, contrasting with the situation in solution. Thus we can speculate that approximately 30% of the PO molecule is hydrophilic and thus exists in the polar phase, while the remainder is compact and submerged into the bilayer. Thus the PO protein can be portrayed as an amphipathic molecule having an exposed polar portion and a buried nonpolar moiety much like a classical membrane protein as pictured by Singer (36). Trypsin can hydrolyze the more polar segment at the NH_2-terminus by cleavage of a lysinyl or arginyl-methionine linkage. Interestingly, the TPO fragment remaining in the bilayer still contains the carbohydrate moiety which is surely exposed to the polar surface. Possibly somewhat more of the PO molecule is actually found at the bilayer surface, but the bulky oligosaccharide may block further action by trypsin.

The position of PO protein in myelin is diagramatically shown in Fig. 11 as spanning the bilayer. Since the lipophilin proteolipid molecule shows a diameter of about 57 Å in liposomes (25), and the PO protein is slightly larger, it is very likely that it also spans the bilayer of 40 Å or so. Both of these proteins are highly hydrophobic and would be expected to exist in a highly globular folded conformation. Trypsin attacks the vulnerable Lys-Met or Arg-Met linkage near the surface leaving TPO embedded in the bilayer and releasing a 80-100 residue peptide which may be further degraded. Further support for this concept comes from the action of BrCN on isolated PO protein which also yields a product of the same size as the TPO protein. Clearly, BrCN treatment must lead to cleavage of the same methionine residue involved in the tryptic attack. There are three and two methionine residues in the PO and TPO proteins respectively. One of these residues is removed in deriving TPO; another occupies the NH_2-terminus of TPO. The third residue may resist cleavage or else is near the COOH-terminus where cleavage leads only to a minor change in size.

This study shows that the use of trypsin on even such a complex structure as PNS myelin can assist our understanding of protein orientation within the membrane. The isolation of the TPO protein provides new insight into the PO protein, the latter being more difficult to purify. This study may also have relevance to our understanding of myelin breakdown in pathologic processes. In Wallerian degeneration, the PO protein is degraded and lost, although the TPO product does not appear (43). Rather, a product of approximately 13,000 molecular weight is seen. Thus, the loss of integrity of the myelin membrane may result from proteolysis of the PO protein regardless of the degradation product, whether TPO or some other unit, depending on the proteinase involved. It is tempting to propose, therefore, that the PO protein is a crucial element in the buildup and maintenance of the myelin membrane. This concept is compatible with recent freeze-fracture studies (7) that show a protein in PNS myelin which spans the bilayer and, moreover, aggregates linearly through numerous lamellae. The most likely candidate for this role in vertical stabilization of the myelin membrane is the PO protein. It would be expected, therefore, that modification of PO protein could adversely affect bilayer stability, and would be agreeable with electron microscopic studies of trypsinized PNS myelin which show swelling at the intraperiod line and splitting at the major period line (28).

Acknowledgements. This work has been supported by a grant from the Medical Research Council of Canada. We are indebted to Professor T. Hoffmann and Mr. S. Rhee for sequence studies, Dr. C. Breckenridge for sugar analysis, and Mr. N. Khan and G. Mason for technical assistance.

REFERENCES

1. Adams, C. and Bayliss, O., Histochemistry of myelin V: trypsin-digestible and trypsin-resistant protein, J. Histochem. Cytochem. 16 (1968) 110-114.
2. Banik, N. and Davison, A.N., Lipid and basic protein in interaction in myelin, Biochem. J.143 (1974) 39-45.
3. Brostoff, S., Burnett, P., Lampert, P. and Eylar, E.H., Isolation and partial characterization of a protein from sciatic nerve myelin responsible for experimental allergic neuritis, Nature 235 (1972) 210-212.
4. Brostoff, S. and Eylar, E.H., The proposed amino acid sequence of the P1 protein of rabbit sciatic nerve myelin, Arch. Biochem. Biophys. 153 (1972) 590-598.
5. Brostoff, S., Karkhanis, Y., Carlo, D., Reuter, W. and Eylar, E.H., Isolation and partial characterization of the major proteins of rabbit sciatic nerve myelin, Brain Res. 86 (1975) 449-458.
6. Buletza, G. and Smith, M.E., Enzymic hydrolysis of myelin basic protein and other proteins in the CNS and lymphoid tissues from normal and demyelinating rats, Biochem. J. 156 (1976) 627-633.
7. DaSilva, P. and Miller, R., Membrane particules on fraction faces of frozen myelin, Proc. Nat. Acad. Sci. U.S.A. 72 (1976) 4046.
8. Dickinson, J., Jones, K., Aparicio, S. and Lumsden, C., Localization of encephalitogenic basic protein in the intraperiod line of lamellar myelin, Nature 227 (1970) 1133-1134.

9. Einstein, E., Csejtey, J. and Marks, N., Degradation of
    encephalitogenic protein by purified brain acid proteinase,
    FEBS Lett. 1 (1968) 191-195.
10. Einstein, E.R., Csejtey, J., Davis, W., Lajtha, A. and Marks,
    N., Enzymatic degration of the encephalitogenic protein,
    Int. Arch. Allergy 36 (1969) 363-375.
11. Everly, J., Brady, R. and Quarles, R., Evidence that the major
    protein in rat sciatic nerve myelin is a glycoprotein, J.
    Neurochem. 21 (1973) 329-334.
12. Eylar, E.H., Brostoff, S., Hashim, G., Caccam, J. and Burnett,
    P., Basic A1 protein of the myelin membrane, the complete
    amino acid sequence, J. Biol. Chem. 246 (1971) 5770-5784.
13. Eylar, E.H., Salk, J. Beveridge, G. and Brown, L., Experimental
    allergic encephalomyelitis: an encephalitogenic basic protein
    from bovine myelin, Arch. Biochem. Biophys. 132 (1969) 34-48.
14. Govindarajan, K., Rauch, H., Clausen, J. and Einstein, E.R.,
    Changes in cathepsins B-1 and D, neutral-proteinase, and
    2',3'-cyclic-nucleotide -3'phosphodydrolase activities in
    monkey brain with experimental allergic encephalomyelitis,
    J. Neurol. Sci. 23 (1974) 295-306.
15. Greenfield, S., Brostoff, S., Eylar, E.H. and Morell, P.,
    Protein composition of myelin of the PNS, J. Neurochem. 20
    (1973) 1207-1216.
16. Hashim, G. and Eylar, E.H., Allergic encephalomyelitis:
    Enzymatic degradation of the encephalitogenic basic protein
    from bovine spinal cord, Arch. Biochem. Biophys. 129 (1969)
    635-644.
17. Herndon, R., Rauch, H. and Einstein, E., Immuno-electron
    microscopic localization of the encephalitogenic basic protein
    in myelin, Immunol. Commun. 2 (1973) 163-172.
18. Ishaque, A., Roomi, M.W., Khan, N. and Eylar, E.H., Myelin
    protein: the composition of the P2 protein from rabbit sciatic
    nerve, Biochem. Biophys. Acta (1977) in press.
19. Jolles, J., Nussbaum, J-L., Schoentgen, F., Mandel, P. and
    Jolles, P., Structural data concerning the major rat brain
    myelin proteolipid P7 apoprotein, FEBS Lett. 74 (1977) 190-
    194.
20. Kies, M., Thompson, E. and Alvord, E., The relationship of
    myelin proteins to experimental allergic encephalomyelitis,
    Ann. N.Y. Acad. Sci. 122 (1965) 148-160.
21. Kitamura, K., Suzuki, M. and Uyemura, K., Purification and
    partial characterization of two glycoproteins in bovine PNS
    myelin membrane, Biochem. Biophys. Acta. 455 (1976) 806-816.
22. Lampert, P.W., Demyelination and remyelination in experimental
    allergic encephalomyelitis, J. Neuropath. exp. Neurol. 24
    (1965) 371-385.
23. Lees, M.B., Messinger, B. and Burnham, J., Tryptic hydrolysis
    of brain proteolipid, Biochem. Biophys. Res. Commun. 28 (1967)
    185-190.

24. London, Y. and Vossenberg, F., Specific interactions of central nervous myelin basic proteins with lipids: Specific regions of the protein sequence protected from the proteolytic action of trypsin, Biochem. Biophys. Acta. 307 (1973) 478-490.
25. Moscarello, M., personal communication.
26. Nakao, A., Davis, W. and Einstein, E., Basic proteins from the acidic extract of bovine spinal cord, Biochem. Biophys. Acta. 130 (1966) 171-179.
27. Norton, W.T., Cammer, W., Bloom, B.R. and Gordon, S., Possible mechanisms of inflammatory demyelination: Macrophage secretion products. Myelination and demyelination: Recent chemical advances, Satellite symposium of the ISN, Helsinki, August 1977.
28. Peterson, R., Electron microscopy of trypsin-digested PNS myelin, J. Neurocyt. 4 (1975) 115-120.
29. Peterson, R.G., Myelin protein changes with digestion of whole sciatic nerve in trypsin, Life Sci. 18 (1976) 845-850.
30. Poduslo, J. and Braun, P., Topographical arrangement of membrane proteins in the intact myelin sheath, J. Biol. Chem. 250 (1975) 1099.
31. Raghavan, S., Rhoads, D. and Kanfer, J., The effects of trypsin on purified myelin, Biochem. Biophys. Acta. 328 (1973) 205-212.
32. Rauch, H., Einstein, E.R., Csejtey, J., Enzymatic degradation of myelin basic protein in central nervous system lesions of monkeys with EAE, Neurobiol. 3 (1973) 195-205.
33. Riekkinen, P., Clausen, J. and Arstila, A., Further studies on neutral proteinase activity of CNS myelin, Brain Res. 19 (1970) 213.
34. Roomi, M.W., Ishaque, A., Breckenridge, W., Khan, N. and Eylar, E.H., The PO protein: A Glycoprotein of PNS myelin, Trans. Am. Neurochem. Soc. 8 (1977) 158.
35. Roomi, M.W., Ishaque, A., Khan, N. and Eylar, E.H., Glycoproteins and albumin in PNS myelin, J. Neurochem. (1977) in press.
36. Singer, S.J., The molecular organization of membranes, Ann. Rev. Biochem. 43 (1974) 805-845.
37. Smith, M., Sedgewick, L. and Tagg, J., Proteolytic enzymes in experimental demyelination in rat and monkey, J. Neurochem. 23 (1974) 965-971.
38. Suzuki, K., Poduslo, S. and Norton, W.T., Gangliosides in the myelin fraction of developing rats, Biochem. Biophys. Acta. 144 (1967) 375.
39. Wisniewski, H., Prineas, J. and Raine, C., An ultrastructural study of demyelination and remyelination, Lab. Invest. 21 (1969) 105-118.
40. Wood, D., Epand, R. and Moscarello, M., Localization of the basic protein and lipophilin in myelin membrane with a non-penetrating reagent, Biochem. Biophys. Acta. 467 (1977) 120-129.
41. Wood, J. and Dawson, R.M.C., A major myelin glycoprotein of sciatic nerve, J. Neurochem. 21 (1973) 717-719.

42. Wood, J.G. and Dawson, R., Some properties of a major struc-
     tural glycoprotein of sciatic nerve, J. Neurochem. 22 (1974)
     627-630.
43. Wood, J. and Dawson, R.M.C., Lipid and protein changes in
     sciatic nerve during degeneration, J. Neurochem. 22 (1974)
     631-635.
44. Wood, J.G., Dawson, R. and Hauser, H., Effect of proteolytic
     attack on the structure of CNS myelin membrane, J. Neurochem.
     22 (1974) 637-643.

CLEARANCE OF MYELIN BASIC PROTEIN FROM BLOOD OF NORMAL AND

EAE RABBITS

L.F. Eng, Y-L. Lee, K. Williams, G. Fukayama, B. Gerstl,
  and M. Kies*
Department of Pathology, Stanford University School of
  Medicine, Stanford, California 94305, and
Veterans Administration Hospital, Palo Alto,
  California 94304, U.S.A.

SUMMARY

The rate of clearance of porcine myelin basic protein (MBP)
from plasma of rabbits was determined following intravenous injection of 20 mg MBP. The MBP level in the plasma was measured by
a 2-site immunoradiometric assay with specific antibody to guinea
pig MBP produced in rabbits. Plasma MBP-antibody levels were determined by competitive binding radioimmune assay (RIA). Unsensitized and those sensitized with complete Freund´s adjuvant (CFA),
with porcine MBP in CFA, and with whole porcine spinal cord in CFA
were studied. Unsensitized and CFA sensitized rabbits exhibited
maximum MBP levels in the plasma within two minutes after injection
with rapid decrease to undetectable levels in one hour. Thirty-nine
of the unsensitized (control) rabbits exhibited normal, rapid
clearance and no subsequent physical signs of EAE while one of the
control rabbits exhibited a slightly retarded clearance rate.
Histologic examination of autopsy tissues from the control group
revealed that five rabbits showed lesions which could be attributed
to Encephalitozoan cuniculi or Toxoplasma and one rabbit autopsied
65 days after clearance had minimal EAE lesions. Rabbits sensitized
with MBP exhibited a retarded rate of clearance at the acute stage
of EAE and following recovery. Rabbits sensitized with whole spinal
cord in CFA also exhibited a retarded rate of MBP clearance. Anti
(MBP) antibodies were detected in the plasma of all rabbits which
exhibited a retarded rate of MBP clearance. Significant rates of

---

*Section on Myelin Chemistry, Laboratory of Cerebral Metabolism,
National Institute of Mental Health, Bethesda, Maryland 20014.

retardation were not detected until approximately three weeks after
sensitization with CFA-MBP or CFA-spinal cord. While MBP antibody
levels in most animals were not detected by the immunodiffusion
technique, antibodies were demonstrated by RIA. The 20 mg MBP given
intravenously is probably in great antigen excess and conducive to
the formation of soluble MBP-anti(MBP) complexes in the blood.

INTRODUCTION

In recent years, the assumption that multiple sclerosis (MS)
is partly or entirely a sequelae of autosensitization has been prom-
ulgated by several authors (13). Consequently, desensitization by
injections of small amounts of myelin basic protein (MBP) or of the
specific immunogenic peptide derived from the intact MBP or prepared by chemical synthesis has been suggested.

Presently, few data are known about the absorption and distribution of MBP when injected without adjuvant into an animal. Large
or repeated doses may occasionally cause experimental allergic
encephalomyelitis (EAE). The experiments reported here were undertaken to study the absorption and clearance of MBP from normal, unsensitized rabbits and rabbits sensitized with complete Freund's
adjuvant (CFA), MBP in CFA, and whole spinal cord in CFA. This
included time sequential determinations of MBP in plasma at various
time intervals following injection of MBP at different stages of
EAE.

While rabbits have been less frequently used for studying EAE
than guinea pigs and rats, they were selected as the experimental
animals because intravenous injection of the MBP was easy and reproducible and sufficient amounts of blood could be obtained at
the various time intervals.

EXPERIMENTAL

Porcine MBP was supplied by Eli Lilly Co., Indianapolis, Ind.,
and porcine whole spinal cord was obtained fresh from our animal
facility. Incomplete Freund's adjuvant (IFA) and M. tuberculosis
(H37Ra) were purchased from Difco.

Antiserum specific against guinea pig MBP was produced in the
rabbit and characterized previously (7).

Adult female white New Zealand rabbits, 3-4 kg body weight,
were purchased locally and kept under observation for two weeks
before immunization. The animals were observed daily.

The immunization procedures are as follows: A total volume
of 300-400 µl of suspension prepared by emulsifying equal volumes
of adjuvant and antigen solution was injected intradermally into 4
footpads. The first group of rabbits received CFA containing 2.1-
2.5 mg H37Ra per animal. The second group received 200-600 µg MBP,

Difco adjuvant, and 2.1-2.5 mg H37Ra per animal. The third group received 40-60 mg whole porcine spinal cord, Difco adjuvant, and 2.1-2.5 mg H37Ra per animal.

Unmodified porcine MBP and 125-iodine-labeled porcine MBP (125-I-MBP) were injected into normal rabbits to determine the optimum doses for subcutaneous and intravenous injections of MBP and to establish the normal rates of MBP clearance from the blood. MBP in 1 ml of physiological saline was injected into the right marginal ear vein and blood was drawn from the left marginal ear vein at various time intervals (2 min to 48 h following MBP injection; a 27-gauge needle was used for injection; blood was collected in heparin).

A 2-site immunoradiometric assay (IRMA) for MBP similar to that developed for the glial fibrillary acidic (GFA) protein (6) and Moore's S-100 protein (10) has been developed for the MBP. MBP immunoadsorbent, purified 125-I-labeled rabbit anti(guinea pig MBP) and 125-I-MBP were prepared using procedures identical to that described for the assay of GFA and S-100 proteins. BSA buffer denotes 0.05 M sodium phosphate buffer, pH 8.0, containing (per liter) 4.5 g NaCl, 200 mg sodium azide, and 1 g bovine serum albumin (Sigma Chemical Co., St. Louis, Mo.).

The 2-site IRMA of MBP was carried out as follows: The standard solutions contained 0.0, 0.4, 1.0, 4.0, 10.0, 40.0, 100.0, 400.0 and 1000.0 ng of porcine MBP protein per 0.1 ml. The assay is performed by pipetting 0.2 ml of diluted MBP standard (prepared by diluting the MBP standard with an equal volume of 1:25 diluted pre-MBP injection plasma) or 0.2 ml of 1:50 dilution of freshly drawn plasma in 0.2 M sodium bicarbonate buffer, pH 9.2, into the bottom of an antibody coated polystyrene tube or an uncoated tube (for the "sticky tube" assay, ref. 11). The tubes were left at room temperature for 24 h (reaction 1), aspirated and washed 2 times with 2 ml BSA-buffer. 0.2 ml (20,000 cpm) of rabbit 125-I-anti(MBP) in BSA-buffer was added and the tubes were left at room temperature for a further 48 h (reaction 2). The tubes were then aspirated, washed three times and counted for 4 min in an automatic gamma counter (Searle Model 1185).

The standard curve is constructed by plotting the radioactivity in the solid-phase (tube radioactivity) against the logarithm of the dose (ng/0.2 ml incubation). Typical standard curves are shown in Figs.2 and 3. Dose interpolation was carried out using a 4-parameter logit-log method which uses variable weighting (15).

Plasma MBP antibody levels were determined by radioimmune assay (competitive binding of 125-I-MBP, ref. 5).

The rate of clearance of 20 mg of MBP from plasma was determined in rabbits at various time intervals following sensitization with CFA, MBP in CFA, and porcine spinal cord in CFA. The clearance study was performed on rabbits which had been sensitized 6, 12, 17, 27 and 60 days with CFA and MBP in CFA. The rabbits sensitized with porcine spinal cord were used when acute clinical EAE symptoms were apparent (15-39 days following sensitization). Three to 5 sensitized

and 2 unsensitized (normal) rabbits were used for each experiment.
    A complete autopsy for each rabbit was performed and nervous
tissue as well as peripheral organs were fixed in 10% formalin.
Hematoxylin and eosin stained sections of the various paraffin-
embedded tissues have been prepared and examined for a majority of
the experimental rabbits. A detailed histopathologic study of the
remaining rabbits is still in progress. A separate report on the
pathology of EAE in our large series of rabbits will be forth-
coming. The numerical indices suggested by Alvord and Kies (1)
for quantitating the extent of EAE were used in this study. Clinical diagnosis was based on the following symptoms: hind leg paralysis, fecal impaction, and loss of weight.

RESULTS

    Electrophoretic comparison at two different hydrogen ion con-
centrations (pH) of porcine MBP provided by Eli Lilly Co. with
bovine MBP is shown in Fig. 1. This analysis which demonstrates
that the porcine MBP is essentially homogeneous was performed in
the research laboratory of Dr. M. Kies.
    A 2-site IRMA similar to that developed for the GFA protein
(6) has been developed for MBP which minimizes the problems encountered in the conventional radioimmune assays (RIA) that have

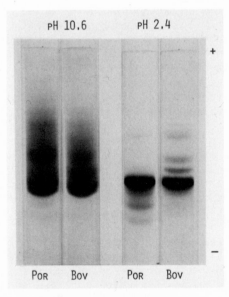

Fig. 1. Polyacrylamide gel electrophoresis of porcine and bovine
central nervous system myelin basic protein at pH 10.6 and pH 2.4.

been used for MBP (2-5, 8, 9). RIA uses 125-I-MBP and the competitive binding reaction (competitive inhibition or sequential saturation principle). MBP in dilute solutions (nanogram range) tends to
bind to glass, plastic, certain brain proteins, and red cells and
is very susceptible to degradation by proteinases at neutral pH.
A typical standard curve for the 2-site IRMA using rabbit MBP is
shown in Fig. 2. Similar dose-response curves are obtained when
purified MBP from brains of humans, monkeys, guinea pigs, rats and
mice are used. It is evident that MBP is lost when the same MBP
solutions are reassayed after 5 days of storage in the frozen state
(Fig. 2). Histones also bind to our MBP antibody. We have developed
an assay which takes advantage of the "sticky" binding of the MBP
to glass and plastic. Instead of using a solid-phase anti-MBP in
the first reaction (i.e., plastic tube coated with anti-MBP antibody), an uncoated plastic tube is used to bind the MBP in the
sample solution. It was determined that other proteins including
histones did not interfere with this specific binding of MBP. Fig.
3 illustrates a standard curve for the "sticky" tube assay. 10,000
ng of histone gives a response of less than 1 ng MBP.

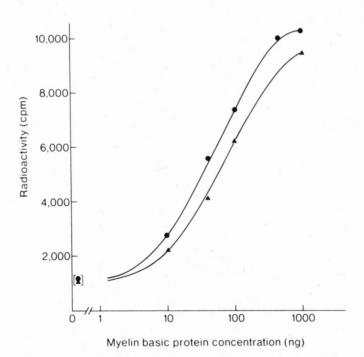

Fig. 2. 2-site IRMA dose-response curves for rabbit myelin basic
protein. ● MBP standards were prepared and used immediately.
▲ The same MBP standards at -20°C for 5 days before use.

The stability of MBP in plasma and serum was examined by injecting a normal rabbit intravenously with 20 mg MBP and taking a
bleed 5 minutes later. Nine aliquots of blood were mixed with
heparin and 9 aliquots were allowed to clot. At 10, 20, 30, 40,
and 50 min, 1, 2, 4, and 8 h intervals following the bleed,
aliquots of plasma and serum were prepared and assayed for MBP.
The plasma content remained at 125 ng per ml from 10 to 30 min
and decreased to a level of 98 ng per ml at 8 h. The serum content
was 100 ng/ml at 10 min, 56 ng/ml at 30 min, and decreased rapidly
to only 2 ng per ml at 8 h. In another experiment, 2 rabbits were
each injected intravenously with 20 mg MBP and blood taken 5 min
later. Plasma was immediately prepared and 8 aliquots stored at
4°C. At time intervals between 30 min and 8 h following the preparation of the plasma, aliquots were analyzed for MBP. The MBP
level remained constant during the initial 60 min and decreased
to half of the initial concentration by 8 h after the blood was
taken. It is evident that immunologically assayable MBP was rapidly lost during preparation of serum possibly due either to hydrolyses
by proteinases involved in the clotting of the blood or to adsorption

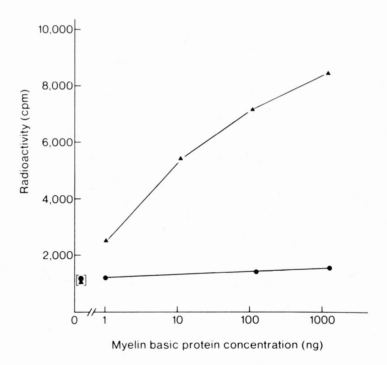

Fig. 3. "Sticky-tube" 2-site IRMA for the measurement of myelin
basic protein showing the failure to recognize cross-reacting
histone. Solid-phase antibody was not used. ▲ Myelin basic protein;
● histone. Zero dose-response is included within brackets.

to blood proteins or cells in the clot. The MBP activity in plasma, however, was stable for at least 1 h after preparation. Therefore, the entire study utilized only freshly prepared plasma. The MBP standard dose-response curve was determined individually for each rabbit by using freshly drawn plasma prior to injection of MBP.

In order to establish the optimum dose of MBP and route of injection, rabbits were injected intravenously and subcutaneously with 125-I-MBP (10, 20, 50, and 100 mg doses) and the clearance determined at intervals extending to 48 h after injection. The MBP content of whole blood, serum, and plasma was estimated by counting the 125-I; the content in the plasma was also determined by the 2-site IRMA. Table 1 and Fig. 4 summarize the results obtained with the rabbits which received subcutaneous injections of MBP.

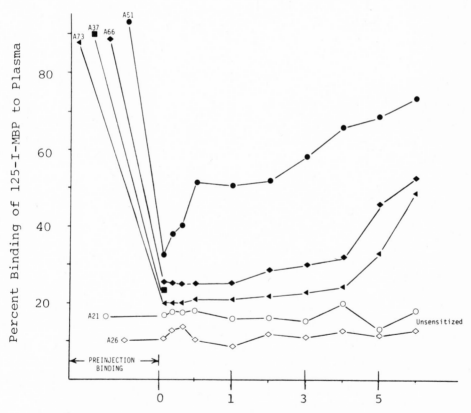

Time (Hours) Following the Injection of 20 mg MBP

Fig. 4. Percent binding of 125-I-MBP to plasma of rabbits following injection of MBP. Rabbits A73, A37, A66 and A51 were proven antibody producers; A21 and A26 were unsensitized, normal controls.

Table 1. Clearance rate of myelin basic protein (µg MBP per ml) from whole blood, red cells, and plasma in rabbits subcutaneously injected with 10, 20, 50, and 100 mg of iodine-125 labelled MBP.

Time following MBP injection (min)	10 mg MBP dose				20 mg MBP dose			
	Determined by I-125 MBP*			2-site IRMA**	Determined by I-125 MBP			2-site IRMA
	Whole	Red cells	Plasma	Plasma	Whole	Red cells	Plasma	Plasma
5	0.9	0.1	1.2	0.0	1.7	0.3	2.0	0.0
15	1.7	0.4	2.3	0.0	3.9	0.8	6.6	0.0
30	3.2	1.2	3.9	2.5	5.7	2.1	7.1	4.5
60	3.9	1.9	5.0	2.1	7.4	3.0	8.4	4.0
120	5.4	2.8	6.0	6.0	7.7	3.9	9.0	10.0
240	5.7	3.2	6.0	6.8	6.9	3.6	7.8	11.0
360	4.9	3.8	5.8	7.2	5.5	2.9	6.2	14.0
480	5.6	3.2	5.6	6.0	4.9	3.1	5.1	11.0
720	4.9	2.8	5.6	5.8	3.0	1.8	3.5	10.0
1440	4.6	2.3	4.9	3.0	2.4	1.1	1.8	7.0
2880	3.6	2.0	4.1	0.0	0.7	0.6	1.0	0.0

Time following MBP injection (min)	50 mg MBP dose				100 mg MBP dose			
	Determined by I-125 MBP			2-site IRMA	Determined by I-125 MBP			2-site IRMA
	Whole	Red cells	Plasma	Plasma	Whole	Red cells	Plasma	Plasma
5	5.3	1.1	6.2	0.0	11.4	2.8	14.7	0.0
15	11.9	2.8	14.7	0.0	21.5	5.0	28.2	1.0
30	16.2	5.1	19.1	1.5	28.4	8.2	34.2	2.5
60	22.4	8.1	30.1	7.5	34.7	13.4	43.7	13.2
120	22.8	13.1	25.8	8.0	38.4	20.3	46.4	15.1
240	22.2	13.9	24.0	12.0	39.2	24.8	44.3	30.1
360	21.1	11.6	21.5	21.5	35.4	23.0	40.5	20.2
480	18.6	13.1	21.6	23.6	30.2	20.3	36.0	23.5
720	17.5	11.7	19.9	18.0	27.1	16.3	31.0	20.0
1440	17.2	9.0	17.2	12.0	23.9	15.4	24.2	16.3
2880	12.3	8.1	13.7	0.0	14.6	8.3	17.2	0.0

* The MBP content was determined by comparing the radioactivity of the sample with that of the specific activity of the injected I-125-labelled MBP. **The MBP content of the plasma was determined by the 2-site IRMA.

Table 2. Clearance rate of myelin basic protein (μg MBP per ml) from whole blood, red cells and plasma in rabbits intravenously injected with 10, 20, 50, and 100 mg iodine-125 labelled MBP.

Time following MBP injection (min)	10 mg MBP dose				20 mg MBP dose			
	Determined by I-125 MBP*			2-site IRMA**	Determined by I-125 MBP			2-site IRMA
	Whole	Red cells	Plasma	Plasma	Whole	Red cells	Plasma	Plasma
5	7.0	1.9	8.7	8.1	15.1	4.3	18.2	23.3
15	5.6	2.0	6.6	4.2	12.0	4.4	14.5	5.1
30	5.1	2.8	5.7	1.4	11.3	5.7	14.0	1.5
60	5.1	3.3	6.0	0.8	11.6	6.6	12.9	1.0
120	4.7	2.0	5.5	0.0	11.0	6.5	12.6	0.0
240	4.2	2.7	4.8	0.0	9.0	6.4	11.3	0.0
480	3.7	2.9	4.8	0.0	8.8	5.8	9.7	0.0
720	3.0	2.2	3.9	0.0	8.5	5.2	11.1	0.0
1440	2.7	1.5	3.0	0.0	8.0	4.0	8.4	0.0
2880	1.6	0.9	2.0	0.0	5.6	6.5	6.5	0.0

Time following MBP injection (min)	50 mg MBP dose				100 mg MBP dose			
	Determined by I-125 MBP			2-site IRMA	Determined by I-125 MBP			2-site IRMA
	Whole	Red cells	Plasma	Plasma	Whole	Red cells	Plasma	Plasma
5	47.6	12.6	62.1	58.6	78.8	20.3	96.3	101.0
15	31.2	12.3	41.6	42.0	52.0	19.1	64.5	68.0
30	32.5	18.0	40.0	12.0	48.0	22.8	54.5	20.0
60	28.9	18.8	35.5	1.5	40.2	20.2	48.3	3.0
120	28.7	20.1	34.6	0.4	37.9	24.5	43.1	1.2
240	28.2	17.6	31.8	0.0	34.6	23.3	40.5	0.0
480	25.8	17.1	30.5	0.0	31.1	20.2	35.7	0.0
720	24.9	18.0	29.7	0.0	30.7	15.9	33.2	0.0
1440	23.4	14.0	26.4	0.0	24.4	12.1	28.6	0.0
2880	18.4	10.4	20.1	0.0	19.1	9.8	21.4	0.0

*MBP content was determined by comparing the radioactivity of the sample with that of the specific activity of the injected I-125-labelled MBP. **The MBP content of the plasma was determined by the 2-site IRMA.

Table 3. Clearance of myelin basic protein from the blood of
normal, unsensitized rabbits.

Rabbit number	2-site IRMA Clearance of 20 mg MBP Normal (−) Delayed (+)	RIA MBP-Antibody in the plasma % 125-I MBP binding	EAE diagnosis Positive (+) Negative (−) Histologic	Clinical
1	−	3	ND	−
2	−	5	±(E)*	−
3	−	6	ND	−
4	−	6	ND	−
5	−	6	±(T)‡	−
6	−	7	ND	−
7	−	8	±(T)‡	−
8	−	9	−	−
9	−	10	ND	−
10	−	10	−	−
11	−	13	ND	−
12	−	13	ND	−
13	−	13	ND	−
14	−	14	ND	−
15	−	15	−	−
16	−	15	−	−
17	−	15	−	−
18	−	15	−	−
19	−	15	ND	−
20	−	16	−	−
21	−	16	−	−
22	−	17	−	−
23	−	17	−	−
24	−	18	−	−
25	−	19	ND	−
26	−	19	ND	−
27	−	21	ND	−
28	−	21	−	−
29	−	22	±(E)*	−
30	−	22	−	−
31	−	22	ND	−
32	−	23	ND	−
33	±	24	−	−
34	−	24	±	−
35	−	24	−	−
36	−	25	ND	−
37	−	25	−	−
38	−	25	±(T)‡	−
39	−	27	−	−
40	−	27	−	−

*Encephalitozoan cuniculi infection; ‡ Toxoplasma infection;
ND = not determined.

Table 4. Clearance of myelin basic protein from the blood of rabbits sensitized with complete Freund's adjuvant.

Rabbit number	Clearance date Days following sensitization	2-site IRMA Clearance of 20 mg MBP Normal (-) Delayed (+)	RIA MBP-Antibody in the plasma % 125-I MBP binding	EAE diagnosis Positive (+) Negative (-) Histologic	EAE diagnosis Positive (+) Negative (-) Clinical
41	6	-	4	-	-
42	6	-	5	-	-
43	6	-	8	-	-
44	6	-	11	-	-
45	12	-	4	-	-
46	12	-	6	-	-
47	12	-	17	-	-
48	12	-	18	-	-
49	17	-	4	-	-
50	17	-	4	-	-
51	17	-	8	-	-
52	17	-	10	-	-
53	27	-	4	-	-
54	27	-	5	ND	-
55	27	-	8	ND	-
56	60	-	4	ND	-
57	60	-	7	ND	-
58	60	-	7	ND	-
59	60	-	9	ND	-

The maximum level of MBP in the plasma as determined by the
2-site IRMA was between 4 and 6 h. MBP as determined by 125-I
radioactivity was detected in the blood throughout the experimental
period. The subcutaneous injection route was not selected for
further consideration because of the larger amounts of MBP required (50-100 ng/rabbit) and the extended length of time required
to sample the blood.

Table 2 summarizes the results obtained with rabbits which
received intravenous injections of MBP. MBP as determined by
125-I was also detected in the blood throughout the experimental
period.   MBP as determined by the 2-site IRMA was essentially
cleared from the blood within one hour after injection. Either
the 125-I-MBP was bound to blood components which no longer could
react with MBP antibody or the 125-I-MBP fragments were no longer
immunologically reactive in the 2-site IRMA. 20 mg MBP and the
intravenous injection route were selected for the clearance study.

Forty normal, unsensitized rabbits were each cleared with 20
mg of porcine MBP (Table 3). Thirty-nine of these rabbits exhibited
normal, rapid clearance of MBP, and showed no subsequent physical
symptoms of EAE. One rabbit (Nr. 33) exhibited a slightly retarded
clearance rate. Histologic examination of autopsy tissues revealed
that 5 rabbits in the normal group showed lesions which could be
attributed to Encephalitozoan (14) or Toxoplasma (16) infections.
One rabbit autopsied 65 days after clearance had minimal EAE lesions.
It was surprising to find that the plasma from the unsensitized
rabbits contained a significant amount of specific MBP binding
factor (3-27%). In order to determine the possibility that this
binding could be due to the heparin used in preparing the plasma,
the following experiment was done with 3 normal rabbits. 125-I-
MBP binding was measured in serum, plasma using heparin as the
anticoagulant, and plasma using ethylenediaminetetraacetate as the
anticoagulant.   For each rabbit the percent 125-I-MBP binding in
the serum was comparable to the two plasma samples.

The MBP clearance rate for all the rabbits that were sensitized
with CFA was normal at time periods examined between 6 and 60 days
following sensitization (Table 4). It is interesting to note that
this group of rabbits exhibited the lowest percent binding to MBP
(4-18%). Histologic examination revealed that 3 rabbits in this
group developed histologic EAE lesions -- 88, 106, and 131 days
after clearance of the MBP.

Table 5 summarizes the clearance results for the MBP-sensitized
rabbits at 6, 12, 16-17, 27 days. Two rabbits tested at 6 days and
2 at 12 days exhibited a retarded clearance rate, but relatively
low binding for MBP. Among the rabbits tested between 16 and 27
days following sensitization, 10 exhibited delayed clearance of
MBP and 9 normal clearance; however, the plasma from this group of
rabbits all showed high percent binding to MBP.

In the group of rabbits that were tested over 60 days after
sensitization with MBP, all showed delayed clearance and a high
percent binding to MBP (Table 6).

Table 5. Clearance of myelin basic protein from the blood of rabbits sensitized with porcine myelin basic protein.

Rabbit number	Clearance date Days following sensitization	2-site IRMA Clearance of 20 mg MBP Normal (−) Delayed (+)	RIA MBP-Antibody in the plasma % I-125 MBP binding	EAE diagnosis Positive (+) Negative (−) Histologic	Clinical
60	6	−	4	ND	−
61	6	−	4	ND	−
62	6	−	8	++	+
63	6	−	10	−	±
64	6	−	11	ND	−
65	6	+	15	ND	−
66	6	+	16	ND	−
67	6	−	19	ND	−
68	12	−	12	ND	−
69	12	−	15	+++	±
70	12	−	16	ND	±
71	12	+++	18	+++	+
72	12	+	23	+++	+
73	12	Subc*	24	ND	
74	12	−	26	−	−
75	12	−	30	−	−
76	12	−	37	+++	−
77	16	Subc*	67	ND	
78	16	++++	71	+++	+
79	16	+++	71	−	±
80	16	++++	72	+++	+
81	16	+++	80	+++	+
82	17	−	36	ND	−
83	17	−	42	+++	+
84	17	−	56	ND	−
85	17	−	62	ND	−
86	17	+++	70	ND	+
87	17	+	75	ND	+
88	17	+	89	ND	+
89	27	−	62	±	+
90	27	−	63	++	+
91	27	−	74	−	+
92	27	−	75	++	+
93	27	+++	75	ND	+
94	27	+++	80	ND	+
95	27	−	85	+++	+
96	27	+	87	ND	−

*The rabbit was injected with MBP subcutaneously in the back rather than the footpads.

Table 6. Clearance of myelin basic protein from the blood of rabbits which had been sensitized with myelin basic protein for more than 60 days.

Rabbit number	2-site IRMA Clearance of 20 mg MBP Normal (−) Delayed (+)	RIA MBP-Antibody in the plasma % I-125 MBP binding	EAE diagnosis Positive (+) Negative (−) Histologic	Clinical
97	+	21	−	±
98	+	31	ND	∓
99	Subc*	42	ND	ND
100	+	49	ND	−
101	+	54	ND	−
102	+	55	ND	+
103	++++	60	ND	−
104	++	63	ND	+
105	Subc*	68	±	±
106	+	71	ND	±
107	++++	71	−	−
108	++++	72	−	−
109	++++	75	−	−
110	+	81	ND	±
111	+	82	ND	+
112	++	83	ND	±
113	++++	84	ND	±
114	+	85	ND	+
115	++	87	ND	+
116	++++	89	ND	+
117	+	91	ND	+
118	++++	91	ND	+
119	++++	92	ND	+

*The rabbit was injected with MBP subcutaneously in the back rather than the footpads.

While all the spinal cord sensitized rabbits were used only after acute clinical symptoms of EAE had developed, 9 of the 22 exhibited normal clearance (Table 7). In the group with normal clearance, four also showed a low percent binding to MBP and five a high percent binding. The majority of the rabbits exhibited a delayed clearance and high percent binding for MBP.

Four rabbits which were initially sensitized with MBP in CFA and used for the clearance study were subsequently given intracutaneuous injections of MBP in CFA and MBP in IFA in order to elicit production of precipitating antibodies to MBP.

Table 7. Clearance of myelin basic protein from the blood of rabbits sensitized with porcine spinal cord and exhibiting acute clinical symptoms of EAE.

Rabbit number	Clearance date Days following sensitization	2-site IRMA Clearance of 20 mg MBP Normal (−) Delayed (+)	RIA MBP-Antibody in the plasma % 125-I MBP binding	EAE diagnosis Positive (+) Negative (−) Histologic	Clinical
120	15	−	9	ND	+
121	20	−	17	ND	+
122	20	−	22	ND	+
123	20	++	23	ND	+
124	18	−	23	+++	+
125	20	++	28	ND	+
126	25	++	42	ND	+
127	20	+	46	−	+
128	25	−	51	+++	+
129	15	+	56	ND	+
130	20	+	59	+++	+
131	30	−	60	ND	+
132	20	++	63	ND	+
133	17	++++	63	ND	+
134	18	−	65	+++	+
135	18	+	67	+++	+
136	25	−	67	ND	+
137	39	++	70	+++	+
138	15	−	71	ND	+
139	30	++++	71	ND	+
140	17	++++	71	ND	+
141	25	++++	72	+++	+
142	20	++++	89	ND	+

After the sera from these rabbits were shown to form immunoprecipi-
tin lines against MBP by immunodiffusion, the rabbits were subjected
to a second clearance study with 20 mg of MBP. Rabbit Nr. 37 went
into convulsion and died immediately following injection of MBP.
Histologic examination of the autopsy tissues showed constriction
of a few pulmonary arterioles which is consistent with that of
anaphylactic shock.

The percent binding of 125-I-MBP to the plasma in the four
experimental animals and two controls are shown in Fig. 4. The
four sensitized rabbits showed high percent binding to MBP prior
to injection of the 20 mg of MBP. A dramatic decrease in MBP
binding occurred immediately after injection of the MBP. The MBP
binding capacity of the three surviving sensitized rabbits remained at a low level for 3 h before rising again. The plasma in
the two control rabbits exhibited a low percent binding to 125-I-
MBP which did not change significantly before or after injection
of the MBP.

DISCUSSION

During the course of this study, several chemical and biological problems were encountered. While the most direct approach to
the MBP clearance study appeared to be the use of 125-I-MBP,
difficulty in assessing the metabolism and catabolism of the labeled
MBP prevented its use. The instability of the MBP in serum required
that only freshly prepared plasma be used. The binding properties
and lability of the MBP, and the cross-reactivity of our MBP antiserum with histones (though minor), necessitated the development of
the 2-site "sticky tube" IRMA. Significant and variable levels
(3-27%) of MBP-binding factor were detected in normal rabbit plasma.
Consequently, plasma was prepared from each rabbit before injection
of MBP and used to measure base-line MBP-binding levels and to add
to the MBP standards in preparing the standard curve.

Biological variations with the rabbits complicated the study.
The response of the rabbits to MBP and whole spinal cord was
variable; some of the rabbits sensitized with MBP in CFA did not
become afflicted with EAE. The time interval between sensitization
and onset of the disease varied from 12 to 46 days. The appearance
of clinical signs of EAE did not always correspond to the appearance
of histologic lesions or the production of MBP antibody.

While the chemical and methodological problems could be minimized, the biological problems were not completely apparent until
the study was well under way. Histopathologic examination of the
rabbit tissues, a very important component of this study, is not
yet complete. Careful examination of tissues from the control
group of rabbits revealed that 5 rabbits which exhibited typical
EAE histologic lesions could be diagnosed as having encephalitozoan
or toxoplasma infections.

Precipitating MBP antibody could not be demonstrated by immuno-diffusion analysis with the majority of plasma samples, however, MBP antibodies were readily detected in many plasma samples by the 125-I-MBP binding technique. It is interesting to note that plasma from the normal, unsensitized rabbits contained significant amounts of MBP binding factor. Whether the binding factor in the control rabbits is MBP antibody, as is likely in the rabbits sensitized for an extend time period (longer than 60 days), is not currently known. The presence of this binding factor may partly explain the variable susceptibility of the rabbits to EAE when the low doses (200 µg) of MBP were injected into the rabbits. More consistent results were obtained when higher doses (600 µg) of MBP were used to sensitize the rabbits. Plasma from the four rabbits which had repeated injections of MBP (Table 7) were shown to form specific immunodiffusion lines against MBP. Demonstration that 125-I-MBP binding decreased immediately following injection of 20 mg MBP strongly indicated that MBP antibody was present in the blood. The immediate death of A37 with classical symptoms of anaphylactic shock further confirmed the antibody-antigen reaction.

The present study demonstrates that immunologically assayable MBP is rapidly cleared from the blood of normal rabbits when in-jected intravenously -- the maximum level detected within 2 min after injection and decreasing to negligible levels after 1 h. Subcutaneously injected MBP reaches the blood stream 30 min follow-ing injection and persists for as long as 8 h. Generally, rabbits at the acute stage of EAE and following recovery exhibited a de-layed clearance of 20 mg of MBP whether they were sensitized with MBP or whole spinal cord in CFA. The retarded clearance rate correlates well with the presence of MBP antibody in the blood. Since the MBP antibody levels are low, the 20 mg MBP is in great antigen excess -- thus favoring the formation of soluble antigen-antibody complexes. The present results and interpretation are in agreement with a similar study using the rat as the test animal (12). Demonstration that a non-encephalitogenic basic protein such as lysozyme does not have a delayed clearance rate in EAE rabbits that exhibit a delayed clearance of MBP would verify our present interpretations.

Acknowledgement. Supported by grant R-1051-A-1 from the National Multiple Sclerosis Society.

REFERENCES

1. Alvord, E.C. and Kies, M.W., Clinico-pathologic correlations in experimental allergic encephalomyelitis. II. Development of an index for quantitative assay of encephalitogenic activity of "antigens", J. Neuropath. Exp. Neurol. 18 (1959) 447-457.
2. Brostoff, S.W., Reuter, W., Hichens, M. and Eylar, E.H., Specific cleavage of the Al protein from myelin with cathepsin D, Biol. Chem. 249 (1974) 559-567.

3. Cohen, S.R., McKhann, G.M. and Guarnieri, M., A radioimmuno-
    assay for myelin basic protein and its use for quantitative
    measurements, J. Neurochem. 25 (1975) 371-376.
4. Day, E.D. and Pitts, O.M., Radioimmunoassay of myelin basic
    protein in sodium sulfate, Immunochem. 11 (1974) 651-659.
5. Driscoll, B.F., Kies, M.W. and Alvord, E.C., Successful
    treatment of experimental allergenic encephalomyelitis (EAE)
    in guinea pigs with homologous myelin basic protein, J.
    Immunol. 112 (1974) 392-397.
6. Eng, L.F., Lee, Y.-L. and Miles, L.E.M., Measurement of glial
    fibrillary acidic protein by a two-site immunoradiometric
    assay, Anal. Biochem. 71 (1976) 243-259.
7. Kies, M.W. and Bump, E.A., A rapid qualitative test for de-
    tection of precipitating antibody to myelin basic protein,
    Res. Comm. in Chem. Path. and Pharm. 4:3 (1972) 569-579.
8. McPherson, T.A. and Carnegie, P.R., Radioimmunoassay with gel
    filtration for detecting antibody to basic proteins of myelin,
    J. Lab. Clin. Med. 72 (1968) 824-831.
9. McPherson, T.A., Gilpin, A. and Seland, T.P., Radioimmunoassay
    of CSF for encephalitogenic basic protein: a diagnostic test
    for MS? CMA Journ. 107 (1972) 856-859.
10. Miles, L.E.M., Lee, Y.-L. and Eng, L.F., Calcium ion dependence
    of the 2-site immunoradiometric assay of Moore's S-100 protein,
    J. Neurochem. 28 (1977) 1201-1205.
11. Miles, L.E.M., Immunoradiometric (IRMA) and 2-site IRMA assay
    systems, Handbook of Radioimmunoassay, Marcel Dekker, New York,
    in press.
12. Ortiz-Ortiz, L. and Weigle, W.O., Cellular events in the in-
    duction of experimental allergic encephalomyelitis in rats,
    J. Exp. Med. 144 (1976) 604-616.
13. Porterfield, J.S. (ed.), Brit. Med. Bull. 33 (1977) 1-83.
14. Robinson, J.J., Common infectious disease of laboratory
    rabbits questionably attributed to encephalitozoan cuniculi,
    Arch. Path. 58 (1954) 71.
15. Rodbard, D. and Hutt, D.M., Radioimmunoassay and Related
    Procedures in Medicine, Vol. I (1974) p. 165, International
    Atomic Energy Agency, Vienna, Austria.
16. Shadduck, J.A. and Pakes, S.P., Encephalitozoonosis (nosemato-
    sis) and toxoplasmosis, Amer. J. Path. 64 (1971) 657-674.

BASIC PROTEIN HYDROLYSIS IN LYMPHOCYTES OF LEWIS RATS WITH

EXPERIMENTAL ALLERGIC ENCEPHALOMYELITIS

Marion Edmonds Smith

Department of Neurology, Veterans Administration
  Hospital and Stanford University School of Medicine
Stanford, California, U.S.A.

SUMMARY

Lymphocytes from lymph nodes of Lewis rats with acute experimental allergic encephalomyelitis (EAE) contain high amounts of
acid and neutral proteinases which hydrolyze myelin basic protein.
The activity at neutral pH is also expressed by whole lymphocytes
in isotonic medium, with about 50% more activity released by homogenization. Neutral proteinase activity in lymphocytes increases
with the onset of acute EAE while the activity of those from
Freund's adjuvant-injected controls increases somewhat later.
The total neutral proteinase activity appears to be membrane-bound,
most likely in the lysosomes, but half the total was associated with
the nuclear fraction.
The basic protein proteinase was compared with an enzyme
described earlier, especially active toward polylysine, and some
differences were noted. It appears that two enzymes may be present
in lymphocytes which hydrolyze basic protein at a neutral pH.
An increase in neutral proteinase activity was observed in
some, but not all, lymphocyte preparations from patients in various
stages of multiple sclerosis.
The finding that whole activated lymphocytes are capable of
hydrolyzing basic protein suggests that these cells which are
believed to be precursors of mononuclear cells migrating into the
central nervous system may be active agents in the early stages
of myelin dissolution in experimental allergic encephalomyelitis.
At present, such a mechanism is only theoretical, and the possibility that activated lymphocytes may be a factor in demyelination
in multiple sclerosis is even more speculative.

INTRODUCTION

Ultrastructural examination of the morphology of invading mononuclear cells and their interactions with the myelin sheath of the central nervous system of the animal with EAE has provided a description of the mechanism of attack on the myelin (5). The mononuclear cell appears to surround the myelin sheath and a vesicular myelinolysis occurs with splitting of the myelin lamellae which are then peeled off. It is believed that the main period and intraperiod lines seen in the ultrastructure of myelin represent proteins. We know that of the five or six myelin proteins presently described, the basic protein is probably the most vulnerable to proteolytic attack. Acid proteinases such as pepsin (4) and cathepsin D (3) hydrolyze basic protein readily as do the more neutral proteases trypsin (2, 10) and elastase (Smith, unpublished observations). It is likely that proteases participate in myelin sheath destruction, and this study is an exploration of the kinds of proteases which might be active.

Because it would be extremely difficult to isolate the invading mononuclear cells from the central nervous system of the rat with EAE, we have chosen to study the lymphocyte from the regional lymph nodes at the site of injection of the encephalitogen. There is much evidence that the regional lymph node is the site of sensitization of lymphocytes to the injected antigen, and that these lymphocytes are the precursors of the mononuclear cells which attack the myelin sheath. Lymphocytes were therefore isolated from the regional lymph nodes, and their proteolytic activity toward myelin basic protein was investigated.

EXPERIMENTAL

Animals. Lewis rats, mostly females were used as host animals in all studies. These were purchased from a local animal supply house when about 100 grams and maintained in our colony until use, usually between 5 and 7 weeks of age, 120-150 grams.

Induction of EAE in Lewis rats. Crude myelin was prepared from guinea pig spinal cord by employing just one discontinuous gradient in a method described previously (6). Material collecting at the interface between 10.5% and 30% sucrose was collected, washed three times with centrifuging between washes, then lyophilized. The rats were injected in the hind foot pads with 0.5 ml Freund's incomplete adjuvant (Difco) to which was added 2 mg lyophilized guinea pig myelin and 1.5 mg Mycobacterium tuberculosis H37Ra. Control rats were injected with 0.5 ml Freund's adjuvant containing the mycobacterium alone.

Preparation of lymphocytes. At the desired time after injection or with the onset of acute symptoms of EAE (usually 12 days), the animals were killed by decapitation and the inguinal and popliteal lymph nodes removed, trimmed of fat, suspended in

phosphate-buffered saline (pH 7.2) and chopped with scissors for
20 min. The finely chopped suspension was teased through nylon
bolting cloth (HC-132, Nitex Bolting, Tetko Inc., Elmsford, N.Y.)
with addition of phosphate-buffered saline and suction until mostly
collagen remained behind. The suspension of cells was then contained in about 20 ml of medium. Lymph nodes from about five rats
were used per preparation. Two ml aliquots of the suspension were
layered over 3 ml of a commercial Ficoll-Hypaque solution (LSM,
Bionetics, Kensington, Maryland) contained in a 10 ml conical
centrifuge tube, the tubes were spun at room temperature for 30-40
min at 400 X g, the lymphocyte layer was removed from the interface,
and pelleted at a low speed in a refrigerated centrifuge. The
lymphocytes were resuspended by gently drawing through a capillary
pipette, then relayered on LSM and the procedure repeated. The
resulting interface material was again collected and centrifuged
into a pellet. Examination of these cells revealed a homogeneous
preparation of small lymphocytes which excluded trypan blue and
less than one per cent of which ingested neutral red. The cell
preparation was divided into half and one-half was homogenized.
     Preparation of basic protein. Beef basic protein was routinely
used as the substrate for proteolytic enzyme assay. This was prepared as previously described (8) from purified myelin either from
frozen beef spinal cord (obtained from Pel-Freeze Biological, Inc.,
Rogers, Arkansas), or from fresh beef brain obtained from a local
slaughter house.
     Analysis of proteolytic activity. Myelin basic protein (2 mg/
ml) was dissolved in phosphate-buffered saline and the pH adjusted
to 7.0. One ml aliquots of the solution were incubated for one
hour in the presence of 0.1 mg or less lymphocyte protein. Aliquots
of the basic protein incubated in buffer alone served as the control.
The reaction was stopped by the addition of 1 ml 16% sucrose, 2%
sodium dodecyl sulfate. This mixture was applied to polyacrylamide
gels (12%), about 50γ protein per gel and separation was by the
method of Weber and Osborne (9). The gels were stained with 1%
Fast green in 10% acetic acid, then destained in 7% acetic acid.
Densitometric scans were made and the amount of breakdown was
estimated by cutting out and weighing the peaks representing the
basic protein and peptide derivatives. Hydrolysis was expressed
as mg basic protein hydrolyzed/mg lymphocyte protein.

RESULTS

     Hydrolysis of myelin proteins. It has been previously shown
that when purified rat myelin is incubated at pH 7 with a 5%
homogenate of inguinal and popliteal lymph nodes from Lewis rats
with acute EAE, a substantial proportion of the basic protein is
lost, seemingly without effect on the proteolipid protein or the
higher molecular weight proteins (Fig. 1). In view of the findings

of others that myelin basic protein is easily hydrolyzed by acid
proteinase, the amount of hydrolysis of basic protein by a homogenate of purified lymphocytes was compared at pH 3.5 and pH 7.0.
Densitometric scans of the polyacrylamide gel separation of the
products of the reaction showed that considerable breakdown
occurred at both the acid and neutral pH regions (Fig. 2). The
degree of hydrolysis of myelin basic protein was analyzed in 0.5
pH steps from pH 3.0 to 7.5 and it was found that considerable
amounts of hydrolysis occurred in all pH regions, but the main
peaks of activity were at pH 3.5 and 7.0-7.5 (Fig. 3). Addition
of pepstatin at 10^{-5} M, a specific inhibitor of acid proteinase
blocked hydrolysis up to about pH 4.5, then the inhibition was
gradually released. The pepstatin curve demonstrates the effective
range of acid proteinase. It was also observed that the amount of
hydrolysis by lymphocytes in the neutral range somewhat exceeded
that in the acid range, thus raising the possibility that if any

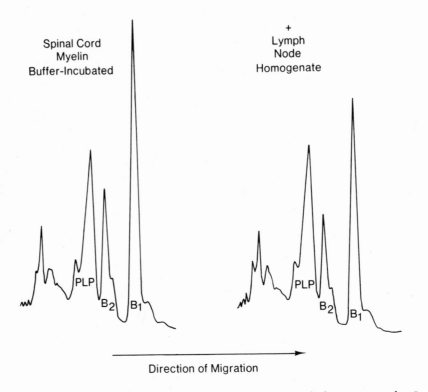

Fig. 1. Densitometric scans of proteins of purified rat spinal
cord myelin incubated 4 h at 37°C in 0.02 M phosphate buffer (left)
and in the presence of 5% lymph node homogenate (right) (8).
Separation was on 12% polyacrylamide-SDS gels (9). B_1, smaller
basic protein; B_2, larger basic protein; PLP, proteolipid protein.

proteases are effective in demyelination, neutral protease is a
distinct candidate as a destructive agent.

A considerable amount of proteolysis occurred when whole unbroken lymphocytes were incubated with purified myelin basic protein. Three or four peptides were produced by the rat lymphocytes
isolated from lymph nodes at 5, 7, 9 and 12 days after injection
with lyophilized meylin in complete Freund´s adjuvant. At 12 days,
the usual time of onset of paralytic symptoms of EAE, proteolytic
activity appeared to increase (Fig. 4a). Somewhat higher proteolytic activity was observed when the lymphocytes were homogenized,
but the same pattern is obvious with an increase in activity at
12 days after injection (Fig. 4b). Lymphocytes from the Freund´s
adjuvant-injected control (FAC) rats also showed considerable
proteolytic activity, but the activity did not increase at 12 days,
and remained at approximately the same level until about 20 days
after injection when some increase was usually seen (Fig. 5). Some
degree of proteolytic activity was observed in lymphocytes isolated
from normal lymph nodes as seen in Fig. 5 as 0 time. (In all cases
the unbroken and homogenized lymphocytes showed parallel activities
with that of the homogenized cells about 50% higher than the whole
cells.)

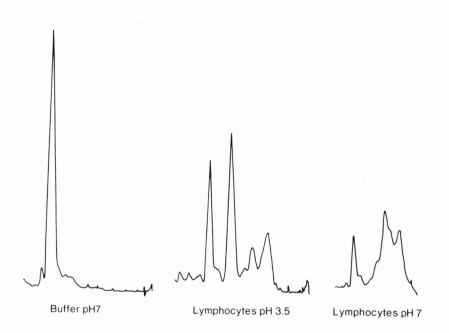

Buffer pH7   Lymphocytes pH 3.5   Lymphocytes pH 7

Fig. 2. Densitometric scans of polyacrylamide gel separation of:
1. Myelin basic protein incubated 1 h in pH 7 buffer alone (left);
2. With lymphocyte homogenate in citrate buffer, pH 3.5 (center);
3. With lymphocyte homogenate in pH 7 buffer (right).

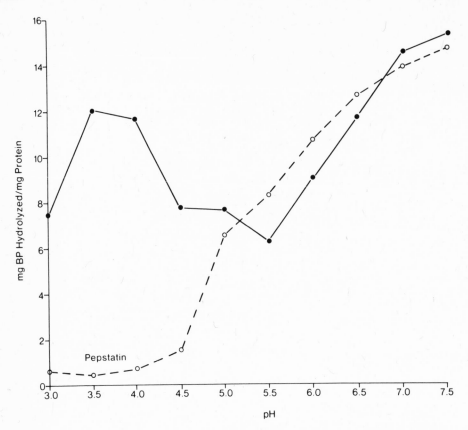

Fig. 3. Specific activity of proteinase in homogenized lymphocytes
with myelin basic protein as substrate. Basic protein (2 mg/ml)
dissolved in phosphate-buffered saline and the desired pH obtained
with addition of acetic acid. Dotted line represents activity in
presence of 10^{-5} M pepstatin.

Fig. 4a. Polyacrylamide gels of myelin basic protein incubated
with whole lymphocytes containing approximately 0.1 mg protein from
lymph nodes of Lewis rats. Gel 1, basic protein incubated in buffer
alone, gels 2, 3, 4,and 5 incubated with lymphocytes obtained 5,
7, 9,and 12 days after immunization with myelin.

Fig. 4b. Polyacrylamide gels of myelin basic protein incubated
with homogenized lymphocytes as above. Gels 1 and 6, basic protein
incubated in buffer alone; gels 2, 3, 4, and 5 with lymphocytes
obtained 5, 7, 9, and 12 days after immunization with myelin.

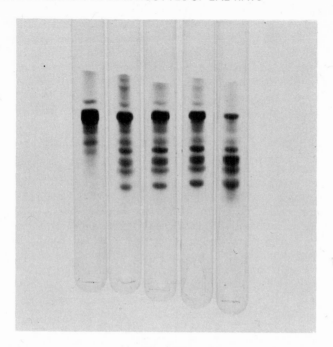

Fig. 4a

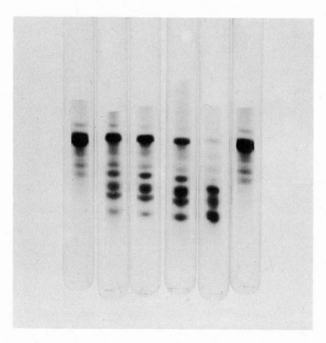

Fig. 4b

Lymphocytes from thymus showed similar relationships (Fig. 6). Due to the acute shrinkage of the thymus with the onset of EAE, it was necessary to measure the proteolytic activity from these animals with a very small amount of lymphocyte protein. In all these experiments it was necessary to use young rats with no infections, otherwise the difference between the lymphocytes of EAE and FAC rats disappeared as the levels of proteolytic enzyme of the control rats increased.

<u>Cellular localization of proteolytic activity</u>. The mechanism of hydrolysis by the whole cells was explored to determine whether proteolytic activity was released into the medium, or whether cellular contact was necessary. Whole lymphocytes were incubated with a small amount of basic protein for about a half hour, then the cells were centrifuged out and the supernatant fluid and the whole cells were incubated separately with additional aliquots of basic protein. Almost no breakdown occurred in basic protein to which the supernatant fluid was added, while a large amount of degradation took place in the mixture to which cells were added (Fig. 7). It appeared that hydrolytic action occurred strictly by contact.

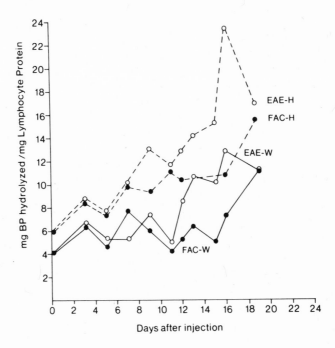

Fig. 5. Specific proteolytic activity of whole and homogenized lymphocytes obtained from lymph nodes of Lewis rats at various times after immunization with myelin or Freund's adjuvant. EAE = Experimental allergic encephalitis; FAC = Freund's adjuvant control; W = Whole lymphocytes; H = Homogenized lymphocytes.

Subcellular fractionation of the lymphocytes was undertaken to determine the site of the neutral proteinase activity. Four fractions were prepared, including a 300 X g fraction, probably nuclear, a 4,000 X g fraction, a 20,000 X g fraction and the supernatant fluid which also contained microsomes (1). Marker enzymes assayed were acid phosphatase (lysosomal), 5'nucleotidase (plasma membrane) and succinic dehydrogenase (mitochondrial). Because of the small amount of material, homogenization was thorough to ensure complete breakage of the cells which are mainly nuclei with a narrow rim of cytoplasm. The distribution of three marker enzymes was somewhat atypical, perhaps due to some solubilization of nuclear material. Succinic dehydrogenase was located predominantly in the 4,000 X g fraction, while acid phosphatase was found in high specific activity in the 4,000 X g, the 20,000 X g and the supernatant material (Table 1).

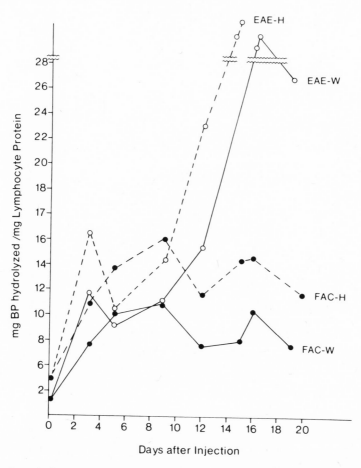

Fig. 6. Specific proteolytic activity of whole and homogenized lymphocytes obtained from the thymus of Lewis rats as in Fig. 5.

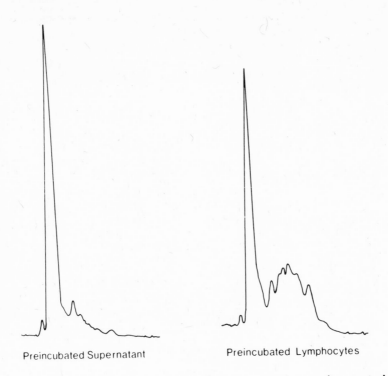

Preincubated Supernatant   Preincubated Lymphocytes

Fig. 7. Scans of polyacrylamide gels of myelin basic protein incubated with: 1. Supernatant fluid from cells preincubated with basic protein (left); 2. Cells removed from the preincubation mixture (right).

Table 1. Specific activities of three marker enzymes in subcellular fractions (1) of homogenized lymphocytes of lymph nodes from Lewis rats with acute EAE. Figures in parentheses indicate per cent of total activity.

	Succinic dehydrogenase O.D. Units reduced INT/ mg protein	Acid phosphatase µMoles P/ mg protein	5'Nucleotidase µMoles P/ mg protein
Homogenate	3.2	2.46	1.7
300 X g	1.57 (27%)	1.28 (21.4%)	0.60 (29%)
4,000 X g	8.15 (65.5%)	4.68 (36.0%)	2.50 (56%)
20,000 X g	None	6.60 (3.0%)	5.46 (7.3%)
Supernatant	None	9.36 (36.6%)	0.64 (7.3%)

Table 2. Specific activities of two lysosomal enzymes and neutral proteinase hydrolyzing myelin basic protein in subcellular fractions (1) of homogenized lymphocytes as in Table 1.

	Acid phosphatase μMoles P/ mg protein	Acid proteinase mg BP hydrolyzed/ mg protein	Neutral proteinase mg BP hydrolyzed/ mg protein
Homogenate	2.46	11.46	8.38
300 X g	1.28 (21.4%)	9.14 (32.0%)	10.71 (52.3%)
4,000 X g	4.68 (36.0%)	18.2 (30.0%)	15.1 (34.2%)
20,000 X g	6.60 (3.0%)	15.7 (1.5%)	8.54 (1.1%)
Supernatant	9.36 (36.6%)	45.2 (37.0%)	10.8 (12.3%)

Most of the total activity was distributed in the 4,000 X g fraction and the supernatant fluid, indicating considerable solubilization of this enzyme under these conditions. 5'Nucleotidase, a plasma membrane marker was present in highest specific activity in the 20,000 X g fraction, but the bulk of the total was in the 4,000 X g fraction. The distribution of two lymphocyte proteinases was compared to that of acid phosphatase (Table 2). The pattern of specific activities of acid proteinase using basic protein as a substrate was approximately similar to that of acid phosphatase, except that the total activity of the former was rather evenly distributed between the 300 X g, the 4,000 X g, and the supernatant fraction. The neutral proteinase which acts on basic protein, however, was rather different in distribution with the highest specific activity in the 4,000 X g fraction, but the bulk of the total was associated with the lower speed (300 X g) fraction, and much less was solubilized. It would appear as if the neutral proteinase is most likely a lysosomal enzyme, but with different solubility characteristics, perhaps located in different kinds of lysosomes, more closely associated with the nuclei. Alternatively, the protein(s) may be more attracted to the nuclear material under conditions of severe homogenization.

Comparison of neutral proteinases acting on basic protein and polylysine. We have previously described a neutral proteinase in lymph nodes of the rat with acute EAE which has a selective substrate specificity for proteins of a basic nature including polylysine, histone, protamine sulfate, and myelin basic protein, but does not hydrolyze many of the common substrates including casein, egg albumin, bovine serum albumin, hemoglobin, or even small basic proteins including cytochrome C and ribonuclease (8). A subcellular distribution of this enzyme was compared to that acting on basic protein (Table 3) and is shown to be much more easily solubilized with the supernatant containing the highest specific activity. A considerable amount, however, is still associated with the 4,000 X g fraction, most probably the lysosomes.

Table 3.   Comparison of specific activities of neutral proteinase
activity using myelin basic protein and polylysine as substrates
in subcellular fractions of lymphocytes as in Table 1.

| | Neutral proteinase | |
| | Basic protein | Polylysine |
	mg BP hydrolyzed/mg protein	μMoles lysine/mg protein
Homogenate	8.38	8.32
300 X g	10.71 (52.3%)	4.41 (23.9%)
4,000 X g	15.1 (34.2%)	11.73 (29.3%)
20,000 X g	8.54 (1.1%)	5.45 (0.8%)
Supernatant	10.8 (12.3%)	36.46 (46.1%)

Table 4.   Specific activity of neutral proteinase hydrolyzing
polylysine in lymph nodes of Lewis rats with EAE and Freund´s
adjuvant-injected controls during purification of the enzyme.

| | Polylysine | |
	EAE (acute) μMoles lysine/ mg protein	Freund´s adjuvant control μMoles lysine/ mg protein
Homogenate (0.1 M phosphate) pH 7	0.931 (0.540-1.13)	0.545 (0.132-1.07)
Supernatant	1.54 (1.21-2.05)	0.893 (0.121-1.78)
0-30% $(NH_4)_2 SO_4$	0.208 (0-0.531	0.204 (0.042-0.635
30-70% $(NH_4)_2 SO_4$	6.08 (3.71-7.7)	3.02 (0.659-6.06)
G-200	20.68 (18.4-23.0)	7.74 (4.4-9.47)
DEAE-Sephadex	66.2 (49.6-82.8)	21.5 (20.2-22.3)

Table 5. Specific activities of neutral proteinase hydrolyzing myelin basic protein as in Table 4.

| | Basic protein | |
	EAE (acute) μMoles lysine/ mg protein	Freund´s adjuvant control μMoles lysine/ mg protein
Homogenate (0.1 M phosphate) pH 7	0.988 (0.778-1.30)	1.04 (0.58-1.94)
Supernatant	0.788 (0.560-0.935)	0.59 (0.253-0.98)
0-30% $(NH_4)_2 SO_4$	0.091 (0 - 0.212)	0.084 (0 - 0.159)
30-70% $(NH_4)_2 SO_4$	2.17 (1.80-2.47)	1.32 (0.725-1.73)
G-200	5.86 (5.8-5.9)	2.15 (1.41-2.52)
DEAE-Sephadex	21.2 (20.2-22.3)	5.98

Table 6. Specific activity of neutral proteinase in blood lymphocytes of normal medical personnel (control), one stroke patient and patients with multiple sclerosis. Myelin basic protein was used as a substrate.

	Whole lymphocytes mg basic protein hydrolyzed/ mg protein	Homogenized lymphocytes mg basic protein hydrolyzed/ mg protein
Control	0.645 0.516 1.71 0.832 0.631 (Stroke)	2.76 2.88 2.85 2.70 (Stroke)
MS-Chronic	7.4 1.2	14.4 5.3
MS-Acute	0.750 1.19 4.0 0.964	6.8 8.3 10.5 2.5

    This enzyme also seems to be especially high in lymphocytes
from lymph nodes of rats with EAE. Various sources such as commercially available lymph nodes from guinea pig, beef, and rabbit
have yielded very little of this enzyme. It is present in much
smaller amounts in lymph nodes of Freund´s adjuvant-injected
animals. A partial purification has been obtained up to about
80 fold. As shown on Table 4, there is some difference between
the activity in the homogenate of lymph nodes from EAE rats and
Freund´s adjuvant controls, but with increasing purification,
much more enrichment was obtained from the EAE lymph nodes than
from those of the controls. This enzyme also appears to hydrolyze
basic protein as shown by a similar scheme on Table 5. The behavior of the polylysine enzyme on Sephadex G-200 is identical to
that hydrolyzing basic protein (Fig. 8), both being eluted very
soon after the void volume and excluded from Sephadex-G-100.

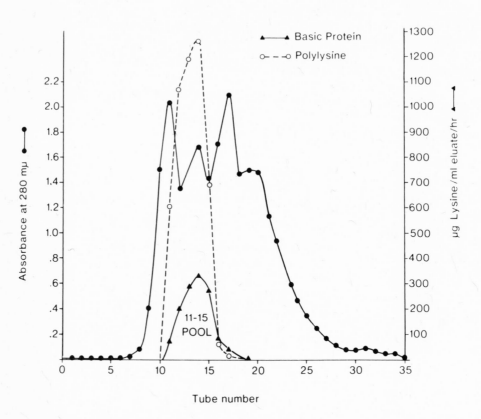

Fig. 8. Elution pattern of neutral proteinase on Sephadex G-200.
Proteinase activity toward myelin basic protein and polylysine
(MW = 230,000) are eluted simultaneously. Assay was by ninhydrin
determination of the TCA-soluble fraction.

Similarly, the elution of the polylysine enzyme from DEAE-52 is at
a fairly high salt concentration, with the activity also identical
for hydrolysis of basic protein (Fig. 9). Thus there may be two
kinds of enzymes acting on basic protein, one of which is solubilized more easily and is active also on polylysine, and one more
tightly bound to membranes which has not yet been solubilized.

Protease activity in lymphocytes from multiple sclerosis
patients. Lymphocytes were separated from blood drawn from normal
medical personnel, one stroke patient, and six patients in various
stages of multiple sclerosis (MS). Dr. Leslie Dorfman, from Stanford University, was instrumental in obtaining patients with previously diagnosed MS. A very low degree of proteolytic activity
toward basic protein was measured in most of these lymphocyte preparations when they were incubated as whole cells (Table 6). When
the isolated lymphocytes were homogenized, however, five out of
six patients showed increases to varying degrees in proteolytic
activity. These ranged in value from 5.3 to 14.4 mg basic protein
hydrolyzed per mg lymphocyte protein per hour compared to the normal
value of about 2.8. These lymphocytes were not tested for their
ability to hydrolyze polylysine.

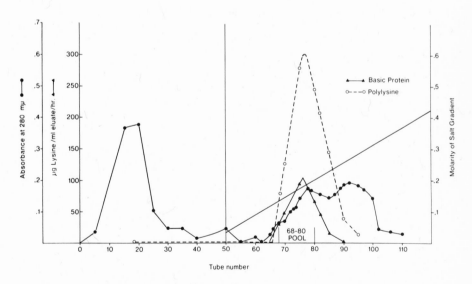

Fig. 9. Elution pattern of neutral proteinase on DEAE-cellulose.
Proteinase activity is shown using basic protein and polylysine as
substrates.

DISCUSSION

It is not likely that with sensitization to basic protein, an enzyme is induced in lymphocytes specifically for basic protein hydrolysis. It is more probable that basic protein happens to be relatively unfolded in structure, and is thereby especially vulnerable to several kinds of proteolytic enzymes. The amount of hydrolysis of basic protein may be considered, therefore, to be the total proteolytic activity at a certain pH. Endopeptidases active at pH 3-4 and at 6.5 to 7.5 seem to be especially active in lymphocytes of lymph nodes, and it appears that at least two neutral proteases may be present. It is unlikely that there are more, in view of the finding that only three main peptides are produced which break down further only after prolonged incubation.

It is also not likely that this protease is only induced in response to basic protein administration. Induction of proteases is more likely a general mechanism in lymphocyte activation of any kind, and the specificity toward myelin in EAE and possibly MS is probably the migration of the lymphoid-derived cells through the blood vessels of the central nervous system to the myelin target.

We were able to find some neutral protease activity in animal lymph nodes purchased commercially, but it was not present in large enough amounts to be useful for enzyme purification. Protease activity in lymphocytes from recently purchased 6-week-old Lewis rats was very low as was that in normal lymph nodes from 6 week Wistar rats born in our colony. On the other hand, lymph nodes from old Wistar rats used as breeders approaching 12 months of age and subjected to repeated onslaughts of outside animals introduced into the room, showed some of the highest activities measured in rats. An activated lymph node taken at autopsy from a cancer patient also showed extraordinarily high activity, about 4 times that of the activated lymph nodes of rats.

The two kinds of neutral proteases differentiated only by subcellular distribution have so far not been identified. Inhibition of basic protein hydrolysis by lymphocytes has been observed with p-chloromercuribenzoate and phenylmethyl sulfonyl fluoride indicating that the enzyme(s) are sulfhydryl-dependent, and are probably serine proteases. These two agents have also been shown to be inhibitory on the purified polylysine enzyme. Further differentiation must await better characterization of the enzyme properties, especially in respect to solubilization of the membrane-bound component.

Acknowledgements. This work was supported by Grant No. NS-02785 from the NINCDS and by the Veterans Administration. The author is grateful to Mr. Paul Somera for scanning the polyacrylamide gels.

REFERENCES

1. Allan, D. and Crumpton, M.J., Preparation and characterization
    of the plasma membrane of pig lymphocytes, Biochem. J. 120
    (1970) 133-143.
2. Banik, N.L. and Davison, A.N., Lipid and basic protein inter-
    action in myelin, Biochem. J. 143 (1974) 39-45.
3. Einstein, E.R., Csejtey, J. and Marks, N., Degradation of en-
    cephalitogen by purified brain acid proteinase, FEBS Letts. 1
    (1968) 191-195.
4. Eylar, E.H., Brostoff, S., Hashim, G., Caccam, J. and Burnett,
    P., Basic A$_1$ protein of the myelin membrane. The complete amino
    acid sequence, J. Biol. Chem. 246 (1971) 5770-5784.
5. Lampert, P.W., Electron microscopic studies in ordinary and
    hyperacute experimental allergic encephalomyelitis, Acta Neuro-
    pathol. 9 (1967) 99-126.
6. Smith, M.E., The turnover of myelin in the adult rat, Biochim.
    Biophys. Acta 164 (1968) 285-293.
7. Smith, M.E. and Chow, S.H., Neutral proteinase in lymp nodes
    specific for basic protein, Trans. Am. Soc. Neurochem. 7 (1976)
    178.
8. Smith, M.E., A lymph node neutral proteinase acting on myelin
    basic protein, J. Neurochem. 27 (1976) 1077-1082.
9. Weber, K. and Osborn, M., The reliability of molecular weight
    determinations by dodecyl sulfate-polyacrylamide gel electro-
    phoresis, J. biol.Chem. 244 (1969) 4406-4412.
10. Wood, J.G., Dawon, R.M.C. and Hauser, H., Effect of proteolytic
    attack on the structure of CNS myelin membrane, J. Neurochem.
    22 (1974) 637-643.

NEUTRAL PROTEINASES SECRETED BY MACROPHAGES DEGRADE BASIC PROTEIN:

A POSSIBLE MECHANISM OF INFLAMMATORY DEMYELINATION

William T. Norton[1], Wendy Cammer[1], Barry R. Bloom[2]
and Saimon Gordon[3]
[1]The Saul Korey Department of Neurology and Departments
of [1]Neuroscience, [2]Microbiology and Immunology, and
[2]Cell Biology, Albert Einstein College of Medicine,
Bronx, N.Y. 10461, U.S.A., and [3]Sir William Dunn
School of Pathology, Oxford University,
Oxford OX1 3RE, England

SUMMARY

In the inflammatory demyelinating diseases, such as multiple
sclerosis, Landry-Guillain-Barré syndrome and experimental allergic
encephalomyelitis, demyelination occurs in the vicinity of infiltrating mononuclear cells. Although the histopathology is characteristic
of each disease, the general observation that myelin destruction in
inflammatory lesions begins prior to phagocytosis suggests a common
mechanism for myelinolysis in these diseases. Recent studies show
that stimulated macrophages secrete several neutral proteinases,
including plasminogen (Plg) activator. We have tested the possibility that these proteinases could, directly or indirectly, initiate
myelin destruction. Isolated brain myelin was incubated with
supernatant media from cultures of stimulated mouse peritoneal
macrophages in the presence and absence of Plg. Cell supernatants
alone caused some degradation of basic protein (BP) in myelin.
The amount degraded was considerably enhanced in the presence of
Plg. The other myelin proteins remained essentially intact. While
the Plg-independent proteolytic activity in the supernatants was
abolished by EDTA, known to inhibit the neutral proteinases, the
Plg-dependent hydrolysis was inhibited by p-nitrophenylguanidinobenzoate, an inhibitor of Plg activator and plasmin. These results

---

Abbreviations used: Plg, plasminogen; BP, myelin basic protein;
MS, multiple sclerosis; EAE, experimental allergic encephalomyelitis;
SDS, sodium dodecyl sulfate; NPGB, p-nitrophenylguanidinobenzoate;
EDTA, ethylenediaminetetraacetic acid.

suggested that the Plg activator secreted by the macrophages generated plasmin, which selectively degraded BP. This interpretation was confirmed by the observation that urokinase, a Plg activator, plus Plg was effective in degrading BP in myelin. We propose that the action of neutral proteinases released by stimulated macrophages, and its amplification by the Plg-plasmin system, may play a significant role in several inflammatory demyelinating diseases; and that the relative specificity of these reactions for myelin lies in the extreme susceptibility of BP to proteolysis.

INTRODUCTION

Primary demyelinating diseases have customarily been classified into two major groups: the acquired inflammatory diseases and the non-inflammatory diseases. However, most neuropathologists now restrict the term, demyelinating diseases, to include only the acquired inflammatory diseases of myelin in which there is loss of myelin with sparing of axons (2, 38, 55). These diseases are characterized by perivenular infiltrates of hematogenous cells in association with areas of demyelination (2, 38, 55). Multiple sclerosis (MS) and the model disease, experimental allergic encephalomyelitis (EAE), are the most extensively studied disorders in this category.

Lesion formation in the inflammatory demyelinating diseases is generally believed to be related to an immunological response, either autoimmune in nature or to a viral antigen. However, the mechanism by which the inflammatory cells, predominantly macrophages and lymphocytes in MS and EAE, may participate in the process of demyelination has not yet been defined. Most of the speculation regarding the biochemical mechanisms of demyelination has focused on the role of the lysosomal proteinases, known to be elevated in and around MS plaques (1, 5, 15, 17, 18, 24-26, 40, 42) and in lesions in animals with EAE (7, 22, 27, 32, 41, 45, 46). The demonstration by Wisniewski and Bloom (56, 57) that myelin can be destroyed as the result of a delayed-type hypersensitivity reaction to non-brain antigens, has shed new light on possible mechanisms. This study confirmed that primary demyelination can occur, in a process morphologically similar to that in EAE, as a non-specific "bystander effect" of a cell-mediated immune reaction to any action. These results suggested that products released by the inflammatory cells may be myelinolytic. Such a process is supported by morphological studies of MS and EAE which show that myelin destruction occurs prior to ingestion by phagocytes.

It is known that stimulated mouse peritoneal macrophages secrete several neutral proteinases (9, 21, 52, 53) including Plg activator (20, 21, 47-49), and that the secretion process can be induced by products of activated lymphocytes (28, 50, 51). Therefore these enzymes become obvious candidates for a role in inflammatory demyelination. If these extracellular proteinases, generated from macrophages activated as a consequence of a reaction of sensitized T-lymphocytes with antigen, were capable of degrading myelin proteins, they could initiate a process of demyelination common to inflammatory and cell-mediated immune reactions occurring in nervous tissue. To demonstrate the feasibility of such a mechanism, we have studied the actions of products of stimulated macrophages on purified myelin in vitro; and have further studied the modulation of their action by added Plg, and by inhibitors of Plg activator and other neutral proteinases.

EXPERIMENTAL

Reagents. Acrylamide and bis-acrylamide were obtained from Eastman Chemical Co., Rochester, N.Y.; Sodium dodecylsulfate (SDS) and Plg ("profibrinolysin") from Sigma Chemical Co., St. Louis, Mo.; glycine from Matheson, Coleman and Bell, Norwood, Ohio; and urokinase (E.C. 3.4.99.26) from Calbiochem, LaJolla, Ca. In most cases immediately before use the Plg was treated with lima bean trypsin inhibitor (Worthington Biochemical Corp., Freehold, N.J.) conjugated to Sepharose (Pharmacia Co., Piscataway, N.J.) (12) in order to remove traces of free plasmin. Ethylene diamine tetraacetic acid (EDTA) was a J.T. Baker reagent (Phillipsburg, N.J.) and p-nitrophenylguanidinobenzoate (NPGB) was a gift from Dr. Daniel Rifkin (Rockefeller University) and can be purchased from ICN Nutritional Biochemical Co., Cleveland, Ohio.

Preparation of myelin. Myelin was prepared from bovine and cat brains by the method of Norton and Poduslo (34). It was stored as a lyophilized powder at $-20^{\circ}C$ over $CaSO_4$. Immediately before use in incubations the myelin was weighed and suspended in distilled water using a Dounce homogenizer.

Preparation of supernatants (conditioned media) from macrophages. Unstimulated and thioglycollate-stimulated macrophages were obtained from Oxford Swiss mice and were plated in minimal essential medium (MEM) plus 5% acid-treated fetal bovine serum (19-21). The cells were washed and fed the same medium at 2 and 24 h. At 48 h the cells were washed three times with serum-free medium and placed in MEM plus 0.17% lactalbumin hydrolyzate (Difco). Supernatants C_A and C_B were from thioglycollate-stimulated cells grown in the presence of 1 and 10 µg Concanavalin A, respectively, added to the last medium. Supernatants U_A and U_B (unstimulated) and T_A, T_B, C_A and C_B (stimulated) were collected after 2 days of growth in serum-free medium, supernatants U_1 and T_1 after 3 days, and U_2 and T_2 after 7 days. All were lyophilized. All activated supernatants contained Plg activator as measured by Plg-dependent fibrinolysis of ^{125}I-fibrin coated plates (21, 36). One unit of activity is defined as the release of 10% of the radioactivity in 4 h. For example, supernatants U_1 and U_2 (unstimulated) had 2.3-4.2 units per 100 µl for both Plg-dependent and Plg-independent fibrinolysis, whereas T_1 had 15 units/100 µl for Plg-independent and 176 units for Plg-dependent fibrinolysis, and T_2 had 6.4 units for Plg-independent and 85 units for Plg-dependent fibrinolysis. Reconstituted lyophilized supernatants from unstimulated and stimulated macrophages contained lysozyme at levels of approximately 5 µg/100 µl and 10 µg/100 µl, respectively.

General method of incubating macrophage supernatants with myelin. Incubation tubes contained 10-40 mM Tris·HCl, pH 7.6, 1.0 mg myelin, added as 100 µl of a 10 mg/ml suspension in water, and, as required by the experiment, one or more of the following: 20-70 µl macrophage supernatant, 5 µg Plg, 10 mM EDTA, 2 µg NPGB, and 0.1-20 µg urokinase, in a total volume of 220 µl. For each experiment control tubes were run with myelin plus buffer alone, and myelin, buffer and Plg. The tubes were incubated for periods varying from 30 to 60 min at 37°C. The reactions were stopped by boiling with SDS as described below.

Gel electrophoresis and quantitation of BP degradation. Polyacrylamide gels (15%) were prepared according to the method of Greenfield et al. (23) using 1% instead of 0.1% SDS in the gels. To each incubation tube of 220 µl containing 1 mg of myelin was added 2 mg SDS powder, and the samples were boiled 2 min. Protein was assayed by the method of Lowry et al. (30), an equal volume of a sample solvent (23) containing 1% SDS and 2% mercaptoethanol was added, and a 100 µl aliquot containing 80-100 µg of protein was placed on the gels. The gels were electrophoresed 18-21 h at 45 volts, and were fixed, stained with fast green and destained as described by Greenfield et al. (23). The stained gels were scanned in a Gilford spectrophotometer at 580 nM, and the protein bands were quantitated by triangulation. The area of the BP was divided by the sum of the areas of all myelin protein bands (BP, intermediate proteins, proteolipid protein and Wolfgram proteins). The percent BP degraded for each incubation was calculated from those values. The control samples incubated with buffer alone were taken as 0% BP degraded.

RESULTS

Degradation of BP by macrophage supernatants plus Plg. An example of the effect of macrophage supernatants on the proteins of myelin can be seen qualitatively in Fig. 1. Note that incubation with Plg alone (gel 2) had no effect. Considerable breakdown of BP was apparent (gel 3) after incubation with the supernatant; and this degradation was increased when Plg was in the incubation mixture (gel 4). Low molecular weight breakdown products can be seen below the BP band in gels 3 and 4. The extra band above Wolfgram protein in these two gels is from the supernatants, and is probably serum albumin. Not all supernatants had this protein. Gels like these were scanned to yield the quantitative data given

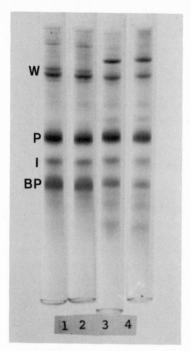

Fig. 1. Effect of incubating myelin with a macrophage supernatant
in the presence and absence of Plg. - Myelin (1 mg) was incubated
for 45 min at 37°C in a total volume of 220 μl containing 18 mM
tris HCl, pH 7.5, plus the following aliquots of supernatant and
Plg: (1) none; (2) 5 μg Plg; (3) 50 μl supernatant T_2; (4) 50 μl
supernatant T_2 plus 5 μg Plg. SDS was added and the samples were
electrophoresed according to the usual procedures. The protein
bands are: W, Wolfgram proteins; P, proteolipid protein; I, intermediate proteins; and BP, basic protein.

in the Tables. In all cases where proteolysis occurred, a preferential loss of BP was seen. In some experiments the Wolfgram
proteins were also diminished slightly (noticeable in Fig. 1), but
the amount was difficult to quantitate because of the relatively
small (approximately 10%) contribution of the Wolfgram protein to
the total myelin protein.
     Because thioglycollate-stimulated, but not unstimulated,
peritoneal macrophages were reported to secrete Plg activator (21,
47, 48) and other neutral proteinases (21, 52, 53), we compared
the effect of supernatants from both types of cells on myelin
(Table 1). Degradation of BP in myelin was most pronounced during
incubation with supernatants from thioglycollate- and Con A-
stimulated macrophages in the presence of Plg (column 4, Table 1;
the total degradation in the presence of Plg is the sum of the Plg-
independent and Plg-dependent degradation). The dramatic increase

of BP degradation when Plg was added to the supernatants, (column
4, Table 1) compared to supernatants alone (column 3, Table 1)
suggested that the Plg activator in the supernatants was cleaving
Plg to plasmin and that the plasmin was hydrolyzing BP. However,
all activated supernatants degraded some BP in absence of Plg,
indicating that neutral proteinases in these supernatants, as well
as plasmin generated by these supernatants, were active in proteolysis of BP. Comparisons with the Plg-independent fibrinolysis data
for these supernatants (see Experimental) suggest that BP in a
myelin suspension may be more susceptible to the neutral proteinases
than is fibrin in a semisolid medium.

Table 1. Effect of incubating macrophage supernatants with myelin
in the presence and absence of plasminogen. - These data are expressed as the percentage of the total amount of BP in 1.0 mg
myelin which was degraded by 50 µl of supernatant at 37°C for 30
min. The data was recalculated in cases where the volume of supernatant was other than 50 µl and the results of several experiments
averaged. The numbers in parentheses represent the number of experiments performed with each supernatant and usually represent
different volumes of the supernatant. If more than two were
averaged the standard deviation is given, otherwise the mean deviation is recorded. The Plg-independent degradation is the amount
of breakdown in the absence of added Plg. The Plg-dependent degradation is the total breakdown in the presence of Plg minus the
Plg-independent degradation   and minus that caused by Plg alone.
This latter value was usually only 1-2%. For example, supernatant
T_B plus 5 µg Plg degraded 32% of the BP, whereas supernatant U_B
degraded only 1-7% of the BP.

Supernatants from unstimulated cells			Supernatants from stimulated cells		
Sup.	Plg-independent deg. of BP	Plg-dependent deg. of BP	Sup.	Plg-independent deg. of BP	Plg-dependent deg. of BP
U_1	13±3 (6)	13±4 (2)	T_1(2)	27±7	23±13
U_2	23±7 (3)	13±9 (2)	T_2(2)	25±5	23±11
U_A	1±1 (2)	5±5 (2)	T_A(2)	13±0	11± 0
			C_A(2)	17±0	16± 1
U_B	0 (2)	3±3 (2)	T_B(1)	9	22
			C_B(1)	4	26

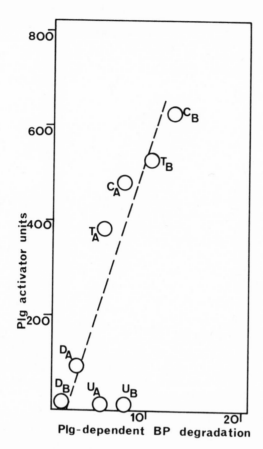

Fig. 2. Comparison between Plg-dependent BP degradation and Plg-dependent fibrin digestion by macrophage supernatants. - Supernatants from thioglycollate-activated macrophages were prepared as described in Experimental, with the following exceptions. To obtain supernatants D_A and D_B, the cultures were fed dexamethasone (10^{-7} M and 10^{-5} M, respectively) at 48 h, and conditioned media were collected two days later. Supernatants U_A and U_B were from unstimulated macrophages, and C_A, C_B, D_A, D_B, T_A and T_B were from thioglycollate-stimulated macrophages. Myelin was incubated with 25 μl of each supernatant, in the absence and in the presence of 5 μg Plg, for 30 min at 37°C. Subsequently, the myelin proteins were quantitated on SDS polyacrylamide gels, as usual. To obtain values for the Plg-dependent BP degradation the percent BP degraded by each supernatant alone and by Plg alone were subtracted from the values for BP degraded by the respective supernatants in the presence of Plg. Plg activator values were obtained by the ^{125}I fibrin plate method and are expressed in units per culture.

Somewhat lower but reproducible Plg-dependent and Plg-independent breakdown of BP was observed with two of the unstimulated macrophage supernatants, U_1 and U_2, although the other two supernatants from normal macrophages, U_A and U_B, had minimal activity. This suggests that some of the mice used had endogenous "activated" cells in the peritoneal macrophage population. This is a common problem in working with macrophages and probably traceable to infections in the mouse colony.

Some idea of the rate of BP degradation by these supernatants can be obtained by converting the data in Table 1 to nmoles. Thus a 25% degradation of BP represents 1.4 nmoles per 30 min per 50 μl of supernatant.

Correlation of Plg-activator activity and Plg-dependent BP degradation. Further confirmation that the Plg-dependent BP degradation by the macrophage supernatants was a function of the secreted Plg-activator is presented in Fig. 2. An excellent correlation was found between the Plg activator content of the supernatants, as measured by the ^{125}I-fibrin plate assay, and Plg-dependent BP degradation. This correlation was not linear if large quantities (50 μl or more) of supernatant were used in the myelin incubation, which caused too great a percentage of the substrate (BP) to be degraded.

Degradation of BP by plasmin. To confirm that plasmin was capable of hydrolyzing BP, the experiment summarized in Table 2 was carried out. Incubation of myelin with the commercially available Plg activator, urokinase (EC 3.4.99.26), plus Plg (tubes 5, 6, 7 and 10) demonstrated that myelin BP was indeed vulnerable to proteolysis by plasmin. Note that in all the experiments described in this paper myelin was not reisolated from the incubation mixtures, but the entire tube contents were electrophoresed after solubilization in SDS. Thus any loss of protein is due to degradation rather than solubilization during incubation. The amount of BP degraded was roughly dependent on the quantity of urokinase used and the incubation time. Up to 10 μg of urokinase alone did not hydrolyze BP in this system (tubes 2, 3 and 4), although 20 μg of urokinase caused some degradation.

It was subsequently found (data not shown) that it was not necessary to preincubate urokinase (or macrophage supernatants) with Plg before adding the myelin suspension, since BP degradation occurred rapidly if Plg, Plg activator and myelin were incubated together. This indicated that conversion of Plg to plasmin was a more rapid reaction than proteolysis of BP. The susceptibility of BP to plasmin appears not to be species specific. Macrophage supernatants plus Plg degraded the BP in bovine, cat and rabbit myelin equally rapidly.

The use of inhibitors to distinguish between Plg activator and other neutral proteinases. The observation of neutral proteinase activities in the macrophage supernatants, as shown by Plg-independent breakdown of BP (Table 1), made it desirable to demonstrate that the plasmin responsible for Plg-dependent degradation of BP was being generated by Plg-activator rather than by cleavage of Plg by

Table 2. Effect of incubating urokinase with myelin in presence or absence of plasminogen. – In this table the raw data for a single experiment are given. Incubation tubes contained 34 mM Tris · HCl, pH 7.6 plus either 5 μg Plg or the indicated amount of urokinase or both, in a volume of 120 μl. After 15 min preincubation at 37°C, to allow the formation of plasmin, 100 μl of a myelin suspension in water, containing 1.0 mg of myelin, was added. The tubes were incubated a further 30 or 60 min as indicated and then the proteins were analyzed as described in the text. The Plg used in this experiment had not been treated to remove plasmin and thus had more blank activity than usual (tubes 1 and 8).

Tube	Incubation time	μg UK added	μg Plg added	% BP degraded
1	30	0	5	9
2	30	0.1	0	0
3	30	1.0	0	3
4	30	10.0	0	0
5	30	0.1	5	13
6	30	1.0	5	18
7	30	10.0	5	26
8	60	0	5	10
9	60	20	0	15
10	60	20	5	70

the other neutral proteinases. Two inhibitors were used for this purpose and their effects are shown in Table 3. NPGB is a known inhibitor of Plg activator and plasmin, whereas EDTA inhibits the neutral proteinases (21).

As expected, EDTA inhibited the Plg-independent degradation of BP almost completely, but had no effect on the Plg-dependent degradation. Conversely, NPGB had no effect on the Plg-independent degradation, but reduced the Plg-dependent degradation to low levels. Although not shown here, when both inhibitors were added, the macrophage supernatants showed no breakdown of BP, either in the presence or absence of Plg. These data show that the EDTA-sensitive neutral proteinases in the supernatants do not activate Plg, although they degrade BP; and they confirm the role of the macrophage Plg-activator in generating plasmin.

Vulnerability of isolated BP. Although all of the results reported in this paper are on proteolysis of BP within isolated myelin, some studies were done on purified BP. These studies showed, as with myelin, that macrophage supernatants degraded isolated BP, and that the rate of proteolysis was increased by including Plg in the reaction mixture.

Table 3. Effects of inhibitors on BP degradation by macrophage supernatants in the presence and absence of plasminogen. Each tube contained 1 mg bovine myelin, 19 mM Tris · HCl, pH 7.6, 50 µl of an activated macrophage supernatant, and, where indicated, 5 µg Plg (Plg-dependent BP deg. column). The top part of the table shows the effect of the presence of 10 mM EDTA (+EDTA columns), while the bottom part of the table shows the effect of adding 2 µg NPGB (+NPGB columns). Tubes were incubated 45 min at 37°C. The data are given as the percent BP degraded, determined as described in the text. Plg-dependent and Plg-independent degradation were calculated as described in Table 1.

	Effect of EDTA			
Supernatant	Plg-indep. BP deg.		Plg-dep. BP deg.	
	-EDTA	+EDTA	-EDTA	+EDTA
T_1	34	0	18	21
T_2	27	1	16	14
	Effect of NPGB			
Supernatant	Plg-indep. BP deg.		Plg-dep. BP deg.	
	-NPGB	+NPGB	-NPGB	+NPGB
T_2	27	25	16	5
T_A	8	8	31	6
T_B	11	8	29	6

DISCUSSION

Our results demonstrate that neutral proteinases secreted by stimulated macrophages degrade BP in myelin, and that this degradation is enhanced by the addition of Plg. It is probable that this Plg-dependent degradation is due to plasmin, produced by the action of a macrophage-secreted Plg activator on Plg. Strong support for this conclusion comes from our observations that BP is degraded by mixtures of urokinase, a Plg-activator, and Plg, but by neither acting alone; and that Plg-dependent BP degradation is blocked by NPGB, a known inhibitor of Plg-activator and plasmin.

The discovery that stimulated macrophages release several neutral proteinases, including Plg activator, suggests that these products may have an important role in causing tissue damage in

inflammation.   Although the Plg-plasmin system has a major role in
the control of blood coagulation and clot lysis and in activating
the complement system, plasmin, a trypsin-like proteinase, is
capable of hydrolyzing a range of protein substrates, including BP
as we demonstrate here.   The high level of plasminogen (0.5 - 1%
of total plasma protein) circulating in the blood could act as a
reservoir of potential proteolytic activity which can be recruited
by cells releasing the activator (47).   Although normally excluded
from the nervous system, Plg would become freely available to the
brain parenchyma in any situation in which the blood-brain barrier
is damaged, e.g. an inflammatory reaction.   The catalytic activity
of Plg activator released from a small number of inflammatory cells
would be sufficient to produce much larger amounts of plasmin, thus
serving to amplify the demyelinating activity of the secreted
proteinases.

The hypothesis proposed here that myelin may be disrupted
either directly or indirectly by products secreted by macrophages
is supported by many pathological and biochemical studies of demyelinating conditions, of which MS and EAE are the most carefully
studied examples.   It has been believed for some time that the
inflammatory cells in these disorders are involved in demyelination,
and of course, in the final clearance of myelin debris by phagocytosis. Many studies have shown that acid proteinases and other
lysosomal enzymes are increased around active MS plaques (1, 5, 8,
14, 15, 17, 18, 24-26, 40, 42).   The increase in acid proteinases
correlates with a decrease of BP (17, 18) a protein known to be
readily digested by these enzymes (31, 40, 45).   Similar elevations
of acid proteinases and lysosomal enzymes have been found in the
central nervous system in EAE (7, 22, 27, 32, 41, 45, 46).   Studies
of both diseases indicate that the increased acid hydrolases are
traceable to the infiltrating hematogenous cells (8, 27, 46).

Although most studies have been concerned with the lysosomal
hydrolases, some investigators have examined the role that neutral
proteinases of the inflammatory cells may play in demyelination.
Buletza and Smith (10) found a greater elevation of neutral
proteinase activity than of acid proteinases in the spinal cord of
rats with EAE.   Lymph node homogenates of these rats were very
active in digesting BP at neutral pH.   Further studies of the
partially purified neutral proteinase from lymph nodes showed that
it could hydrolyze either free BP or BP within myelin, but that
 it was inactive against many other proteins, including casein,
hemoglobin and albumin (44).   Cuzner et al. (13) have found that
rabbit peritoneal macrophages will degrade free BP or BP in intact
myelin most readily at neutral pH.   Lymphocytes had much less
proteolytic activity.   Smith concluded (44) that the neutral
proteinase of the monocyte may be more important for myelin destruction than the lysosomal enzymes.

It is not clear from these studies on proteinases in demyelination, whether the enzymes act on myelin intracellularly or

extracellularly. Analyses of tissue for enzyme activity or the use of homogenates for in vitro studies do not allow this discrimination, nor do they permit identification of the inflammatory cell type which is furnishing the enzyme.

We believe that the lysosomal enzymes are probably not a significant factor in demyelination prior to phagocytosis. Good evidence that the agents which cause myelin destruction are acting extracellularly comes from morphological studies of MS and EAE. In EAE macrophages can be seen penetrating and peeling away the myelin layers (29, 58). Other commonly seen alterations in myelin structure are splitting and loosening of the lamellae and extensive vesicular, honeycomb-like disruptions of the sheath occurring in the vicinity of mononuclear cells (16, 29, 39). An essentially identical morphological picture is seen in the early stages of demyelination occurring as a "bystander effect" to a delayed hypersensitivity reaction to a non-brain antigen in the rabbit eye model (57). Ultrastructural studies of MS show that the early changes in myelin are disintegration of lamellae into granular and lamellar debris. These changes are frequently localized to one side of a sheath and visually occur within a space created by the splitting and opening up of the interperiod line (11). The remainder of the sheath can retain a normal periodicity and appearance. Active stripping of myelin from axons by macrophages has never been seen (4, 35). Prineas claims that a common pattern in demyelination in early lesions is a gradual reduction in the number of myelin lamellae occurring in the vicinity of cells which could be macrophages or microglia, but which have no obvious physical connection with the altered myelin (35). These cells apparently do not participate in phagocytosis until the myelin has been partially degraded (35).

A critical part of our hypothesis is that myelin has a special sensitivity to the enzymes secreted by macrophages and to plasmin. In our incubations of myelin with macrophage supernatants, with or without Plg, only BP was degraded to a measurable extent. We propose that the selective action of macrophage products on myelin is a consequence of the vulnerability of BP to proteinase action. Studies of the digestion of myelin with trypsin (6, 31, 37, 59), cathepsin D (31), Type II collagenase (W. Cammer, unpublished studies) or lymph node neutral proteinase (44) in vitro show BP to be selectively degraded by all of these enzymes. Moreover, of ten substrates tested against the latter enzyme, only two (protamine sulfate and polylysine) were found to be more labile than BP, and five were not hydrolyzed at all under the same conditions. Several studies have shown that BP is selectively depleted in the margins of MS plaques (17, 18, 24), but from this work it was not possible to conclude that BP was decreased more than other myelin constituents. Cuzner et al. (14) have now found that white matter areas adjacent to active plaques showed a preferential loss of BP relative to other proteins, including the principal myelin protein, proteolipid protein.

Our results would lead to the prediction that myelin in the initial stages of degradation in inflammatory lesions would have a deficit of BP. Although most studies of myelin isolated from normal appearing white matter show that it is of normal composition (33), Althaus et al. (3) and Riekkinen et al. (43) found a decreased content of BP in MS myelin, which was more pronounced in myelin isolated from plaques than from normal appearing white matter (3).

The occurrence of myelin fragments in the cerebrospinal fluid (CSF) of patients undergoing inflammatory demyelination would be consistent with a mechanism for extracellular degradation of myelin. Cohen et al. (11) and Whitaker (54) found that in the CSF of MS patients the amount of material reacting with antibodies to BP or its fragments in a radioimmunoassay correlates with the clinical stage of the disease. These data provide the first compelling evidence that exacerbations are related to demyelinating episodes. Of particular significance for our work are Whitaker's data showing that the antigen in CSF may not be intact BP, but rather a fragment of BP. He speculates that such fragments are produced by acid proteinases, but it would be our view that macrophage-initiated extracellular proteolysis might be more significant.

It should be noted that while the mechanism proposed here may be common to many cases of inflammatory demyelination, other mechanisms of tissue destruction may be quantitatively as important or more important in some diseases. An example could be demyelination resulting from oligodendroglial cell death following viral infection.

The mechanism of demyelination proposed here offers some possibilities for intervention. Available inhibitors of the extracellular proteinases will, as we have described, block BP hydrolysis in vitro. It may be possible to employ such a strategy to reduce demyelination in vivo. In addition, secretion of plasminogen activators and neutral proteinases by activated macrophages can be dramatically inhibited in vitro by glucocorticoids such as dexamethasone (49). These findings justify increased effort directed to the definition of biochemical mechanisms of demyelination in vivo, and to the control of these processes.

Acknowledgements. We thank Mrs Lesley Bieler, Mrs Gertrude Sager, Miss Renee Sasso, Mrs Marion Levine, and Mrs Marie Prendergast for their excellent assistance in this study. This work was supported by National Multiple Sclerosis Society grants 1089 and 1006, by grants NS-02476, NS-03356, FD-00787 and AI-07118 from the U.S. Public Health Service, and by a grant from the Sloan Foundation.

REFERENCES

1. Adams, C.W.M., Research on Multiple Sclerosis, Charles C. Thomas, Springfield (1972).
2. Adams, R.D. and Sidman, R.L., Introduction to Neuropathology, McGraw-Hill, New York (1968).

3. Althaus, H.H., Pilz, H. and Müller, D., The protein composition
    of myelin in multiple sclerosis (MS) and orthochromatic leuko-
    dystrophy (OLD), Z. Neurol. 205 (1973) 229-241.
4. Andrews, J.M., The ultrastructural neuropathology of multiple
    sclerosis, in Multiple Sclerosis (F. Wolfgram, G.W. Ellison,
    J.G. Stevens and J.M. Andrews, eds.) Academic Press, New York
    (1972) pp. 23-52.
5. Arstila, A.U., Riekkinen, P., Rinne, U.K. and Laitinen, L.,
    Studies on the pathogenesis of multiple sclerosis - Participa-
    tion of lysosomes on demyelination in the central nervous
    system white matter outside plaques, Eur. Neurol. 9 (1973)
    1-20.
6. Banik, N.L. and Davison, A.N., Lipid and basic protein inter-
    action in myelin, Biochem. J. 143 (1974) 39-45.
7. Boehme, D.H., Fordice, M.W. and Marks, N., Proteolytic activity
    in brain and spinal cord in sensitive and resistant strains of
    rat and mouse subjected to experimental allergic encephalo-
    myelitis, Brain Res. 75 (1974) 153-162.
8. Bowen, D.M. and Davison, A.N., Macrophages and cathepsin A
    activity in multiple sclerosis brain, J. Neurol. Sci. 21 (1974)
    227-231.
9. Boxer, P.A. and Leibovich, S.J., Production of collagenase by
    mouse peritoneal macrophages in vitro, Biochim. Biophys. Acta
    444 (1976) 626-632.
10. Buletza, G.F. and Smith, M.E., Enzymic hydrolysis of myelin
    basic protein and other proteins in central nervous system
    and lymphoid tissues from normal and demyelinating rats,
    Biochem. J. 156 (1976) 627-633.
11. Cohen, S.R., Herndon, R.M. and McKhann, G.M., Radioimmunoassay
    of myelin basic protein in spinal fluid: An index of active
    demyelination, New Eng. J. Med. 295 (1976) 1455-1457.
12. Cuatrecasas, P., Wilchek, M. and Anfinsen, C.B., Selective
    enzyme purification by affinity chromatography, Proc. Nat.
    Acad. Sci. (USA) 61 (1968) 636-643.
13. Cuzner, M.L., Banik, N.L. and Davison, A.N., The metabolism
    of myelin proteins by macrophages and lymphocytes. Abstract,
    Fifth Meeting Int. Soc. Neurochem., Barcelona 1975, p. 417.
14. Cuzner, M.L., Barnard, R.O., MacGregor, B.J.L., Borshell, N.J.
    and Davison, A.N., Myelin composition in acute and chronic
    multiple sclerosis in relation to cerebral lysosomal activity,
    J. Neurol. Sci. 29 (1976) 323-334.
15. Cuzner, M.L. and Davison, A.N., Changes in cerebral lysosomal
    enzyme activity and lipids in multiple sclerosis, J. Neurol.
    Sci. 19 (1973) 29-36.
16. DalCanto, M.C., Wisniewski, H.M., Johnson, A.B., Brostoff, S.W.
    and Raine, C.S., Vesicular disruption of myelin in autoimmune
    demyelination, J. Neurol. Sci. 24 (1975) 313-319.
17. Einstein, E.R., Csejtey, J., Dalal, K.B., Adams, C.W.M.,
    Bayliss, O.B. and Hallpike, J.F., Proteolytic activity and
    basic protein loss in and around multiple sclerosis plaques:

combined biochemical and histochemical observations, J. Neurochem. 19 (1972) 653-662.

18. Einstein, E.R., Dalal, K.B. and Csejtey, J., Increased protease
    activity and changes in basic proteins and lipids in multiple
    sclerosis plaques, J. Neurol. Sci. 11(1970) 109-121.

19. Gordon, S., Todd, J. and Cohn, Z.A., In vitro synthesis and
    secretion of lysozyme by mononuclear phagocytes, J. Exp. Med.
    139 (1974) 1228-1248.

20. Gordon, S., Unkeless, J.C. and Cohn, Z.A., Introduction of
    macrophage plasminogen activator by endotoxin stimulation and
    phagocytosis. Evidence for a two-stage process, J. Exp. Med.
    140 (1974) 995-1010.

21. Gordon, S., Werb, Z. and Cohn, Z.A., Methods for detection of
    macrophage secretory enzymes, in In Vitro Methods in Cell-
    Mediated Immunity (B.R. Bloom and J.R. David, eds.) Academic
    Press, New York (1976) pp. 341-352.

22. Govindarajan, K.R., Rauch, H.C., Clausen, J. and Einstein, E.R.,
    Changes in cathepsins B-1 and D, neutral proteinase, and
    2',3'-cyclic nucleotide-3'-phosphohydrolase activities in
    monkey brain with experimental allergic encephalomyelitis, J.
    Neurol. Sci. 23 (1974) 295-306.

23. Greenfield, S., Norton, W.T. and Morell, P., Quaking mouse:
    isolation and characterization of myelin protein, J. Neurochem.
    18 (1971) 2119-2128.

24. Hallpike, J.F., Enzyme and protein changes in myelin breakdown
    and multiple sclerosis, Prog. Histochem. Cytochem. 3 (1972)
    179-215.

25. Hallpike, J.F., Adams, C.W.M. and Bayliss, O.B., Histochemistry
    of myelin. VIII. Proteolytic activity around multiple
    sclerosis plaques, Histochem. J. 2 (1970) 199-208.

26. Hirsch, H.E., Duquette, P. and Parks, M.E., The quantitative
    histochemistry of multiple sclerosis plaque: acid proteinase
    and other acid hydrolases, J. Neurochem. 26 (1976) 505-512.

27. Hirsch, H.E. and Parks, M.E., Acid proteinases and other acid
    hydrolases in experimental allergic encephalomyelitis: pin-
    pointing the source, J. Neurochem. 24 (1975) 853-858.

28. Klimetzek, V. and Sorg, C., Lymphokine-induced secretion of
    plasminogen activator by murine macrophages, Eur. J. Immunol.
    7 (1977) 185-187.

29. Lampert, P., Demyelination and remyelination in experimental
    allergic encephalomyelitis. Further electron microscopic
    observations, J. Neuropath. Exp. Neurol. 24 (1965) 371-385.

30. Lowry, O.H., Rosebrough, N.J., Farr, A.L. and Randall, R.J.,
    Protein measurement with the Folin phenol reagent, J. Biol.
    Chem. 193 (1951) 265-275.

31. Marks, N., Grynbaum, A. and Lajtha, A., The breakdown of
    myelin-bound proteins by intra- and extracellular proteases
    Neurochem. Res. 1 (1976) 93-111.

32. Marks, N., Grynbaum, A. and Levine, S., Proteolytic enzymes
    in ordinary, hyperacute, monocytic and passive transfer

forms of experimental allergic encephalomyelitis, Brain Res. 123 (1977) 147-157.

33. Norton, W.T., Chemical pathology of diseases involving myelin, in Myelin (P. Morell, ed.) Plenum Press, New York (1977), pp. 383-413.

34. Norton, W.T. and Poduslo, S.E., Myelination in rat brain: method of myelin isolation, J. Neurochem. 21 (1973) 749-757.

35. Prineas, J., Pathology of the early lesion in multiple sclerosis, Hum. Pathol. 6 (1975) 531-554.

36. Quigley, J.P., Ossowski, L. and Reich, E., Plasminogen: the serum proenzyme activated by factors from cells transformed by oncogenic viruses, J. Biol. Chem. 249 (1974) 4306-4311.

37. Raghavan, S.S., Rhoads, D.B. and Kanfer, J.N., The effects of trypsin on purified myelin, Biochim. Biophys. Acta 328 (1973) 205-212.

38. Raine, C.S. and Schaumburg, H.H., The neuropathology of myelin diseases, in Myelin (P. Morell, ed.) Plenum Press, New York (1977) pp. 271-323.

39. Raine, C.S., Snyder, D.H., Valsamis, M.P. and Stone, S.H., Chronic experimental encephalomyelitis in inbred guinea pigs - an ultrastructural study, Lab. Invest. 31 (1974) 369-380.

40. Rauch, H.C. and Einstein, E.R., Specific brain proteins: a biochemical and immunological review, Rev. Neuroscience 1 (1974) 284-343.

41. Rauch, H.C., Einstein, E.R. and Csejtey, J., Enzymatic degradation of myelin basic protein in central nervous system lesions of monkeys with experimental allergic encephalomyelitis, Neurobiology 3 (1973) 195-205.

42. Riekkinen, P.J., Clausen, J., Frey, H.J., Fog, T. and Rinne, U.K., Acid proteinase activity of white matter and plaques in multiple sclerosis, Acta Neurol. Scand. 46 (1970) 349-353.

43. Riekkinen, P., Rinne, U.K., Savolainen, H., Palo, J., Kivalo, E. and Arstila, A., Studies on the pathogenesis of multiple sclerosis. Basic proteins in the myelin and white matter of multiple sclerosis, subacute sclerosing panencephalitis and postvaccinal leucoencephalitis, Eur. Neurol. 5 (1971) 229-244.

44. Smith, M.E., A lymph node neutral proteinase acting on myelin basic protein, J. Neurochem. 27 (1976) 1077-1082.

45. Smith, M.E., The role of proteolytic enzymes in demyelination on experimental allergic encephalomyelitis, Neurochem. Res. 2 (1977) 233-246.

46. Smith, M.E., Sedgewick, L.M. and Tagg, J.S., Proteolytic enzymes and experimental demyelination in the rat and monkey, J. Neurochem. 23 (1974) 965-971.

47. Unkeless, J.C. and Gordon, S., Secretion and regulation of plasminogen activator in macrophages, Cold Spring Hbr. Conf. on Cell Prolif. Vol. 2: Proteases and Biological Control (E. Reich, D.B. Rifkin and E. Shaw, eds.) (1975) pp. 495-514.

48. Unkeless, J.C., Gordon, S. and Reich, E., Secretion of plasminogen activator by stimulated macrophages, J. Exp. Med. 139 (1974) 834-850.

49. Vassalli, J.-D., Hamilton, J. and Reich, E., Macrophage plasmin-ogen activator: modulation of enzyme production by anti-in-flammatory steroids, mitotic inhibitors, and cyclic nucleotides, Cell 8 (1976) 271-281.

50. Vassalli, J.-D. and Reich, E., Macrophage plasminogen activator: induction by products of activated lymphoid cells, J. Exp. Med. 145 (1977) 429-437.

51. Wahl, L.M., Wahl, S.M., Mergenhagen, S.E. and Martin, G.R., Collagenase production by lymphokine-activated macrophages, Science 187 (1975) 261-263.

52. Werb, Z. and Gordon, S., Secretion of a specific collagenase by stimulated macrophages, J. Exp. Med. 142 (1975) 346-360.

53. Werb, Z. and Gordon, S., Elastase secretion by stimulated macrophages, J. Exp. Med. 142 (1975) 361-377.

54. Whitaker, J.N., Myelin encephalitogenic protein fragments in cerebrospinal fluid of persons with multiple sclerosis, Neurology, in press.

55. Wisniewski, H.M., Immunopathology of demyelination, Br. Med. Bull. 33 (1977) 54-59.

56. Wisniewski, H.M. and Bloom, B.R., Primary demyelination as a nonspecific consequence of a cell-mediated immune reaction, J. Exp. Med. 141 (1975) 346-359.

57. Wisniewski, H.M. and Bloom, B.R., Experimental allergic optic neuritis (AEON) in the rabbit, J. Neurol. Sci. 24 (1975) 257-263.

58. Wisniewski, H.M., Prineas, J. and Raine, C.S., An ultra-structural study of experimental demyelination and remyelina-tion. I. Acute experimental allergic encephalomyelitis in the peripheral nervous system, Lab. Invest. 21 (1969) 105-118.

59. Wood, J.G., Dawson, R.M.C. and Hauser, H.H., Effect of proteo-lytic attack on the structure of CNS myelin membrane, J. Neuro-chem. 22 (1974) 637-643.

VIRUS INFECTION IN DEMYELINATING DISEASES

V. ter Meulen and H. Wege

Institute of Virology and Immunobiology,
  University of Würzburg
8700 Würzburg, G.F.R.

SUMMARY

Several animal and human demyelinating diseases of the central
nervous system (CNS) are associated with RNA or DNA viruses. These
viruses infect CNS cells lytically or persistently. They mainly
belong to the group of envelope viruses which derive their envelope
partly from the host cell membrane. The process of virus release
may result in the appearance of new antigens of virus-infected cells
or the incorporation of cell membrane material into the viral
envelope. These changes may lead to an immune response which selectively injures the CNS. These alterations of host cell membranes
and host cell functions, together with the immune mechanism, are
central to many of the hypotheses regarding virus-induced demyelination. The role of virus infection in progressive multifocal leukoencephalopathy, subacute sclerosing panencephalitis, visna and
mouse hepatitis virus infections, is discussed in relation to the
demyelinating process of these diseases.

INTRODUCTION

Demyelination is a common neuropathological feature of certain
CNS diseases associated with virus infections. The detection of
virus particles in brain tissue has led to the assumption that the
destruction of brain cells by the viruses responsible for maintaining the myelin sheaths may possibly be the underlying mechanism

Part of this work was supported by the Deutsche Forschungsgemeinschaft, Schwerpunkt "Multiple Sklerose und verwandte Erkrankungen",
Az. Me 270/16.

of demyelination. However, the available laboratory evidence
suggests that the events leading to virus-induced demyelination are
probably of a more complex nature. It has been shown that a large
number of DNA and RNA viruses, especially enveloped RNA viruses, not
only induce an acute infection with a marked cytopathic effect but
also establish a persistent infection with no immediate destruction
of the host cell. The following viruses are included in this group:
herpes, varicella-zoster, measles, canine distemper (CDV), parainfluenza, mumps, rabies, Japanese encephalitis, western equine
encephalitis and mouse hepatitis (25). The majority of these virus
strains are neurotropic and can induce a CNS disease which is often
accompanied by demyelination.

     Of particular interest for the discussion of virus-induced
demyelination is the group of enveloped viruses which are released
by a budding process. In the course of virus replication, viral
proteins are incorporated into the cell membrane which allows the
immune surveillance system to recognize such a cell as being infected. Consequently, a chain of events start which eventually lead
to cell destruction. This communication briefly describes the
virological and immunological findings in some demyelinating diseases
in animals and human paradigmatically and discusses the possible
mechanisms of virus-induced demyelination in these diseases.

THE ROLE OF VIRAL INFECTION IN DEMYELINATING DISEASES OF ANIMALS

     Visna. Visna is a naturally occurring disorder of the CNS in
sheep which can be transmitted experimentally from animal to animal
(6). This disease belongs to the group of slow virus infections
(SVI) and is characterized by an aberration in the gait followed by
paraplegia or total paralysis. As the name SVI indicates, these
symptoms appear after an incubation period ranging from months to
years. In the CNS of the diseased animals an increase in protein
and cell count is found. In addition, serum and CSF specimens reveal
anti-visna-antibodies which already can be detected during the incubation period. Neuropathologically, a meningitis and perivascular
cuffing consisting of lymphocytes and macrophages is found as early
lesions which are most intense in the white matter. These changes
are followed by patchy demyelination most prominent in a subependymal
distribution.

     During the last years laboratory investigations have shed some
light on the pathogenicity of this disease. Data have been provided
which offer an explanation for visna virus persistency and focus on
the role of the immune response in the development of neuropathological changes. Visna virus is an enveloped RNA virus which morphologically resembles oncorna viruses (12). This virus contains an RNA-
dependent DNA polymerase which allows the virus to transfer its
genetic information into a DNA intermediate or provirus. In this
way the virus is able to persist in a cell without being recognized

by the immune surveillance system. Such visna-proviruses have been
detected in infected tissue cultures as well as in visna-infected
brain material (7). Haase and co-workers demonstrated visna DNA
by in situ hybridization techniques in visna infected brain
material. They were able to show that the majority of visna-DNA-
containing cells did not produce viral antigen which indicates a
restriction in virus gene expression (7). In this respect, the
virus resembles RNA tumor viruses, in other aspects, however, visna
virus exhibits properties which RNA tumor viruses lack. For example,
visna virus induces an inflammatory reaction in infected organs, is
capable of lysing infected cells and has a prominent cell fusion
activity. Moreover, there is no antigenic relationship or nucleic
acid sequence homology between RNA tumor viruses and visna viruses.
However, whether cell lysis or cell fusion occurs in the animal
has still not been demonstrated in infected brain.

Preliminary observations suggest that cell damage could occur
by immunopathological mechanisms. Nathanson and co-workers were
able to demonstrate that the early lesion of visna can be prevented
by immunosuppression (22). Visna sheep, treated with anti-thymocyte
serum, did not develop the typical neuropathological changes. EAE
sheep were used as controls to demonstrate the effectiveness of
immunosuppression. Moreover, visna virus does obviously escape
neutralization in animals. Gudnadottir and co-workers (6) and
Narayan and co-workers (21) have shown that an antigenic shift
occurs in visna after virus inoculation. They observed that
isolated visna virus strains from experimentally infected animals
differ in their antigenicity to the virus inoculum. In addition,
propagation of visna virus in tissue cultures in the presence of
antibodies yielded an infectious virus which was antigenically
different from the parent strain. This antigenic shift allows the
virus to escape the immune defense mechanism and may help to per-
petuate the infection. There remains little doubt that in visna a
very complex relationship between the virus and the immune system
may be the pathogenetic mechanism of this disease.

Canine distemper. Canine distemper is a widespread disease
naturally occurring in dogs and other members of the canine family
associated with a paramyxovirus and is biochemically and antigenically related to measles and rinderpest virus (3). This acute
or subacute disease is clinically characterized by pyrexia, exanthema
and signs of respiratory and gastrointestinal infection. Some dogs
develop demyelinating encephalomyelitis with severe neurological
symptoms of tremor, paralysis and convulsion. This symptomatology
may appear weeks or months after recovery from the acute infection.
Demonstrating the great variety of neuropathological lesions found,
the CNS disorder observed in dogs has been described as post-dis-
temper encephalitis, subacute diffuse sclerosing encephalitis and
old dog encephalitis (3). In general, the neuropathological changes
are either demyelinating or necrotic, affecting primarily the white
matter of the cerebellum, brainstem and spinal cord. The demyelinating areas are characterized by loss of myelin with relative sparing

of axons and presence of gitter cells. In the neighborhood of
demyelinating plaques perivascular cuffings consisting of lymphocyte and macrophages can often be observed. The necrotic plaques
frequently resemble a glial scar with astrocytes forming a network
in which macrophages are detectable. In addition, intranuclear
inclusion bodies of Cowdry type A containing distemper virus
nucleocapsids can be observed (16).

Virological studies on brain material from diseased animals
revealed the presence of CDV antigen in neuronal glial cell elements.
In addition, these cells contained canine gammaglobulin which
suggests an immunopathological phenomenon. Attempts to isolate
infectious canine distemper virus from brain material was only
successful when co-cultivation methods were applied on brain tissue
culture cells (5). Studies on this CNS disorder in experimentally
infected dogs have proved to be difficult, since the available virus
strains rarely induced such a disease. However, after isolation of
a canine distemper virus from a naturally occurring case of demyelinating distemper, a CNS infection could be produced in about
50% of animals without inducing a lethal respiratory infection (16).
After an incubation period of 45 to 60 days, animals, infected by
intracerebral inoculation or contact, developed either an acute or
subacute encephalomyelitis. The acute form was characterized by
focal demyelination without perivascular cuffing but with presence
of intranuclear inclusion bodies. All of these animals exhibited
sustained lymphopenia throughout the course of the disease and
died within six days. Animals having subacute encephalomyelitis
with prolonged clinical course, ranging up to a period of 12 weeks,
revealed only a transient lymphopenia. The neuropathological
changes in this group consisted of multifocal areas of demyelination
with perivascular cuffing and viral inclusion bodies. Immunological
studies on these animals revealed a depression of peripheral blood
lymphocyte mitogen response probably as a result of lymphocyte infection by CDV. CDV-antibodies as well as antibodies to CNS myelin
could be detected in the serum and in CSF specimens. In addition,
an elevation of plasmalogenase activity in the CNS was already
found before clinical symptoms were detectable (16).

CVD-infection in dogs, complicated by CNS disorder, has proven
to be an interesting model for the study of the mechanism by which
the CNS changes are induced. Whether the demyelination observed
with this infection results from a direct virus effect on the oligodendroglial cells or from an immunopathological response to this
infection has not been unraveled. More detailed studies on the
immune response to CNS infections have to be carried out, and experiments in animals in which the immune reactions have been
suppressed are also required.

THE ROLE OF VIRAL INFECTIONS IN HUMAN DEMYELINATING DISEASES

Subacute sclerosing panencephalitis (SSPE). SSPE is a rare, slowly evolving disease of the CNS which has been found primarily in children and young adults. Clinically, the condition begins with subtle intellectual deterioration, gradual appearance of inco- ordination and other motor abnormalities followed by myoclonal jerks, coma and death. The course of the disease varies from months to years. Pathognomonic findings include: classic EEG abnormalities, known as burst suppression patterns, an increase in the IgG fraction of gammaglobulin of the cerebrospinal fluid (CSF), and the detection of high measles antibody titers in serum and CSF specimens through- out the disease (1, 20).

Light microscopic studies of the brain reveal diffuse enceph- alitis of varying severity in both the gray and white matter through- out the brain. The encephalitic process is characterized by peri- vascular cuffing consisting of lymphocytes and plasma cells and by a diffuse infiltration of the gray and white matter by these cells. The most striking features of SSPE brain material are the enormous increase in hypertrophic astrocytes which form a dense network of fibres within both the gray and white matter, demyelination as well as the presence of intranuclear inclusion bodies of Cowdry type A. The latter formations are most frequently seen in the oligodendro- glial cells and contain paramyxovirus nucleocapsid structures which have been identified as measles virus nucleocapsids. Measles anti- gen is not only present in cells which reveal intranuclear inclusion bodies but also in the cytoplasm of many neurons and oligodendroglial cells which do not reveal morphological changes. In addition, it is noteworthy that measles antibodies and complement can be detected on cell membranes as well as within disrupted cells which are in- fected by measles virus. This observation suggests that cell- mediated immune reactions may possibly destroy infected cells (20).

The humoral immune response in SSPE is very pronounced and re- veals a state of hyperimmune reactions against all antigenic com- ponents of measles virus. In addition, measles IgM has been de- monstrated to be present in serum and CSF specimens of SSPE patients underlying the fact of measles virus persistency in this disease (15). Detailed immunological studies have shown that oligoclonal measles-specific antibodies appear in the CSF which probably origi- nated in the lymphocytes invading the CNS. Studies on cell-mediated immune reactions in these patients yielded a disparity in results. Some laboratories found minor defects in cell-mediated immunity which have not yet been confirmed by other groups (1). SSPE patients seem to have a fairly normal response to mitogens and to many other specific antigens both in vivo and in vitro. The cell- mediated immune response (CMI) to measles virus antigen, expressed by skin reactions, is apparently absent whereas the ability of SSPE lymphocytes to respond and kill measles infected target cells in vitro is not impaired (18).

The failure to incriminate the immune system in SSPE as major factor in the pathogenicity of this disease has turned the research interest back to the infectious agent and its host relationship in the CNS. The fact that SSPE results from a chronic measles virus infection has been accepted and the isolation of measles-like virus (referred to as SSPE virus) from SSPE brain material has been accomplished by different laboratories (1). So far, morphological analysis and antigenic studies of measles and SSPE viruses did not reveal any major differences among these virus strains. However, detailed biochemical analysis showed distinct differences between these viruses and has provided the basis for the characterization of SSPE and measles virus.

By comparing the RNA homology of SSPE with measles virus we found that SSPE virus not only shows differences to measles virus but also contains additional genomic information over and above those contained in measles virus (9). To verify this finding, the experiments were extended to the analysis of messenger RNA (mRNA) synthesis in infected cells. Our studies revealed that the smallest mRNA, probably the message coding for the virus membrane (M) protein, migrates slower in the systems of SSPE viruses (8). This observation led to a detailed study of the SSPE and measles virus M proteins. The M proteins of both viruses were isolated and their physical and chemical properties determined. Rabbits were subsequently immunized with the isolated proteins and the antigenicity of the two M proteins analyzed. The M proteins of SSPE and measles virus are antigenically unrelated. In immunodiffusion studies and immuno-electrophoresis, precipitation lines were obtained only in the homologous system. The antisera obtained did not reveal any activities against biologically active measles or SSPE antigens. These results indicate that SSPE viruses are related to measles virus but are not identical viruses (10).

The presence of a different M protein in SSPE virus raises the question of how this difference occurs. One possibility would be that the SSPE viruses develop from measles virus as a result of modification or mutation in that part of the genome which codes for the M protein. The question whether this mutation occurs in the host or whether the host is initially infected by the SSPE virus can still not be decided upon. However, these findings could imply that during mutation the production of a non-functioning or defective M protein occurs resulting in a non-productive persistent infection. This infection is probably the main underlying mechanism of virus-host relationship in SSPE.

Progressive multifocal leukoencephalopathy (PML). PML is a rare subacute demyelinating disease with multiple and different neurological symptoms depending on the location of the CNS infection. The neurological signs such as paralysis, mental deterioriation, visual loss, sensory abnormalities or ataxia take a progressive course and the disease usually leads to death in less than one year. No signs of an inflammatory infection are found in the patients, and

their CSF is also normal. This disease is considered to be an
opportunistic infection of some underlying disorders such as
reticuloendothelial diseases, carcinomas, granulomatous and inflammatory diseases associated with a state of secondary immunodeficiency (14). The pathological changes consist, in contrast to
the other diseases discussed in this paper, of a non-inflammatory
demyelinating process associated with human papova viruses. Demyelinating plaques are found throughout the white matter. The
demyelinating areas reveal loss of oligodendroglial cells and
myelin sheaths sparing the axon cylinders. The oligodendroglial
cells surrounding the plaques are often enlarged and contain intranuclear inclusion bodies which are filled with papova-like particles.
These cells are considered permissive for the human papova virus
infection. Within the foci of demyelination, the astrocytes are
abnormal with mitotic figures, bizarre chromatin patterns and
multinucleation. In certain ways, their forms resemble neoplastic
cells. Two different virus strains have been isolated from PML
brain by cell fusion techniques or by transferring brain material
to human fetal spongioblast cultures (24, 27). The viruses were
identified as human papova viruses JC and SV40 PML virus. These
viruses share capsid antigens and reveal a cross reaction of their
T-antigen to the known SV40 T-antigen. In addition, hyperimmune
sera showed cross reactions of hemagglutinating, fluorescing and
neutralizing antibodies. Epidemiological studies demonstrated antibodies to JC virus in humans only. It could be shown that already
at the age of 14 up to 80% of the population exhibit antibodies
to this virus, supporting the ubiquity of this agent. In contrast,
antibodies to SV40 can only be detected in 2-4% of humans. The
pathogenicity of this disease is unknown and the critical question
of whether this agent assumes residence in normal brain and starts
a disease process by specific triggering events, such as immunodeficiency, cannot be answered; moreover, these viruses contain
oncogenic properties as has been shown in studies with hamsters.
The fact that giant astrocytes in PML cannot be morphologically
distinguished from malignant astrocyte of pleomorphic glioblastoma
deserves further investigation.

DISCUSSION

From a virological and immunological point of view, the three
main conceivable mechanisms by which a virus infection may lead to
demyelination as a result of the destruction or functional impairment of glial cells are: a) direct effect of virus infection, b)
immune reactions against virus-induced glial membrane changes, and
c) autoimmune reaction triggered by the virus infection (Table 1).
Direct effects of virus replication within glial cells can produce
demyelination without involving the immunopathological mechanism.
Acute diseases of the CNS associated with mouse hepatitis virus

Table 1. Possible mechanisms of virus-induced demyelination.

I. Viral infection of glial cells:
    Acute infection   - destruction of the cell
    Chronic or latent   - destruction or functional
     infection   impairment of the cell

II. Immune reactions to virus-infected glial cells:
    Cell-mediated immune reactions against membrane components
     of infected glial cells

III. Demyelination resulting from virus-induced autoimmune
     reactions.

(see the paper of Nagashima et al., in this volume) or canine distemper virus are types of infections which lead directly to cell destruction. The same situation may occur in the chronic infection of PML and SSPE. In PML, the infection usually occurs as an opportunistic infection in an immunodeficient host. The oligodendroglial cells contain infectious virus indicating that these cells are permissive for human papova virus. Such an infection leads to morphological changes of these cells followed by demyelination. In SSPE, morphological changes in glial cells can also be observed. In contrast to PML, SSPE patients do exhibit a humoral hyperimmune reaction, which has been interpreted by some investigators as an immunopathological phenomenon for this disease (26). The available laboratory data suggest, however, that the detectable antibodies are only directed against viral antigens and not against the brain cell membrane as one would expect in a case where virus-induced membrane changes lead to a situation of an immunopathological phenomenon (1). In addition, the possible pathogenetic role of antibodies or antigen-antibody complexes is complicated by reports that SSPE has been observed in patients with hypogammaglobulinemia and combined immunodeficiency syndrome (2, 11). Moreover, immunosuppressive treatment of SSPE patients does not alter the course of this CNS disease.

The interesting aspect of the functional impairment of virus infected cells has so far been neglected. Only recently have studies been carried out in tissue cultures to investigate the effect of viruses such as LCM-virus (23) in neuroblastoma cells. Cells persistently infected with LCM virus revealed a decrease in the concentration of choline acetylcholine-transferase and acetylcholine esterase without visible morphological changes. Moreover, alterations in the vital functions of the cells such as growth rate, RNA, or protein synthesis could not be detected. Events similar to those observed in tissue cultures occurred also in animals.

These cell lines offer the possibility to investigate some aspects of cell function with virus-infected cells. It is possible that such a persistent infection of glial cells may lead to demyelination.

The possibility that an interaction between a viral infection of the CNS and an immune response may lead to demyelination has been suggested for visna (22). This infection in sheep reveals a unique virus-host relationship which has not been described for any other virus infection. The virus is biochemically equipped to transfer its genetic information into the DNA intermediate which allows it to persist in a host cell indefinitely. Moreover, the occurrence of an antigenic shift in the process of virus replication permits the persistence of extracellular infectious virus; a phenomenon known only in chronic protozoal infections and in equine infectious anemia (EIA) virus infections of horses (4, 17). The latter disease is characterized by hemolysis and fever which occurs during viremia. Development of neutralizing antibodies leads to remission of the disease which relapses when antigenically altered virus appears in the blood stream. EIA is also a retravirus. Whether this virus persistency occurs through the mechanism described for visna virus has still to be demonstrated. Visna in sheep, however, does not appear to be a remitting or relapsing disease. Its course is of a progressive nature. The effect of immuno-suppression on the early lesions of visna infection suggests an immunopathological mechanism participating in the neuropathological changes observed in this disease. In this connection two other CNS diseases could serve as a model; EAE in a variety of animals, and LCM infection in mice. In both diseases, a T-cell mediated immunopathology has been clearly demonstrated. Suppression of T-cells prevents these CNS disorders. Sensitized T-cells transfer to normal recipients in EAE and infected LCM-tolerant mice transmit the disease. Similar events may be involved in visna. However, more information is needed before the role of the immune system can be defined in this disease.

On the basis of circumstantial evidence, the postinfectious encephalomyelitides in humans could also belong to the group of virus infections where an immune reaction may play a pathogenetic role. These CNS diseases sometimes occur as a complication of measles, varicella, mumps, influenza, rubella and non-specific upper respiratory tract infections. They usually follow either a respiratory infection or develop after or at the time of virus-induced general exanthema. This observation and the neuropathological changes characterized by perivenular demyelination, not usually seen in a primary viral encephalitis, as well as the similarities of these diseases with EAE or rabies vaccine encephalitis have suggested an immunopathological phenomenon. However, laboratory evidence to support this hypothesis is lacking. No experimental animal is available for the investigation of the pathogenesis of postinfectious encephalomyelitides. Only in few instances, such as measles encephalitis, could a virus be isolated from brain

specimens (19). So far, no immune reactions directed against host
cell membranes have been reported in this disease.

From a hypothetical point of view, the possibility that a virus
infection within or outside the CNS might indirectly start a process
of demyelination by inducing an autoreactivity should be considered.
Several mechanisms have been suggested by which viruses may initiate
an autoimmune phenomenon: release of sequestered antigens from virus
infected cells, virus-induced alterations of the host cell membrane
antigens, immunological cross-reactivity between viral and host
antigenic determinants, and direct or indirect alterations of immunocytes by the virus infection (13). Although none of these mechanisms
has been shown to be operating in demyelinating diseases until now,
these conjectures provide useful models for investigation of these
diseases. Especially, the possibility of immunological cross-
reactivity between viral and myelin antigens merits attention.
Since viruses, particularly budding viruses, probably incorporate
host antigens into the viral envelope, it is possible that a close
association of a weak autoantigen and a strong viral antigen may
result in the presentation of a self-determinant in an immunogenic
form. If an antigenic relationship to myelin exists in such a
situation, an autoimmune reaction against myelin would occur.

At present, little is known about immune reactions in the CNS.
From an immunological point of view, the CNS is considered to be a
privileged site to which the immune system does not have easy access.
Little information on the flow of antibodies, lymphoid cells, macrophages, antigens and antigen-antibody complexes in and out of the
CNS is available. In the case of demyelinating diseases associated
with virus infections, many virological and immunological problems
have to be studied and solved before the mechanism by which such a
process occurs can be answered.

REFERENCES

1. Agnarsdottir, G., Subacute sclerosing panencephalitis, in
    Recent Advances in Clinical Virology (A.P. Waterson, ed.)
    Churchill Livingstone, London (1977).
2. Allison, A.C., J. Clin. Pathol. 25 (1972) 121-131.
3. Appel, M.J.G. and Gillespie, J.H., Canine distemper virus,
    Virology Monographs 11 (1972) 1-96.
4. Brown, J.N., Brown, K.N. and Hills, L.A., Immunity to malaria:
    The antibody response to antigenic variation by plasmodium
    knowlesi, Immunol. 14 (1968) 127.
5. Confer, A.W., Kahn, D.E., Koestner, A. and Krakowka, S.,
    Biological properties of a canine distemper virus isolate
    associated with demyelinating encephalitis, Infect. Immunol.
    11 (1975) 835-844.
6. Gudnadottir, M., Visna-Maedi in sheep, Progr. Med. Virol. 18
    (1974) 336-349.

7. Haase, A.T., Stowring, L., Narayan, O., Griffin, D. and Prince, D., Slow persistent infection caused by visna virus: role of host restriction, Science 195 (1977) 175-177.

8. Hall, W.W., Kiessling, W.R. and ter Meulen, V., Biochemical comparison of measles and subacute sclerosing panencephalitis (SSPE)-viruses, in Negative Strand Virus and the Host Cell (B. Mahy and R. Barry, eds.) Academic Press, in press.

9. Hall, W.W. and ter Meulen, V., RNA homology between subacute sclerosing panencephalitis and measles viruses, Nature 264 (1976) 474-477.

10. Hall, W.W., Nagashima, K., Kiessling, W.R. and ter Meulen, V., Isolation and properties of the membrane (M) protein of measles virus, in Negative Strand Virus and the Host Cell (B. Mahy and R. Barry, eds.) Academic Press, in press.

11. Hanissian, A.S., Jabbour, J.T., de Lamerens, S., Garcia, J.H. and Horta-Barbosa, L., Subacute encephalitis and hypogamma-globulinemia, Amer. J. Dis. Child. 123 (1972) 151-155.

12. Harter, D.H., Sheep progressive pneumonia viruses, in Slow Virus Infections of the Central Nervous System (V. ter Meulen and M. Katz, eds.) Springer, New York (1977).

13. Hirsch, M.S. and Proffitt, M.R., Autoimmunity in viral infections, in Viral Immunology and Immunopathology (A.L. Notkins, ed.) Academic Press, New York (1975) pp. 419-434.

14. Johnson, R.T., Narayan, O., Weiner, L.P. and Greenlee, J.E., Progressive multifocal leukoencephalopathy, in Slow Virus Infections of the Central Nervous System (V. ter Meulen and M. Katz, eds.) Springer, New York (1977).

15. Kiessling, W.R., Hall, W.W., Yung, L.L. and ter Meulen, V., Measles-virus-specific immunoglobulin-M-response in subacute sclerosing panencephalitis, Lancet I (1977) 324-327.

16. Koestner, A. and Krakowka, S., A concept of virus-induced demyelinating encephalomyelitis relative to an animal model, in Slow Virus Infections of the Central Nervous System (V. ter Meulen and M. Katz, eds.) Springer, New York (1977).

17. Kono, Y., Kabayashi, K. and Fukunaga, Y., Antigenic drift of equine anemia virus in chronically infected horses, Arch. Ges. Virusforsch. 41 (1973) 1.

18. Kreth, W.H., Käckell, M.Y. and ter Meulen, V., Demonstration of in vitro lymphocyte-mediated cytotoxicity against measles virus in SSPE, J. Immunol. 114 (1975) 1042-1046.

19. Meulen, V. ter, Käckell, Y., Müller, D., Katz, M. and Meyer-mann, R., Isolation of infectious measles virus in measles encephalitis, Lancet II (1972) 1171-1175.

20. Meulen, V. ter, Katz, M. and Müller, D., Subacute sclerosing panencephalitis: a review, Current Trends in Microbiology 57 (1973) 1-38.

21. Narayan, O., Griffin, D.E. and Silverstain, A.M., Slow virus infection: replication and mechanisms of persistence of visna virus in sheep, J. Infec. Dis. 135 (1977) 800-806.

22. Nathanson, N., Panitch, H., Palsson, P.A., Petursson, G. and
    Georgsson, G., Pathogenesis of visna. II. Effect of immuno-
    suppression upon early central nervous system lesions,
    Laboratory Investigation 35 (1976) 444-451.
23. Oldstone, M.B., Holmstoen, J. and Welsh, R.M. Jr., Alterations
    of acetylcholine enzymes in neuroblastoma cells persistently
    infected with lymphocytic choriomeningitis virus, J. Cell.
    Physiol. 91 (1976) 459-472.
24. Padgett, B.L., Walker, G.M., zu Rhein, G.M. and Eckroade, R.J.,
    Cultivation of papova-like virus from human brain with pro-
    gressive multifocal leukoencephalopathy, Lancet I (1971)
    1257-1260.
25. Rima, B.K. and Martin, S.J., Persistent infection of tissue
    culture cells by RNA viruses, Med. Microbiol. Immunol. 162
    (1976) 89-118.
26. Sever, J.L. and Zeman, W. (eds.), Conference on measles virus
    and subacute sclerosing panencephalitis, J. Amer. Acad. Neurol.
    18 (1968) No. 1, Part 2.
27. Weiner, L.P. and Narayan, O., Virologic studies of progressive
    multifocal leukoencephalopathy, Prog. Med. Virol. 18 (1974)
    229-240.

EARLY AND LATE CNS-EFFECTS OF CORONA VIRUS INFECTION IN RATS[+]

K. Nagashima, H. Wege and V. ter Meulen

Institute of Virology and Immunobiology,
  University of Würzburg
8700 Würzburg, G.F.R.

SUMMARY

The mouse hepatitis virus strain JHM was injected intra-cerebrally into newborn and weanling rats. Three types of diseases were observed:

1. Acute panencephalitis: Almost all suckling rats became moribund within 6 days. Histologically severe panencephalitis with demyelinating foci was noticed; the foci were similar to those found in mice. Virus was easily detectable in the oligodendroglial cells and neurons both by immunofluorescence and electron microscopy. Infectious virus could be isolated.

2. Subacute demyelinating encephalomyelitis (SDE): Three weeks after infection of weanling rats, about 35% of the animals developed paralysis. Neuropathologically, demyelination with a striking predilection for white matter was observed in the brain stem, optic nerve and spinal cord. Virus was detectable by electron microscopy in degenerating oligodendroglial cells only, which corresponded to the results obtained by the immunofluorescent techniques. Infectious virus could be recovered.

3. Chronic progressive paralysis: Inoculated weanling rats without SDE developed 6 to 8 months later a slowly progressing paralysis of the legs. Hydrocephalus and myelomalacia were present. Viral "footprints" could not be detected.

[+]Supported by the Deutsche Forschungsgemeinschaft, Schwerpunkt "Multiple Sklerose und verwandte Erkrankungen", Az. Me 270/16.

INTRODUCTION

The neuropathological finding of demyelination accompanying virus infections of the central nervous system (CNS) in human and animals is a common feature of acute and chronic diseases. So far, the pathogenetic mechanism by which such demyelination is induced is for most of these infections unknown. From a virological point of view it is of particular interest to study the virus-host relationship which is responsible for these changes. Such studies have been carried out with JHM virus infection in mice (2, 9, 16, 17). This murine corona virus causes an acute disseminated encephalomyelitis with destruction of the myelin, which results from infection of the myelin supporting oligodendroglial cells (9, 17). However, investigations in chronic viral infections of the CNS in small laboratory animals, with demyelination, have not been reported, since proper animal models are not available.

The present communication describes the neuropathological findings of three different CNS diseases obtained in rats after intracerebral JHM virus infection. Depending on the age of the animal an acute panencephalitis, a subacute demyelinating encephalomyelitis or a chronic progressive paralysis was observed. These experimentally induced diseases with a more subacute and chronic nature offer the possibility to analyze the virus and host factors, which play a role in the process of demyelination in persistent viral infections.

EXPERIMENTAL

<u>Animals</u>. Specific pathogen-free pregnant or weanling (20-25 days old) rats, strain CHBB/THOM, were purchased from Thomae, Biberach, Germany, and used for the experiments. The animals did not reveal neutralizing antibodies against JHM virus.

<u>Virus</u>. The original stock virus of JHM, a homogenate of suckling mouse brain, was kindly obtained from Dr. L.P. Weiner, Johns Hopkins University, Baltimore, U.S.A. The virus was passaged in our laboratory by intracerebral inoculation of suckling mice and was adapted also to grow in L-929 cells and Sacc(-)-cells. Both, 20% brain suspension or clarified supernatant of infected culture cells, were used as inoculum for the experiment. Depending on the experiment the virus preparation contained between 5×10^5 - 1×10^7 ID50/ml.

<u>Animal inoculation</u>. Weanling and newborn rats were inoculated into the left brain hemisphere. Newborn rats received 0.01 ml and weanling rats 0.03 ml of the desired virus suspension.

<u>Immunofluorescence studies</u>. Antiserum against JHM in mice was prepared by weekly intraperitoneal inoculations of brain suspension containing virus (0.5 ml/animal) over a period of six weeks. Animals were exsanguinated two weeks after the last injection. For the

detection of JHM antigen in CNS-tissue, cryostat sections were
fixed for 10 min in acetone and stained with the specific antiserum
applying the indirect immunofluorescent technique. FITC labeled
anti-mouse globulin was obtained from Microbiological Ass., Maryland, U.S.A. Anti-JHM serum and FITC labeled anti-mouse globulin
were used only after absorption with brain powder of control rat
brain. Cryostat sections stained for viral antigens were further
examined by hematoxylin-eosine staining to correlate the virological
findings with the histological changes.

Virus isolation. The animals were dissected under aseptic
conditions. After several washings in cold PBS with antibiotics
specimens were homogenized in a glass douncer to give a 15% (w/v)
suspension. Crude homogenates were adsorbed on monolayers of L-
cells (0.3 ml/petridish 20 ccm) for one hour. The monolayers were
washed and overlaid with 5 ml MEM containing 5% fetal calf serum
and antibiotics. Cultures, which did not show a JHM-CPE after 48 h
were passaged two times before a negative result was accepted.

Histology and electron microscopy. For histological and ultrastructural examinations tissue blocks were taken from animals
perfused with 2.5% glutaraldehyde, 2% paraformaldehyde in 0.1 M
phosphate buffer solution at 37°C. Paraffine embedded specimens
were stained with hematoxylin-eosine (HE), Klüver-Barrera method for
staining of myelin (KB) and Glees and Marsland´s method for staining
of axons. Blocks for electron microscopy were postfixed in 1%
osmium tetroxide, stained with 2% uranyl acetate in 70% alcohol,
dehydrated and embedded in epon. Thick sections, cut with a
Reichert microtome, were stained with toluidine blue or paraphenylene
diamine (PPD). Thin sections from selected blocks were cut with a
diamond knife. The sections were stained with lead citrate and
examined with a Zeiss 10B electron microscope.

RESULTS

Acute panencephalitis. Intracerebral inoculation of JHM virus
in newborn rats led to a hindleg paralysis within 3 to 4 days after
virus infection (Table 1). The animals died one to two days after
onset of the disease. Neuropathologically the following changes
were observed. In the cerebral cortex and hippocampal gyrus (Fig. 1)
foci of fresh necrosis were present. In these necrotic areas
pyknotic neurons were found surrounded by nuclear debri and polymorphonuclear leukocytes. Glial nodules (Fig. 1b) were often encountered in the hippocampal gyrus and basal ganglia. Meningitis
had developed in all cases and ependymitis was found in a few rats.
Perivascular areas of the cortex and white matter were infiltrated
by polymorphonuclear leukocytes and small lymphoid cells. A few
multinucleated giant cells were found in the perivascular areas
and meninges. No inclusion bodies were detected.

Table 1.   Acute encephalitis in newborn rats. - The incubation
period ranged from 3 to 7 days. Virus could be isolated from the
brain material of all animals tested.

No. of animals infected (I.C.)	No. of diseased animals
12	5
9	7
15	13
38	32

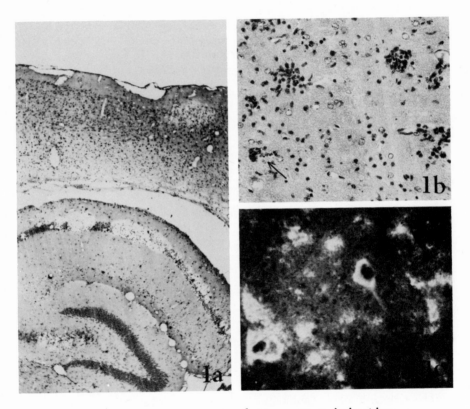

Fig. 1.   Cerebrum of newborn rats 6 days after injection.
    1a.   Patchy circumscribed fresh necrosis found in hippocampal
          gyri. HE x 120.
    1b.   Scattered glia-mesenchymal nodules in basal ganglia. Note
          polymorphonuclear infiltration and multinucleated giant
          cell (↖). HE x 300.
    1c.   Immunofluorescent staining of brain stem. JHM antigen
          detectable in glial cells and large neurons. x 600.

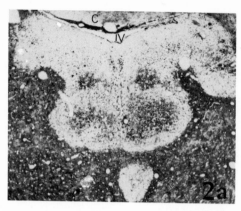
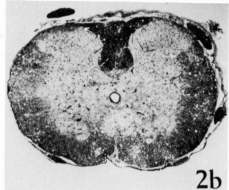

Fig. 2. Myelin stained preparations of pons and spinal cord of
newborn rats 6 days after injection.
2a. Almost symmetrically distributed large circumscribed
spongy lesions. Note the relatively well remaining neurons
in lesions. C: cerebellar cortex, IV: fourth ventricle
(vessels were dilated due to perfusion). x 60.
2b. Spongy state in the white matter of spinal cord. Advanced
lesions were found deep in the anterior column. Note cell
infiltration in the gray matter. x 60.

In the brain stem many sharply circumscribed lesions were
found, which consisted of a spongy and rarified ground substance
(Fig. 2a). The neurons in these areas were relatively unaltered
although staining with HE was very pale. Myelin sheaths were
completely destroyed and in addition to some extent axons. However, in some areas axons were relatively well preserved in contrast to the severe destruction of myelin sheaths.

In the gray matter of the spinal cord glial nodules and a few
mononuclear cell infiltrations were detectable whereas the white
matter revealed lesions of demyelination unrelated to specific
tracts (Fig. 2b). The pronounced white matter lesions lacked myelin
sheaths completely and were filled with large amounts of macrophages.
The early lesions of demyelination showed the beginning of a spongy
degeneration. Spinal ganglia and peripheral nerves were histologically normal.

By immunofluorescence technique JHM antigen could be demonstrated in neurons and glial cells. In the cerebrum, the pyramidal
cells of hippocampal gyrus were constantly affected. In the
cerebral white matter antigen-positive small cells were arranged
in parallel to the myelin sheaths. The Purkinje cells of the
cerebellum were stained positive up to their dendrites. Large
neurons as well as glial cells in the brain stem showed positive
immunofluorescence (Fig. 1c). In the spinal cord antigens were

found both in the gray and white matter. It is of particular
interest that in the white matter of the spinal cord the antigen
present in cells was arranged in a triangular shape pointing to the
center of the spinal cord. This suggests that the virus infection
proceeds from the periphery to the center. Viral antigen could also
be found in some meningeal cells, however, ependymal cells, nerve
roots, spinal ganglia and peripheral nerves were negative.

     Electron microscopy revealed virus particles in the neurons,
astrocytes and oligodendroglial cells. In the cytoplasmic vacuoles
of large neurons in brain stem many virus particles were found
(Fig. 3). Some were seen in the vesicles near the Golgi apparatus
(Fig. 3). The particles were also detectable outside the neuron

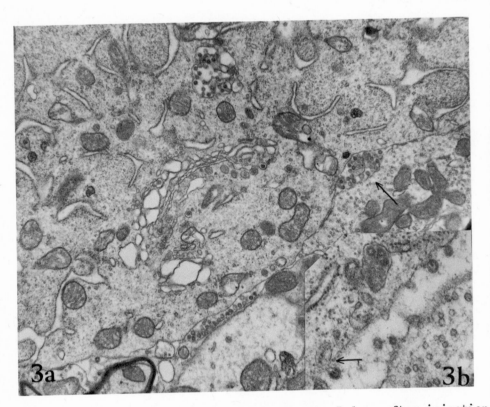

Fig. 3. Neuron in brain stem of newborn rats 5 days after injection.
     3a. Virus particles observed in the vacuoles and vesicles
         around Golgi apparatus as well as in the synaptic cleft
         (↖). x 20,000.
     3b. Neuronal cytoplasm on left upper side and synapse on right
         lower side. Virus particles found in the vacuoles and
         synaptic cleft. One vacuole adjacent of cell membrane
         releasing a particle into the cleft (↖). x 40,000.

in the synaptic cleft (Fig. 3a). A vacuole just beneath the cell
membrane contained many virus particles (Fig. 3b) and in another
vacuole attached to the cell membrane it seemed that a particle was
released into the synaptic cleft (Fig. 3b). The virus particle had
a diameter of 60-80 mμ. In the early lesions of the spinal white
matter scattered degenerating cells containing virus particles were
observed (Fig. 4a). These cells were considered to be oligodendroglia because of their location within the white matter and lack of
glial fibrils. Moreover, in the cytoplasmic processes extending
along the myelin sheaths viruses budding into the vacuole were detectable (Fig. 4b).

    Virological studies revealed infectious virus present in the
area of the brain and spinal cord which showed histological changes.
From all animals tested infectious virus could be isolated. Histological studies of extraneural tissue revealed foci of necrosis in
the liver of some animals.

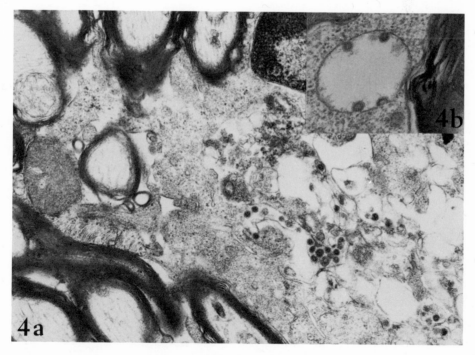

Fig. 4. Degenerating cell in the spinal white matter of a weanling
         rat 5 days after injection.
    4a. Virus particles found in the vacuoles. x 28,000.
    4b. A vacuole in the cytoplasm adjacent of myelin sheath.
        Note budding process. x 44,000.

Table 2. Subacute demyelinating encephalitis in weanling rats.
- The incubation period ranged from 2 to 10 weeks with an average
of 3 weeks. Virus could be isolated from the brain material up to
45 days after inoculation.

No. of animals infected (I.C.)	No. of diseased animals
12	6
10	4
32	12
45	15

     Subacute demyelinating encephalomyelitis. A total of 99
weanling rats were intracerebrally inoculated with JHM virus (Table
2). Thirty-five rats developed hindleg paralysis between the 14th
to the 24th day after inoculation, two rats showed the first symptoms
on 45th and 66th day respectively, and the other animals remained
clinically well. The incubation period ranged from 2 to 10 weeks
after inoculation with an average incubating period of 3 weeks
(Table 2). Clinically the rats showed signs of a spastic paralysis
with hunched backs and a ruffled fur. Infectious JHM virus could
be isolated from brain and spinal cord specimens up to 45 days after
virus inoculation. A precise account of this subacute encephalomyelitis will be published elsewhere (13). The results are briefly
summarized here: Histologically, acute lesions such as fresh
necrosis or polymorphonuclear infiltration, observed in the suckling
rats, were absent. The prominent lesions were present in the brain
stem, optic chiasma and spinal cord. The lesions showed a more
striking predilection for the white matter. The large circumscribed
patchy lesions in the brain stem were partly similar to those of
suckling rats with regard to complete loss of the myelin sheath.
The neurons and axons, however, were far better preserved than those
in acute cases. Moreover, neither polymorphonuclear infiltration
nor multinucleated giant cells were observed. Lesions in the spinal
cord were strictly confined to the white matter. Early or more
pronounced demyelinating areas were found without connection to
specific tracts (Fig. 5a).
     In the advanced areas many gitter cells were detectable (Fig.
5b). In the early areas spongy stages were noticed, which consisted
of the two types of vacuoles, one surrounded by myelin sheath and
the other containing amorphous flocculent material (Fig. 5c).
     Like in the acute panencephalitis the spinal ganglia and periph-
eral nerve were histologically normal.
     The liver of a few animals revealed scattered nodules of small,
round cells; foci of necrosis were absent.
     Immunofluorescent studies revealed JHM antigen in the white
matter of the cerebrum, brain stem and spinal cord (Fig. 5d). The
neurons of the cerebral cortex, brain stem and spinal cord remained

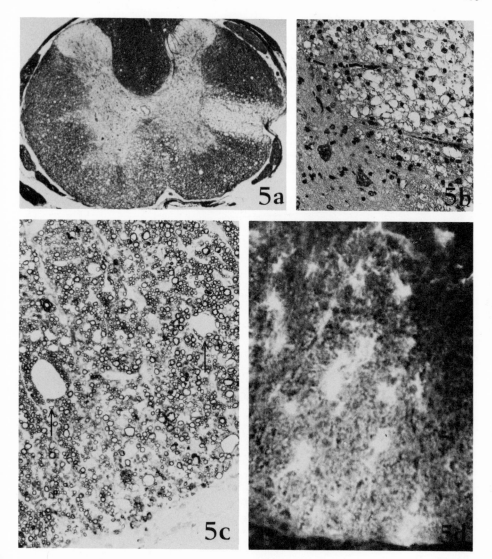

Fig. 5. Subacute demyelinating encephalomyelitis.
5a. Well circumscribed advanced demyelinating lesion found in
    the left lateral column. Early spongy state found in other
    white matter. KB x 60.
5b. Advanced demyelinating area near gray matter. Many gitter
    cells found in the lesions. Note small round cell in-
    filtrations in the gray matter. HE x 300.
5c. Early spongy area in the white matter. Note lipid-loaded
    macrophage near the arachnoidea. PPD x 600.
5d. Immunofluorescent staining of the spinal white matter,
    only oligodendroglial cells contain JHM antigen. x 900.

negative. In the spinal cord, viral antigen was only found in the
early spongy areas and not in or around advanced demyelinating
lesions.

By electron microscopy, the virus particles were detected only
in the hypertrophically degenerating cells in the early spongy
state of spinal white matter, which seemed to correspond to the
vacuoles containing amorphous material in the histological preparations. The cells were highly degenerated but particles were still
found within the vacuoles (Fig. 6a). Around the vacuoles there was
a large amount of microtubules, characteristic for oligodendroglia
(Fig. 6b).

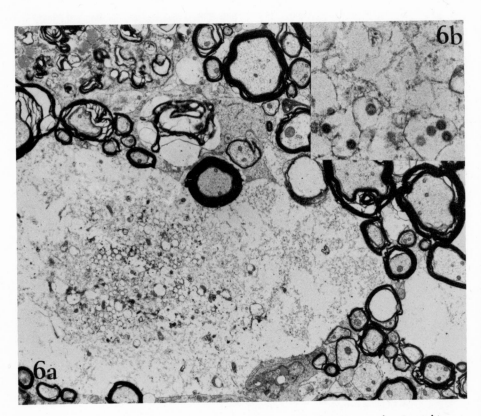

Fig. 6. Hyperthropically degenerating cell in the spinal white
          matter, corresponding to "marked" cell in Fig. 5c.
       6a. Vacuoles containing virus particles. Abundant microtubules
           are seen. Myelin sheaths are degenerating but axons are
           still preserved. Macrophage containing myelin debris
           found on the left upper corner. x 5,000.
       6b. Higher magnification of Fig. 6a. Virus particles and
           microtubules. x 44,000.

Table 3.   Chronic progressive paralysis in weanling rats.   - The incubation period ranged from 6 to 8 months.   No infectious virus or viral antigen was detected in brain tissue.

No. of animals infected (I.C.)	No. of diseased animals
17	4
24	6

Chronic progressive paralysis. Weanling rats, which did not exhibit subacute demyelinating encephalitis, developed 6 to 8 months later a slowly progressive paralysis of the legs (Table 3). Four rats were neuropathologically examined. Hydrocephalus was found in all rats and in three of them also myelomalacia. Hydrocephalus consisted of an enlargement of the lateral ventricles as well as of the fourth aqueduct (Fig. 7). The aqueductus Sylvii was not closed. The leptomeninges showed diffuse fibrous thickening. Fibrosis was most prominent around the cerebrospinal junction. Cerebral cortices became thin and the white matter was partly degenerated with gliosis along the ventricles. No inflammatory changes were found throughout the central nervous system. In the cerebro-cerebellar cortices and spinal cord scattered calcospherite deposition was found. Myelomalacia consisted of the rarefactive degeneration partly involving

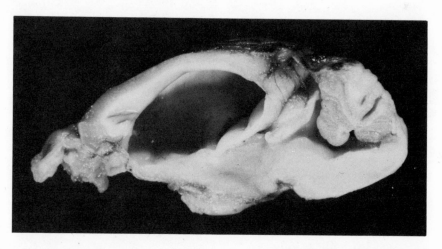

Fig. 7. Sagittal section of the brain from an animal with chronic progressive paralysis. Lateral ventricle as well as fourth ventricle are dilated. Note the thickened meninges. x 5.

the gray matter (Fig. 8a). It was most prominent in the upper
cervical cord and gradually less marked down to the thoracic cord.
The central canal was neither obstructed nor dilated. In less
affected areas, gray matter was in a spongy state (Fig. 8c). In
these areas neurons remained relatively unaltered. No ballooning
nerve cells were found. The wall of the anterior spinal artery was
thickened but the lumen was not closed (Fig. 8b). Severe arachnoid
fibrosis with partial calcification was observed (Fig. 8d). The
liver of two rats revealed few nodules of inflammatory cells.

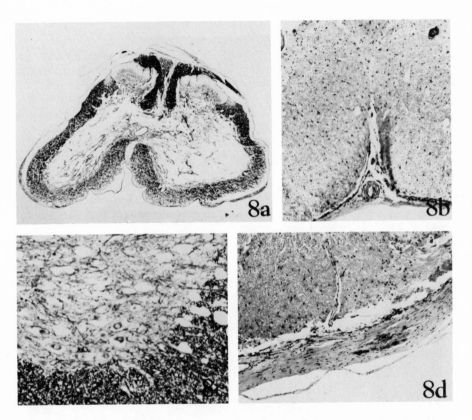

Fig.   8. Spinal cord of a case of chronic progressive paralysis.
       8a. Gray matter of cervical cord showing advanced rarefactive
           degeneration. KB x 60.
       8b. Thickened wall of the anterior spinal artery. Calcospherite
           deposition found on the right upper corner. HE x 150.
       8c. Early spongy state of the gray matter, partly extending to
           the white matter. Note the well preserved anterior horn
           cells. KB x 150.
       8d. Fibrously thickened arachnoid of the spinal cord. Note
           the calcification (the cleft between the cord and arachnoid
           is an artifact). HE x 150.

Attempts to isolate JHM virus were unsuccessful despite the fact that methods of isolation were applied which yielded infectious virus in subacute sclerosing panencephalitis. Moreover, JHM virus antigen could not be demonstrated in brain or spinal cord material by conventional immunofluorescent techniques.

DISCUSSION

In our experiments with JHM infections in rats three types of diseases were observed: acute panencephalitis, subacute demyelinating encephalitis and chronic progressive paralysis. The lesions of acute panencephalitis produced in newborn rats are comparable to those in mice. Studies carried out in mice have shown that JHM virus, independent of the age of the inoculated animals, affects the gray and white matter (2, 9, 16, 17). The neuropathology consists of an acute encephalomyelitis with patchy demyelinating lesions in the brain stems and spinal cord. Like in newborn rats, neurons and oligodendroglial cells are infected by JHM virus as it has been demonstrated by immunofluorescent techniques (17). The demyelination occurring in mice is interpreted as a result of oligo-dendroglial cell destruction by JHM virus infection (9, 17). Similar virus-host relationships probably account for the neuropathological changes in JHM infected newborn rats.

In contrast to the findings reported in mice, inoculated weanling rats revealed a different neuropathological picture. Sub-acute encephalomyelitis was observed, which showed the most striking changes in the white matter. Demyelination was very marked without destruction of axons. Electron microscopic examination of this sub-acute form showed that virus particles were found only in the hyper-trophically degenerated cells in the white matter.

The co-presence of microtubules in these cells may support the contention that the cells are oligodendroglia by origin. These degenerated oligodendroglial cells were only found in the slightly spongy areas of the white matter, where the myelin sheaths and axons were spared and only few macrophages had infiltrated. The demyelination may be caused by the death of oligodendroglia in this subacute form, a mechanism that was suggested from experiments with mice (9).

It is noteworthy that the CNS diseases in rats by JHM virus are apparently influenced by host factors. In mice, regardless of the age of the animals, JHM virus always causes an acute encephalo-myelitis. In weanling rats, however, a subacute encephalomyelitis or a chronic paralysis is observed, suggesting that the host's defense mechanisms play a role in the development of these diseases.

Chronic progressive paralysis in JHM virus infection has so far not been reported. Herndon et al. (6) examined mice without any clinical signs at 16 months after inoculation and reported that small foci of active myelin degeneration were found by electron microscopy. In our experiments in rats, hydrocephalus and myelo-malacia were found with corresponding clinical symptoms. No in-flammatory signs were noticed. The most frequent cause of virus-induced hydrocephalus is acute aqueductal stenosis caused by viral ependymitis (5, 7, 14). In our cases no aqueductal stenosis was found. Instead, marked meningeal fibrosis was observed, resembling the picture of hydrocephalus caused by polyoma virus inoculation (10).

Since the meningeal or arachnoid fibrosis is the common cause of hydrocephalus of human infants (4) we suggest that in our cases the thickened meninges gradually obstructed the lateral apertulas of medulla oblongata, resulting in chronic hydrocephalus. Prior to meningeal fibrosis, diffuse meningitis might have been present, which was caused by JHM virus inoculation. Myelomalacia found in our rats represented not necrotic but spongy degenerations, almost confined to gray matter. Marked arachnoid fibrosis was observed. The histology of this myelomalacia, however, is quite different from those found in spinal adhesive arachnoiditis (3, 11, 15), because neither cavitations and slit-like defects nor marginal white matter involvement were observed in our cases. Although the walls of anterior spinal arteries were thickened, the pathology of insufficient arterial blood supply for spinal cord is dissimilar to this myelomalacia.

It must be taken into consideration that cultured L cells used for JHM virus propagation contain endogenous C type virus (13). Andrews and Gardner (1) reported a lower motor neuron degeneration associated with oncorna virus infection in mice. The spongy de-generation of gray matter is similar to our myelomalacia but the predilection for the spinal segment is different; C type virus affects the lumbosacral cord, while myelomalacia was found in the upper cervical cord. Moreover, the cytoplasmic vacuolization in neurons was not observed in the remaining neurons in myelomalacia. The actual cause of myelomalacia in this chronic progressive paral-ysis of rats remains to be discovered.

The neuropathological description of the three diseases associated with JHM virus in the rat suggests the importance of host factors in the development of CNS changes. It is evident that the mechanisms responsible for the three diseases differ from each other. Detailed virological and immunological studies are necessary to unravel the pathogenicity of these diseases. Hopefully, the subacute encephalomyelitis and the chronic paralysis will provide an animal model to understand CNS changes induced by persistent viral infections.

REFERENCES

1. Andrews, J.M. and Gardner, M.B., Lower motor neuron degeneration associated with type C, RNA virus infection in mice: neuro-pathological features, J. Neuropath. Exp. Neurol. 33 (1974) 285-307.

2. Bailey, O.T., Pappenheimer, A.M., Cheever, F.S. and Daniels, J.B., A murine virus (JHM) causing disseminated encephalomyelitis with extensive destruction of myelin. II. Pathology, J. Exp. Med. 90 (1949) 195-212.

3. Dohrmann, G.J., Cervical spinal cord in experimental hydrocephalus, J. Neurosurg. 37 (1972) 538-542.

4. Fried, R.L., Hydrocephalus - Special Pathology. Developmental Neuropathology, Springer, Wien (1975) pp. 214-229.

5. Friedman, H.M., Gilden, D.H., Lief, F.S., Rorke, L.B., Santoli, D. and Koprowski, H., Hydrocephalus produced by the 6/94 virus: A parainfluenza type I isolated from multiple sclerosis brain tissue, Arch. Neurol. 32 (1975) 408-413.

6. Herndon, R.M., Griffin, D.E., McCormick, U. and Weiner, L.P., Mouse hepatitis virus-induced recurrent demyelination. A preliminary report, Arch. Neurol. 32 (1975) 32-35.

7. Johnson, R.T., Johnson, K.P. and Edmonds, J.C., Virus induced hydrocephalus: Development of aqueductal stenosis in hamsters after mumps infection, Science 157 (1967) 1066-1067.

8. Kersting, G. and Pette, E., Zur Pathohistologie und Pathogenese der experimentellen JHM-Virus Encephalomyelitis des Affen, Dtsch. Z. Nervenheilk. 174 (1956) 238-304.

9. Lampert, P.W., Sims, J.K. and Kinazeff, A.J., Mechanism of demyelination in JHM virus encephalomyelitis. Electron microscopic studies, Acta neuropath. (Berl.) 24 (1973) 76-85.

10. Li, C.P. and Jahnes, W.G., Hydrocephalus in suckling mice inoculated with SE polyoma virus, Virology 9 (1959) 489-492.

11. McLaurin, R.L., Bailey, O.T., Schurr, P.H. and Ingraham, F.D., Myelomalacia and multiple cavitations of spinal cord secondary to adhesive arachnoiditis. An experimental study, Arch. Pathol. 57 (1954) 138-146.

12. Nagashima, K., Wege, H. and ter Meulen, V., Corona virus induced subacute demyelinating encephalomyelitis in rats, in preparation.

13. Nagashima, K., Wege, H. and ter Meulen, V., Corona virus in cultured cell: ultrastructural and immunofluorescent studies on L-cell infected with JHM strain, in preparation.

14. Nielsen, S.L. and Baringer, J.R., Reovirus induced aqueductal stenosis in hamsters. Phase contrast and electron microscopic studies, Lab. Invest. 27 (1972) 531-537.

15. Solov'ev, V.N., Changes in the spinal cord in so-called spinal ossifying arachnoiditis, Arkh. Pathol. 35 (1973) 48-54.

16. Waksman, B.H. and Adams, R.D., Infectious leukoencephalitis. A critical comparison of certain experimental and naturally occurring viral leukoencephalitides with experimental allergic encephalomyelitis, J. Neuropath. Exp. Neurol. 21 (1962) 491-518.

17. Weiner, L.P., Pathogenesis of demyelination induced by a mouse hepatitis virus (JHM virus), Arch. Neurol. 28 (1973) 298-303.

A SEARCH FOR THE "MULTIPLE SCLEROSIS VIRUS" - LACK OF EFFECT OF BRAIN EXTRACTS ON MYELIN DEVELOPMENT IN CHICKENS, MICE AND RATS

N.R. Sims, C.C.A. Bernard[*][1], L. Horvath, I.R. Mackay[*]
and P.R. Carnegie
Russell Grimwade School of Biochemistry, University of
Melbourne, and [*]Walter and Eliza Hall Institute of
Medical Research
Parkville, Vic. 3052, Australia

SUMMARY

Attempts were made to transmit possible infectious agents from tissue of MS patients into three animal species, under conditions designed to enhance the development of such an agent. Myelination was monitored by measuring CNPase activity and myelin basic protein. Although no significant effects were observed, the usefulness of a new assay for CNPase was demonstrated. Nude mice were found to have a lower level of CNPase than their heterozygous littermates.

INTRODUCTION

The use of 2',3'-cyclic 3'-phosphodiesterase (CNPase) as a marker of myelination has been widely adopted (22). This enzyme is of particular value in the study of diseases and other conditions affecting myelin as it allows a simple and quantitative comparison of samples. A decrease in CNPase levels has been demonstrated in several conditions including neonatal undernutrition (17), subacute sclerosing panencephalitis (18), some cases of multiple sclerosis (18) and Schilder's disease (7). The recently developed precipitation assay for CNPase is particularly suitable for routine application (22). A study was undertaken to determine if the development of myelin could be influenced by the injection of tissue extracts from MS patients into chickens, mice and rats.

---

[1]Present address: Roche Institute for Immunology, Basel, Switzerland.

Transmissible agents in multiple sclerosis. Various theories
have been proposed for MS involving transmissible agents as causative factors. The evidence that a transmissible agent may be involved in the disease is indirect and definitive demonstration of
such an agent is lacking. However, there have been occasional reports in which direct evidence for a transmissible agent was claimed
(for reviews, see 4, 14).

In 1972, Carp and coworkers (2) reported that injection of mice
with serum, cerebrospinal fluid, spleen and brain material from patients with multiple sclerosis (MS) produced a depression in the
polymorphonuclear (PMN) leucocyte levels in blood. A similar effect
was also reported for mice injected with material from animals with
scrapie (12). Initial attempts to reproduce these studies were
not successful (1, 15). The technique for repetitive PMN leucocyte
determination has been shown to be difficult to standardize, and
results are dependent upon the mouse strain used and a number of
other characteristics (19). The findings of Carp's group on PMN
leucocyte depression in mice was recently confirmed (6) and extended (5); again the difficulty in standardizing PMN leucocyte
levels was recorded. The PMN leucocyte depression was observed in
other rodents and the effect could be removed by centrifugation of
brain homogenates for 1 h at 105,000 g, but not at 50,000 g.

In previous attempts on transmission of infectious agents from
MS material, scant attention was paid to the age of the animals
used. Two periods in development stand out as being of particular
interest. The first is the period just prior to and during rapid
myelination when the myelin is particularly susceptible to changes
from the normal situation, e. g. loss of CNPase and other myelin
components which occurs in neonatal protein deficiency, hypothyroidism, zinc and copper deficiencies (for references see review, 23). Introduction of an agent at this stage, capable of
affecting either the oligodendroglial cell or myelin itself could
produce marked changes. A further advantage of examining myelin
during this period is that injections are able to be performed at
times when immune defence mechanisms and the blood-brain barrier
are incompletely developed (8), and the chances are maximal for infectious material reaching the brain. The second period of interest for studying infection is from the end of rapid myelination to
early adult life. This is analogous to the situation proposed for
MS, for which migration studies suggest that the trigger (be it infection or other environmental factor) occurs in the mid-teens
whilst the symptoms commonly first appear 10 or more years later.
Thus, we attempted to influence myelination by injection of MS
material into experimental animals at these two periods of particular interest.

Animals chosen were chickens, with injections being made into
the allantoic fluid of embryos, and rats and mice, both being injected intraperitoneally. The mice selected for examination were
homozygote and heterozygote carriers of the nude allele (nu/nu and
nu/+ respectively). Animals which are homozygous for this allele
are hypothymic, whereas heterozygotes are phenotypically normal,

although there is some debate as to whether these animals behave
as normal mice under all conditions (2). The hypothymic condition
in nude mice results in a lack of T-cell mediated immunity and
these animals are far more susceptible to disease. However, it
should be pointed out that if a disease were dependent upon the
involvement of the animals' immune system, as has been demonstrated
for Theiler's virus (13), these animals would in fact be less susceptible.

EXPERIMENTAL

Preparation of Brain Homogenates

Extracts for injection were prepared by the procedure used by
Carp (2) and Koldovsky et al. (6). MS material was obtained from
a male patient (aged 42 years) who had the disease for 18 years
prior to death from cerebral haemorrhage. Cerebral cortex was obtained within 8 h of death and stored at-70°C until required.
Cerebral cortex from a 70-year-old male who died from myocardial
infarction was similarly stored and used as control material.
Material (10 g) from these brains was homogenized on ice for 4 min
in 40 ml cold sterile phosphate-buffered-saline (PBS) in a Sorvall
omni-mixer and transferred to sterile bottles for centrifugation
at 10,000 g for 1 h. The resultant supernatant was divided into
small aliquots and stored at -70°C until required for injection.

Treatment of Animals

Chickens. Eggs from White Leghorn-Austrolope hens (Research
Poultry Farm, Research, Victoria) were obtained one day after
laying and maintained at 38°C in an incubator. At day 9, eggs
were numbered and treatments randomized amongst the eggs. Injection
was made into allantoic fluid with 0.1 ml of MS brain or control
brain homogenate, injection holes were covered with adhesive tape
and eggs returned to the incubator. At 2 days prior to normal
hatching eggs were separated according to treatment into containers
so that identification after hatching was possible, and positions
of the containers in the incubator were rotated every 12 h until
hatching was complete. Embryos or chickens were killed at days 17,
19, 21 (hatching) and 23 (2 days post hatching) and brains removed
into liquid nitrogen rapidly (less than 2 min for embryos, less
than one min for chickens) and stored at -70°C until homogenized
and examined.

Mice. Inbred mice of the strain BALB/c Wehi nu [18] (from the
specific pathogen-free facility, Walter and Eliza Hall Institute,
Parkville, Victoria) which were either heterozygous (nu/+) or
homozygous (nu/nu) for the nude allele were used in all studies.

All litters were distributed immediately after birth for care by
foster mothers. Homogenate (0.1 ml) was injected intraperitoneally
within 6 h of birth and animals killed with ether between days 18
and 30. Brains were rapidly removed into liquid nitrogen and stored
at -70°C until tested. In one experiment animals were injected at
day 30 and killed at day 70. In all experiments body weights of
mice were recorded at 5 day intervals.

Rats. Neonatal buffalo rats (bred in the School of Biochemistry, University of Melbourne, Parkville, Victoria) were retained
with their natural mothers. Half the litter received MS-derived
material and the remainder control material; injections (0.1 ml)
were made intraperitoneally within 6 h of birth. In two litters
brain homogenates (MS and normal) were injected, whilst in the
other five litters serum samples from different MS and control patients were used. Body weights of all animals were recorded at five
day intervals. A few animals died or were killed by their mothers
within two days of birth. All other animals survived to day 26
when they were killed with ether and brains removed to liquid nitrogen within one min of death.

Treatment and Analysis of Animal Brains

In all cases whole brains were removed from cold storage,
allowed to thaw at room temperature, and homogenized on ice in 4
ml of cold (4°C) 0.2 M Tris-HCl (pH 7.3) for three min in a Sorvall
omni-mixer with a micro-attachment. Homogenates were left for one
min to allow froth to settle and a 2 ml sample removed and added
to 2 ml of cold (4°C) 5% Triton X-100 in 0.1 M imidazole-HCl (pH
6.2) and mixed by inversion. Further dilutions in water were performed prior to assay of CNPase (22) and protein in triplicate (11).
One unit of CNPase activity equals 1 μmole 2',3'-cyclic AMP hydrolysed per min at 37°C. Myelin basic protein in the chicken and
mouse brain homogenates was assayed by a radioimmunoassay (3)
using antibody to human myelin basic protein prepared in a sheep.
This batch of antibody appeared to react with the sequence Ser-Arg-
Phe-Ser-Trp-Gly in myelin basic protein (Carnegie and Horvath, unpublished). Statistical analysis was by "Students" t-test where
comparison of two groups was involved, and by parametric analysis
of variance techniques where more than two groups were compared.

RESULTS

Chickens. Figure 1 shows the appearance of CNPase between days
16 and 23 in animals treated with MS and control material. This is
the pooled result of two experiments, the first between days 16 and
21 in which PBS injection was used as control, and the second for
days 21 to 23 in which both normal brain and PBS were used. There
was no difference between these two control groups and results are

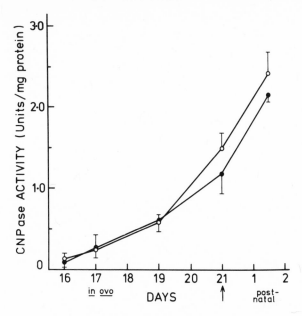

Fig. 1. Development of CNPase activity in chickens injected with MS brain homogenates (●) and control material (0). Error bars show standard deviations; 3 to 6 chickens per point.

represented for convenience as only a single control point. There was no significant difference (p > 0.05) between MS and control-injected animals at any age.

The increase in myelin basic protein paralleled that for CNPase in the development of the chicken brain. There was no significant difference between the embryos injected with MS and normal brain extracts.

Mice. In a trial experiment nu/nu and nu/+ animals were injected at day 0 with MS material or PBS (as control) and all animals killed on day 26. Treatments were distributed so that only one treatment type was given within a litter which contained both nu/nu mice and heterozygous littermates (nu/+) (Table 1). For neither the nu/nu nor nu/+ mice were there significant differences although the difference between the two groups for the nu/+ animals approached significance (0.05 < p < 0.1). For this reason, study of these nu/+ animals was extended further and treatments randomized between animals within litters so that any effect induced by differences between the litters was removed. PBS was used as control for all days and normal brain homogenates were also injected as controls for animals killed on days 18 and 26. Results are presented in Table 2 and as is readily apparent there was no difference at any of the ages studied.

Table 1.   Specific activity of CNPase in brains of 26-day old mice following injection of MS brain and control material within 6 h of birth.

Group	Material injected	Number of animals	CNPase specific activity [+]
nu/nu	MS brain PBS	5 4	1.3±0.29 1.2±0.27
nu/+	MS brain PBS	5 5	1.4+0.18 1.8±0.07

[+]Units/mg protein (± SD).

Table 2.   Specific activity of CNPase in developing nu/+ mouse brain following injection of MS brain and control material within 6 h of birth.

Age (days)	Material injected	Number of animals	CNPase specific activity [+]
18	MS brain PBS Control brain	9 8 5	1.4±0.17 1.4±0.13 1.4±0.12
22	MS brain PBS	4 3	1.7±0.22 1.7±0.20
26	MS brain PBS Control brain	10 7 5	1.7±0.12 1.7±0.16 1.6±0.10
30	MS brain PBS	3 3	1.9+0.12 2.0±0.09

[+]Units/mg protein (± SD).

A further group of mice (nu/nu and nu/+) were injected with MS and control material (PBS and normal brain) at day 30 and caged in treatment groups until day 70. By this age one of the nu/nu mice injected with MS material had died and several appeared very weak and emaciated. The body weights for this group were significantly lower than for the control groups ($0.025 > p > 0.01$) but there was no significant difference in brain weight. There was no difference ($p > 0.05$) in the CNPase levels between all three of the groups (Table 3). Histological examination revealed the presence of inclusions in samples from several tissues taken from the sick animals but the nature of these inclusions could not be established. The experiment was repeated with a new group of animals but treatments were randomized within cages and all animals were maintained under strictly sterile conditions. No disease was observed in any of the animals although these were retained until 120 days of age. It seems that the illness observed in the original experiment was the result of accidental infection of the vulnerable nu/nu mice and not due to the treatment given. Similar symptoms have been previously observed among infected nude mice (20).

From the data, a significant difference was observed between the nude mice and littermates in CNPase levels at both day 26 ($0.02 > p > 0.01$) and day 70 ($p < 0.01$), a difference which had not previously been reported. Brain weights of the nude mice were also significantly lower than those of the littermates at these two days ($0.02 > p > 0.01$, day 26; $p < 0.01$, day 70).

A selection of homogenates from different groups of mice were assayed for myelin basic protein. No significant difference was

Table 3. Specific activity of CNPase in brains of 70-day old mice following injection of MS brain and control material at day 30.

Group	Material injected	Number of animals	CNPase specific activity[+]
nu/nu	MS brain	5	2.6+0.23
	PBS	5	2.5+0.15
	Normal brain	5	2.3+0.25
nu/+	MS brain	5	3.0+0.17
	PBS	5	3.0+0.01
	Normal brain	5	2.8+0.25

[+] Units/mg protein (+ SD).

Table 4. Specific activity of CNPase in brains of 26-day-old rats following injection within six hours of birth of MS or control sera, or MS or control brain homogenates.

Litter No.	Material injected Tissue		Source	No. of animals	CNPase specific activity+
	Serum				
1		A	MS exacerbation	5	2.3+0.20
		B	CVA	4	2.0+0.24
2		C	MS exacerbation	4	2.0+0.24
		D	CVA	4	1.9+0.22
3		E	MS remission	2	1.7
		F	CVA	3	1.6+0.25
4		G	MS remission	5	2.2+0.33
		H	Pituitary tumour	3	2.2+0.28
5		I	MS exacerbation	3	1.9+0.37
		J	Cerebral haematoma	1	2.0
6 & 7	Brain Homogenate	X	MS	6	2.2+0.17
		Y	Normal	7	2.0+0.22

+Units/mg protein (+ SD).

found between the control and MS groups. Because of the need for
extensive dilution of the particulate material in the homogenates,
radioimmunoassay of myelin basic protein was found to be less reliable than CNPase as measure of myelin content.

Rats. Despite the use of sera from five different MS patients
at various stages of the disease, and treatment with MS and control
brain homogenates, no differences were observed between the test
and control groups within a litter (Table 4). There was no difference in body weights for the groups and no other evidence of
disease in any animal.

When the CNPase levels were compared between the seven litters,
without taking account of the treatments given, significant differences (p <0.01) were observed.

DISCUSSION

Despite the use of three animal species and conditions conducive
to the development of infectious agents, no evidence of changes in
myelination or of observable disease was found after injection of
MS tissue. That this and other attempts to produce transmission
have been unsuccessful in inducing pathological changes in animals
does not necessarily negate hypotheses proposed for transmissible
agents producing MS. For instance, the agent may be highly host
specific, only producing observable changes in humans.

A criticism possible with the study presented here is that
only one MS brain and five MS serum samples were tested for effects
on myelination. Whilst it would perhaps have been desirable to
examine other brains, positive effects were claimed for all brain
homogenates tested in the studies of the Carp and Henle groups
(2, 5, 6). The brains in their studies were stored and treated by
methods very similar to those used in this work. Furthermore,
positive results were obtained in the PMN depression test with 73%
of serum from patients in active disease and 31% of those in remission (6). It would seem unlikely therefore that the "agent"
responsible for PMN depression was not present in at least some of
the samples tested here.

Since the experiments reported here were performed, some dis-
turbing results have appeared in relation to the "Carp-Henle agent",
in that several groups have been unable to confirm the original
findings (16, 21, Clausen et al., personal communication) or
results have been equivocal (Mackay and Bernard, unpublished).

The new assay for CNPase provided accurate and reproducible
data and no difficulties were experienced in handling the large
numbers of samples examined. The time course obtained for the
chicken shows a pattern of increase between days 16 and 23 similar
to that reported by Kurihara and Tsukada (10), although the
absolute values obtained in this study are somewhat higher,
probably because Triton X-100 rather than sonication was used to
activate CNPase.

The CNPase levels obtained for the mice samples at day 70 (2.9 units/mg protein) compared favourably with those previously reported (9).

For the rat samples it was observed that at day 26 there was a highly significant difference between the average CNPase levels in the different litters. It seems that these differences may arise from variations in the nursing abilities of the mothers. It has been demonstrated that nutritional deprivation affected subsequent myelination, and CNPase was reduced by 44% in rats at 22 days of age (17). Whatever the cause of these differences, it would be necessary to ensure that they would not influence results in studies where changes were being sought during myelination. It is likely that such variation between litters was responsible for the small differences for the groups at day 26 in the initial mouse experiment. In subsequent experiments where treatments were randomised within litters no differences were seen.

A significant difference was also observed between CNPase levels of nude mice and heterozygous littermates at both 26 and 70 days. These results are worthy of further investigation as they may be a direct consequence of the thymus deficiency in these animals.

In the design of subsequent experiments it would be essential to maintain both the nude mice and littermates in a pathogen-free environment.

Acknowledgements. We thank the National Multiple Sclerosis Society New York (Grant Nos. RG 1022-A-7, 887-B-3), Australian Research Grants Committee and the National Health and Medical Research Council for financial support. C.C.A.B. was supported by the Canadian Multiple Sclerosis Society. Ms. G. Jackson and Ms. J. Leydon are thanked for technical assistance.

REFERENCES

1. Brown, P. and Gajdusek, D.C., No mouse PMN leukocyte depression after inoculation with brain tissue from multiple sclerosis or spongiform encephalopathies, Nature 247 (1974) 217-218.
2. Carp, R.I., Licursi, P.C., Merz, P.A. and Merz, G.S., Decreased percentage of polymorphonuclear neutrophils in mouse peripheral blood after inoculation with material from multiple sclerosis patients, J. Exp. Med. 136 (1972) 618-629.
3. Cohen, S.R., McKhann, G.M. and Guarnieri, M., A radioimmuno-assay for myelin basic protein and its use for quantitative measurements, J. Neurochem. 25 (1975) 371-376.
4. Fraser, K.B., Multiple sclerosis: a virus disease? Br. Med. Bull. 33 (1977) 34-39.
5. Henle, G.,Koldovsky, U., Henle, W., Ackermann, R. and Haase, G., Multiple sclerosis-associated agent: neutralization of the agent by human sera, Inf. Imm. 12 (1975) 1367-1374.

6. Koldovsky, U., Koldovsky, P., Henle, G., Henle, W., Ackermann, R. and Haase, G., Multiple sclerosis-associated agent: transmission to animals and some properties of the agent, Inf. Imm. 12 (1975) 1355-1366.

7. Komiya, Y. and Kasahara, M., 2',3'-cyclic nucleotide 3'-phosphohydrolase activity in myelin fractions from one patient with Schilder´s disease, J. Biochem. 70 (1971) 371-374.

8. Kristensson, K., Olsson, Y. and Sourander, P., Virus encephalitis: pathogenesis in the immature brain, Develop. Med. Child Neurol. 16 (1974) 382-394.

9. Kurihara, T., Nussbaum, J.L. and Mandel, P., 2',3'-cyclic nucleotide 3'-phosphohydrolase in brains of mutant mice with deficient myelination, J. Neurochem. 17 (1970) 993-997.

10. Kurihara, T. and Tsukada, Y., 2',3'-cyclic nucleotide 3'-phosphohydrolase in the developing chick brain and spinal cord, J. Neurochem. 15 (1968) 827-832.

11. Lees, M.B. and Paxman, S., Modification of the Lowry procedure for the analysis of proteolipid protein, Analyt. Biochem. 47 (1972) 184-192.

12. Licursi, P.C., Merz, P.A., Merz, G.S. and Carp, R.I., Scrapie-induced changes in the percentage of polymorphonuclear neutrophils in mouse peripheral blood, Inf. Imm. 6 (1972) 370-376.

13. Lipton, H.L. and Dal Canto, M.C., Theiler´s virus-induced demyelination: prevention by immunosuppression, Science 192 (1976) 62-64.

14. Lumsden, C.E., The clinical pathology of multiple sclerosis, in Multiple Sclerosis, a Reappraisal (D. McAlpine, C.E. Lumsden and E.D. Acheson, eds.) Churchill, Livingstone, Edinburgh (1972) pp. 311-621.

15. McNeill, T.A., Killen, M. and Trudgett, A., Mouse granulocyte precursors and multiple sclerosis, Nature 249 (1974) 778.

16. Madden, D.L., Kreslewicz, A., Gravell, M. and Sever, J.L., Multiple sclerosis associated agent: failure to confirm an association, Neurology 27 (1977) 371.

17. Nakhasi, H.L., Toews, A.D. and Horrocks, L.A., Effects of a postnatal protein deficiency on the content and composition of myelin from brains of weanling rats, Brain Res. 83 (1975) 176-179.

18. Riekkinen, P.J., Rinne, U.K., Arstila, A.U., Kurihara, T. and Pelliniemi, T.T., Studies on the pathogenesis of multiple sclerosis: 2',3'-cyclic nucleotide 3'-phosphohydrolase as marker of demyelination and correlation of findings with lysosomal changes, J. Neurol. Sci. 15 (1972) 113-120.

19. Russell, E.S., Neufeld, E.F. and Higgins, C.T., Comparison of normal blood picture of young adults from 18 inbred strains of mice, Proc. Soc. Exp. Biol. Med. 78 (1951) 761-766.

20. Rygaard, J., Thymus and self, Immunobiology of the mouse mutant nude (1973) F.A.D.L. Copenhagen.

21. Sever, J.L., Fuccillo, D.A., Madden, D.L. and Castellano, G.A.,
     Multiple sclerosis: attempts to demonstrate altered immune
     responses and viruses, Neurology 26 (6, part 2) (1976) 72-74.
22. Sims, N.R. and Carnegie, P.R., A rapid assay for 2',3'-cyclic
     nucleotide 3'-phosphohydrolase, J.Neurochem. 27 (1976) 769-
     772.
23. Sims, N.R. and Carnegie, P.R., 2',3'-cyclic nucleotide 3'-
     phosphodiesterase, Advances in Neurochem. 3 (1977) in press.

PLASMALOGENASE IS ELEVATED IN EARLY DEMYELINATING LESIONS

Lloyd A. Horrocks[1], Sheila Spanner[2], Rita Mozzi[1,5];
Sheung Chun Fu[1], Robert A. D'Amato[3] and
Steven Krakowka[4]

[1]Department of Physiological Chemistry, 1645 Neil Ave.,
The Ohio State University, Columbus, Ohio 43210, U.S.A.
[2]Department of Pharmacology (Pre-Clinical), University
of Birmingham, Birmingham, U.K.
[3]Department of Pathology, The Ohio State University
[4]Department of Veterinary Pathobiology, The Ohio State
University, U.S.A.
[5]Permanent address: Istituto di Chimica Biologica,
Universita di Perugia, 06100, Perugia, Italy

SUMMARY

Plasmalogenase catalyzes the hydrolysis of ethanolamine plasmalogens to long-chain aldehydes and 2-acyl-$\underline{sn}$-glycero-3-phospho-
ethanolamines. During development, plasmalogenase activity parallels myelination. The enzyme is most concentrated within oligodendroglial cells and is absent from myelin. The normal function
of plasmalogenase in white matter may be related to its specificity
for plasmalogens that contain most of the thromboxane and prostaglandin precursors.

Plasmalogenase activities are elevated in demyelinating CNS
tissues including canine white matter with lesions due to distemper
virus. Elevated plasmalogenase activity precedes cellular invasion
and lysosomal activation as indicated by β-glucuronidase, acid
proteinase and neutral proteinase activities. The elevation of
plasmalogenase activity was 4.9-fold greater than normal in an
early demyelinating lesion caused by the Snyder-Hill strain of distemper virus. Phospholipases acting on phosphatidyl ethanolamine
were not activated in this tissue and have activities much lower
than plasmalogenase in control tissues. Plasmalogenase activities
are also elevated after intracerebral injections of complement-
dependent anti-myelin antibody and after ischemia. Plasmalogenase

acting on the oligodendrocyte plasma membrane may be responsible
for necrosis of the oligodendrocyte that results in demyelination.

INTRODUCTION

In white matter and myelin, the most prevalent phospholipid
type is ethanolamine plasmalogen which accounts for one-third of
the phospholipids (15, 16). In many studies of demyelination, the
first change in myelin lipid composition is a loss of ethanolamine
plasmalogens and the earliest enzyme change that has been detected
is an increase in plasmalogenase activity. Ansell and Spanner (1)
discovered this enzyme which is capable of cleaving the alk-1-enyl-
ether moiety of ethanolamine plasmalogens. The reaction catalyzed
by plasmalogenase, 1-alk-1'-enyl-2-acyl-sn-glycero-3-phospho-
ethanolamine alk-1'-enylhydrolase, EC 3.3.3-., produces long-chain
aldehydes and lysophosphatidyl ethanolamines. Choline plasmalogens
are also good substrates and diacyl forms of choline and ethanolamine phosphoglycerides are competitive inhibitors (7). Plasmalogenase has been purified more than 300-fold (17). It is probably
a small protein because it is soluble in saturated ammonium sulfate
solutions, is present in particulate fractions of rat brain (3),
and is destroyed by heating for 10 min at $60-70^{\circ}C$.

Plasmalogenase increases markedly in activity during development (Table 1). About one-third of the adult concentration of
plasmalogenase is present at 8 days of age (2) and 63% is present
at 15 days of age in the rat brain. Plasmalogenase levels in mouse
brain increase similarly (9). Increases of plasmalogenase activity
seem to precede increases in plasmalogen content during myelination.

White matter has much more plasmalogenase activity than gray
matter (3). Within white matter, plasmalogenase is absent from
purified myelin preparations but is very active in preparations of
oligodendroglial cell bodies (8). The activity in oligodendroglia

Table 1. Plasmalogenase activities, expressed as μmol (g tissue)$^{-1}$
(h)$^{-1}$, in rat brain during development (29). Plasmalogenase activities were assayed by the method of Ansell and Spanner (1).

Age (days)	Activity
5	not detected
8	0.91
10	0.84
15	1.53
20	2.29
27	2.38
34	2.64

is 10-fold greater than in neuronal perikarya and 6-fold greater than in the astroglia (8). The coincidence of increases of plasmalogenase activity with myelination is also consistent with a primary localization of plasmalogenase in oligodendroglia. Metabolic activities of oligodendroglia are deficient in brains of jimpy mice (23). At 25 days of age, jimpy brains contain only 43% of the plasmalogenase activity observed in control brains (9).

Plasmalogenase must be involved in the turnover of ethanolamine plasmalogens. Even in the myelin sheath, plasmalogens and other phosphoglycerides have a substantial rate of turnover (16, 19, 28). A relatively high level of plasmalogenase in oligodendroglia must be required for catabolism of the large amounts of plasmalogens in the myelin. Most of the prostaglandin precursors, arachidonate (20:4) and adrenate (22:4), in white matter are in the ethanolamine plasmalogens. We have proposed (17) that plasmalogenase also has the function of initiating the release of prostaglandin precursors by way of lysophosphatidyl ethanolamine and a lysophospholipase (7).

Plasmalogenase may be located on the cytoplasmic side of the plasma membrane together with the ethanolamine plasmalogens. The enzyme is not present in the cytosol or in lysosomes, but 60% is in the crude mitochondrial fraction with the remainder in microsomes (3). This distribution together with plasmalogenase activation by antigen-antibody reactions suggests a plasma membrane localization. The requirement for Mg^{2+} and the lack of activity with Ca^{2+} suggest that plasmalogenase is not an ecto enzyme.

A lipolytic agent which destroys myelin was proposed as part of the pathogenesis of demyelination in the early part of this century (24). Phospholipase A catalyzed production of lysolecithin has been a popular hypothesis (31). Phospholipase A_2 and lysolecithin cause demyelination when injected into peripheral nerve or spinal cord (13, 14). However, all measurements of phospholipase A activity in demyelinating lesions have shown rather small elevations during the early stages of demyelination (34, 35, 37). Often, the only change in myelin composition detected before demyelination is a decrease in the proportion of ethanolamine plasmalogens (18, 30, 38).

EXPERIMENTAL

Plasmalogenase assays may be done by several methods as reviewed recently (17). In these investigations we have extracted all phospholipases from acetone-dried powders (1). Unless specified otherwise, plasmalogenase activities were assayed by measuring the loss of plasmalogens at several time points during the course of incubation (7). Phosphatidyl ethanolamines containing [^{14}C]palmitoyl groups at the 1-position or [^{14}C]linoleoyl groups at the 2-position were prepared (36). Phospholipases were assayed in dispersions

(32, 36) and in extracts from acetone-dried powders (6). Lysophosphatidyl ethanolamine for the assay of lysophospholipase was
prepared from phosphatidyl ethanolamine with [^{14}C]palmitoyl groups
at the 1-position by treatment with snake venom phospholipase A$_2$.
The release of radioactive fatty acid was taken as a measure of
the phospholipase activity. Other experimental methods are summarized in the text.

RESULTS AND DISCUSSION

<u>Plasmalogens in white matter injury</u>. Rapid changes in myelin
take place after ischemia. In the rat with unilateral vascular
occlusion and anoxia, at one hour the stainability of myelin is
reduced. At three hours, autolytic changes are found in oligodendroglia and swelling of myelin is seen after four hours (5). In
the gerbil brain with ligation of both carotid arteries, plasmalogenase activity reaches 235% of control values at 20 minutes
(Fig. 1). No differences from controls are found for β- glucuronidase, acid proteinase and neutral proteinase at one hour after
arterial ligation (26). Thus only plasmalogenase is elevated prior

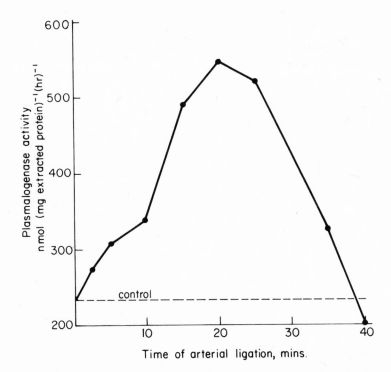

Fig. 1. Plasmalogenase activity in whole brains of gerbils after
bilateral ligation of carotid arteries. Plasmalogenase activities
were assayed with extracts from acetone-dried powders (7).

to the time that irreversible injury takes place in ischemic brain.
Plasmalogenase activities correlate very well with the development
of edema (33).

Plasmalogenase activities were assayed in two white matter
samples obtained at autopsy from a subject with multiple sclerosis
(3). On a fresh weight basis, the activity in these samples was
twice that in normal white matter (Table 2). Plasmalogenase activities were also markedly elevated in spinal cord tissue from monkeys
that had demyelination due to vitamin B_{12} deficiency (3).

Table 2. Plasmalogenase activities, expressed as μmol $(g \ tissue)^{-1}$
$(h)^{-1}$, in normal and demyelinating human white matter. The results
for multiple sclerosis and the assay method are from Ansell and
Spanner (3). Results are given as means $\pm$ SD.

	Activity
Normal, corpus callosum	0.90
Normal, frontal lobe	0.85-0.90
Multiple sclerosis, corpus callosum	1.90
Multiple sclerosis, frontal lobe	1.81
Alzheimer's disease, frontal lobe	1.92$\pm$0.26 (5)

Biopsy samples were obtained from frontal lobe white matter of
five patients with Alzheimer's disease. These tissues also had
twice as much plasmalogenase activity as was found in the control
white matter (Table 2). White matter from Alzheimer's disease had
38% lower plasmalogen concentration than was found in normal tissues
(Table 3). Presumably, the lower plasmalogen concentration in
white matter from Alzheimer's disease is due to the increased
activity of plasmalogenase. Plasmalogen concentrations were not
decreased in white matter from subjects with senile dementia or
cerebral atrophy without Alzheimer's disease. The pathogenesis of
Alzheimer's disease is not yet established but the demyelination
that may be mediated by plasmalogenase should be involved in the
dementia by disruption of neuronal connections.

Table 3. Plasmalogen concentrations, expressed as μmol $(g \ tissue)^{-1}$,
in human frontal lobe white matter. Assays (11) are reported as
means $\pm$ SD.

	Plasmalogen
Normal	28
Alzheimer's disease	17.3$\pm$4.2 (6)
Senile dementia	31.9, 29.5 (2)
Cerebral atrophy	26.0

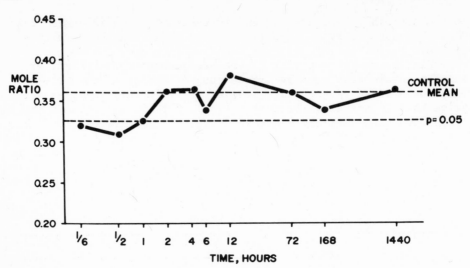

Fig. 2.   The mole ratio of ethanolamine plasmalogens to total
phospholipids in myelin isolated from spinal cords of monkeys at
various times after trauma (18).

Table 4.   Plasmalogenase activities, expressed as μmol (g tissue)$^{-1}$
(h)$^{-1}$, in control and scrapie-infected mouse brains. Plasmalogenase
was assayed (3) four months after inoculation when the mice displayed distinct signs of scrapie. Values are means $\pm$ SD (number
of female mice).

	Activity	
Normal whole brain	1.06$\pm$0.05	(6)
Scrapie-infected whole brain	0.80$\pm$0.07	(6)

        The loss of myelin frequently observed after injury of the
spinal cord may also be mediated by plasmalogenase (18). Experimental spinal cord injury was caused by dropping a weight onto the
exposed cord of rhesus monkeys. The quantity of myelin that was
isolated from the crude mitochondrial plus nuclear fraction was
half of the control value at two hours after trauma. The only
abnormality in chemical composition of the isolated myelin fractions
was a significant decrease in the proportion of plasmalogens before
the decrease in quantity of isolated myelin (Fig. 2).
        Brain samples from mice infected with scrapie have plasmalogen-
ase activities, brain weights and protein contents that are lower
than control values (Table 4). Perhaps the decreased plasmalogenase
activity reflects a lower content of oligodendroglia in mice with

scrapie.

　　Plasmalogenase in canine distemper. McMartin et al. (27)
assayed plasmalogenase in brain samples from dogs with canine distemper encephalomyelitis and age-matched control dogs (Fig. 3).
Plasmalogenase activity was 67% greater in samples from distemper
dogs than in samples from control dogs. Activities were highest
in samples with the least demyelination and were below the control
value in samples with the most extensive demyelination. The
decrease in plasmalogenase activity during the course of the disease
may be due to the disappearance of the oligodendroglia. Several
other hydrolytic enzymes were also assayed (26). Neutral proteinase,
acid proteinase and β-glucuronidase increased with increasing demyelination as illustrated by the values for β-glucuronidase in
Fig. 3. Thus the increase in plasmalogenase activity preceded
phagocytic activity.

　　Further experiments with demyelination induced by canine distemper virus have been done with dogs infected at a known time.

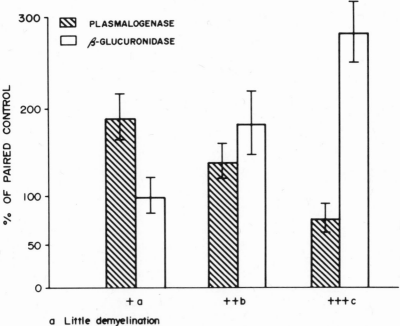

a Little demyelination
b Demyelination covered about 3 to 10% of white matter area
c Demyelination covered about 15 to 25% of white matter area

Fig. 3. Plasmalogenase and β-glucuronidase activities in white
matter from brain of dogs infected with distemper (26, 27).
Activities are given as the percentage of the age-matched control
value, mean ± SEM.

Surgically derived colostrum-deprived gnotobiotic dogs were raised
by the technique of Griesemer and Gibson (12). Intracerebral
inoculation was described by McCullough et al. (25). Two control
dogs received a suspension of normal cerebellum and an experimental
dog received a suspension of cerebellum infected with R252 canine
distemper virus. Five weeks after inoculation, the experimental
dog had an early demyelinating lesion in the white matter surrounding the fourth ventricle. No lesions were found in other white
matter areas. Results of plasmalogenase assays (7) are shown in
Table 5. The plasmalogenase activity in the area with the early
demyelinating lesion was 91% greater than in the same area in the
controls (P < 0.01) and was also 80% higher than the mean of all
control samples (P < 0.001). In the infected canine brain, only
the area with the lesion had a significant increase in activity.

Table 5. Plasmalogenase activities, expressed as nmol (mg protein)$^{-1}$
(h)$^{-1}$, in white matter from gnotobiotic dogs. Rest is remaining
white matter. Values are means (number of determinations).

	Activity		
	Control dogs		Inoculated dog (Canine distemper virus)
	1	2	
White matter surrounding 4th ventricle	270 (2)	275 (2)	520 (4)
Optic tract	280 (2)	283 (2)	320 (2)
Corpus callosum	260 (2)	272 (2)	296 (2)
Brain stem	225 (2)	232 (2)	220 (2)
Rest No. 1	275 (2)	280 (2)	294 (2)
Rest No. 2	278 (2)	273 (2)	296 (2)

Since other phospholipases have been implicated in the pathogenesis of demyelination, we carried out another experiment with
measurements of phospholipase A_1 (EC 3.1.1.32) and A_2 (EC 3.1.1.4)
activities at pH 4.3 and 6.8 for comparison with plasmalogenase
activities. Gnotobiotic dogs were vaccinated with the Snyder-Hill
strain of canine distemper virus. Of the four dogs used in this
study one showed no signs of illness and was used as a normal control.
Two dogs had a depressed episode but then recovered. The fourth
dog displayed neurological symptoms of distemper encephalomyelitis
before it was killed. White matter samples were taken from the
area of the fourth ventricle.

Phospholipase A_1 and A_2 activities in dispersions were somewhat
lower for the dog with distemper than for the normal dog (Fig. 4).
Generally, the activities found in dispersions of tissue from the
recovered dogs were intermediate between the normal and distemper

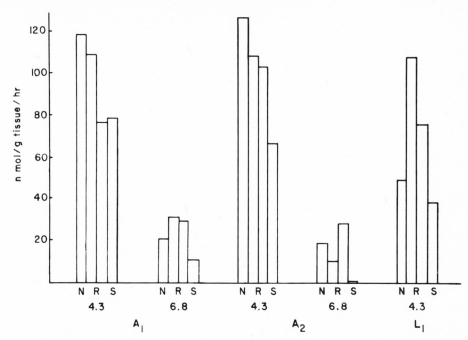

Fig. 4. Phospholipase activities in dispersions of white matter
from brains of dogs challenged with Snyder-Hill canine distemper
virus. Phospholipases A_1, A_2, and lysophospholipase L_1, were
assayed at the indicated pH values. One dog was normal (N), two
dogs recovered (R) and one dog was sick with distemper (S).

tissue. Lysophospholipase activities were highest in the tissues
from recovered dogs. If lysophosphoglycerides are damaging to
cells, the higher lysophospholipase activities in tissues from recovered dogs may have aided in the recovery. Since endogenous
substrates are present in tissue dispersions, extracts from acetone-
dried powders were also assayed (Fig. 5). Sufficient tissue was
available from only the normal and distemper dogs. The values for
phospholipase A_1 and A_2 activities were comparable for the two
procedures and again no marked elevations of phospholipase activities were found in the tissue from the dog with distemper. No
phospholipase A_1 activity was found in the extract from the normal
tissue and the value for the distemper tissue was only 25 nmol
$(g\ tissue)^{-1}(h)^{-1}$. Very little lysophospholipase activity was found
in the extracts. The extract from the normal dog did not contain
detectable plasmalogenase activity whilst the extract from the dog
with distemper had an extremely high value for plasmalogenase. This
value was 4.9-fold greater than the plasmalogenase activity found
for controls with no exposure to distemper virus.
        Thus, plasmalogenase activities in the tissue from the two
dogs that were challenged with distemper virus were in parallel with

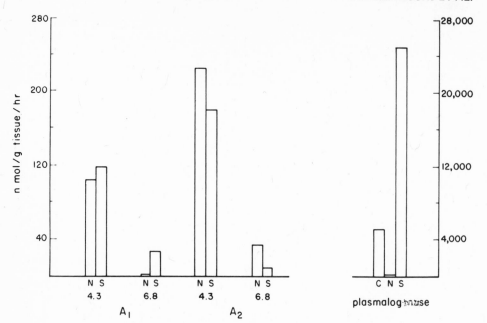

Fig. 5. Phospholipase and plasmalogenase activities in extracts
of acetone-dried powders prepared from white matter of dogs
challenged with Snyder-Hill canine distemper virus. Phospholipases
A_1 and A_2 were assayed at the indicated pH values. The scale for
plasmalogenase activity is 100-fold greater than the scale for the
other phospholipases. Two dogs were unchallenged controls (C),
one was normal (N) and one dog was sick with distemper (S).

the clinical course. The normal dog had a plasmalogenase activity
lower than controls and the sick dog had a plasmalogenase activity
much greater than the controls. All other phospholipase activities
in the tissue from the sick dog were at least two orders of magnitude
lower than the plasmalogenase activity. Therefore we believe that
plasmalogenase is the only phospholipase that is important in the
pathogenesis of demyelinating lesions.

Cerebrospinal fluid samples from other gnotobiotic dogs were
obtained by cisterna magna -puncture and then frozen. Coded
samples were freeze-dried and redissolved in the glycerol-bicarbo-
nate mixture used for extraction of acetone-dried powders. Plasmalogenase and protein were assayed (7). The activity of the plasmalogenase was quite high in the CSF and was significantly higher
($P < 0.05$) in the CSF from distemper dogs than in the CSF from
control dogs (Table 6). There was no significant difference in the
protein content of the CSF, indicating a normal blood-brain barrier
in the infected dogs.

Plasmalogenase and antibodies. The role of the immune response
in the etiology of demyelinating diseases such as canine distemper

Table 6. Plasmalogenase activity, expressed as μmol $(ml\ CSF)^{-1}(h)^{-1}$, in CSF from control and distemper dogs. Each value is the mean of two determinations.

	Activity				
	1	2	3	4	Mean $\pm$ SD
Normal	3.05	2.54	3.32		2.97$\pm$0.32
Distemper	7.82	5.36	3.87	3.13	5.02$\pm$1.80

and multiple sclerosis remains to be elucidated. Complement-dependent serum demyelinating factors in the sera have been described by using the cerebellar explant culture technique and sera from cases of experimental allergic encephalomyelitis, multiple sclerosis and Guillain-Barré syndrome (10, 20). Koestner et al. (21) reported that some distemper sera were capable of demyelinating explant cultures of canine cerebellum in vitro. The myelinolytic effect was complement dependent.

Complement-fixation and indirect immunofluorescent methods were used to examine sera from dogs with spontaneously occurring and experimentally produced canine distemper (22). Complement-fixing immunoglobulin M antibodies and non-complement-fixing immunoglobulin G antibodies were found in 97% of the spontaneous cases. In contrast, only 28% of the control sera contained these antibodies. Complement-fixing antimyelin antibodies were also found in the sera of gnotobiotic dogs with experimentally induced distemper virus-associated demyelination. These results indicate that demyelination in canine distemper may have an immune mechanism.

Hyperimmune antimyelin serum was prepared in rabbits by bimonthly injections of 10 mg myelin emulsified in complete or incomplete Freund's adjuvant. The myelin was freshly prepared (4) from dog brains. Antibody activity in the antisera was quantified by complement-fixation (22). The indirect immunofluorescent antibody method was used to confirm the myelin-binding capacity of these antibodies.

Two experiments with similar results were done with intracerebral injections of CNS-myelin specific antibody. The plasmalogenase activity was 25% higher in brains injected with normal rabbit serum than in non-injected control brains, presumably due to the trauma of injection. In the brains exposed to the CNS-myelin antibody, the plasmalogenase activity had increased by 45% at 70 hours after injection and reached a peak increase of 102% at 140 hours after injection (Fig. 6). Since these antibodies are complement-dependent, we suggest that one or more components of complement activate plasmalogenase.

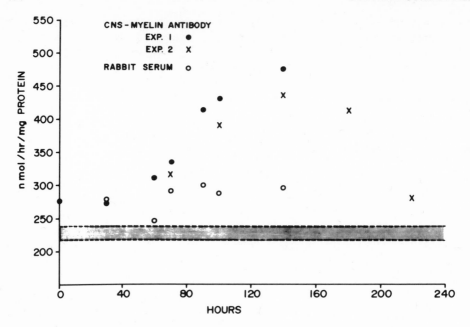

Fig. 6.   Increase of plasmalogenase activity by myelin-specific
antibodies.   Sprague-Dawley rats were given an intracerebral injection of 100 μl control rabbit serum with a titer of 1:276 against
CNS myelin.   The area between the dashed lines represents the mean
± SD of non-injected controls.

   Hypothesis.   The following is our present working hypothesis
for the involvement of plasmalogenase in demyelination:
   1.   Plasmalogenase is located primarily in oligodendroglia,
        probably on the interior of the plasma membrane.
   2.   Injury of the white matter produces an activator of oligo-
        dendroglial plasmalogenase.
   3.   Prostaglandin precursors and lysophosphatidyl ethanol-
        amines are formed.
   4.   These products disrupt the oligodendroglial plasma membranes
        and produce inflammation.
   5.   Myelin that was maintained by the necrotic oligodendroglia
        is then removed.
   Elevation of plasmalogenase activity in white matter is an
early response to injury and may represent the first common denomi-
nator in the irreversible injury to oligodendroglia that results
from ischemia, complement-mediated antigen-antibody reactions,
trauma, vitamin B_{12}-deficiency, and acute inflammation.   Many causes
of elevated plasmalogenase activity are possible.   In each situation,

the subsequent injury to the oligodendrocyte may be mediated by prostaglandins or related compounds produced from the arachidonate, $20:4$ (n-6), and adrenate, $22:4$ (n-6), that was released from ethanolamine plasmalogens by plasmalogenase and lysophospholipase.

Acknowledgements. This research was supported in part by research grants AI-09022, NS-08291 and NS-10165 and training grant FR-05409 from the U.S. Public Health Service and by the Multiple Sclerosis Society of Great Britain. Part of the research was done during the tenure of a NATO Fellowship (R.M.). One of us (S.S.) would like to thank Dr. G.D. Hunter for providing facilities for the study on scrapie at the Agricultural Research Council Institute for Research on Animal Diseases, Compton, Newbury, U.K., and Mr E.A. Turner of the Department of Neurosurgery, Medical School, Birmingham, U.K., for the human biopsy samples. We are grateful for the assistance of Marilyn Waugh, Arrel D. Toews, Robert V. Dorman, William R. Snyder, Alan D. Edgar, Jeffrey W. Cox and Gianfrancesco Goracci.

REFERENCES

1. Ansell, G.B. and Spanner, S., The magnesium ion-dependent cleavage of the vinyl ether linkage of brain ethanolamine plasmalogen, Biochem. J. 94 (1965) 252-258.
2. Ansell, G.B. and Spanner, S., The activity of plasmalogenase in brain of developing rat, in Variation in Chemical Composition of Nervous System (G.B. Ansell, ed.) Pergamon Press, Oxford, 7 (1966).
3. Ansell, G.B. and Spanner, S., Plasmalogenase activity in normal and demyelinating tissue of the central nervous system, Biochem. J. 108 (1968) 207-209.
4. Autilio, L.A., Norton, W.T. and Terry, R.D., The preparation and some properties of purified myelin from the central nervous system. J. Neurochem. 11 (1964) 17-27.
5. Clendenon, N.R., Allen, N., Komatsu, T., Liss, L., Gordon, W.A. and Heimberger, K., Biochemical alteration in anoxic-ischemic lesion of rat brain, Arch. Neurol. 25 (1971) 432-448.
6. Cooper, M.F. and Webster, G.R., The differentiation of phospholipase A_1 and A_2 in rat and human nervous tissues, J. Neurochem. 17 (1970) 1543-1554.
7. D'Amato, R.A., Horrocks, L.A. and Richardson, K.E., Kinetic properties of plasmalogenase from bovine brain, J. Neurochem. 24 (1975) 1251-1255.
8. Dorman, R.V., Toews, A.D. and Horrocks, L.A., Plasmalogenase activities in neuronal perikarya, astroglia and oligodendroglia isolated from bovine brain, J. Lipid. Res. 18 (1977) 115-117.
9. Dorman, R.V., Freysz, L., Mandel, P. and Horrocks, L.S., Plasmalogenase activities in the brains of Jimpy and Quaking mice, J. Neurochem., in press.

10. Dowling, P.C., Kim, S.U. and Murray, M.R., Serum 19S and 7S
    demyelinating antibodies in multiple sclerosis, J. Immunol. 101
    (1968) 1101-1104.
11. Gottfried, E.L. and Rapport, M.M., The biochemistry of plasma-
    logens. I. Isolation and characterization of phosphatidal
    choline, a pure native plasmalogen, J. Biol. Chem. 237 (1962)
    329-333.
12. Griesemer, R.A. and Gibson, J.P., The gnotobiotic dog, Lab.
    Animal Care 13 (Suppl.) (1963) 643-648.
13. Hall, S., The effect of injections of lysophosphatidyl choline
    into white matter of the adult mouse spinal cord, J. Cell. Sci.
    10 (1972) 535-546.
14. Hall, S. and Gregson, N.A., The in vivo and ultrastructural
    effects of injection of lysophosphatidyl choline into myelin-
    ated peripheral nerve fibres of the adult mouse, J. Cell. Sci.
    9 (1971) 769-789.
15. Horrocks, L.A., The alk-1-enyl group content of mammalian
    myelin phosphoglycerides by quantitative two-dimensional thin-
    layer chromatography, J. Lipid Res. 9 (1968) 469-472.
16. Horrocks, L.A., Content, composition and metabolism of mammalian
    and avian lipids that contain ether groups, in Ether Lipids -
    Chemistry and Biology (F. Snyder, ed.) Academic Press, New
    York (1972) pp. 177-272.
17. Horrocks, L.A. and Fu, S.C., Pathway for hydrolysis of plasma-
    logens in brain, in Enzymes of Lipid Metabolism (S. Gatt, L.
    Freysz and P. Mandel, eds.) Plenum Press, New York, in press.
18. Horrocks, L.A., Toews, A.D., Locke, G.E. and Yashon, D.,
    Changes in myelin following trauma of spinal cord in monkey,
    Neurobiology 3 (1973) 256-263.
19. Horrocks, L.A., Sun, G.Y. and D'Amato, R.A., Changes in brain
    lipids during aging, in Neurobiology of Aging (J.M. Ordy and
    K.R. Brizzee, eds.) Plenum Press, New York (1975) pp. 359-
    369.
20. Hughes, D. and Field, E.J., Myelotoxicity of serum and spinal
    fluid in multiple sclerosis: a critical   assessment, Clin.
    Exp. Immunol. 2 (1967) 295-309.
21. Koestner, A., McCullough, B., Krakowka, G.S., Long, J.F. and
    Olsen, R.G., Canine distemper: A virus induced demyelinating
    encephalomyelitis in slow virus diseases, in Symposium on
    Slow Viruses (W. Zeman and E.H. Lennett, eds.) Williams and
    Wilkins, Baltimore (1974) pp. 86-101.
22. Krakowka, S., Mc.Cullough, B., Koestner, A. and Olsen, R.,
    Myelin-specific autoantibodies associated with central nervous
    system demyelination in canine distemper virus infection,
    Infection and Immunity 8 (1973) 819-827.
23. Mandel, P., Nussbaum, J.L., Neskovic, N.M., Sarlieve, L.L.,
    Farkas, E. and Robain, O., in Proceedings, Symposium of the
    International Union of Biochemistry (Y. Pollak and J.W. Lee,

eds.) Australian and New Zealand Book Co., Sidney (1973) pp. 410-422.

24. Marburg, O., The so-called acute multiple sclerosis, J. Psychiat. Neurol. 27 (1906) 213-312.

25. McCullough, B., Krakowka, S. and Koestner, A., Experimental canine distemper virus-induced demyelination, Laboratory Investigation 31 (1974) 216-222.

26. McMartin, D.N., Koestner, A. and Long, J.F., Enzyme activities associated with the demyelinating phase of canine distemper. I. Beta-glucuronidase, acid and neutral proteinase, Acta Neuropath. (Berl.) 22 (1972) 275-287.

27. Mc Martin, D.N., Horrocks, L.A. and Koestner, A., Enzyme activities associated with the demyelinating phase of canine distemper. II. Plasmalogenase, Acta Neuropath. (Berl.) 22 (1972) 288-293.

28. Miller, S.L., Benjamins, J.A. and Morell, P., Metabolism of glycerophospholipids of myelin and microsomes in rat brain, J. Biol. Chem. 252 (1977) 4025-4037.

29. Spanner, S., Ph.D. Thesis (1966) University of Birmingham, England.

30. Suzuki, Y., Tucker, S.H., Rorke, L.B. and Suzuki, K., Ultrastructural and biochemical studies of Schilder's disease, J. Neuropath. Exper. Neurol. 29 (1970) 405-419.

31. Thompson, R.H.S., Myelinolytic mechanisms, Proc. Roy. Soc. Med. 54 (1961) 30-33.

32. Webster, G.R. and Cooper, M., On the site of action of phosphatide acylhydrolase activity of rat brain homogenates on lecithin, J. Neurochem. 15 (1968) 795-802.

33. Wise, G., Stevens, M.E., Shuttleworth, E.C., Donahue, T. and Allen, J.N., An experimental model for the evaluation of ischemia of the cerebral hemispheres, submitted for publication (1977).

34. Woelk, H. and Kanig, K., Phospholipid metabolism in experimental allergic encephalomyelitis - activity of brain phospholipase A_1 toward specifically labelled glycerophospholipids, J. Neurochem. 23 (1974) 739-744.

35. Woelk, H. and Peiler-Ichikawa, K., Zur Aktivität der Phospholipase A_2 gegenüber verschiedenen 1-Alk-1'-enyl-2-acyl- und 1-Alkyl-2-acyl-verbindungen während der Multiplen Sklerose, J. Neurol. 207 (1974) 319-326.

36. Woelk, H. and Porcellati, G., Subcellular distribution and kinetic properties of rat brain phospholipases A_1 and A_2, Hoppe-Seyler's Z. Physiol. Chem. 354 (1973) 90-100.

37. Woelk, H., Kanig, K. and Peiler-Ichikawa, K., Phospholipid metabolism in experimental allergic encephalomyelitis - activity of mitochondrial phospholipase A_1 of rat brain toward specifically labelled 1,2, diacyl-, 1-alk-1'-enyl-2-acyl- and 1-alkyl-2-acyl-sn-glycero-3-phosphorylcholine, J. Neurochem. 23 (1974) 745-750.

38. Yanagihara, T. and Cumings, J.N., Alterations of phospholipids,
     particularly plasmalogens, in the demyelination of multiple
     sclerosis as compared with that of cerebral oedema, Brain 92
     (1969) 59-70.

EFFECT OF DIPHTHERITIC DEMYELINATION ON AXONAL TRANSPORT IN THE SCIATIC NERVE AND SUBSEQUENT MUSCLE CHANGES IN THE CHICKEN

Antony D. Kidman[1], William de C. Baker[2] and
    H. Jane Sippe
Neurobiology Unit, School of Life Sciences,
    The N.S.W. Institute of Technology
Gore Hill, N.S.W. 2065, Australia

SUMMARY

Chicken sciatic nerves undergo demyelination following intra-neural injection of diphtheria toxin and subsequent atrophy of some muscular cells. Paresis occurs after one week and lasts approximately three weeks; at the height of the lesion C^{14}-leucine was injected into the ventral horn cells of the spinal cord. The axonal transport of fast flowing labelled proteins was followed down the sciatic nerve axons and flow rates at two different times were measured. Muscle cells were stained for succinic dehydrogenase and ATPase; fibre diameters, total protein, and total radioactivity associated with the nerves were also measured. The results showed that the fast flowing labelled proteins accumulated at the demyelination site while the muscle cells supplied by these nerves showed reduction of fibre diameter and evidence of degeneration. Further studies are in progress on slow moving proteins and muscle cells.

[1]Supported by grants from the Australian National Health & Medical Research Council and the N.S.W. Muscular Dystrophy Association. We would like to thank Dr. G. Morgan for helpful comments.
[2]Dr. Baker's address is Dept. of Pediatrics, Prince of Wales Hospital, Randwick, N.S.W. 2031, Australia.

INTRODUCTION

Centrifugal or orthograde axonal transport of metabolites in peripheral nerves was originally shown by Weiss and Hiscoe (18) and subsequently confirmed by a variety of methods including labelling of transported macromolecules by a radioactive precursor (9). Flow rates have been determined for mitochondria (8), catecholamines (11), proteins (4) and, in the case of latter, divided into slow (2-3 mm/day) and fast ($2.5 - 3.5 \times 10^2$ mm/day) rate in the chicken sciatic nerve (4). Centripetal or retrograde axonal flow has also been demonstrated for specific enzymes (13).

Peripheral neuropathies can occur as disease states or can be induced experimentally by injection of chemical agents such as diphtheria toxin (5).

The relationship of the satellite cell to the neuron has only been partly explained. In the peripheral nervous system the Schwann cell is necessary for the relatively rapid conduction of nerve impulses via saltatory conduction but the influence of this cell on axonal metabolism is not clear.

Intraneural injection of diphteria toxin into the sciatic nerve produces demyelination in a localised region by interfering with the synthesis of the myelin sheath (16). We have used this system to study whether myelin is necessary for the axonal transport of metabolites from the nerve cell body to the nerve ending and the subsequent effect of demyelination of the nerve supply on the muscle cells.

Adult chickens were chosen to analyse the effect of experimental demyelination on the metabolism of axons and muscle cells because of the evidence of axonal transport in the sciatic nerve already available together with the detailed histological studies of diphtheritic demyelination on the same nerve (5, 17).

EXPERIMENTAL

Diphtheria toxin, 10 µl in physiological saline at a concentration of 1.25×10^6 Lf/µl (low) or 1.25×10^{-5} Lf/µl (high), was injected into each bundle of the sciatic nerve of white Leghorn chickens at a point 5 ± 1 cm from the spinal cord and an equal volume of saline was injected on the contralateral side. This toxin was supplied by the Commonwealth Serum Laboratories, Melbourne. (The Lf unit of toxin is the antigen content determined by incubating serial dilutions of diphtheria antitoxic horse serum of known international antigen with a fixed quantity of toxin - or toxoid - and the equivalence point is determined as the most rapidly flocculating mixture of antigen and serum using a test such as the Ramon Flocculation Test.) Paresis was evident one week after injection and lasted for a further three weeks before recovery. The chickens were killed and the nerves processed at 16 ± 4 days, unless

otherwise stated, after injection of the toxin when the paresis was
at its height.

Six μc of C^{14}-leucine (270 μc/μmole and 324 μc/μmole) was injected into the ventral horn motoneurons. At 5 h and 6 h after
injection, the sciatic nerve was excised, cut into 1 cm segments
and the labelled protein extracted according to the method of Bray
and Austin (4). The protein extract was counted in a Packard Tri-
Carb scintillation counter model 3320 and the amount of protein per
segment was determined by the method of Lowry et al. (12).

Results, expressed as DPM/mg protein, were normalised as
follows to eliminate the effects of slight variations in the amount
of label injected and the site of the injection. The first segment
was excluded in the calculation as it always showed a relatively
high count due to diffusion of label from the cord.

$$\text{Normalised count} = \frac{\text{DPM per segment/mg protein per segment}}{\Sigma \text{ DPM per segment/mg protein per segment}} \times 100$$

Mean total protein per segment and the mean DPM per segment were
determined in both normal and demyelinated nerves.

Nerves were divided into five regions 0.25 cm, 0.7 cm and 1.5
cm on either side of the injection site. Firstly, some injected
nerves were placed in 1% osmium tetroxide for 24 h, then in 33.3%
glycerol for 24 h, and the fibres were teased out from each region
using fine sewing needles under a dissecting microscope. They were
mounted and examined; damage was assessed using an eyepiece with a
scale and was graded as follows: no damage, (+) damage to nodal or
paranodal regions not extending beyond 40 μ from the node, (++)
partial breakdown of the internode being greater than 40 μ from the
node but not affecting the whole internode, (+++) complete inter-
nodal breakdown (10).

Secondly, 1 mm lengths of the two separated bundles of the
sciatic nerve were taken from each of the five regions, fixed in
glutaraldehyde and Dalton's osmium and treated with 2.5% uranyl
acetate. They were embedded in Spurrs resin and 1 μ sections were
cut and stained with 0.5% toluidine blue for examination by light
microscopy.

Conduction along the nerve in vivo was tested by placing a
stimulating probe at sites above and below the demyelinated region
in the exposed sciatic nerve. A response from the gastrocnemius
pars externa muscle was shown by a displacement transducer operating a pen in a conventional chart recorder. Stimuli between 300
and 1000 mV were used.

The peroneus longus, gastrocnemius interna and gastrocnemius
externa were examined histologically in 6 birds. Two birds had
sciatic nerve section 30 and 27 days respectively prior to examination. Four birds had a demyelinating injection of diphtheria toxin
into the sciatic nerve 24 days, 30 days, 31 days and 63 days respectively prior to examination. The latter was reinjected 36
days after the first injection. The contralateral normal muscles

were used as controls.

After removal of the muscles under general anaesthetic the birds were killed. The muscles were immediately blocked for frozen sections and frozen in isopentane cooled with liquid nitrogen. Tissue for paraffin sections was fixed in Helly's fixative for 4 h, washed in 70% alcohol and stored in formal saline until processing commenced. Frozen sections were cut at 10 μ and stained for myosin ATPase at pH 9.3 (15) and succinic dehydrogenase (7). Frozen sections at 7 h were stained with haematoxylin and eosin. Paraffin sections were cut at 5 μ and stained with haematoxylin and eosin. Muscle fibre diameters were measured on the sections stained for myosin ATPase by using a camera lucida, outlining the fibres and measuring the minimum diameter. Whenever possible 100 Type II fibres were measured (minimum 85 fibres). Type I fibres were relatively infrequent and a minimum of 33 fibres were measured.

RESULTS

The flow results for the C^{14} labelled protein are shown in Fig. 1. The data show that a 3 cm segment of demyelination produced a block of fast flowing protein with either a high or low dose of toxin. A fast flow rate of 3.4×10^2 mm per day based on peak height movement was calculated for the control sciatic nerve and this falls within the range of fast flow rates in the chicken sciatic nerve stated earlier (4).

Mean total DPM per segment and mean total protein per segment were calculated to establish if demyelination caused any change in the total amount of protein or the total amount of labelled protein in the sciatic nerve. The results are shown in Table 1 and no significant differences from the control nerves were found.

Fig. 1. Distribution of protein bound radioactivity along the sciatic nerve of the chicken and normalised as explained in the text. Each point is the mean and the bars represent the standard error of the mean, ——— is the saline injected nerve (10 μl per bundle) and - - - - - is the toxin injected nerve (10 μl per bundle). "A,B" show the distribution following injection with 1.25×10^{-4} Lf of diphtheria toxin per bundle (high dose). "C,D" show the distribution of label following injection with 1.25×10^{-5} Lf of diphtheria toxin per bundle (low dose). "A" shows the movement of labelled protein 5 h after injection, each point on the saline injected side represents the mean of six nerves while on the toxin injected side each point is the mean of four nerves. "B" shows the position 6 h after injection, each point represents the mean of four nerves unless otherwise noted. Similarly "C" represents the mean of four nerves and "D" the mean of five nerves unless otherwise noted.

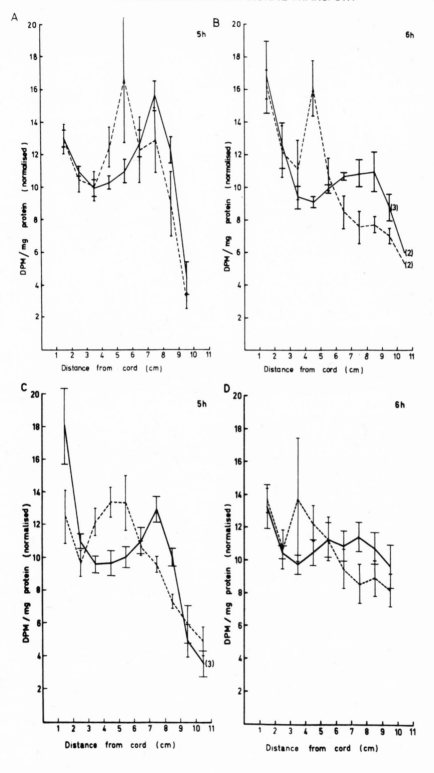

Nerve fibres were teased and examined and the results are summarised in Table 2. Significant demyelination over the injected region was found. Photographs of transverse sections of the normal and demyelinated sciatic nerves (Fig. 2) show disruption of the myelin sheath following high and low dose injections.

Conduction was observed on the control side when stimuli of 300 mV were applied to the nerve. On the treated side (high dose) conduction occurred below the demyelinated region but was blocked when the stimulus was applied above this. Preliminary conduction velocity experiments on excised sciatic nerves maintained at constant temperature in Ringer's solution and in a low dose treated nerve confirmed the previous observations and will be the subject of a separate report.

Because the low dose of toxin produced paresis, blockage of fast flowing protein, blockage of conduction and obvious disruption to the myelin sheath it was decided to carry out further experiments using this amount of toxin as this would minimise direct damage to the axons.

The histological changes in muscle cells under low dose conditions are qualitatively similar in the muscles having a demyelinated or severed nerve supply. The specific changes are as follows.

In both types of lesion the muscle nuclei are larger with more prominent nucleoli than in normal control muscle. There was also a reduction in muscle fibre diameter compared to controls. The mean muscle fibre diameters in the three types are shown in Table 3. The diameters following nerve section are smaller than those following demyelination. However, the period of about 7 days between injection of the toxin and the start of paresis makes it difficult to assess the difference between these groups.

The histochemistry showed that both types of lesions developed a reduced and irregular staining for succinic dehydrogenase and for many fibres the types became indistinguishable. Fig. 3 shows light micrographs of normal peroneus longus and the contralateral muscle following 31 days demyelination.

Three fibre types are distinguishable with ATPase (pH 9.4): type I - pale, type IIA - dark, and type IIB - intermediate. Following both types of lesion type IIA and B became indistinguishable but type I remained clearly distinguishable. Fig. 4 shows light micrographs of normal and contralateral peroneus longus stained for ATPase.

In the preparation 63 days post injection, reinjected at 36 days to maintain demyelination, many muscle fibres appeared normal but there were variable numbers of small angular fibres, some showing grouped atrophy. This is evidence of continued degeneration in some fibres while others have recovered.

Table 1. Mean total radioactivity and protein per segment in control and demyelinated nerves.

Nerve	HIGH DOSE		LOW DOSE	
	DPM/segment	Protein(mg)/segment	DPM/segment	Protein(mg)/segment
Control nerve	175±25 (4)^x	2.23±0.21 (4)	234±61 (5)	2.29±0.16 (5)
Demyelinated nerve	238±80 (4)	2.41±0.44 (4)	228±51 (5)	2.43±0.14 (5)

^{x}Mean ± SEM (no. of determinations)

Table 2. Extent of demyelination in single fibres due to diphtheria toxin.

Region	HIGH DOSE					LOW DOSE				
	No.of fibres	No damage^x	+	++	+++	No.of fibres	No damage^x	+	++	+++
+2	86	1	13	26	60	60	32	23	23	23
+1	82	4	11	20	65	60	39	18	10	33
0	143	2	11	15	72	74	13	1	19	67
-1	100	7	4	22	67	58	5	2	26	67
-2	113	2	4	17	77	44	18.5	18.5	11	52

^{x}These figures represent the percentage of fibres in each of the four categories as defined in the text.

Table 3. Mean muscle fibre diameters in micrometers, with normal, demyelinated and sectioned nerve supply.

Nerve supply	Mean diameter of fibre types I and II
Normal Demyelinated[+] Resectioned[+]	69.4+5.9 (4) [++] 45.6+4.5[x] (6) 26.3+3.9[xx] (4)

[+] Nerves were treated or resectioned $28+4$ days before the muscle was excised.

[++] This represents the mean $\pm$ SEM with the number of values in parentheses. These values are each the mean of at least 85 fibres (type II) or 33 fibres (type I). Half the values were of type II and half of type I.

[x] $p < 0.05$.

[xx] $p < 0.001$.

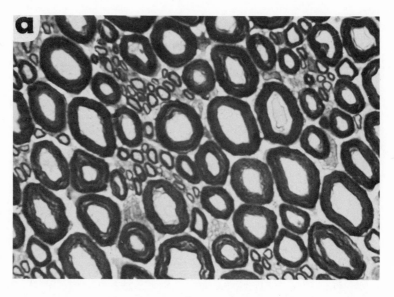

a

Fig. 2. Transverse sections of sciatic nerve fibres x 1000. "a" is a control nerve that has been injected with normal saline, 10 µl per bundle. "b" is a demyelinated nerve that has been injected with 1.25×10^{-5} Lf of diphteria toxin per bundle (low dose). "c" is a demyelinated nerve that has been injected with 1.25×10^{-4} Lf of toxin per bundle (high dose).

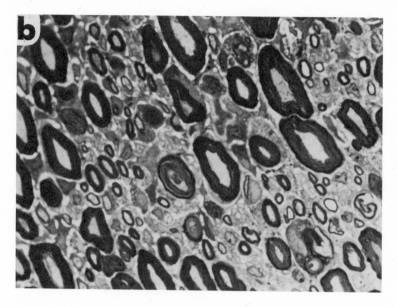

b

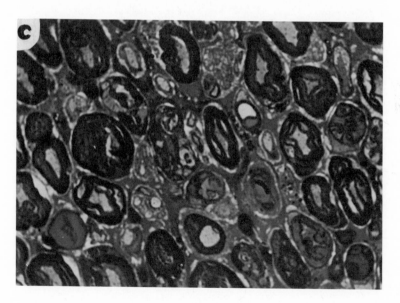

c

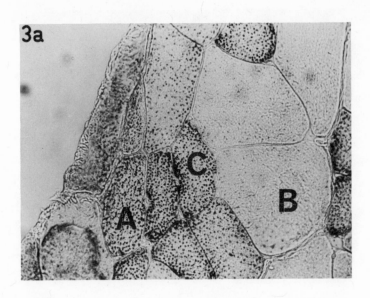

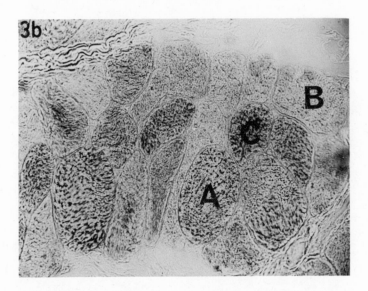

Fig. 3. Normal (a) and demyelinated (b) peroneus longus muscle
(x 300) stained for succinic dehydrogenase. Type I fibres are
designated A, type IIA fibres as B, and type IIB which are smaller,
as C.

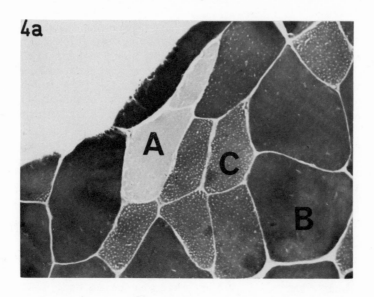

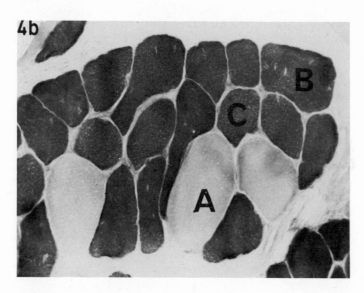

Fig. 4. Normal (a) and demyelinated (b) peroneus longus muscle
(x 300) stained for myosin ATPase. Type I fibres are pale and
designated A, type IIA fibres are dark and large and shown as B
and type IIB which are intermediate in staining and smaller as C.
However, in the demyelinated preparation type IIA and IIB cannot
be distinguished.

DISCUSSION

A metabolic dependence of the axon upon the Schwann cell has been demonstrated in this report by the accumulation of rapidly transported axonal proteins at high and low doses of diphteria toxin in the chicken sciatic nerve. Paresis occurs under these conditions together with changes in the muscle supplied by the impaired nerve when compared to normal. We had shown in an earlier report a characteristic lactic dehydrogenase isoenzyme profile in demyelinated murine leg muscles (6).

Fig. 1 shows the movement of proteins 5 h and 6 h post injection of the label. Radioactively labelled protein accumulates at the fifth and sixth segments, the site of the demyelinating lesion.

Total radioactivity incorporated into protein and total protein as shown in Table 1 does not demonstrate any significant differences between normal and demyelinated sciatic nerves. We expected an increased protein concentration in the proximal region of the demyelinated sciatic nerve; the failure to observe this may be due to increased degradation of protein in this region or changes in retrograde flow due to the lesion. Further analysis of total protein above and below the site of the lesion is being done following longer periods of demyelination.

Thus the Schwann cell disruption besides blocking the action potential under these conditions causes an accumulation of fast flowing axonal proteins. The passage of these proteins appears to require an intact myelin sheath in the sciatic nerve. However, we have assumed that the axons have not been damaged directly by the toxin but only the Schwann cells. Allt and Cavanagh (2) claim no damage to the fine structure of unmyelinated axons in the rat following endoneural injection of diphteria toxin while Bradley and Jennekens (3) showed that if the dose of toxin is high enough axonal damage will occur.

We stimulated the axon on the side of the lesion distal to the spinal cord and found the same response as in the control. Conduction velocity can still be close to normal in degenerating axons provided demyelination has not occurred (14).

We would expect some eventual impairment of the axons if fast flowing proteins are blocked by the diphtheritic lesion. The muscle histology (Figs. 3, 4) following demyelination and denervation when compared to normal muscle indicates degeneration of axons and consequent reduction in muscle fibre diameter although not to the same extent as the sectioned nerves (Table 3).

A recent review of the pathology of the peripheral nerve by Allt (1) concludes that the Schwann cell does not support the axon in its trophic, ionic or energy requirements from studies of experimental pathology. Our data suggest that the Schwann cell is necessary for the intra-axonal transport of fast flowing proteins and that muscle cell changes reflect the axonal damage due to this blockage.

Further studies are necessary to clarify the effects of demyelination and remyelination on slow moving axonal proteins.

REFERENCES

1. Allt, G., in The Peripheral Nerve (D.N. Landon, ed.), Chapman
   and Hall (1976) London, pp. 666-739.
2. Allt, G. and Cavanagh, J.B., Ultrastructural changes in the
   region of the node of Ranvier in the rat caused by diphtheria
   toxin, Brain 92 (1969) 459-468.
3. Bradley, W.G. and Jennekens, F.G.I., Axonal degeneration in
   diphtheritic neuropathy, J. Neurol. Sci. 13 (1971) 415-530.
4. Bray, J.J. and Austin, L., Axoplasmic transport of ^{14}C proteins
   at two rates in chicken sciatic nerve, Brain Res. 12 (1969)
   230-233.
5. Cavanagh, J.B. and Jacobs, J.M., Some quantitative aspects of
   diphtheritic neuropathy, Brit. J. Exp. Path. 45 (1964) 309-
   322.
6. Dolan, L., Chew, L., Morgan, G. and Kidman, A.D., Enzyme
   studies of skeletal muscle in mice with different types of
   neural impairment and muscular dystrophy, Exp. Neurol. 47
   (1975) 105-117.
7. Harrison, W.A., Unpublished observations.
8. Jeffrey, P.L., James, K.A.C., Kidman, A.D., Richards, A.M.
   and Austin, L., The flow of mitochondria in chicken sciatic
   nerve, J. Neurobiol. 3 (1972) 199-208.
9. Jeffrey, P.L. and Austin, L., Axoplasmic transport, Prog. in
   Neurobiol. 2 (1973) 205-255.
10. Jacobs, J.M., Experimental diphtheritic neuropathy in the rat,
    Brit. J. Exp. Path. 48 (1967) 204-216.
11. Livett, B.G., Geffin, L.B. and Austin, L., Axoplasmic trans-
    port of (^{14}C)-noradrenaline and protein in sympathetic nerves,
    Nature 217 (1968) 931-939.
12. Lowry, O.H., Rosebrough, N.J., Farr, A.L. and Randall, R.J.,
    Protein measurement with the Folin phenol reagent, J. Biol.
    Chem. 193 (1951) 265-275.
13. Lubinska, L., Axoplasmic streaming in regenerating and in
    normal nerve fibres, Prog. Brain Res. 13 (1964) 360-377.
14. McDonald, I., Pathophysiology in multiple sclerosis, Brain 97
    (1974) 179-196.
15. Padykula, H.A. and Herman, E., Factors affecting the activity
    of adenosine triphosphatase and other phosphatases as measured
    by histochemical techniques, J. Histochem. Cytochem. 3 (1955)
    161-169.
16. Pleasure, D.E., Feldmann, B., and Prockop, D.J., Diphtheria
    toxin inhibits the synthesis of myelin proteolipid and basic
    proteins by peripheral nerve in vitro, J. Neurochem. 20 (1973)
    81-90.

17. Weller, R.O. and Mellick, R.S., Acid phosphatase and lysosome in diphtheritic neuropathy and Wallerian degeneration, Brit. J. Exp. Path. 47 (1966) 425-434.
18. Weiss, P. and Hiscoe, H.B., Experiments of the mechanism of nerve growth, J. Exp. Zool. 107 (1948) 315-395.

MYELIN DEFICIENCY IN EXPERIMENTAL PHENYLKETONURIA:

CONTRIBUTION OF THE AROMATIC ACID METABOLITES OF PHENYLALANINE

Yen Hoong Loo, Joseph Scotto and Henryk M. Wisniewski

New York State Institute for Basic Research in Mental
    Retardation
Staten Island, New York 10314

SUMMARY

    Retarded body and brain growth and a deficit of myelin in
the cerebral hemispheres and the cerebellum were observed in an
animal model of phenylketonuria, the p-chlorophenylalanine and
L-phenylalanine treated preweanling rat. These manifestations of
phenylketonuria were reproduced in rats treated with phenylacetate
in amounts approximating those likely to be produced in phenylketonuria. Young rats treated with equivalent amounts of other
metabolites of phenylalanine, namely, phenylpyruvate, phenyllactate,
and mandelate, which also accumulate in the brain during hyperphenylalaninemia, did not exhibit any toxic effects. Phenylpyruvate did not give rise to phenylacetate in the brain, but a
small percentage was converted to phenyllactate. The gross composition of myelin isolated from the brains of saline and phenylacetate treated animals was similar.
    At various time intervals after subcutaneous injection,
phenylacetate in the brain reached levels thirty times those of
phenylpyruvate and phenyllactate, although animals received
equivalent amounts of the three metabolites. The retarded growth
of the body and brain of the young animal treated with phenylacetate may be attributed to the formation of phenylacetylcoenzyme
A in the tissues. The site of action is very likely linked to
acylcoenzyme A metabolism, i.e., the synthesis and utilization of
acetylCoA and acetoacetylCoA, which are involved in reactions
generating ATP and energy and in the synthesis of cholesterol and
fatty acids. Results of this investigation indicate that growth
retardation induced by phenylacetate during the period of very
rapid development of the brain is responsible for the mental
retardation in phenylketonuria.

INTRODUCTION

The neurochemist continues to seek an answer to the question, to what extent is behavior determined by the molecular composition of the brain? Studies of the nature of the brain damage in inborn errors of metabolism and the mechanisms by which this brain damage is caused may contribute to an answer. We have, therefore, focused our attention on phenylketonuria which specifically and irreversibly affects central nervous system function and produces a severe mental deficit.

Because of a deficiency of the enzyme phenylalanine hydroxylase (EC 1.99.1.2) in the liver of phenylketonurics (26), the major normal pathway of phenylalanine metabolism, the hydroxylation to tyrosine, is blocked. Consequently tissue levels of phenylalanine become elevated to 20-40 times that of normal, and the amino acid undergoes decarboxylation to β-phenylethylamine (15, 43, 46) and transamination to phenylpyruvic acid (27). The amine is further metabolized to phenylacetic (15) and mandelic (5)acids, while the ketoacid is converted to phenyllactic (27) and o-hydroxyphenylacetic (1, 6) acids.

Little is known of the neuropathology of phenylketonuria (11) aside from the reports of microcephaly (11), of alterations in cerebral lipids (12, 13, 21, 40, 41) and of a myelin deficit (47, 51, 57). Persistent hyperphenylalaninemia induced in the developing rat brain produces similar changes (8, 10, 24, 48, 50). The lipids in myelin isolated from the phenylketonuric patient and from the hyperphenylalaninemic rat were found to have a normal gross composition but decreased proportions of long chain (29, 30) and unsaturated (18, 19, 29, 30) fatty acids.

Of all the metabolites derived from phenylalanine, phenylpyruvate has most frequently been suggested to contribute to the brain damage in phenylketonuria. This aromatic keto acid has been found to have an inhibitory effect, in vitro, on enzymes catalyzing reactions involved in the production of ATP and energy for cellular processes and in acetyl group transfer, which would diminish cholesterol and lipid synthesis (4, 7, 9, 20, 22, 31, 32, 33, 44, 45, 49, 55).

To assess the possible toxic effects of the metabolic products of phenylalanine on neuronal maturation, we first determined the pattern of aromatic acid metabolites and the extent of their accumulation in the developing brain when tissue levels of phenylalanine simulated those reported for uncontrolled phenylketonuria. The predominant metabolite found under these conditions was phenylacetate, with decreasing amounts of phenylpyruvate, phenyllactate and mandelate (35). We are at present investigating the pattern of changes brought about by the action of each one of these metabolic products. In this communication we report on the effects on body weight, brain weight, myelination, and the composition of purified myelin.

EXPERIMENTAL

L-phenylalanine and reagents for its estimation, L-phenyl-lactic acid, sodium phenylpyruvate, lactose, cholesterol, and orcinol were purchased from Sigma Chemical Co., St. Louis, MO; DL-p-chlorophenylalanine and beef serum albumin, from Nutritional Biochemicals Corp., Cleveland, O.; phenylacetic and L-mandelic acids from Aldrich Chemical Co., Milwaukee, WI; Triton X-100 from Packard Instrument Co., Inc., Downers Grove, IL; platinum oxide from ICN Pharmaceuticals, Inc., Cleveland, O. The silylating reagents bis-(trimethylsilyl)trifluoroacetamide (BSTFA) and bis-(trimethylsilyl)acetamide (BSA) and the column stationary phase and packing, 5% OV-1 on Chromosorb W-HP, were obtained from Regis Chemical Co., Chicago, IL; Sylon (a mixture of hexamethyldisilazane and trimethylchlorosilane), methylesters of fatty acids C-15-C-24, free fatty acids C-15-C-24, and a α-hydroxy fatty acids, C-18 and C-24 from Supelco, Inc., Bellefonte, PA, borontrichloridemethanol esterification kit from Applied Science Lab., Inc., State College, PA. We used organic solvents distilled in glass from Burdick and Jackson Labs, Inc., Muskegon, MI. Tanks of highly purified dry hydrogen, helium, compressed air, and nitrogen were purchased from the Matheson Co., East Rutherford, NJ. All other chemicals were of the highest purity available from Fisher Scientific Co., Fair Lawn, NJ.

Animal experiments. Rats of the Sprague-Dawley strain, pregnant for two weeks, were obtained from the Charles River Farms and maintained on a diet of Purina chow. Neonates of both sexes from 3-4 litters were mixed and each mother nursed a litter of eight. The regimen of injections was started on the 4th postnatal day and ended on the 21st, when the animals were weaned and fed Purina chow. All injections were administered subcutaneously at the back of the neck. Animals were weighed daily.

Induction of hyperphenylalaninemia. Hyperphenylalaninemia was induced by treatment with the hydroxylase inhibitor, DL-p-chloro-phenylalanine (p-CPA) and L-phenylalanine (Phe). The chloro-derivative was washed with ethanol and distilled water before use. Uniform suspensions of each of the amino acids and of a mixture of the two were prepared by sonication in 0.9% saline containing 0.5% starch and 0.1 ml of a 10% solution of triton X-100 per 10 ml of suspension. On the 4th and 5th postnatal days, the experimental group received one injection of p-CPA only (0.9 µmol/g). Thereafter, daily injections of a mixture of p-CPA (0.45 µmol/g) and Phe (2.2 µmol/g) were given in the morning and Phe only (2.2 µmol/g) 7-8 hours later. The control group received injections of the vehicle twice daily.

For the estimation of brain levels of phenylalanine, animals of different ages were killed at varying time intervals after the injections. To correct for the contribution of p-chlorophenyl-alanine a parallel experiment was carried out with another group of

animals which received only p-CPA at the same dosage and were killed
at the same time intervals after the injection. The fluorimetric
method developed by McCaman and Robins (39) was employed.

For myelin preparations, animals were killed at 35 days of
age.

Treatment with the aromatic acid metabolites of phenylalanine.
The sodium salt of each of the acids, phenylacetic, phenylpyruvic,
L-phenyllactic, and L-mandelic, was dissolved in 0.9% saline, and
each solution was adjusted to pH 7.2-7.4 if necessary. Injections
of the compounds were given twice daily, spaced 7-8 hours apart.
Phenylacetate, phenylpyruvate, L-phenyllactate were administered at
the same dosage (μmol/g) as follows: 4-6 d old, 1.2; 7-14 d, 2.1;
15-21 d, 3.0. Mandelate was administered in the same manner at half
the dosage of the other compounds. The control group received injections of 0.9% saline.

The concentrations of the metabolites in the brains of animals
of different ages at varying time intervals after the injection
were monitored by the gas chromatographic method developed by Loo
et al. For the estimation of myelin, animals were killed at 35 days
of age.

Isolation and purification of myelin. Animals were killed by
decapitation and the brains were removed. The olfactory lobes were
discarded. For the isolation of myelin, three different areas were
separated by dissection; the cerebral hemispheres including the
basal ganglia and thalamus, the cerebellum, and the pons-medulla.
Tissues from four animals were pooled for preparations from the
cerebellum and from the medulla-pons. Tissues from two animals
were pooled for preparations from the cerebral hemispheres. Myelin
was purified by the procedures described by Suzuki et al.(52) and
by Norton (42).

Composition of myelin. Myelin, dried by lyophilization, was
extracted three times with chloroform:methanol, 2:1 (v/v) and the
pooled extracts were diluted to a final volume of 10 ml (17).
Aliquots of the extracts were removed for analyses.

Total lipid. Proteins in the chloroform-methanol extract were
removed by repeatedly drying and redissolving the lipids (17). The
final chloroform-methanol solution was dried in a tared vial and the
residue of lipids was weighed.

Total protein. Protein was determined by Lowry's method (37)
in the residues that were soluble and insoluble in 2:1 chloroform-
methanol. The residues were incubated with 0.1N NaOH at 37°C for
30-45 min, and the clear solutions were used for assay. Beef serum
albumin served as a standard.

Total phospholipids. Aliquots of the chloroform-methanol
extract were hydrolyzed and phosphorus was determined by the method
of Bartlett (2), using monopotassium dihydrogen phosphate as a
standard. A factor of 25 was used to convert P to phospholipid,
and an average molecular weight of 808 was used to calculate molar
concentrations.

Total cholesterol. The ferric chloride-sulfuric acid reaction
described by Glick et al. (23) was applied.

Cerebrosides and sulfatides. The total amount of galactose in
the chloroform-methanol extract was used as a measure of the content
of cerebrosides plus sulfatides. The orcinol reaction of Svennerholm (53) as modified by Hess and Lewin (25) was applied, using
lactose as a standard. A factor of 4.6 was used to convert galactose to galactolipid, and an average molecular weight of 846 was
used for the calculation of molar concentrations.

Fatty acids. The major fatty acids of myelin with a chain
length of 16, 18, 20, 22, and 24 carbon atoms were estimated as
fully saturated acids by gas chromatography of their methylesters-
trimethylsilyl ethers. Internal standards, C-15 and C-17 acids
were added to myelin (3-4 mg) before saponification in equal volumes of 40% KOH and ethanol (total volume, 0.5 ml) at 80% for 2 h.
A mixture of pure, authentic samples of C-16, C-18, C-20:6, C-22,
C-24, and α-hydroxy-C-24 acids was also carried through the entire
procedure.

Ethanol was removed from the hydrolysate under a stream of
nitrogen and was replaced by an equal volume of distilled water.
Amines and sterols were removed by extraction with petroleum ether
and diethylether. The combined organic layers were washed once
with 0.4 ml of distilled water, which was pooled with the alkaline
hydrolysate. The fatty acids were extracted at pH 2 into chloroform, then hydrogenated in alcohol solution with platinum oxide
as catalyst at 50-60°C for 15-20 min. The catalyst was removed
by filtration and washed twice with alcohol, containing 0.01
N HCl and once with chloroform. The filtrate and washings were
combined and concentrated under nitrogen, then dried in vacuo
over NaOH pellets.

The methyl esters were prepared by reaction of the fatty
acids with a mixture of B Cl_3-methanol (0.15 ml) at 65-70°C for
3-5 min. Distilled water (0.3 ml) was added to the cooled
solution and the esters were removed with hexane. After evaporation of the hexane under N_2, the residue of esters from 1-2 mg
of myelin was reacted with a mixture of 45 µl of BSA and 5 µl of
Sylon at 70°C for 50 min.

The Varian gas chromatograph, Model 2100, with a hydrogen
flame ionization detector was used. The methylesters of the fatty
acids and methylesters-trimethylsilyl ethers of hydroxy-fatty
acids were separated on a 6 ft. x 0.25 cm glass U column packed
with 5% OV-1 on Chromosorb W-HP 80/100 mesh. Injector port
temperature was 275°C and that of detector cell 300°C. Flow
rate of carrier gas helium was 45 ml/min. Separations were
carried out by temperature programming from 140-260°C at 2°C/min.
Chart speed was 50 in/h. The C-16, C-18, C-20, C-22, and C-24
acids as their methylesters and the α-hydroxy C-24 acid as the
methylester-trimethylsilyl ether were identified by their positions on the chromatogram and quantitated by comparison of their

peak areas with those of the internal standards. The distance
between fatty acids differing in 2C atoms on the chromatogram was
constant. The recovery of the internal standards added to myelin
samples and of the mixture of standard acids carried through the
entire procedure ranged from 80-90%.

RESULTS

Clinical observations. Animals treated with phenylpyruvate,
phenyllactate, and mandelate appeared as healthy and tame as the
control group injected with saline or the vehicle. In contrast,
the p-CPA + Phe and the phenylacetate treated animals were smaller
in body size, had a dull, thin coat of fur, and became irritable
and difficult to handle as they passed 18 days of age. Although
these animals seemed to nurse normally, their delayed development
may possibly be due to a poor appetite and underfeeding. It was
not feasible to accurately assess their intake of milk. Ongoing
studies on neurological development and learning ability of these
animals have revealed deficits in these areas (H. Kaplan et al.,
in preparation).

Effects of hyperphenylalaninemia. Treatment with p-CPA
+ L-Phe elevated phenylalanine in the brain of the very young rat
(5-12 d old) to levels reported for plasma of phenylketonuric
patients. Hyperphenylalaninemia was sustained over a 24 h period.
In the older animal (17-21 d), however, brain levels of phenylalanine were only 3-4 times that of the normal (Table 1).

Table 1. Phenylalanine levels in the developing rat brain after
subcutaneous injections of p-chlorophenylalanine and L-phenylalanine.

Age d	Time after 1st injection h	Concentration of phenyl- alanine (corrected for p-CPA) μmol/g wet brain
6-12	7-8 12 24	1.46 1.82 0.98
17-21 21	7-8 12 24 0	0.54 0.62 0.43 0.15

Values represent an average of 2-3 animals. See text for details
of the schedule of injections.

Although a simulation of phenylketonuria was induced during a
limited period of postnatal cerebral development, noticeable effects
on growth and myelin levels were still observed in the 35-day-old
animals. The experimental animals showed a decrease of approximately 24% in body weight, 18% in the weight of cerebral hemi-
shperes, and 31% in the weight of the cerebellum, but the weight
of the pons-medulla was normal (Table 3). Less myelin was formed
in the cerebral hemispheres (25%) and in the cerebellum (32%).
However, myelination in the medulla-pons was not affected (Table 4).

Table 2. Transport of aromatic acid metabolites of phenylalanine
into the developing rat brain after subcutaneous injections.

Age	Time after 1st injection	Concentration of metabolite in whole brain (nmol/g wet tissue)			
d	h	Phenyl-acetate	Phenyl-pyruvate	Phenyl-lactate	Mandelate
4-6	7	52			20
	12	180			22
	24	7			16
7-11	7	920	19	20	
	12	1390	36	46	
	24	9	22	17	
12-15	2	1660			
	4	920			
	7	730	20	16	15
	12	1070	32	17	20
	24	9	20	15	12
16-21	7	780	26	7	16
	12	1640	41	11	13
	24	9	20	6	8

All injections of the metabolites were given twice daily, 7-8
h apart, at the same dosage with the exception of mandelate, which
was given at half the amount of the others. Animals 4-6 d old
received 1.2 μmol/g; 6-15 d, 2.1; 16-21, 3.0. Phenylacetate was
not detected in the brain after the injection of phenylpyruvate,
but phenyllactate was found in low concentrations, ranging from
2-5 nmol/g.

Effects of the aromatic acids derived from phenylalanine.
The four metabolic products of phenylalanine that accumulate in
the brain of the preweanling, phenylketonuric rat are phenylacetate,
phenylpyruvate, phenyllactate, and mandelate, in decreasing order
of concentration (35). All four of these metabolites were transported into the brain of the young rat after peripheral injection.
Over a 12 h period after subcutaneous injection of approximately
the same dosage, phenylacetate concentration in the brain ranged
from 52-1660 nmol/g, phenylpyruvate, 20-40 nmol/g; and phenyllactate, 20-46 in the very young and 7-17 in the older animal.
Mandelate, administered at half the dosage of the other three
acids, reached levels of 13-22 nmol/g in the brain (Table 2).

No phenylacetate but small amounts of phenyllactate were
detected in the brain after peripheral injection of phenylpyruvate.

Of the four acids tested, only phenylacetate mimicked the
effects of p-CPA + L-Phe-treatment. A decrease of 29% in body
weight, 18% in the weight of the cerebral hemispheres, 27% in the
weight of the cerebellum, and 16% in the weight of the medulla-pons
was observed (Table 3). A marked deficit of myelin (Table 4) was
observed in the cerebral hemispheres (35%) and in the cerebellum
(28%), but a normal amount of myelin was found in the pons-medulla.

Composition of myelin. The yield of myelin purified from the
brains of 35 day old rats by the method of Norton (42) was quantitative and consistent, in accord with published results of other
investigators (16, 52). The usual criteria of purity (42) were
also satisfied. At least 95% of the dried myelin was soluble in
2:1 (v/v) chloroform:methanol. Total lipid content was 78-79%
and protein, 20-23%. The molar ratio of cholesterol:galactolipid
was approximately 1.8:1.

No differences were observed in the gross composition of the
myelin prepared from control, p-CPA + L-Phe, and phenylacetate
treated animals. Total cholesterol, total phospholipid, and total
galactolipid (Table 5) content was similar.

The total amount of each of the hydrogenated fatty acids, C-16,
C-18, C-20, C-22, C-24, and hydroxy C-24 in myelin preparations
from control and phenylacetate treated animals was also not significantly different (Table 6).

Table 3. Effect of hyperphenylalaninemia and phenylalanine metabolites on growth of the young rat.

Treatment	Body wt (g)	Brain area Wet wt. of tissue (g)		
		Cerebral hemispheres	Cerebellum	Medulla-pons
Saline or vehicle	147± 5 (18)	1.34±0.04 (18)	0.26±0.01 (18)	0.20±0.01 (18)
p-CPA + Phe	112±11 (16)+	1.10±0.05 (16)+	0.18±0.01 (16)+	0.19±0.008 (16)
Phenylacetate	104± 7 (16)+	1.10±0.03 (16)+	0.19±0.008(16)+	0.16±0.008 (16)+
Phenylpyruvate	147±11 (14)	1.27±0.04 (14)	0.24±0.01 (14)	0.19±0.004 (14)
Phenyllactate	156±12 (16)	1.28±0.03 (16)	0.24±0.005(16)	0.19±0.008 (16)
Mandelate	144± 7 (16)	1.32±0.04 (16)	0.25±0.01 (16)	0.19±0.005 (16)

Each value represents the mean ± S.D. of the number of animals or tissues shown in parentheses. +Differences between these groups and the controls are statistically significant, $p < 0.001–0.01$ (student's t-test, Fisher probability table). p-CPA, DL-p-chlorophenylalanine; Phe, L-phenylalanine.

Table 4. Effect of hyperphenylalaninemia and phenylalanine metabolites on myelination in different areas of the rat brain.

| | Brain area | | |
| Treatment | Cerebral hemispheres | Cerebellum | Medulla-pons |
	Wt. of dried myelin (mg/tissue)		
Saline or vehicle	28.0 ± 1.5 (7)	2.9 ± 0.3 (7)	10.6 ± 1.5 (4)
p-CPA + Phe	21.0 ± 1.2 (8)+	1.8 ± 0.2 (4)+	11.0 ± 1.6 (4)
Phenylacetate	18.2 ± 2.1 (8)+	2.1 ± 0.3 (5)+	9.4 ± 0.6 (4)
Phenylpyruvate	27.4 ± 1.0 (7)	2.8 ± 0.6 (6)	12.0 ± 1.9 (4)
Phenyllactate	25.4 ± 2.5 (4)	3.0 ± 0.3 (4)	10.3 ± 0.6 (4)
Mandelate	25.3 ± 1.3 (7)	2.8 ± 0.4 (4)	11.0 ± 1.4 (4)

Values represent the mean + S.D. of the number of preparations shown in parentheses.
+Differences between these groups and the controls are significant, p 0.001-0.01 (student's t-test, Fisher probability table). p-CPA, DL-p-chlorophenylalanine; Phe, L-phenylalanine.

Table 5. Gross composition of cerebral myelin from control and experimental rats.

Group	Total lipid (%)	Total protein (%)	Total cholesterol	Total galactolipids	Total phospholipids
			μmol/mg dried myelin		
Control	79 ±2.6	20.5±2.7	0.42±0.01	0.22±0.01	0.45±0.02
p-CPA + Phe	78.2±2	20.4±1.8	0.45±0.02	0.25±0.02	0.48±0.01
Phenylacetate	79 ±1.0	22.8±1.0	0.43±0.02	0.23±0.01	0.47±0.02

Each value represents the mean + S.D. of three samples of purified dried myelin from cerebral hemispheres of 35 d old rats. p-CPA, DL-p-chlorophenylalanine; Phe, L-phenylalanine. An average molecular weight of 387 for cholesterol, 848 for galactolipids, and 808 for phospholipids was used to calculate the molar concentrations.

Table 6. Hydrogenated fatty acids in cerebral myelin from control and phenylacetate treated rats.

Group	C-16	C-18	C-20	C-22	C-24	H-C-24
		Fatty acids (μmol/mg dry myelin)				
Control	0.11±0.009	0.37±0.008	0.093±0.005	0.086±0.006	0.059±0.002	0.054±0.003
Phenyl-acetate	0.12±0.005	0.37±0.009	0.10 ±0.01	0.093±0.004	0.057±0.001	0.053±0.001

Values represent the mean ± S.D. of three samples of purified myelin from cerebral hemispheres of 35-day-old rats. See text for details of procedures. H, hydroxy.

DISCUSSION

For many years, the question has persisted whether the brain damage that occurs in phenylketonuria is due to the extremely high levels of phenylalanine <u>per se</u>, or to the high concentrations of metabolic products. Of the four phenylalanine metabolites tested in this investigation, only phenylacetate produced the microcephaly and myelin deficit observed in phenylketonuria (11) and in hyperphenylalaninemia induced by p-CPA + Phe. It should be noted, however, that other biochemical changes as depressed serotonin and elevated phenylethylamine levels in the brain of the p-CPA + L-Phe treated animal (36) may also contribute to the deficiencies observed in this group. We should also point out that during the course of our experiments we have observed individual variations in response to phenylacetate treatment among animals in the same litter. Approximately 10% were much more severely affected while 2-5% were only slightly affected.

The myelin deficit and microcephaly appear to be closely related. It is of interest that in the medulla-pons, which exhibited either no change or only a slight decrease in weight (16%), the amount of myelin was normal. In the cerebral hemispheres and the cerebellum, where larger decrements of retarded growth occurred, a myelin deficit was observed. In the rat brain, myelin is formed at a rapid rate from the 15th - 30th postnatal day (3). Although phenylacetate was withdrawn on the 21st day, retarded growth and a deficiency of myelin were still evident in the 35-day-old rat. Whether the myelin deficiency is a result of hypomyelination or the presence of fewer axons is not clear at present. However, it is apparent that interruption by phenylacetate of a chronological sequence of biochemical events during the period of rapid development of the brain caused an irreversible arrest of brain development. A similar course of events following malnutrition during the critical period of postnatal development has been described by Winick (56). It is logical to deduce that in phenylketonuria, mental retardation is caused primarily by growth retardation during the critical period of CNS maturation.

In our experiments, rats were treated with the aromatic acid metabolites of phenylalanine in amounts approximating those found in untreated phenylketonuria. Phenylpyruvate levels in the blood of patients with classical phenylketonuria range from 20-120 nmol/ml (28). We were able to produce in the developing rat brain concentrations of phenylpyruvate in this range, 20-40 nmol/g, by subcutaneous injection of 1-3 μmol/g body wt. Since the urinary pattern of metabolites reflects the overall metabolic activity of the tissues, the dosage of phenylacetate and phenyllactate relative to that of phenylpyruvate was determined on this basis. Large variations in the urinary excretion of these compounds have been reported; the relative amounts were observed to depend in part on tissue levels of phenylalanine (5, 54). Quantitative analyses of

urine from 11 untreated patients fed the same diet revealed wide
variations in the amounts of the metabolites excreted as follows:
phenylpyruvate, 1-7 µmol/mg creatinine; phenylacetate, 1-6 µmol;
phenyllactate, 0.5-4 µmol; and mandelate, 0.02-0.17 µmol (36).
Since roughly similar amounts of phenylpyruvate, phenylacetate,
and phenyllactate are apparently produced by the tissues in phenylketonuria, we decided to test these compounds at the same dosage.
Calculated on this same basis, the dosage of mandelate should be
0.1 as much. We employed a large excess, 0.5 the dosage of the
others, in order to simulate phenyllactate concentrations in the
brain.

Peripheral administration of phenylpyruvate did not produce
detectable quantities of phenylacetate in the brain. This finding
supports the conclusion reached by other investigators (15) that
phenylethylamine is the major source of phenylacetate in the
tissues.

Clearly the noxious effects of phenylacetate are unique to
this metabolite and are not shared by the other aromatic acid
metabolites of phenylalanine, found in the brain in experimental
phenylketonuria. The unique properties of phenylacetate are its
very ready penetration into the developing brain of the young
animal and its metabolism to phenylacetylcoenzyme A (38).

Brain levels of phenylacetate were extremely high in contrast
to those of phenylpyruvate and phenyllactate, although equivalent
amounts of the three compounds were injected (Table 2). Phenylacetate was found to be uniformly distributed through the cerebral
hemispheres, the cerebellum, and the pons-medulla. On subcellular
fractionation of the whole brain, it was found mainly in the soluble supernatant fraction (unpublished results). We have no evidence for the synthesis of unstable myelin of abnormal composition
in the phenylacetate treated animals (Tables 5, 6). Rather, the
deficit of myelin appears to be closely tied to growth retardation
of the brain. Phenylacetate has been reported to inhibit the utilization of ketone bodies (4) which are known to be precursors of
fatty acids and of cholesterol synthesized in the developing brain
(14).

Although we have been mainly concerned with the effects of
phenylacetate on the developing brain, it should be emphasized
that other tissues of the young animal undoubtedly were affected
as well, since body growth was observed to be retarded. After
subcutaneous injection, the concentration of phenylacetate
(µmol/g) in other tissues as spleen, kidney, liver, heart, and
spinal cord was higher than that in the brain (unpublished results). Since no significant differences in body weight and brain
weight were observed between the control rats and those treated
with phenylpyruvate, phenyllactate and mandelate, the concentrations of these metabolites in peripheral tissues were not measured.

The primary biochemical action of phenylacetate may well be
interference with either the synthesis and/or the utilization of
acetyl CoA and acetoacetylCoA. As a consequence, ATP and energy

production would decline, and the biosynthesis of cholesterol and lipids required for the formation of myelin and other structural elements would be curtailed. The morphological and functional consequences of the growth retardation produced by phenylacetate during early development of the brain are under investigation.

Acknowledgements. This investigation was supported by the New York State Department of Mental Hygiene. The authors thank the Institute's staff for their cooperation, in particular, the Animal Colony staff. The authors acknowledge the support of a grant from the National Institute of Child Health and Human Development, HD 06843-02A2.

REFERENCES

1. Armstrong,M.D., Shaw, K.N.F. and Robinson, K.S., Studies on phenylketonuria. II. The excretion of o-hydroxyphenyl-acetic in phenylketonuria, J. biol. Chem. 213 (1955) 797-804.
2. Bartlett, G.R., Phosphorus assay in column chromatography, J. biol. Chem. 234 (1959) 466-468.
3. Bass, N.H., Netsky, M.G. and Young, E., Microchemical studies of postnatal development in rat cerebrum: Formation of myelin, Neurology 19 (1969) 405-414.
4. Benavides, J., Gimenez, C., Valdivieso, F. and Mayor, F., Effect of phenylalanine metabolites on the activities of enzymes of ketone-body utilization in brain of suckling rats, Biochem. J. 160 (1976) 217-222.
5. Blau, K., Aromatic acid excretion in phenylketonuria.Analysis of the unconjugated aromatic acids derived from phenyl-alanine, Clin. Chim. Acta 27 (1970) 5-18.
6. Boscott,R. J. and Bickel, H., Detection of some new abnormal metabolites in the urine of phenylketonuria, Scan. J. clin. lab. Invest. 5 (1953) 380-382.
7. Bowden, J.A., Dikeman, R.N., Helmer Jr., G. and Broussard, J., Phenylketonuria: The effect of phenylpyruvic acid on lipid biosynthesis in rat liver and brain, Fed. Proc. 33 (1974) 1525.
8. Chase, H.P. and O'Brien, D., Effect of excess phenylalanine and of other amino acids on brain development in the infant rat, Pediat. Res. 4 (1970) 96-102.
9. Clark, J.B. and Land, J.M., Differential effects of α-oxoacids on pyruvate utilization and fatty acid synthesis in rat brain, Biochem. J. (1974) 25-29.
10. Clarke, J.T.R. and Lowden, J.A., Hyperphenylalaninemia: Effect on the developing rat brain, Canad. J. Biochem. 47 (1969)
11. Crome, L., The morbid anatomy of phenylketonuria, in Phenyl-ketonuria and Some Other Inborn Errors of Amino Acid Metab-olism (H. Bickel, F.P. Hudson and L.I. Woolf, eds.), pp. 126-131, Georg Thieme Verlag, Stuttgart (1971).

12. Crome, L., Tymms, V. and Woolf, L.I., A chemical investigation of the defects of myelination in phenylketonuria, J. Neurol. Neurosurg. Psychiatry 25 (1962) 143-148.
13. Cumings, J., Grundt, I. and Yanagihara, T., Lipid changes in the brain in phenylketonuria, J. Neurol. Psychiatry 31 (1968) 334-337.
14. Edmond, J., Ketone bodies as precursors of sterols and fatty acids in the developing rat, J. biol. Chem. 249 (1974) 72-80.
15. Edwards, D.J. and Blau, K., Phenylethylamines in brain and liver of rats with experimentally induced phenylketonuria-like characteristics, Biochem. J. 132 (1973) 95-100.
16. Einstein, E.R., Protein and enzyme changes with brain development, in Advances in Behavioral Biology 8 (1974), Drugs and the Developing Brain (A. Vernadakis and N. Weiner, eds.) pp. 375-393, Plenum Press, New York.
17. Folch, J., Lees, M. and Sloane-Stanley, G.H., A simple method for the isolation and purification of total lipids from animal tissues, J. biol. Chem. 226 (1957) 497-509.
18. Foote, J.L., Allen, R.J. and Agranoff, B.W., Fatty acids in esters and cerebrosides of human brain in phenylketonuria, J. Lipid Res. 6 (1965) 518-523.
19. Foote, J.L. and Tao, R.V.P., The effects of p-chlorophenyl-alanine and phenylalanine on brain ester-bound fatty acids of developing rats, Life Sci. 7,Part II (1968) 1187-1192.
20. Gallagher, B.B., The effect of phenylpyruvate on oxidative-phosphorylation in brain mitochondria, J. Neurochem. 16 (1969) 1071-1076.
21. Gerstl, B., Malamud, N., Eng, L.F. and Hayman, R.B., Lipid alterations in human brains in phenylketonuria, Neurology 17 (1967) 51-57.
22. Glazer, R.I. and Weber, G., The effects of L-phenylalanine and phenylpyruvate on glycolysis in rat cerebral cortex, Brain Res. 33 (1971) 439-450.
23. Glick, D., Fell, B.F. and Sjølin, K-E.,Spectrophotometric determination of nanogram amounts of total cholesterol in microgram quantities of tissue or microliter volumes of serum, Analyt. Chem. 36 (1964) 1119-1121.
24. Grundt, I.K. and Hole, K., p-Chlorophenylalanine treatment in developing rats: Protein and lipids in whole brain and myelin, Brain Res. 74 (1974) 269-277.
25. Hess, H.H. and Lewin, E., Microassay of biochemical structural components in nervous tissues - II. Methods for cerebrosides, proteolipid proteins and residue proteins, J. Neurochem. 12 (1965) 205-211.
26. Jervis, G.A., Studies on phenylpyruvic oligophrenia. The position of the metabolic error, J. biol. Chem. 169 (1974) 651-656.
27. Jervis, G.A., Excretion of phenylalanine and derivatives in phenylpyruvic oligophrenia, Proc. Soc. exp. Biol. Med. 75 (1950) 83-86.

28. Jervis, G.A. and Drejza, E.J., Phenylketonuria: Rlood levels
     of phenylpyruvic and o-hydroxyphenylacetic acids, Clin. Chim.
     Acta 13 (1966) 435-441.
29. Johnson, R.C. and Shah, S.N., Effect of hyperphenylalaninemia
     on fatty acid composition of lipids of rat brain myelin, J.
     Neurochem. 21 (1973) 1225-1240.
30. Johnson, R.C., McKean, C.M. and Shah, S.N., Fatty acid compo-
     sition of lipids in cerebral myelin and synaptosomes in phenyl-
     ketonuria and Down syndrome, Arch. Neurol. 34 (1977) 288-294.
31. Land, J.M. and Clark, J.B., Effect of phenylpyruvate on
     enzymes involved in fatty acid synthesis in rat brain,
     Biochem. J. 134 (1973) 545-555.
32. Land, J.M. and Clark, J.B., Inhibition of pyruvate and β-
     hydroxybutyrate oxidation in rat brain mitochondria by phenyl-
     pyruvate and α-ketoisocaproate, FEBS Letters 44 (1974) 348-
     351.
33. Land, J.M., Mowbray, J. and Clark, J.B., Control of pyruvate
     and β-hydroxybutyrate utilization in rat brain mitochondria
     and its relevance to phenylketonuria and maple syrup urine
     disease, J. Neurochem. 26 (1976) 823-830.
34. Loo, Y.H., Scotto, L. and Horning, M.G., Gas chromatographic
     determination of aromatic acid metabolites of phenylalanine
     in brain, Analyt. Biochem. 76 (1976) 111-118.
35. Loo, Y.H., Scotto, L. and Horning, M.G., Aromatic acid metabo-
     lites of phenylalanine in the brain of the hyperphenylala-
     ninemic rat: Effect of pyridoxamine, J. Neurochem. (1977)
     in press.
36. Loo, Y.H., Jervis, G.A. and Horning, M.G., Possible role of
     β-phenylethylamine in the pathology of the central nervous
     system, in Phenylethylamine: Biological Mechanisms and Clinical
     Aspects (A.D. Mosnaim, ed.), Marcel Dekker, New York (1977)
     in press.
37. Lowry, O.H., Rosebrough, N.J., Farr, A.L. and Randall, R.J.,
     Protein measurement with the Folin phenol reagent, J. biol.
     Chem. 193 (1951) 265-275.
38. Mahler, H.R. and Wakil, S.J., Studies on fatty acid oxidation.
     1. Enzymatic activation of fatty acids, J. biol. Chem. 204
     (1953) 453-467.
39. McCaman, M.W. and Robins, E., Fluorimetric method for the
     determination of phenylalanine in serum, J. lab. clin. Med.
     59 (1962) 885-890.
40. Menkes, J.H., Cerebral lipids in phenylketonuria, Pediatrics
     37 (1966) 967-978.
41. Menkes, J.H., Cerebral proteolipids in phenylketonuria,
     Neurology 18 (1968) 1003-1008.
42. Norton, W.T., Recent developments in the investigation of
     purified myelin, in Adv. in exp. Medicine Biology 13 (1971),
     Chemistry and Brain Development (R. Paoletti and A.N. Davison,
     eds.) Plenum Press, New York, pp. 327-337.

43. Oates, J.A., Nirenberg, P.Z., Jepsin, J.B., Sjoerdsma, A. and Udenfriend, S., Conversion of phenylalanine to phenylethylamine in patients with phenylketonuria, Proc. Soc. exp. Biol. Med. 112 (1963) 1078-1081.

44. Patel, M.S., Grover, W.D. and Auerbach, V.H., Pyruvate metabolism by homogenates of human brain: Effects of phenylpyruvate and implications for the etiology of the mental retardation in phenylketonuria, J. Neurochem. 20 (1973) 289-296.

45. Patel, M.S. and Owen, O.E., Effect of hyperphenylalaninemia on lipid synthesis from ketone bodies by rat brain, Biochem. J. 154 (1976) 319-325.

46. Perry, T.L., Urinary excretion of amines in phenylketonuria and mongolism, Science 136 (1962) 879-880.

47. Prensky, A.L., Carr, S. and Moser, H.W., Development of myelin in inherited disorders of amino acid metabolism, Arch. Neurol. 19 (1968) 552-558.

48. Prensky, A.L., Fishman, M.A. and Daftari, B., Differential effects of hyperphenylalaninemia on the development of the brain in the rat, Brain Res. 33 (1971) 181-191.

49. Shah, S.N., Peterson, N.A. and McKean, C.M., Inhibition of sterol synthesis in vitro by metabolites of phenylalanine, Biochim. Biophys. Acta 187 (1969) 236-242.

50. Shah, S.N., Peterson, N.A. and McKean, C.M., Impaired myelin formation in experimental hyperphenylalaninemia, J. Neurochem. 19 (1972) 479-485.

51. Shah, S.N., Peterson, N.A. and McKean, C.M., Lipid composition of human cerebral white matter and myelin in phenylketonuria, J. Neurochem. 19 (1972) 2369-2376.

52. Suzuki, K., Poduslo, S.E. and Norton, W.T., Gangliosides in the myelin fraction of developing rats, Biochim. Biophys. Acta 144 (1967) 375-381.

53. Svennerholm, L., The quantitative estimation of cerebrosides in nervous tissue, J. Neurochem. 1 (1956) 42-53.

54. Wadman, S.K., vanSprang, F.J., van der Heiden, C. and Ketting, D., Quantitation of urinary phenylalanine metabolites in phenylketonuria, in Phenylketonuria (H. Bickel, F.P. Hudson and L.T. Woolf, eds.), pp. 65-72, G.T. Verlag, Stuttgart (1971).

55. Weber, G., Inhibition of human brain pyruvate kinase and hexokinase by phenylalanine and phenylpyruvate: Possible relevance to phenylketonuric brain damage, Proc. Natl. Acad. Sci. (USA) 63 (1969) 1365-1369.

56. Winick, M., Nutrition and mental development, Medical Clinics of North America 54 (1970) 1413-1429.

57. Woolf, L.I., Myelin deficiencies related to inborn errors of human metabolism, in Myelination (A.N. Davison and A. Peters, eds.), pp. 183-190, C.C. Thomas, Springfield, IL (1970).

PERIPHERAL NERVES AS TARGET TISSUE OF THE IMMUNE RESPONSE IN EAN.

A NEUROCHEMICAL AND MORPHOLOGICAL STUDY

G.K. Molnár and P.J. Riekkinen

Departments of Neurology and Medical Microbiology,
    University of Turku
Turku, Finland

SUMMARY

The final steps of immune response against the peripheral nerve myelin, the target tissue in EAN, are incompletely known. To find out whether the target tissue is intact or worked up before the arrival of sensitized lympocytes into the venules of the nerve roots the activities of acid proteinase and acid phosphatase were determined in pieces taken from different sites of nerves supplying the muscles of forelimbs and hindlegs of rabbits. The samples were taken daily from the day before the manifestation of clinical signs of the disease to the third day after the day when the experimental animals seemed to become ill and every second day thereafter. The total observation period was 15 days. For the neurochemical data light microscopical references were used. There was a clear-cut increase in the activity of acid proteinase in the nerve roots during the first three days of observation. The morphological findings, the increase of macrophages and demyelination, were in good correlation with the increase of acid proteinase in the same area but also with the progress of the clinical signs. The increase of acid phosphatase activity was less marked and did not follow the proximodistal distribution observed in the morphological changes and in the acid proteinase activity. The results of the study give us data for the timetable of the different events during the acute stage of EAN but our original question still remains without answer.

INTRODUCTION

The idea that the peripheral nerve is the primary lesion site in Guillain-Barré syndrome (GBS) has been presented on several occasions. Already Waksman and Adams (7) and later others have

described the histopathology of experimental allergic neuritis
(EAN), which serves as a model for GBS, and it is well known that
the histopathological pictures of these two conditions are quite
similar. In general, EAN is produced in experimental animals with
a supposedly intact nervous system.

While it seems to be clear that the crucial point in mediating
the disease is either the production of lymphocytes sensitized to
an antigenic protein from the peripheral nervous system or a sufficient increase in their number, one further question deserves
special interest: How can a sensitized lymphocyte, traveling in
a venule within the peripheral nerve, recognize an important target
tissue on the other side of the vascular endothelium? This question
has already been discussed (1) and a very simple explanation may
exist: There may be a minimal stream or leak of the antigenic protein - or protein which has a similar antigenic determinant as the
antigenic protein - through the walls of the venule. But is this
phenomenon physiological or is it a consequence of the underlying
immune response? In other words: Is the target tissue intact or is
it already worked up when the sensitized lymphocyte arrives in the
venule of the target tissue?

The purpose of the present work was to illuminate this question
by studying the activity of lysosomal hydrolases in the target
tissue before, during and soon after the manifestation of the
clinical signs of EAN in rabbits.

EXPERIMENTAL

EAN was produced by a conventional method. The antigen was
human whole nerve in complete Freund's adjuvant. More than half of
the experimental animals had the first and well-known symptoms of
the disease on the 12th day after the inoculation of the antigen.
The disease was most severe in the animals which became ill earlier,
and the symptoms appeared to increase to their maximum within 2-3
days after the onset. At that stage they were totally unable to
move forward, the function of the sphincters was lost, and considerable dyspnoe was apparent.

Various groups of animals were chosen to represent the different stages of the pathogenesis and samples from the nerve roots,
spinal nerves and three different sites of the sciatic nerve were
taken on the day when the first signs of the disease manifested
(0-day), 1 day before it (-1 day), and several days after it (+1,
+2, +3, +5, +7 and +9).

The specific activity of acid proteinase (pH 3.6) (EC 3.4)
and p-nitrophenylphosphatase (pH 4.8) (EC 3.1.3.3.) was determined
by the method described by Riekkinen and Clausen (6) in the whole
nerve homogenate in water. Total protein was measured by the
method of Lowry et al. (4) using L-tyrosine as a standard.

For the light microscopy the nerve pieces were fixed in neutral

buffered formalin, embedded into gelatin blocks and the frozen
sections were stained with a myelin staining method (Luxol fast blue)
originally described by Klüver and Barrera (5). The counterstain
was neutral red.

RESULTS

Morphology. The purpose of this part of the study was to
serve as a morphological reference for the neurochemical results.
In general, the distribution and nature of the histopathological
changes agreed with the earlier description of the histopathology
of EAN in rabbits (1). However, it was possible to distinguish
three types of foci which differed from each other in regard to the
cell composition and demyelination. In addition, a certain quantitative relation in the occurrence of the foci in different stages
of the pathogenesis was characteristic to some extent. The three
types presumably represented different consecutive ages of the foci.
The three types of foci were as follows: 1. Acute foci were
characterized by perivenular cellular infiltrations with blast
cells, lymphocytes and polymorphonuclear leucocytes some of which
seemed to phagocytize myelin. 2. The predominating cell type
during the subacute stage was the macrophage which could occasionally
be the only cell type encountered in a distinctly demyelinating
focus. 3. Typical feature of the chronic phase was the proliferation
of Schwann cells.
The number of acute and especially subacute lesions increased
during the days around the manifestation of the clinical signs of
the disease. On the third day after this critical moment the number
of subacute foci with macrophages and massive demyelination, especially in the nerve roots, reached the maximum and thereafter the
picture became more diffuse. When the clinical signs of the disease
had been visible for 5-7 days a new period could be established
during which acute and subacute foci occurred simultaneously. Proliferating Schwann cells could not be seen before 5-7 days of the
manifested EAN. Proliferation of Schwann cells, coinciding with a
few acute foci, could be observed on the 7th to 9th day after the
onset of clinical symptoms.
Enzyme activities. Comparison between the enzyme activities
of EAN and control animals is presented in Fig. 1. An example of
the absolute specific activities of acid proteinase is given in
Table 1. The nerve root area showed the most marked changes so
that even before the onset of the clinical symptoms the enzyme activity was about 50% higher than that in the controls. On the day
of onset the percentage was about 80 and after that the activity
increased in a linear fashion until the 3rd day on which it was
3.5-fold higher than the normal value. The activity then decreased
conspicuously until the 9th day. In the more distal parts of the

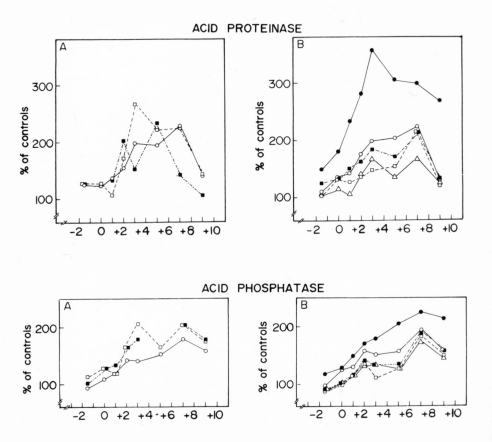

Fig. 1. Enzyme activity changes in various parts of the peripheral
nerves of the rabbit during the pathogenesis of EAN (time points
-1, 0, +1, +2, +3, +5, +7 and +9 days). The results are expressed
as percents of the enzyme activities in corresponding anatomical
structures of normal rabbits. Figures A represent the nerves of
forelimbs and figures B those of hindlegs. The individual anatomical
structures are as follows: nerve roots ●————●, spinal nerves
○————○, proximal parts of the sciatic nerve or cord of the
brachial plexus ■—·—·—■ , medial parts of the sciatic nerve or
median nerves of forelimbs □— — — —□ , and distal parts of the
sciatic nerve △————△.

Table 1. Specific activities of acid proteinase (nmoles/mg protein/h) in samples collected from peripheral nerves of hindlegs of the rabbits 3 days after the manifestation of the clinical signs of EAN.

Anatomical site	Enzyme activity $\pm$ SEM		
	EAN	Controls	
		Normal	FCA
Nerve root	302.71$\pm$22.82***	83.29$\pm$ 8.16	73.67$\pm$26.76
Spinal nerve	239.00$\pm$29.73***	112.57$\pm$ 9.92	95.00$\pm$ 6.12
Proximal part of the sciatic nerve	160.50$\pm$18.42*	109.00$\pm$ 9.32	88.75$\pm$12.33
Middle part of the sciatic nerve	173.63$\pm$26.61**	94.25$\pm$ 7.45	74.25$\pm$10.23
Distal part of the sciatic nerve	184.17$\pm$28.77*	110.86$\pm$10.75	88.00$\pm$16.26

  *when compared with normal $p < 0.05$
  **when compared with normal $p < 0.01$
***when compared with normal $p < 0.001$

Table 2. Specific activities of p-nitrophenylphosphatase (nmoles/mg protein/min) in samples collected from peripheral nerves of hindlegs of the rabbits 3 days after the manifestation of the clinical signs of EAN.

Anatomical site	Enzyme activity $\pm$ SEM		
	EAN	Controls	
		Normal	FCA
Nerve root	10.50$\pm$1.07***	5.24$\pm$0.55	3.9$\pm$0.61
Spinal nerve	9.33$\pm$0.73**	6.13$\pm$0.57	4.70$\pm$0.16
Proximal part of the sciatic nerve	6.78$\pm$1.42	6.18$\pm$0.74	4.55$\pm$0.35
Middle part of the sciatic nerve	7.28$\pm$0.83	5.46$\pm$0.68	3.38$\pm$0.56*
Distal part of the sciatic nerve	8.18$\pm$0.50*	6.09$\pm$0.68	4.57$\pm$0.67

  *when compared with normal $p < 0.05$
  **when compared with normal $p < 0.01$
***when compared with normal $p < 0.001$

peripheral nerve the increase was less apparent. No other differences between the proximal and distal parts could be demonstrated,
only in the spinal nerves of the lumbar segments the activity appeared to be higher than in the more distal parts. The first significant changes appeared on the 2nd and 3rd day after the onset of
the symptoms in the main nerve trunks of both anterior and posterior
extremities.   The maximum changes, about 50% higher activities
than in the controls, declined on the 5th to 7th day, i.e. slightly
later than in the nerve roots. Even here the activity began to
decrease 9 days after the onset of the symptoms.

An example of the absolute specific activities of acid phosphatase is given in Table 2. At the onset of the clinical symptoms
the activity was not significantly higher than in the controls.
The differences became significant two days after the onset and
appeared to be of similar intensity in posterior and anterior extremities. The highest enzyme activities were found in the rabbits
which were sacrificed 7 days after the onset of the symptoms. No
significant differences between the enzyme activities in various
parts of the nerves could be demonstrated during the observation
period.

                              DISCUSSION

The evolution of a target tissue lesion as a result of an inflammatory process is a highly complex event. The origin of enzyme
activities in the tissue homogenates may be normal endogenic,
pathological endogenic and pathological exogenic. The increase of
acid proteinase activity had the best correlation with the amount
of inflammatory cell infiltration and demyelination. Macrophages
seem to be the most potent source of exogenic enzyme activity in
these processes (7). The correlation was so evident that the role
of endogenic proteinase, emphasized in Wallerian degeneration (2,
5), seems to be of minor importance during the first few days of
the pathogenesis of EAN. If the second peak in the activity curve
of this enzyme in the nerve root area reflects the same process
seen in the morphological study, namely a new period of acute and
subacute foci in the target tissue, the observation is the first
biochemical evidence that the nature of this disease is not mono-
phasic.

Although both acid proteinase and acid phosphatase are lysosomal
hydrolases, their patterns differed from each other especially in
the area of nerve roots. The increase in the activity of acid
phosphatase was slower and not as high as in the activity of acid
proteinase. These findings suggest that their origin or function
in this experimental model might be partly different. However,
the original problem still remains obscure and more specific methods
are needed before the pathogenesis of EAN is clarified.

REFERENCES

1. Åström, K.E., Webster, H. de F. and Arnason, B.G., The initial
   lesion in experimental allergic neuritis. A phase and electron
   microscopic study, J. Exp. Med. 128 (1968) 469-485.
2. Hallpike, J.F. and Adams, G.W.M., Proteolysis and myelin breakdown. A review of recent histochemical and biochemical studies,
   Histochem. J. 1 (1969) 559-578.
3. Klüver, H. and Barrera, E., Method for combined staining of
   cell fibers in nervous system, J. Neuropath. Exp. Neurol, 12
   (1953) 400-403.
4. Lowry, O.H., Rosebrough, N.J., Farr, A.L. and Randall, R.J.,
   Protein measurement with the Folin phenol reagent, J. Biol.
   Chem. 193 (1951) 265-275.
5. Porcellati, G., Studies on proteinase enzymes during Wallerian
   degeneration, in Protein metabolism of the nervous system
   A. Lajtha, ed.) Plenum Press, New York (1970) pp. 601-620.
6. Riekkinen, P.J. and Clausen, J., Proteinase activity of myelin,
   Brain Res. 15 (1969) 413-430.
7. Steinman, R.M. and Cohn, Z.A., The metabolism and physiology
   of the mononuclear phagocytes, in Inflammatory process I
   (B.W. Zweifach, L. Grant and R.T. McCluskey, eds.) Academic
   Press, New York (1974) pp. 450-510.
8. Waksman, B.H. and Adams, R.D., Allergic neuritis: An experimental disease of rabbits induced by the injection of peripheral nervous tissue and adjuvants, J. Exp. Med. 102 (1955)
   213-235.

BIOCHEMICAL STUDIES OF CNS AND PNS IN HUMAN AND EXPERIMENTAL DIABETES

J. Palo, Edith Reske-Nielsen[*] and P. Riekkinen[**]

Department of Neurology, University of Helsinki, Finland
[*]Department of Neuropathology, Aarhus University School
of Medicine, Denmark, and
[**]Third Clinical Institute of Medicine/Neurology
University of Turku, Finland

SUMMARY

Neuropathological evidence of encephalopathy and neuropathy has been found in all autopsied patients with long-term juvenile diabetes. Earlier biochemical studies of human post mortem specimens indicated extensive biochemical damage of the diabetic peripheral nerve but not of the brain. The activities of acid proteinase and phosphatase, β-glucosidase, β-glucosaminidase, glucose-6-phosphatase, succinyl dehydrogenase (SDH), and 2',3'-cyclic nucleotide-3'-phosphohydrolase (CNP) were now measured from the brain homogenates of rats made diabetic with streptozotocin at the age of 1 month and killed after 1, 3, 6 and 15 months. The activities of acid proteinase and β-glucosidase decreased and that of SDH increased at the beginning of the experiment. A slight increase of acid phosphatase was noted at the end and a slight decrease of β-glucosaminidase at the beginning. The activities of SDH and CNP increased throughout the experiment both in the diabetic and control animals, probably due to maturation. In general, experimental streptozotocin diabetes induced few, transient and not very significant changes in enzymes known to be connected with myelination and demyelination in the CNS. The findings agree with those obtained previously for human diabetic specimens.

INTRODUCTION

Neuropathological studies of the central nervous system (CNS) of autopsied diabetic patients have been conducted for years at the

Department of Neuropathology, Aarhus University School of Medicine.
In a series of 47 patients with long-term juvenile diabetes narrowed brain cortex and enlarged ventricular system, both due to
neuronal loss, were observed (7). In addition, pseudocalcinosis
of the vessels in the globus pallidus and severe degeneration of
the dentate nucleus of the cerebellum were common findings. The
vessel alterations often caused typical malacia with phagocyte and
lymphocyte accumulation. The other findings included selective
degeneration and loss of myelin sheaths in the posterior column of
the spinal cord, severe demyelination of the spinal roots and
peripheral nerve, and neurogenic atrophy of the striated muscle.
These changes in the CNS and peripheral nervous system (PNS) seem
to be the result of juvenile diabetes and develop together with
pathological process in the blood vessels but they can be found
already before angiopathy.

A biochemical investigation was recently carried out on <u>post</u>
<u>mortem</u> CNS and PNS specimens taken from diabetic patients (5).
The activities of four enzymes, acid and neutral proteinase, β-
glucuronidase and CNP were largely normal in the brain gray and
white matter but appeared increased in the sciatic nerve of diabetic
patients. The amount of total protein was decreased in the diabetic
PNS myelin. The basic proteins of PNS myelin also appeared decreased
in a number of diabetic patients. On the basis of these findings
it was suggested that extensive biochemical damage occurs in the
peripheral nerve in diabetes.

The purpose of the present study was to compare biochemical
findings possibly observed in experimental diabetes of the rat to
those reported previously for human patients who died from clinical
diabetes. It was also of interest to investigate whether the findings showed any similarity to those reported for MS (see for example
ref. 1).

EXPERIMENTAL

Experimental diabetes was produced in male Sprague-Dawley-rats
by giving streptozotocin injections into the tail vein. The first
injection, 60 mg/kg, was given at the age of 1 month and the second
injection, 40 mg/kg, at 1.5 months. At 2 weeks after the first injection the blood glucose level ranged from 6.0 to 7.9 mM/l, and 2
weeks after the second injection from 7.8 to 21.9 mM/l with a mean
($\pm$S.E.M.) at 12.4$\pm$3.43 mM/l. The normal level in healthy rats is
4.0 mM/l. After that, glucosuria was controlled with Clinistix^{R}.
Blood glucose was measured from the oldest group of diabetic animals
again after 15 months. It ranged from 4.1 to 6.9 mM/l indicating
at least partial recovery of the animals. The control group received
no injections. Both groups lived in the same conditions and were
given the same standard laboratory diet.

The experimental and control animals were killed by decapitation in groups of ten at 1, 3, 6 and 15 months after the induction of diabetes. The brains were removed immediately and frozen at -22°C. Small pieces of the brain and sciatic nerve were also fixed with glutaraldehyde-osmium tetroxide for future morphological studies. The activities of acid proteinase (pH 3.6), acid phosphatase, β-glucosidase, β-glucosaminidase, glucose-6-phosphatase (8), SDH (2) and CNP (3) were measured from total brain homogenates. No attempt was made to separate gray and white matter from each other as was done previously for human brains (5).

RESULTS

The weights of the diabetic animals remained at the same level as those of the controls (Table 1) with rather great individual variations. The greatest differences in the activities of the various enzymes between the two groups were measured at the beginning of the experiment. The activities of acid proteinase and β-glucosidase were decreased and the activity of SDH was increased in the diabetic animals (Tables 2 and 3). However, the differences were not highly significant ($P < 0.01$). The activity of acid phosphatase was slightly increased ($P < 0.05$) at the end of the experiment, and β-glucosaminidase slightly decreased ($P < 0.05$) at the beginning. It is interesting to note that the activity of acid proteinase was low in the diabetic brain still at 3 months but reached the control level by the end of the experiment. Furthermore, SDH appeared high at 15 months, after being at the normal level at 3 and 6 months.

Table 1. Weights of the diabetic and control rats (grams $\pm$ SEM). The number of animals in each group is given in parentheses.

Duration of diabetes	Diabetic	Control
1 month	240 ± 29 (10)	228 ± 16 (10)
3 months	321 ± 55 (10)	304 ± 45 (10)
6 months	387 ± 50 (10)	414 ± 45 (10)
15 months	452 ± 35 (10)	458 ± 43 (10)

Table 2. The activities of acid proteinase, acid phosphatase, β-glucosidase and β-glucosaminidase in the brains of diabetic and control rats. The number of animals in each group is given in parentheses.

Duration of diabetes	ENZYME							
	Acid proteinase (nM/mg protein/min)		Acid phosphatase (nM/mg protein/min)		β-glucosidase (nM/mg protein/h)		β-glucosaminidase (nM/mg protein/min)	
	Diabetic	Control	Diabetic	Control	Diabetic	Control	Diabetic	Control
1 month	3.81±0.27** (10)	4.17±0.32 (10)	46.7±1.25 (10)	47.2±2.25 (10)	42.7±3.01** (10)	45.8±1.30 (10)	10.4±0.34* (10)	10.8±0.61 (10)
3 months	3.27±0.36* (10)	3.63±0.29 (10)	37.7±1.28 (10)	36.9±1.07 (10)	44.3±3.39 (9)	45.2±2.03 (10)	9.22±0.41 (10)	9.17±0.30 (10)
6 months	3.97±0.19 (10)	4.17±0.33 (10)	47.3±1.46 (10)	47.1±2.02 (10)	51.7±2.50 (10)	50.3±2.39 (10)	9.81±0.40 (10)	10.2±0.44 (10)
15 months	5.19±0.39 (8)	5.04±0.28 (10)	52.3±1.39* (8)	49.9±2.22 (10)	41.3±0.70 (8)	42.5±2.00 (10)	10.2±0.60 (8)	10.5±0.63 (10)

*p $<$ 0.05
**p $<$ 0.01

Table 3. The activities of glucose-6-phosphatase, SDH and CNP in the brains of diabetic and control rats. The number of animals in each group is given in parentheses.

Duration of diabetes	Glucose-6-phosphatase (nM/mg protein/min)		ENZYME SDH (nM/mg protein/min)		CNP (U/mg protein)	
	Diabetic	Control	Diabetic	Control	Diabetic	Control
1 month	2.45+0.26 (10)	2.38+0.39 (9)	72.8+9.36** (10)	61.6+4.05 (10)	3.75+0.17 (4)	3.70+0.08 (4)
3 months	2.30+0.25 (10)	2.44+0.13 (10)	96.5+8.48 (10)	99.4+10.1 (10)	3.95+0.17 (4)	4.03+0.10 (4)
6 months	2.31+0.24 (10)	2.31+0.22 (10)	198+4.73 (10)	203+10.9 (10)	4.28+0.22 (4)	4.50+0.24 (4)
15 months	2.54+0.34 (8)	2.61+0.31 (10)	239+12.6* (7)	222+9.47 (9)	5.03+0.30 (7)	5.04+0.27 (8)

*p $<$ 0.05
**p $<$ 0.01

In general, the activities of most enzymes remained rather
stable throughout the experiment. The most marked changes in the
controls were observed in SDH with an increase from 61.6 ± 4.05 to
222 ± 9.47 nM/mg protein/min, and in CNP with an increase from $3.70\pm$
0.08 to 5.04 ± 0.27 U/mg protein. These changes were most probably
due to the increasing age and maturation of the animals.

DISCUSSION

Alloxan is the best known agent to induce experimental diabetes.
A number of neurophysiological and neuropathological studies have
documented its effect on the peripheral nerve where it causes, for
example, segmental demyelination and axonal abnormalities. In an
electron microscopic study of the alloxan diabetic neuropathy
demyelination and remyelination, axonal degeneration and regenera-
tion as well as onion bulb formation by proliferated Schwann cells
were found in rats rendered diabetic two years before sacrifice (6).
In another study on the PNS of rats made diabetic by streptozotocin
and alloxan no morphological changes were seen after 6 months to 1
year after the beginning of the experiment (9). The present investigation was more concerned with the CNS which has received
little attention in studies of experimental diabetes. It is also
difficult to carry out biochemical investigations on very small
quantities of nervous tissue, as in the case of the rat sciatic
nerve.

A marked hyperglycaemia was induced in the animals after the
second streptozotocin injection but the blood glucose level approached normal by the end of the experiment. Because all experimental animals were already diabetic at the age of 1.5 months
(blood glucose ≥ 6.0 mM/l) and the condition became worse after the
second injection (blood glucose ≥ 7.8 mM/l) it is obvious that the
data obtained at 1 month and 3 months represent values characteristic
of diabetic metabolism. Although the diabetic rats excreted glucose
throughout the experiment the level of blood glucose is not known
at 6 months. However, the results obtained at 15 months indicate
that the condition of the animals improved considerably with time.
This finding warrants careful monitoring of the glucose and insulin
metabolism in future experiments.

Increased proteinase activities have been measured at the
borders of MS plaques (1). The activity of acid proteinase appeared slightly increased in the brain white matter of a series of
diabetic patients but it was not increased in the gray matter (5).
Since neutral proteinase was normal it was concluded that the
proteinase activities are not significantly increased in diabetes
and that there is considerable overlapping between the diabetic
and control patients. The activity of acid proteinase was even
lower in the diabetic rats than in the controls of the present
study and the difference was still seen after 3 months. In both

groups of animals the activity remained essentially unchanged with increasing age thus confirming the result of an earlier study on guinea-pigs (2). The activity of acid phosphatase also remained on the same level in both groups.

Despite slightly decreased activities at 1 month both β-glucosidase and β-glucosaminidase remained essentially unchanged throughout the experiment. The same applies to glucose-6-phosphatase which, at least in the cerebellum of the rat, is known to reach its maximum activity already on the 8th postnatal day of life (4). The absence of developmental changes in these three enzymes may therefore be due to the fact that the first measurements were carried out at the age of 2 months when the most dramatic maturational changes had already disappeared. The activities of SDH and CNP are known to increase parallel to myelination (2, 10) and this was also observed in the present study. Because SDH is connected with oxidative mitochondrial activity experimental diabetes appears to stimulate this activity.

It can be concluded that experimental streptozotocin diabetes induced few, transient and not very significant changes in enzymes known to be connected with myelination and clinical demyelination in the CNS. These findings agree with those obtained previously for diabetic human patients whose greatest biochemical changes were found in the PNS (5). They also give indirect support to the role of inflammatory cells which are present in the demyelinated CNS areas of MS patients but absent in diabetics with the exception of malacia areas (7). It is unkown why the PNS appears so much more vulnerable to diabetes than the CNS although its resistance and good recovery is well documented in many other neurological conditions.

Acknowledgements. We thank Mrs Leena Lehikoinen, Miss Kaarina Lindberg and Mrs Leena Sajama for technical assistance, and the National Research Council for Medical Sciences for financial support.

REFERENCES

1. Einstein, E.R., Dalal, K.B. and Csejtey, J., Increased protease activity and changes in basic proteins and lipids in multiple sclerosis plaques, J. neurol. Sci. 11 (1970) 109-121.
2. Frey, H., Enzymes of central nervous system myelin with special reference to maturation. An experimental study on guinea-pigs, Doctoral thesis, University of Turku 1971.
3. Kurihara, T. and Tsukada, Y., The regional and subcellular distribution of 2',3'-cyclic nucleotide-3'-phosphohydrolase in the central nervous system, J. Neurochem. 14 (1967) 1167-1174.
4. Lehrer, G.M. and Bornstein, M.B., Carbohydrate matabolism of the developing brain in vivo and in vitro, in Abstracts of the International Neurochemical Conference, Oxford (1965) p. 68.

5. Palo, J., Reske-Nielsen, E. and Riekkinen, P., Enzyme and pro-
    tein studies of demyelination in diabetes, J. neurol. Sci. 33
    (1977) 171-178.
6. Powell, H., Knox, D., Lee, S., Charters, A.C., Orloff, M.,
    Garrett, R. and Lampert, P., Alloxan diabetic neuropathy:
    Electron microscopic studies, Neurology 27 (1977) 60-66.
7. Reske-Nielsen, E., Pathology of the nervous system in diabetes,
    Meeting of the Scandinavian Diabetes Society, Aarhus 1973.
8. Riekkinen, P. and Clausen, J., Proteinase activity of myelin,
    Brain Res. 15 (1969) 413-430.
9. Sharma, A.K. and Thomas, P.K., Peripheral nerve structure and
    function in experimental diabetes, J. neurol. Sci. 23 (1974)
    1-15.
10. Yonezawa, T., Bornstein, M.B., Peterson, E.R. and Murray, M.R.,
    A histochemical study of oxidative enzymes in myelinating
    cultures of central and peripheral nervous tissue, J. Neuro-
    path. exp. Neurol. 21 (1962) 479-487.

THE EFFECT OF INTOXICATION WITH ALKYLNITROSOUREA DERIVATIVES ON CEREBRAL MYELIN*

M. Wender, Z. Adamczewska-Goncerzewicz, O. Mularek and
B. Zgorzalewicz

Department of Neurology, Medical Academy
Poznań, Poland

SUMMARY

Adult BD IX rats were injected with methylnitrosourea and pregnant mice on the 15th day of gestation with a single intravenous dose of ethylnitrosourea. The cerebral myelin fraction of adult BD IX rats and of the mice offsprings was studied.

It was found that a part of the rats intoxicated with methylnitrosourea developed spongious changes in the cerebral and cerebellar white matter. The myelin fraction of intoxicated rats also showed severe losses of sphingomyelin with a steady increase in the cholesterol ester content. The myelin fraction from mice intoxicated during the foetal development appeared deficient with respect to galactolipids and plasmalogen. It is concluded that, besides the carcinogenic effect, alkylnitrosourea derivatives effectively disturb the lipid metabolism of membrane structures of the central nervous system.

INTRODUCTION

Studies of the biological effects of alkylnitrosourea derivatives have been concerned mainly with their direct or indirect carcinogenic action, predominantly in the nervous system. Some experimental studies have disclosed also other effects of alkylnitrosoureas on the metabolism and structure of the nervous system. The studies of Kroh (3, 4) have shown that ethylnitrosourea (ENU)

*This investigation was supported by the Polish Academy of Sciences (No. 10.4.2.02.3.3.).

affects the cerebral white matter of litter mice also when administered to their pregnant mothers. The affected animals showed multifocal demyelination without any relationship to the vascular system, and without notable cellular response around the demyelination foci. In her next investigation Kroh (5) reported also a delayed appearance of multiple demyelinating foci and axonal lesions with the presence of typical products of myelin catabolism in brains of some mothers, injected during pregnancy with ENU.

The demyelinating process described by Kroh bore some resemblance to that observed in human pathology, in cases where disseminated lesions of the central myelin sheaths are found. However, the pathomechanism of demyelination brought about by alkylnitrosoureas is entirely obscure and the elucidation of this question could obviously contribute to the understanding of essential aspects of demyelination in general. The aim of our experimental work was therefore to determine both the long-term effect of methylnitrosourea (MNU) on the central myelin of adult animals and of the litter of mothers intoxicated with ENU during pregnancy.

EXPERIMENTAL

The first experimental group consisted of adult BD IX rats injected with 60 mg MNU per kg of body weight for 6 consecutive days. The lipid and protein composition of the myelin fraction obtained from animals sacrificed 2, 3, 4, 6, 8 and 12 weeks following the last injection of MNU was investigated.

In the second part of the studies, pregnant mice were injected on the 15th day of gestation with a single intravenous dose of 80 mg of ENU per kg of body weight and their offsprings were investigated after reaching the postnatal age of 20, 40 and 70 days, respectively. The animals were sacrificed by decapitation and the lipid composition of the cerebral myelin was determined.

The myelin fraction was isolated according to the method of Norton and Poduslo (6). The identity and purity of the fraction was checked by means of electron microscopy. Several brains of the immature animals were pooled for a single isolation procedure. The total lipids extracted were further separated by means of combined column and thin-layer chromatography as described previously (9). The myelin proteins were separated using polyacrylamide gel electrophoresis (8).

RESULTS

Histological staining revealed in all experimental groups of adult BD IX rats intoxicated with MNU considerable dilatation of perivascular spaces along with spongious changes which were located almost exclusively in the cerebral and cerebellar white matter (Fig. 1). The spongious vacuoles were sharply demarcated from the

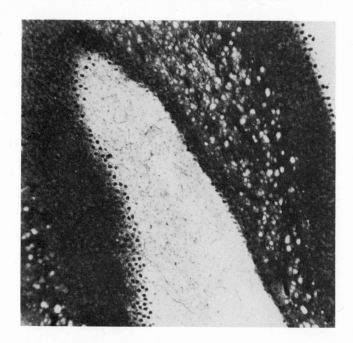

Fig. 1. The spongious degeneration of the white matter in a rat intoxicated with methylnitrosourea.

neighbourhood and were not accompanied by a marginal glial reaction. Myelin stains revealed no demyelinating foci, and staining with Sudan III failed to demonstrate sudanophilic deposits.

A number of quantitative changes were found in the lipid composition of myelin preparations isolated from the intoxicated BD IX rats. Some of them were restricted only to particular experimental groups and some others persisted throughout the whole period of investigation. The most impressive change was the severe loss of sphingomyelin to about 50% of the control values throughout the whole period of 2 to 12 weeks after intoxication (Fig. 2). The myelin fraction from rats sacrificed 2 weeks after MNU treatment was deficient also with respect to plasmalogen, phosphatidyl serine, and inositol phosphatides.

When the lipid composition was expressed in percentage of total myelin lipids a significant increase of the cholesterol ester content, ranging from 100 to 300%, was also found in all experimental groups from the 4th until the 12th week after the intoxication (Figs. 3 and 4).

The proportions of the two main glycolipid classes, cerebrosides and sulfatides, showed a tendency towards and increase of the relative percentage of cerebrosides on the expense of sulfatides in all experimental groups from the 2nd to the 8th week.

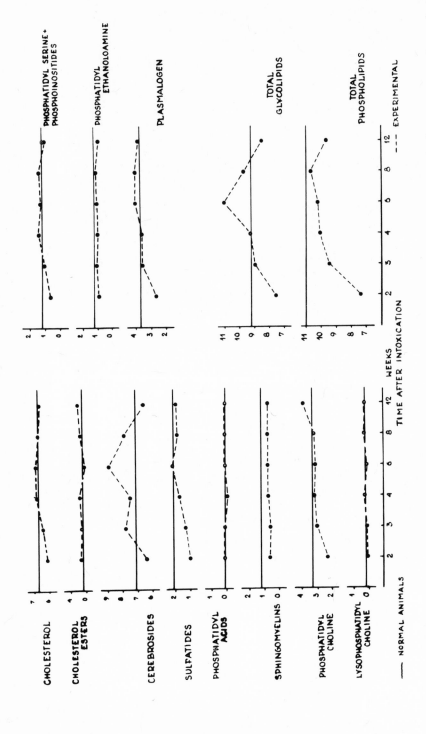

Fig. 2. Lipid composition of brain myelin in experimental MNU intoxication (g/100 g dry tissue).

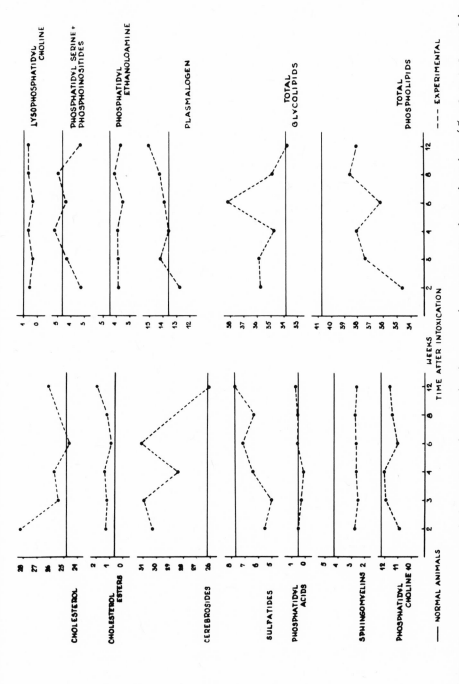

Fig. 3. Lipid composition of brain myelin in experimental MNU intoxication (% of total myelin lipids).

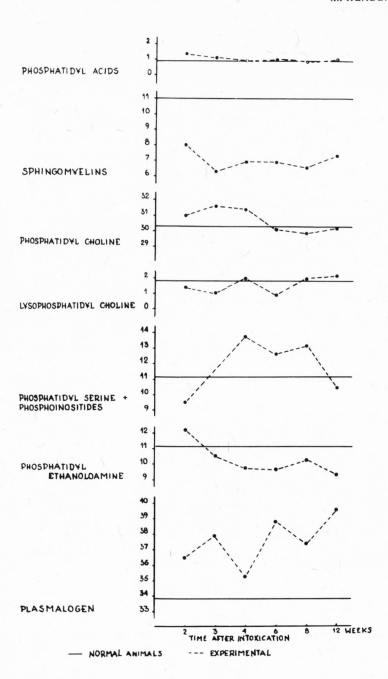

Fig. 4. Phospholipids of brain myelin in experimental MNU intoxication (% of total myelin phospholipids).

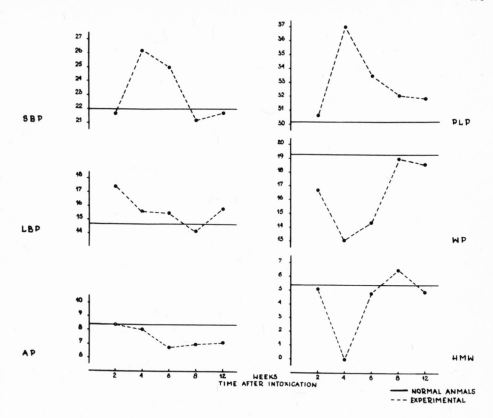

Fig. 5. Protein composition of brain myelin in experimental MNU intoxication (% of total proteins).

The electrophoretic pattern of myelin proteins from adult BD IX rats sacrificed at various time intervals following MNU administration remained essentially unchanged, the apparent deviations not exceeding the dispersion of control values (Fig. 5).

The myelin fractions of mice intoxicated transplacentally with ENU during their foetal life also displayed significant changes in their lipid composition (Figs. 6,7,8). First of all, both the absolute and relative contents of myelin galactolipids and plasmalogens were severely reduced. The two individual galactolipids, i.e. the cerebrosides and sulfatides, contributed almost equally to the total loss of glycolipids. As far as the phospholipids are concerned plasmalogen was the only lipid which was significantly decreased.

The considerable increase of lysophosphatides, mainly of lysolecithin, in the brains of the 40-day-old animals should also be mentioned. The content of both free and esterified cholesterol remained essentially unchanged.

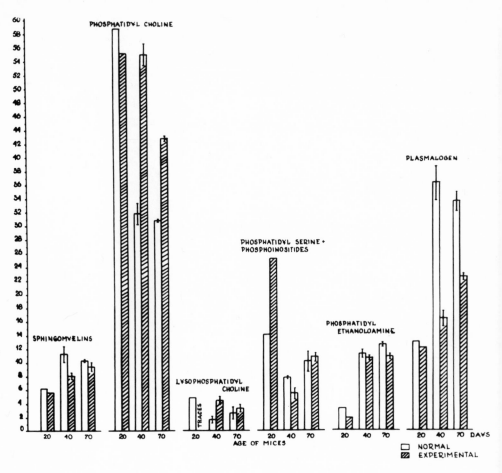

Fig. 6. Phospholipids of brain myelin in transplacental ENU
intoxication (% of total myelin phospholipids).

DISCUSSION

     Considerable morphological alterations in the myelin sheath
of adult BD IX rats treated with MNU were found in the present
study. These changes resemble to some degree those seen after
triethyl tin—intoxication. However, they are not identical with
changes observed in genuine demyelinating processes, neither
primary nor secondary demyelination. Also the chemical changes
which were most striking in the present experimental condition —
the massive loss of sphingomyelin from the affected sheaths —
has so far not been reported in typical demyelinating processes.

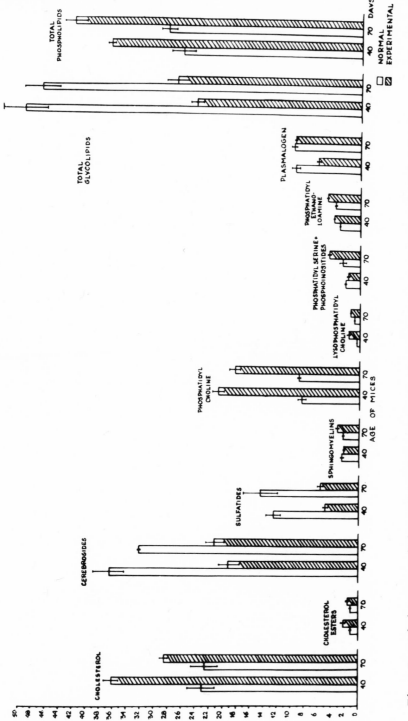

Fig. 7. Lipid composition of brain myelin in transplacental ENU intoxication (% of total myelin lipids).

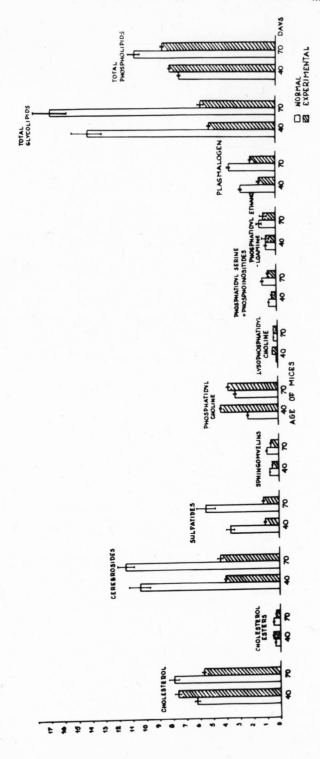

Fig. 8. Lipid composition of brain myelin in transplacental ENU intoxication (g/100 g dry tissue).

Less characteristic was the increased cholesterol ester content of the myelin fraction obtained from the intoxicated animals.

The transplacental effect of ENU on mouse myelin was different. The essential finding in the myelin fraction of the intoxicated offsprings was a reduction of the galactolipid and plasmalogen content. This clearly indicates that animals intoxicated transplacentally with ENU produce chemically defective myelin. Both the influence of MNU on adult rats and the effects of ENU on foetal mice evidently show that, besides the carcinogenic effect, the alkylnitrosourea derivatives effectively disturb the lipid metabolism of CNS membrane structures. Almost all studies which deal with these compounds have been concerned with their strong neurotropic carcinogenicity as an indication of their metabolic effectiveness.

The mechanisms by which alkylnitrosourea derivatives induce neoplastic growth of neuroglial or Schwann cells are currently under discussion. It has been suggested that alkylnitrosoureas become somehow metabolically activated to yield final or intermediate carcinogenic compounds which then affect the metabolism of target cells.

Druckrey et al. (1) have shown that intravenously injected MNU gives rise to diazomethane, which is a strong alkylating agent and capable of methylating guanine, thus changing the genetic code of nucleic acids. However, according to Viale (7), the question of whether alkyl derivatives of nitrosourea affect selectively the metabolism of nucleic acids, or by virtue of their alkylating activity affect the overall protein metabolism more or less specifically, remains unsolved. Anyhow, Kleihues and Magee (2) have proved that administration of N-methyl-N-nitrosourea to experimental animals has a prompt effect on the degree of methylation of the RNA and DNA of the nervous tissue.

There exists evidence that the increase of methylation of RNA during ontogenic development is related to stages of cell organisation. The molecular and biological modifications effected in t-RNA´s are considered to take place during the process of cell differentiation.

In view of the anticipated influence of t-RNA´s on either the synthesis or translation of messenger-RNA, modifications such as overmethylation or alkylation of specific t-RNA´s should lead to a defect in the regulation of protein synthesis. Such modifications occurring in the course of ontogenic development could eventually explain the independence of early protein synthesis and - in mature animals - the qualitative shift of specific protein synthesis.

It would thus be conceivable to assume that alkylation or overmethylation of the t-RNA´s induced by alkylnitrosourea could disturb the metabolism of interfascicular oligodendroglia, which in turn could affect the metabolism of myelin lipids.

REFERENCES

1. Druckrey, H., Ivankovic, S. and Preussmann, R., Selektive Erzeugung maligner Tumoren im Gehirn und Rückenmark von Ratten durch N-methyl-N-nitrosoharnstoff, Z. Krebsforsch. 66 (1965) 389-394.

2. Kleihues, P. and Magee, P., Alkylation of rat brain nucleic acids by n-methyl-n-nitrosourea and methyl methanesulfonate, J. Neurochem. 20 (1973) 595-606.

3. Kroh, H., Ethylnitrosourea - induced microcephaly in Swiss mice and Wistar rats, in Aktuelle Probleme der Neuropathologie (K. Jellinger, ed.) Facultas-Verlag, Wien (1973) pp. 29-35.

4. Kroh, H., Demyelination in mice brain resulting from transplacental action of ethylnitrosourea (ENU). IIIrd Neuropathological Conference, Warsaw 1975.

5. Kroh, H., Multiple demyelinating foci induced with ethylnitrosourea (ENU) in mouse brain, International Symposium on Chemical brain injuries and brain tumors, Warsaw 1976, p. 21.

6. Norton, W. and Poduslo, S., Myelination in rat brain: method of myelin isolation, J. Neurochem. 21 (1973) 749-757.

7. Viale, G., Nucleic acid composition and metabolism in brain tumors, in Experimental Biology of Brain Tumors (W. Kirsch, E. Grossi-Paoletti and P. Paoletti, eds.) Thomas, Springfield (1972) pp. 357-403.

8. Waehneldt, T.V. and Mandel, P., Isolation of rat brain myelin, monitored by polyacrylamide gel electrophoresis of dodecyl sulfate-extracted proteins, Brain Res. 40 (1972) 419-436.

9. Wender, M., and Adamczewska, Z., Lipidveränderungen im Gehirn bei Krankheiten, die mit Myelinschädigung verbunden sind, in Neue Forschungsergebnisse des Hirnstoffwechsels und der Entmarkungsenzephalomyelitis, R. Schmidt, Halle-Wittenberg (1974) pp. 248-255.

DEMYELINATION

Clinical Demyelination

CELLULAR AND HUMORAL RESPONSES TO MYELIN BASIC PROTEIN IN MULTIPLE SCLEROSIS: A DICHOTOMY

William Sheremata[+], Montreal Neurological Institute,
   Montreal, and
Denise D. Woods and Mario A. Moscarello,
   Research Unit, Sick Children's Hospital, University
   of Toronto, Toronto, Ontario, Canada

SUMMARY

The macrophage migration inhibition factor (MIF) assay and a counterimmunodiffusion assay were utilized to measure immune responses to human myelin basic protein in 75 patients with multiple sclerosis (MS) and in 120 control subjects. Eight out of ten MS patients in acute exacerbation and one out of seventeen convalescent, but none of chronically ill MS patients gave positive results in the MIF test. Forty-six percent of the patients with negative MIF assays but only 22% of those with positive assays had positive antibody results. In the counterimmunodiffusion assay, myelin basic protein antibody was demonstrated in almost 2/3 of patients during convalescence but it was not present in those whose illness had been stable for 6 months or longer. While no correlation with the stage or duration of the illness was present in other disorders, in MS an inverse correlation with clinical activity and in vitro evidence of cellular sensitization to encephalitogenic basic protein was apparent.

INTRODUCTION

Immune responses to brain antigens have been implicated in multiple sclerosis (MS) by many investigators over the last half century. The original finding of complement fixing anti-brain antibody in MS serum by Sachs and Steiner (24) has not been confirmed. Subsequently, a wide variety of techniques have reportedly detected antibody to brain or its sole encephalitogenic constituent,

---

[+]Present address: Department of Neurology, University of Miami, School of Medicine, Miami, Florida, U.S.A.

myelin basic protein, but confirmation has generally been lacking
(14).   A recent finding of anti-myelin basic protein antibody in
experimental allergic encephalomyelitis (EAE) employing newer
techniques by Lisak et al. (11), McPherson and Carnegie (16), and
Woods et al. (30) has led to the application of these techniques
in the search of antibody in MS.

Using these techniques, Lisak et al. (11) and McPherson and
Carnegie (16) could not detect such antibodies in MS.   Recently,
however, McPherson et al. (17) and Sheremata et al. (29) have obtained preliminary evidence that such antibody is present, especially
during convalescence.   In our present report we have extended our
earlier studies reporting the detection of specific antibody which
appears to bear an inverse correlation with the appearance of
cellular immune responses.

EXPERIMENTAL

Seventy-five patients with multiple sclerosis and 120 control
subjects of similar age and sex were studied (Table 1).   Fifty-five
controls were normal, ten had optic neuritis, ten encephalitis and
fifteen had miscellaneous central nervous system (CNS) disorders.
In addition, 30 patients with peripheral nervous system (PNS)
disease were studied.   This group was composed of 4 patients with
polyneuropathy, 16 with mononeuritis, and 10 with myasthenia.   All
MS patients were diagnosed as such by at least three neurologists,
using the Schumacher criteria (26).   Twenty-five patients were in
acute exacerbations of illness (0-3 weeks), 25 were 4-24 weeks after
onset (convalescent) and 25 others more than 24 weeks (stable).
Comparative antibody and macrophage migration inhibition factor
(MIF) assays were performed in 33 MS patients and 34 control subjects.   Twelve controls were normals, 6 were myasthenics, 7 had
encephalitis, and 9 others had miscellaneous disorders.   Five had
neuropathies and 4 had optic neuritis.

Antigen

Human myelin basic protein was prepared by the method of
Lowden et al. (13).   The antigen was used in both counterimmunodiffusion assays and MIF assays.

Macrophage Migration Inhibition Factor Assay

Lymphocyte cultures.   Fifty milliliters of peripheral venous
blood are collected by venipuncture into a heparinized plastic
syringe and sedimented with 0.6% dextran (v/v) for 1 h at 37°C.
The buffy coat was expressed via canula into a sterile 50 ml test
tube containing non-absorbent cotton and incubated for 60 min to
remove the polymorphonuclear leukocytes, monocytes and B-cells.

Table 1. The presence of myelin basic protein antibody in controls and in patients with central nervous system and peripheral nervous system diseases.

Diagnosis	Total number		Number positive
Controls		55	2
CNS-diseases:			
Multiple sclerosis		75	18
acute	25		2
convalescent	25		16
stable	25		0
Encephalitis		10	1
Optic neuritis		10	2
Miscellaneous		15	6
stroke	4		2
ALS	5		0
SSPE	4		3
Metastatic carcinoma	2		1
PNS-diseases:			
Polyneuritis		4	1
Mononeuritis		16	1
Myasthenia gravis		10	4

The purified lymphocyte suspension is expressed through a second butterfly anchored in the cotton. The cotton is washed twice with approximately 120 ml of tissue culture medium TC199. The washes, together with the collected lymphocytes, are centrifuged in a 250 ml round bottom flask for 15 min at 650 x g. The supernatant is discarded and the cells resuspended in TC199, transferred to a 15 ml conical centrifuge tube and centrifuged at 650 x g for 15 min. The latter procedure is repeated and the cells are counted in a hemacytometer. Triplicate 1.5 ml cultures prepared to contain 3×10^6 lymphocytes/ml are incubated with or without antigen for 72 h. Cultures containing tissue culture medium only or medium plus antigen are included to control for non-specific effects of antigen toxicity. Each 24 hours the supernatants are pooled and replenished with fresh medium containing antigen. The pooled supernatants are dialyzed against physiological saline for 24 h and against distilled water for 48 h. They are then lyophilized and stored at $-20^\circ C$. Supernatants are reconstituted to 1/5 of their original volume with TC199 containing 15% guinea pig serum, 1% glutamine, and pen/strep 50 units/ml for cell migration assays.
    Preparation of guinea pig macrophages. Hartley guinea pigs (Canadian Breeding Farms) weighing 375-400 g are injected intra-peritoneally with 30 ml of Marcol 50 oil (Esso) and sacrificed by cardiac puncture at five days. The skin is incised from the

sternum to the pelvis and a trocar, attached to a drainage tube,
is inserted into the peritoneal cavity. The peritoneal cavity is
lavaged twice with 100 ml of Hanks' balanced salt solution (BSS),
and the fluid collected in a 250 ml separatory funnel. The aqueous
layer is eluted and centrifuged at 650 x g for 15 min. The cell
pellet is washed once in Hanks' BSS and the supernatant is discarded. Osmolality is adjusted to 0.4% with sterile water and
TC199 to lyse red blood cells, allowed to stand at room temperature
for 5 min and centrifuged at 650 x g for 15 min. Supernatants are
discarded and the cells resuspended in TC199 containing 15% guinea
pig serum, 1% glutamine and pen/strep 50 units/ml to give a 10%
cell suspension. Capillary tubes, filled with the cell suspension,
are sealed with warm paraplast and centrifuged at 108 x g for 5
min. The tubes are cut at the cell-liquid interface and two cell
containing portions are anchored with a sterile silicone grease in
each small Mackaness tissue culture chamber which is then closed
with a 22 mm glass cover slip and sealed with paraplast. Reconstituted concentrated supernatants from the human lymphocyte cultures
are added and the chamber is sealed. Cultures are incubated without
disturbance for 24 h at $37^{\circ}C$ and migrations are measured by projection and planimetry.

$$\text{Migration Index (M.I.)} = \frac{X}{Y} \times 100$$

where $X = \dfrac{\text{Migration in supernatant with antigen}}{\text{Migration in supernatant without antigen}}$

and $Y = \dfrac{\text{Migration in medium with antigen}}{\text{Migration in medium without antigen}}$

Antibody Assays

Preparation of antibasic protein antibody. Monkey anti-human
basic protein antibody as well as rabbit and guinea pig antisera
against human basic protein were used.

Gel electrophoresis. Polyacrylamide gels (0.5 x 8.0 cm) containing 1.0% SDS are prepared according to the method of Eng et al.
(8). Two mg of protein are taken up in 1.0 ml of phosphate buffer
(0.1 M, pH 7.4) containing 1% SDS, 1.5% Cleland's reagent and
16% sucrose. The solution is heated at $100^{\circ}C$ for 2-5 min. An
aliquot containing 150 μg myelin basic protein is applied to each
gel. Electrophoresis is carried out at 4mA/tube for 90 min. One
gel is fixed and a densitometric tracing made using a Joyce Loebl
U.V. scanner (Translab Type D8 MK2) in order to locate the position
of the protein. The unfixed gels are used for the disc immunodiffusion experiments.

Immunodiffusion plates. An agar solution (1.5% special NOBLE
agar in 0.15 M NaCl containing 0.02% sodium azide) is used to
prepare the plates for disc immunodiffusion (19). Routinely 500 ml
of agar are prepared and stored in 12 ml aliquots at $4^{\circ}C$. Each

12 ml aliquot was sufficient for one plate (10 x 8 cm).

Disc immunodiffusion. The protein bands from the acrylamide gels are cut into 1-2 mm slices which are then placed in wells 6 mm in diameter and covered with aliquots of phosphate-Sarkosyl buffer. Wells 4 mm in diameter are filled with 20 µl (200 µg) of the appropriate control or test 7S protein. The plates are kept in a moist chamber at 4°C and observed daily (x3) for the appearance of precipitation lines.

Immunoabsorption. One mg of antigen and 1 ml of the 7S fraction are suspended in 200 µl of the phosphate-Sarkosyl buffer, incubated at 37°C for 60 min and centrifuged at 2,000 rpm for 30 min. Aliquots of 20 µl of the resultant supernatant are used to test for antibody activity against basic myelin protein.

Immunoelectrophoresis. Immunoelectrophoresis was carried out by the method of Scheidegger (25).

RESULTS

Antibody. Assay results are shown in Table 1. Two of the 55 normals, 27 of 110 subjects with CNS, and 6 of 30 subjects with PNS disease were positive. Only 2 (8%) of the acute MS group, but 16 of 25 (64%) of those in the convalescent and none of the stable group were positive. Two of 10 optic neuritis cases, and 6 of the miscellaneous group also gave significant results. Of the 30 patients with PNS disease, only one patient with Guillain-Barré and one Bell's palsy, but 4 of 10 myasthenics were positive. No relationship between duration or activity of disease was obvious in myasthenics. The precipitation band seen with MS sera was similar to that seen with the 7S antibody from immunized monkeys. In addition, the responsible serum component was shown to be a 7S immunoglobulin. Preliminary studies have identified it as IgG.

Macrophage migration inhibition assays. Mean of MIF values in normals was 113±17. It was 98±23 in encephalitides, 107±13 in myasthenics, 99±21 in the miscellaneous group and 88±22 in MS. Patients in acute exacerbations gave a mean of 68±26 and those between 4 and 24 weeks gave a mean of 96±7. Patients stable more than 6 months gave a mean of 100±16. Values 2 S.D. below normal migration of 79.4 were considered to be significant. One myasthenic and one of 9 miscellaneous patients, with optic neuritis, gave positive MIF results. Eight of 10 patients in acute exacerbations of multiple sclerosis, and one of 17 convalescent, but none of 6 chronically ill patients gave positive results. 11/24 (46%) of these patients with negative MIF assays had positive antibody results whereas 2/9 (22%) of those with positive MIF assays gave positive results. Correlation of MIF and antibody data are shown in Figures 1 and 2.

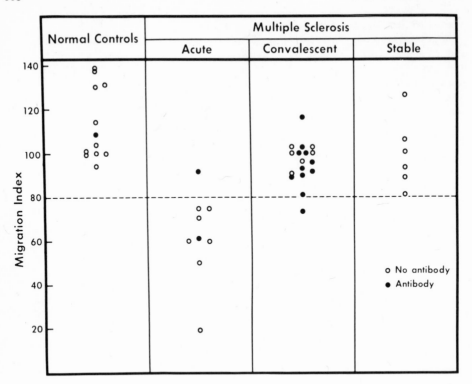

Fig. 1.   Immune responses to myelin basic protein.   MIF production related to antibody reaction.

DISCUSSION

Myelin basic protein antibody has been demonstrated in MS sera using an adaptation of a counterimmunodiffusion assay. Antibody is present in one-quarter of the patients. However, it is found in almost 2/3 of patients during convalescence. In contrast it is not present in those with illness stable for 6 months or longer. While no correlation with the stage or duration of illness was present in other disorders, in MS an inverse correlation with clinical activity and in vitro evidence of cellular sensitization to encephalitogenic basic protein was apparent.

Serum complement fixing anti-brain antibody in MS patients was reported in 1934 by Sachs and Steiner (24). The use of crude brain antigens in a variety of assay systems (hemagglutinin, precipitin, and anti-human globulin assays) has failed to give consistent results (see the review by Lumsden, ref. 14). However, there has been little attempt to relate these studies to disease activity. Berg and Källen (3) have shown that MS serum is cytotoxic to glial tissue culture. Bornstein and Appel (4) and

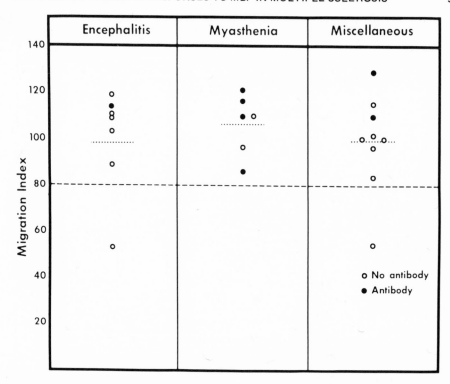

Fig. 2.   Immune responses to myelin basic protein.   MIF production related to antibody detection.

Lumsden (14) demonstrated positive myelinotoxicity assays in EAE and MS.   Recently, Brosman et al. (5) demonstrated antibody-dependent cell-mediated demyelination in an in vivo system – rabbit eye model.   However, Seil et al. (27) have shown that sera of animals with this EAE induced by sensitization to purified myelin basic proteins are not myelinotoxic.   It is therefore unlikely that in vitro demyelinating activity is due to sensitization to encephalitogenic basic protein.   Nevertheless, it is possible that other anti-myelin antibodies could play a role in demyelination, especially in sites where previous impairment of the blood–brain barrier has occurred, i.e. as with a cellular immune response.
     Lisak et al. (11) using radio-immunoelectrophoresis showed that animals with EAE produced small quantities of anti-myelin basic protein antibodies, but similar results could not be found subsequently in MS patients (12).   McPherson and Carnegie (16) also obtained similar data in EAE using a different type of radio-immunoassay.   Woods et al. (30) using the counterimmunodiffusion technique employed in the present study also demonstrated the presence of such antibody.   While there is no doubt that specific

antibody to myelin basic protein is present in EAE sera, the time
of appearance of antibody in relation to cellular immune events has
been incompletely studied (15).

Despite the failure of earlier studies, McPherson et al. (17)
have shown that convalescent MS serum will decrease binding of
radioisotopically labelled basic protein to normal sheep lymphocytes.
This data suggests that specific antibody may be present in convalescence, but does not specifically identify this responsible
factor as antibody. Their results, however, are similar to those
seen in the present study. The reason for the apparent discrepancy
between previous studies and the results of McPherson et al. (17)
and those of the present study may be related to the use of gel
separation of intact basic protein from degradation products usually
present in such preparations. Peptide fragments may block antibody
receptors without causing precipitation of protein. The results of
the present investigations suggest that negative assays in previous
studies may simply reflect the study of patients only during the
acute phase of their illness.

Patterson and others have convincingly shown that mechanisms
of cellular immunity are primarily responsible for disease production in EAE (20). In vitro correlates of EAE have been shown in
other studies using MIF (2, 7). In addition, MIF assays in patients
with MS have demonstrated findings similar to those presented here
(1, 6, 20, 22, 27). In these studies, hypersensitivity to a myelin
basic protein was most evident at the time of exacerbation (6, 21,
28).

The importance of our observations that a small amount of
specific anti-myelin basic protein antibody is produced in MS is
difficult to interpret. Antibody has been found in some patients
with repeated stroke, SSPE and myasthenia. It is occasionally present
in apparently normal and other subjects. Our studies, while identifying the material in the precipitin bands as a 7S globulin, and
probably IgG, do not indicate the subclasses of antibody involved.
Hence, we cannot ascertain whether any or all of the demonstrated
antibody to myelin basic protein are demyelinating or blocking in
nature (10). In MS, the observed antibody response could be an
additional factor in inducing demyelination. Alternatively, such
antibody might be a factor in blocking a specific cellular immune
response, or it may simply be a concomitant of some other B-cell
function regulating the T-cell response. It is possible, however,
that antibody production and MIF elaboration in vitro may be
epiphenomena secondary to CNS tissue damage. Further characterizatio
of the antibody demonstrated in MS and other disorders will be necessary. Although Offner et al. (18) have reported binding of
serum β-lipoprotein to myelin basic protein, the serum factor
appearing in the precipitation bands is not β-lipoprotein.

Acknowledgements. This investigation was supported by the
Medical Research Council of Canada, and the Multiple Sclerosis
Society of Canada, St. Mary's Foundation, and Endowment Funds of

the Montreal Neurological Institute.

The assistance of Dr. J.B.R. Cosgrove and Dr. Sabah Bekhor in referring and evaluating patients is acknowledged. The encouragement and support of Dr. William Feindel, director of the Montreal Neurological Institute, is gratefully acknowledged. The work presented would not have been possible without the understanding and support of my wife Leah.

REFERENCES

1. Bartfeld, H., Atoynatan, T. and Donnenfeld, H., In vitro cellular immunity to central nervous system antigens in multiple sclerosis, in Multiple Sclerosis: Immunology, Virology and Ultrastructure (F. Wolfgram, G.W. Ellison, J.G. Stevens, J.M. Andrews, eds.) Academic Press, New York (1972) pp. 333-364.
2. Behan, P.O., Kies, M.W., Lisak, R.P. and Sheremata, W., Immunological mechanisms in experimental encephalomyelitis in non-human primates, Arch. Neurol. 29 (1973) 4-9.
3. Berg, O. and Källen, B., Effect of mononuclear blood cells from multiple sclerosis patients of neuroglia in tissue culture, J. Neuropath. Exp. Neurol. 23 (1964) 550-559.
4. Bornstein, M.B. and Appel, S.H., Tissue culture studies of demyelination, Ann. N.Y. Acad. Sci. 122(1965) 280-286.
5. Brosman, C.F., Stoner, G.L., Bloom, B.R. and Wisniewski, H.M., Studies on demyelination by activated lymphocytes in the rabbit eye. Antibody-dependent cell-mediated demyelination, J. Immunol. 6 (1977) 2103-2110.
6. Colby, S., Sheremata, W., Bain, B. and Eylar, E.H., Cellular hypersensitivity in attacks of multiple sclerosis. A comparative study of MIF production and lymphoblastic transformation, Neurology 27 (1977) 132-139.
7. David, J.R. and Patterson, P.Y., In vitro demonstration of cellular sensitivity in allergic encephalomyelitis, J. Exp. Med. 122 (1965) 1161-1171.
8. Eng, L.F., Choa, F.C., Gerstl, B., Pratt, D. and Tavaststjerna, M.G., The maturation of human white matter myelin. Fractionation of the myelin membrane proteins, Biochem. 7 (1968) 4455-4465.
9. Kies, M.W. and Alvord, E.C., Encephalitogenic activity in guinea pigs of water soluble protein fractions of nervous tissue, in Allergic encephalomyelitis (M.W. Kies and E.C. Alvord, eds.) Thomas, Springfield (1959) pp. 293-299.
10. Lebar, R., Boutry, J.-M., Vincent, C., Robineaux, R. and Voisin, G.A., Studies on autoimmune encephalomyelitis in guinea pig. II. An in vitro investigation on the nature, properties and specificity of the serum-demyelinating factor, J. Immunol. 116 (1976) 1439.
11. Lisak, R.P., Heinze, R.G., Kies, M.W. and Alvord, E.C., Antibodies to encephalitogenic basic protein in experimental allergic encephalomyelitis, Proc. Soc. Exp. Biol. Med. 130 (1969) 814-818.

12. Lisak, R.P., Heinze, R.G., Falk, G.A. and Kies, M.W., Search
    for anti-encephalitogen antibody in human demyelinative
    disease, Neurology 18 (1968) 122-128.
13. Lowden, J.A., Moscarello, M.A. and Morecki, R., The isolation
    and characterization of an acid-soluble protein from myelin,
    Can. J. Biochem. 44 (1966) 567-577.
14. Lumsden, C.E. Jr., The clinical pathology of multiple sclerosis,
    in Multiple Sclerosis. A reappraisal.(D. McAlpine, C.F. Lums-
    den, E.D. Acheson, eds.) Churchill-Livingstone, Edinburgh
    (1972) pp. 311-621.
15. MacKay, I.R., Carnegie, P.R. and Coates, A.S., Immunopathologi-
    cal comparisons between experimental autoimmune encephalo-
    myelitis and multiple sclerosis, Clin. Exp. Immunol. 15 (1973)
    471-482.
16. McPherson, T.A. and Carnegie, P.R., Radioimmunoassay with gel
    filtration for detecting antibody to basic proteins of myelin,
    J. Lab. Clin. Med. 72 (1968) 824-831.
17. McPherson, T.A., Liburd, E.M. and Seland, T.P., Binding of
    125 I-labelled encephalitogenic basic protein to normal lympho-
    cytes. Inhibition with multiple sclerosis serum. Clin. Exp.
    Immunol. 19 (1975) 451-458.
18. Offner, H., Clausen, J. and Fog, T., Precipitation of myelin
    basic protein by β-lipoprotein of human serum, Acta Neurol.
    Scand. 50 (1974) 221-227.
19. Ouchterlony, O., Diffusion-in-gel methods for immunological
    analysis, in Progress in Allergy, vol. 5 (P. Kallos, ed.)
    Karger, Basel and New York (1958) pp. 1-78.
20. Patterson, P.Y., Transfer of allergic encephalomyelitis in
    rats by means of lymph node cells, J. Exp. Med. 111 (1960)
    119-136.
21. Pekarek, J., Jedlicka, P. and Svejcar, J., Production of mig-
    ration inhibitory factor by lymphocytes of patients with
    multiple sclerosis to brain antigens, Clin. Exp. Immunol.,
    in press.
22. Rocklin, R.E., Meyers, O.L. and David, J.R., An in vitro assay
    for cellular hypersensitivity in man, J. Immunol. 104 (1970)
    95-102.
23. Rocklin, R.E., Sheremata, W., Feldman, R.G. et al., The
    Guillain-Barré syndrome and multiple sclerosis. In vitro cel-
    lular responses to nervous tissue antigens, N. Engl. J. Med.
    284 (1971) 803-808.
24. Sachs, H. and Steiner, G., Serologische Untersuchungen bei
    multipler Sklerose, Klin. Wochenschr. 13 (1934) 1714-1717.
25. Scheidegger, J.J., Une micro-méthode de l´immuno-électro-
    phorèse, Int. Arch. Allergy Appl. Immunol. 7 (1955) 103-110.
26. Schumacher, G.A., Beebe, G., Kibler, R.F., Kurland, L.T.,
    Kurtzke, J.F., McDowell, F., Nagler, B., Sibley, W.A.,
    Tourtellotte, W.W. and Willman, T.L., Problems of experimental
    trials in multiple sclerosis, Ann. N. Y. Acad. Sci. 122 (1965)
    552-568.

27. Seil, F.J., Falk, G.A., Kies, M.W. et al., The in vitro de-
     myelinating activity of sera from guinea pigs sensitized with
     whole CNS and with purified encephalitogen, Exp. Neurol. 22
     (1968) 545.
28. Sheremata, W., Cosgrove, J.B.R. and Eylar, E.H., Cellular
     hypersensitivity to basic myelin (A1) protein and clinical
     multiple sclerosis, N. Engl. J. Med. 291 (1974) 14-17.
29. Sheremata, W., Wood, D.D., Moscarello, M.A. and Cosgrove,
     J.B.R., Multiple sclerosis: An inverse correlation between
     antibody and MIF production to myelin basic protein, J. Neurol.
     Sci., in press.
30. Wood, D.D., Orange, E.P. and Moscarello, M.A., The interaction
     of antibodies to two myelin proteins, Immunol. Commun. 4
     (1975) 17-27.

CEREBROSPINAL FLUID MYELIN BASIC PROTEIN AND MULTIPLE SCLEROSIS

Steven R. Cohen, Mary Jane Brune, Robert M. Herndon
  and Guy M. McKhann
Department of Neurology, Johns Hopkins University
  School of Medicine
Baltimore, Maryland 21205, U.S.A.

SUMMARY

We have previously reported that myelin basic protein appears in CSF during acute attacks of multiple sclerosis. These studies have been extended to over 700 patients, 91 with multiple sclerosis. The data continues to indicate that myelin basic protein is released into cerebrospinal fluid during acute attacks of multiple sclerosis. We are currently characterizing the basic protein in the CSF.

INTRODUCTION

Myelin basic protein (MBP) comprises approximately 10% of the dry weight of the myelin membrane. This major structural protein has been well characterized in terms of its biochemical and immunological properties. Thus, in order to study the biochemistry of myelin development and degeneration, we selected basic protein as a marker in the membrane and a radioimmunoassay for MBP was developed (3). This assay has been used to monitor the pattern of myelin synthesis in various areas of developing rat brain (1), including the optic nerve (7).

In 1969, Herndon and Johnson (4) using electron microscopic techniques described the presence of myelin fragments in the cerebrospinal fluid (CSF) of multiple sclerosis patients undergoing acute exacerbations. This led to the development of radioimmunoassays for MBP by several laboratories in an attempt to find a diagnostic test for multiple sclerosis. These initial assays for myelin basic proteins in CSF either did not detect any myelin basic protein in the CSF (5) or yielded non-specific results (6). This led us to

513

develop a more sensitive assay for the MBP. When this sensitive
(4 ng/ml) specific method was applied to spinal fluids of actively
demyelinating multiple sclerosis patients, significant levels
(10-100 ng/ml) of basic protein were found. In contrast, spinal
fluid from non-demyelinating patients did not have significant
levels of MBP (< 4 ng/ml) (2).

The original report described results from approximately 300
patients. Since that time, we have assayed an additional 400 spinal
fluid samples for MBP and we now have a basis for suggesting   the
clinical value of the test.   These studies have been successful
largely due to the nature of the antibodies in use. In this report,
we describe results on our latest patients and the method of antibody production.

EXPERIMENTAL

Patients. All patients except some of those with optic neuritis
were from Johns Hopkins Hospital. Approximately half of the optic
neuritis CSF samples came from Dr. Shirley Wray of the Massachusetts
General Hospital.

We have divided our patients into the following categories:
1. Classical multiple sclerosis - at least two attacks occurring in different parts of the nervous system more than 1 month
apart and not explainable on the basis of other disease processes.
Age between 10 and 50 years.
a. Active - within 1 week of the onset of new neurological
symptoms.
b. Inactive (remission) - patients more than 1 month from the
onset of any new neurological symptoms or change in existing symptoms.
2. Chronic multiple sclerosis - a progressive disease of more
than 6 months duration affecting more than one area of the central
nervous system (this may occur in the absence or presence of previous exacerbations and remissions). Typical remitting disease
which has become progressive is included in this category for pur-
poses of this study.
3. Optic neuritis - without evidence of other nervous system
involvement.
4. Myelinopathy - demyelinating diseases other than multiple
sclerosis.
5. Non-demyelinating neurological disease.
Assay of CSF. All samples were stored at -10°C until assay.
The spinal fluid basic protein appears to be stable as identical
values for CSF basic protein were obtained on a sample before and
after incubation for 1 week at room temperature.

For the assay, 0.05 ml of a 10-fold concentrated assay buffer
(2 M **Tris**-acetate, pH 7.5, containing 10 mg of histone per ml) and
antiserum at the appropriate concentration was added directly to

0.5 ml of spinal fluid. This mixture was incubated for 1 hour at 37°C, 15,000 cpm of ^{125}I-labelled basic protein (specific activity 3407 mCi/µg) were added, and the mixture was incubated for an additional 10 to 24 hours at 4°C. The antibody-basic protein complex was then precipitated with cold ethanol, the pellet and supernatant fraction were separated by centrifugation, and each was assayed for radioactivity. The percentage of ^{125}I basic protein bound (i.e. in the pellet) was then determined.

Production of antiserum. The best method for producing an antiserum that will react with cerebrospinal fluid MBP is first to inoculate rabbits with 250 mg of guinea pig spinal cord homogenized in 0.250 ml of 0.9% NaCl and emulsified with 0.5 ml of complete Freund's adjuvant containing 10 mg/ml of $H_{37}Ra$ myobacterium tuberculosis (Difco Labs., Detroit, Mi.). When the animals show symptoms of experimental allergic encephalomyelitis they are treated by daily intravenous injection of 1 mg of basic protein in 1 ml of 0.9% NaCl until the symptoms disappear. They are then given monthly boosters of pure basic protein (1-2 mg) in incomplete Freund's adjuvant (1 ml) and bled.

RESULTS

Subjects are grouped into three classes based on the content of basic protein in the CSF. Less than 5 ng/ml is negative; between 6 and 15 ng/ml is weakly positive; and greater than 16 ng/ml is positive. Samples have been assayed from 697 patients (Fig. 1). These include 91 samples from multiple sclerosis patients, 6 from patients with other active demyelinating diseases, and 600 from patients with non-demyelinating neurological diseases.

The 42 multiple sclerosis patients in acute exacerbation had CSF basic protein levels greater than 16 ng/ml. Sixteen of 22 patients with the slowly progressive form of the disease had CSF basic protein levels between 6 and 15 ng/ml. The patients with inactive disease all had levels below 5 ng/ml (Fig. 1).

Serial samples were obtained from patients before, during, and 10 to 30 days after attacks (Table 1). The CSF basic protein levels rose and fell with the exacerbation. Generally, as the patient improved, the CSF myelin basic protein returned to normal levels.

The category of "myelinopathies" included patients with transverse myelitis, metachromatic leukodystrophy, central pontine myelinolysis, adrenal leukodystrophy, and an unknown hereditary leukodystrophy. These also had elevated CSF basic protein (Table 2).

So far, 25% of the patients with optic neuritis have had basic protein in the CSF (Table 2). All these patients are being followed to determine the outcome of this first attack. All but 3 of the 600 controls had less than 6 ng basic protein per ml of CSF.

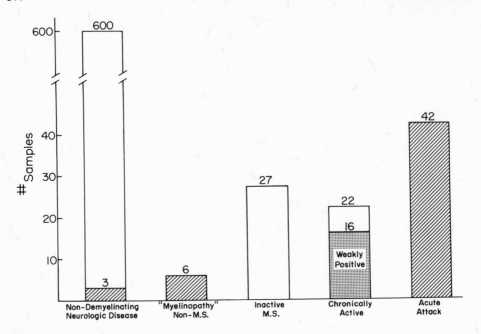

Fig. 1. Presence of myelin basic protein in CSF. The patients are grouped into five clinical categories as shown. The shaded area represents the number of samples in each group with myelin basic protein in the CSF. The myelinopathies and positive non-demyelinating neurologic diseases are in Table 2.

Table 1. Changes in level of CSF myelin basic protein after acute attack of demyelination. (The values of CSF myelin basic protein for six multiple sclerosis patients are shown during, after, and, in one case, prior to an exacerbation. The value over the arrow represents the time between the serial spinal taps.)

Before attack ng/ml	Acute stage ng/ml	Recovery ng/ml
8.5 $\xrightarrow{\text{30 days}}$	60 $\xrightarrow{\text{14 days}}$	0
	60 $\xrightarrow{\text{10 days}}$	0
	60 $\xrightarrow{\text{10 days}}$	0
	15 $\xrightarrow{\text{7 days}}$	10
	30 $\xrightarrow{\text{16 days}}$	10
	38 $\xrightarrow{\text{10 days}}$	17

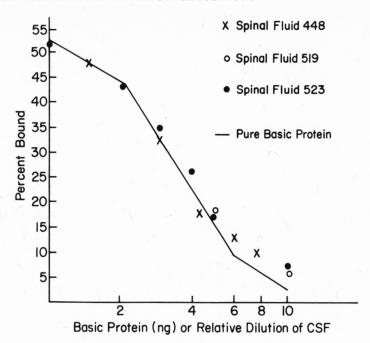

Fig. 2. Displacement of ^{125}I basic protein from its antibody by
CSF basic protein. Different dilutions of spinal fluid from three
patients (numbers 448, 519, 523) were assayed for MBP by radioimmunoassay. Spinal fluid 448 was assayed at concentrations of
10, 20, 30, 40 and 50 percent; X represents the relative dilutions.
Number 519 (open circles) was assayed at 10 and 20 percent. Spinal
fluid 523 (closed circles) was assayed at 10, 20, 30, 40, 50 and
100 percent. The solid line is the standard value for basic
protein.

        In collaboration with Drs. Marion Kies and Bernard Driscoll
of the National Institutes of Health, we have found that our antiserum to myelin basic protein is directed against two antigenic
sites in the middle portion of the molecule (residues 37-88 and
89-115). With this antiserum, the basic protein measured in the
CSF is antigenically identical to purified basic protein, as shown
in Fig. 2, since parallel displacement curves are obtained for CSF
and pure basic protein.
        It should be noted that not all antisera to MBP will react
with the CSF myelin basic protein. This is probably due to masked
or missing antigenic sites in the CSF myelin basic protein. These
possibilities are currently under investigation.

Table 2. Levels of CSF myelin basic protein in patients without
multiple sclerosis.

	ng/ml
Neurological disease - non-demyelinating	
Lateral medullary infarction	60
Cerebellum infarction	50
Radiation necrosis, pt. 1	12
Radiation necrosis, pt. 2	0
Neurological disease - myelinopathies	
Transverse myelitis and systemic lupus erythematosis	100
"Hereditary leukodystrophy"	23
Metachromatic leukodystrophy	12
Central-pontine myelinolysis	50
Adrenal leukodystrophy	8
Adrenal leukodystrophy	10
Optic neuritis (4)	5-12
Optic neuritis (12)	0

DISCUSSION

These results on an additional 500 patients have confirmed
the earlier finding that myelin basic protein is present in the
spinal fluid of patients undergoing active demyelination. This
includes multiple sclerosis patients and those with other demyelinating diseases.

It is important to distinguish between a diagnostic test and
a test for active demyelination. Radioimmunoassay for MBP is one
measurement of active demyelination rather than a diagnostic test
for multiple sclerosis. This is because CSF myelin basic protein
levels rise and fall with the exacerbations and remissions that
are typical of multiple sclerosis. This is constantly observed
although there are variations in the amount of spinal fluid basic
protein at the height of the attack. This probably reflects the
amount of tissue undergoing demyelination. Thus in some optic
neuritis patients where the area of demyelination is probably very
small, myelin basic proteins cannot be detected in the CSF.

We are currently using the test as an aid in determining
whether or not a patient is having an active demyelinating episode.
Because the test is used clinically as an index of activity of the
disease, it may be a useful method for assessing the efficacy of
potential treatments for multiple sclerosis as they become available.

REFERENCES

1. Cohen, S.R. and Guarnieri, M., Immunochemical measurement of myelin basic protein in developing rat brain: An index of myelin synthesis, Devel. Biol.49 (1976) 294-299.
2. Cohen, S.R., Herndon, R.M. and McKhann, G.M., Radioimmunoassay of myelin basic protein in spinal fluid: An index of active demyelination, New Engl. J. Med.295 (1976) 1455-1457.
3. Cohen, S.R., McKhann, G.M. and Guarnieri, M., A radioimmuno-assay for myelin basic protein and its use for quantitative measurements, J. Neurochem. 25 (1975) 371-376.
4. Herndon, R.M. and Johnson, M., A method for the electron microscopic study of cerebrospinal fluid sediment, J. Neuropath. Exp. Neurol. 29 (1970) 320-330.
5. Lennon, V. and Macay I.R., Binding of ^{125}I myelin basic protein by serum and cerebrospinal fluid, Clin. Exp. Immunol. 11 (1972) 595-603.
6. McPherson, T.A., Gilpin, A. and Seloved, T.P., Radioimmuno-assay of CSF for encephalitogenic basic protein: A diagnostic test for MS?, Canad. Med. Assoc. J. 4 (1972) 856-859.
7. Tennekoon, G.I., Cohen, S.R., Price, D.L. and McKhann, G.M., Myelinogenesis in optic nerve, a morphological, autoradiographic and biochemical analysis, J. Cell. Biol. 72 (1977) 604-616.

PROTEOLYTIC ACTIVITY IN CSF

P.T. Richards and M. Louise Cuzner

Department of Neurochemistry, Institute of Neurology,
    The National Hospital
Queen Square, WC1N 3BG, U.K.

SUMMARY

Proteolytic enzyme activity, present at both acid and neutral
pH values, in cerebrospinal fluid, can be measured by a sensitive
assay, which monitors the rate of ^{125}I-basic protein breakdown on
polyacrylamide gel electrophoresis. CSF cellular neutral proteinase
and supernatant acid proteinase are increased in acute multiple
sclerosis and in CNS infections.

INTRODUCTION

In the cellular immune response, T-lymphocytes, stimulated by
antigen, produce lymphokines which recruit the auxiliary cells of
the immune system, the polymorphonuclear (PMN) cells and macrophages. The presence of phagocytic cells in any inflammatory
lesion is marked by increased levels of lysosomal hydrolases, particularly of neutral proteinase in PMN cells and of acid proteinase
in macrophages (5). Cellular infiltration and perivascular cuffing
are features of the multiple sclerosis (MS) lesion and there is a
predilection for plaques to be located around the ventricles (1).
The suggestion that there are factors in the cerebrospinal
fluid (CSF) which contribute to the demyelinating process is further
strengthened by the finding of a moderate pleocytosis in the CSF of
patients with multiple sclerosis (11). The results of a study by
Allen et al. (3) of the T-and B-lymphocyte profiles in CSF in
temporal relationship to exacerbations of multiple sclerosis indicated that the percentage of T-cells is 65% in the acute stage of
a relapse, as compared to 30% in stable patients. Evidence for

the production of lymphokines in the CSF of multiple sclerosis
patients comes from a report of increased CSF lysozyme levels,
which have been attributed to the production of the enzyme by PMN´s
and macrophages within the meninges (6). A sensitive enzyme assay
has been developed to quantitate levels of other proteolytic enzymes
in small volumes of CSF at acid and neutral pH, in MS patients with
stable and relapsing disease.

EXPERIMENTAL

Proteolytic enzyme activity was measured in the cellular and
supernatant fraction of the CSF in four groups of patients:
1. Neurological controls with bacterial or viral meningitis or
   encephalitis
2. Neurological controls with disease of non-infectious origin
   excluding tumours
   e.g. motor neurone disease, disc disease, subarachnoid haemorrhage
3. Multiple sclerosis in remission
4. Multiple sclerosis in exacerbation
   CSF samples (1-3 ml) were centrifuged at 1000 g for 20 min
and the supernatant carefully removed with a Finn pipette. The
sedimented fraction was suspended in 200 µl of 0.9% (w/v) NaCl and
all samples were frozen at -70°C until analysis. Neutral and acid
proteinase activities were assayed in the samples by measuring the
rate of digestion of ^{125}I-basic protein. The incubation medium
consisted of 40 µl of supernatant or cell homogenate and 20 µl of
0.167 M acetate (pH 3.6) or Tris-HCl (pH 7.6) buffer, containing
40 µg ^{125}I-basic protein. Basic protein was prepared from human
white matter (4) and radiolabelled with Na ^{125}I by the lactoperoxidase method (7). The enzyme reaction was terminated after 4 h
with 40 µl of SDS buffer and 50 µl aliquots were separated by PAGE
(2). The basic protein band was cut from the gel and the radioactivity determined in an LKB Wallac gamma counter. Routine cell
counts and cell cytology were carried out on all CSF´s analysed.

RESULTS

Neutral proteinase activity of CSF polymorphonuclear cells
was basically the same as that of circulating cells with either
haemoglobin or basic protein as substrate (Table 1), and the same
three characteristic high molecular weight peptides were seen
(Fig. 1). Since myelin basic protein is selectively attacked in
demyelinating disease in the CNS and is a preferential substrate
for neutral proteinase, it was routinely used as the substrate in
the present assay system. Minimal activity was found in CSF
lymphocytes, whereas the enzyme activity of the PMN´s was

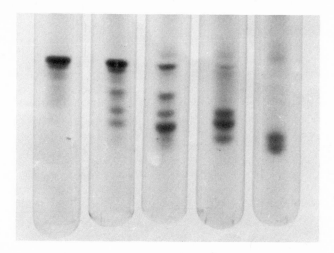

Fig. 1. High molecular weight peptide products of basic protein (BP) proteolysis. From left to right: (1) BP; (2) and (3) BP + incubation at pH 3.6 with brain homogenate for 3 and 18 h; (4) and (5) BP + incubation at pH 7.6 with PMN homogenate for 20 min and 3 h.

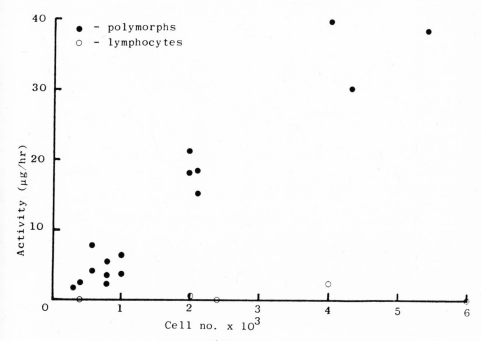

Fig. 2. Rate of I^{125} basic protein digestion.

proportional to the cell count (Fig. 2). The assay method was
sensitive enough to measure the activity of PMN's to a lower limit
of 1-2 cells per mm^3 CSF.

The cellular neutral proteinase of the CSF in the different
disease groups is shown in Table 2 and Fig. 3. Patients with CNS
infections had elevated values, which correlated with the PMN cell
count. In the second group of neurological controls, the highest
w.b.c. (white blood cell) count was 73/mm^3 CSF, and exclusively
mononuclear. Only one of the eight CSF's in this series had any
significant cellular neutral proteinase activity. In both groups
of MS patients, the maximum w.b.c. count of any CSF was 8 mononuclear
cells/mm^3. Nevertheless the mean CSF cellular neutral proteinase
activity of MS patients with an exacerbation was significantly
higher than that of MS patients in remission, and of neurological

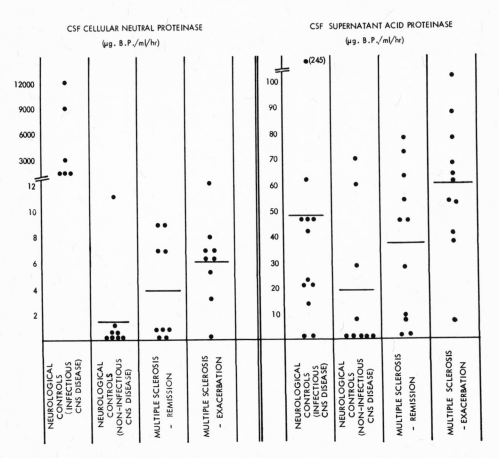

Fig. 3. Proteolytic activity in cerebrospinal fluid (CSF) in the
different disease groups. Horizontal bars indicate mean values.

Table 2. CSF neutral and acid proteinase (μg basic protein/h/ml CSF) in the different disease groups.

Subjects	Number of observations	Cell-bound neutral proteinase[+]	Supernatant acid proteinase[++]
1. Multiple sclerosis acute exacerbation	10	6.11±3.34	60.2±26.8
2. Multiple sclerosis remission	10	3.87±4.17	36.8±29.0
3. Neurological controls (infectious disease)	12	4500 (mean) 1.78-12,711 (range)	47.6±65.5
4. Neurological controls (non-infectious disease)	8	1.55±3.93	18.5±28.1

[+] Significant difference (P<0.001) for group 1 vs. 4 and (P<0.01) for group 2 vs. 1 and 4.

[++] Significant difference (P<0.001) for group 4 vs. 1 and 2 and for group 1 vs. 2; other differences not significant.

Table 1.   Neutral proteinase (pH 7.6) activity of polymorphonuclear
cells.

	Haemoglobin	I^{125} -basic protein
	(μmol. tyrosine/mg protein/h)	(μg lost/10^3 cells/h)
Blood	0.44	4.7
CSF	0.13	6.0

controls with disease of non-infectious origin, despite the wide
scatter of the values. Significant levels of both acid and neutral
proteinase were found in CSF supernatant but only acid proteinase
levels were investigated in detail. The mean value for neurological
controls, with non-infectious disease was significantly lower than
that for the other three groups of patients (Table 2, Fig. 3).

                              DISCUSSION

        There is a direct correlation between the neutral proteinase
activity of the cellular fraction of the CSF and the PMN cell count
in infectious diseases of the CNS. In the remaining three groups
of patients in this study, the CSF w.b.c. count was very low and
exclusively mononuclear. But the neutral proteinase activity in
the CSF of nine multiple sclerosis patients, with an exacerbation
of the disease, was significantly increased in comparison to patients in remission and to other neurological controls. The increased activity corresponded to 1-2 polymorphs/mm^3 CSF, which
may be below the limit of sensitivity of the cell counting method.
Alternatively, the activity could be attributed to histiocytes
(macrophages) which were identified in the CSF of 6 out of 10 MS
patients in relapse. The raised acid proteinase activity in the
CSF supernatant in CNS infections and in acute MS could be due to
release from infiltrating cells but a more likely explanation is
that damage to the myelin sheath results in the release of brain
acid proteinase into the CSF (10).
        Cellular infiltration and perivascular cuffing are features
of the MS lesion; macrophages are seen (1) but the presence of
PMN´s has been reported only rarely (9). Entry into an early MS
lesion, depending on its location, could result in the presence of
the cells in CSF. The localization of antigen-antibody complexes
in a demyelinating lesion would recruit phagocytic cells (8), and
infiltrating lymphocytes, stimulated by antigen, secrete factors

chemotactic for PMN´s and macrophages. Thus, the finding of raised
proteolytic activity in the CSF of MS patients in exacerbation
lends further support to the implication of the immune response
in the pathogenesis of multiple sclerosis.

REFERENCES

1. Adams, C.W.M., Pathology of multiple sclerosis: Progression
    of the lesion, Brit. Med. Bull. 33 (1977) 15-20.
2. Agrawal, H.C., Burton, R.M., Fishman, M.A., Mitchell, R.F. and
    Prensky, A.L., Partial characterization of a new myelin protein
    component, J. Neurochem. (1972) 2083-2089.
3. Allen, J.C., Sheremata, W., Cosgrove, J.B.R., Osterland, K.
    and Shea, M., Cerebrospinal fluid T and B lymphocyte kinetics
    related to exacerbations of multiple sclerosis, Neurology 26
    (1976) 579-583.
4. Banik, N.L. and Davison, A.N., Isolation of purified basic
    protein from human brain, J. Neurochem. 21 (1973) 489-494.
5. Davison, A.N. and Cuzner, M.L., Immunochemistry and biochemis-
    try of myelin, Brit. Med. Bull. 33 (1977) 60-66.
6. Hansen, N.E., Karle, H., Jensen, A. and Bock, E., Lysozyme
    activity in cerebrospinal fluid, Acta Neurol. Scand. 55 (1977)
    418-424.
7. Morrison, M., Bayse, G.S. and Webster, R.G., Use of lacto-
    peroxidase catalyzed iodination in immunochemical studies,
    Immunochemistry 8 (1971) 289-297.
8. Movat, H.Z., Pathways to allergic inflammation: The sequelae
    of antigen-antibody complex formation, Fedn. Proc. 35 (1976)
    2435-2441.
9. Peters, G., Klinische Neuropathologie; Spezielle Pathologie
    der Krankheiten des zentralen und peripheren Nervensystems,
    2nd Ed. Thieme, Stuttgart (1970).
10. Rinne, U.K. and Riekkinen, P., Esterase, peptidase and protein-
    ase activities of human cerebrospinal fluid in multiple scle-
    rosis, Acta Neurol. Scand. 44 (1968) 156-167.
11. Sandberg-Wollheim, M., Optic neuritis: Studies on the cerebro-
    spinal fluid in relation to clinical course in 61 patients,
    Acta Neurol. Scand. 52 (1975) 167-178.

THE IMMUNE RESPONSE IN HUMAN DEMYELINATING DISEASES

Hans Link

Department of Neurology, University Hospital

S-581 85 Linköping, Sweden

SUMMARY

Lymphocytes present in the brain, meninges and cerebrospinal fluid (CSF) in multiple sclerosis (MS) are capable of synthesizing IgG. The CSF in MS contains more T-lymphocytes and fewer B-lymphocytes compared to blood. The reactivity of CSF lymphocytes in MS to T-cell mitogens and probably also to a combined B-and T-cell mitogen is absent or heavily reduced. This unresponsiveness of CSF lymphocytes may be a consequence of their previous activation. The blood lymphocytes in MS are not altered regarding distribution of B-and T-cells, nor regarding responsiveness to mitogens, when compared with healthy controls. An asynchronous synthesis of heavy and light immunoglobulin chains occurs within the CNS in many MS patients, giving rise to oligoclonal band patterns on electrophoresis and abnormal kappa/lambda light chain ratios of CSF. The synthesized immunoglobulins are most probably antibodies which may play a role in the pathogenesis and course of human demyelinating diseases. The brain must be regarded, from an immunological point of view, as a privileged site with its own immune system and its characteristic immune reactions, and future research concerning demyelinating diseases should, if possible, include investigations of these reactions.

INTRODUCTION

From an immunological point of view the human central nervous system (CNS) must be regarded as a separate entity, with its own immune system and its characteristic immune reactions. A number of

abnormalities in the humoral immune response has been described in
human demyelinating disorders, of which multiple sclerosis (MS) is
the most common and important, and therefore also the most thoroughly
investigated. Despite our increasing knowledge regarding various
abnormal humoral immune reactions within the CNS, their importance
for the pathogenesis in e.g. MS has not been elucidated.

It is only in the last few years that the central role of the
lymphocyte in antibody mediated immunity and also in cellular
immunity has been established. Developmentally and functionally
lymphocytes can be divided into two types: bursa-equivalent B-cells
which are concerned with antibody formation, and thymus-dependent
T-cells which are responsible for cell-mediated immunity (CMI).

Immunologically competent B-lymphocytes and their plasma cell
derivatives are concerned with the synthesis of antibodies with the
ability to combine specifically with the provocative antigen. T-
lymphocytes have been found to carry a variety of immunological
functions, such as helper as well as suppressor activity in various
types of immune response, mixed lymphocyte culture (MLC) reactivity,
and reactivity in CMI responses. Different functions are probably
carried out by different sublines of T-lymphocytes, and immunological
research is currently focused on specification of such sublines.

T-lymphocytes seem to have an important role in the development
of autoimmune diseases, when e.g. a loss of tolerance for antigenic
substances of a specific tissue or organ, such as the myelin sheath
of nerves, occurs. Classical examples of autoimmune diseases involving the nervous system are experimental allergic encephalitis
and polyneuritis which are produced by injecting emulsions of brain
or nerve into animals, together with Freund´s adjuvant, which is an
emulsion of <u>Mycobacterium tuberculosis</u>. Under these conditions T
lymphocytes become sensitized to injected antigen, which is thought
to be myelin basic protein. Sensitized lymphocytes invade the
nervous tissue and destroy myelin sheaths on direct contact. In
addition they release biological substances that are lytic, attract
inflammatory cells, and probably modify endothelial cell continuity.

The present paper deals with analysis of the immune response
within the human CNS in comparison to blood. The following parameters have been studied:

1. The CSF and blood lymphocyte function in patients with MS
   and acute aseptic meningitis, as reflected by lymphocyte
   proliferation after stimulation with the mitogens
   phytohaemagglutinin (PHA), concanavallin A (Con A), and
   poke weed mitogen (PWM);

2. B and T lymphocytes in CSF and blood in MS and acute mumps
   meningitis patients;

3. The clinical value of determination of the CSF-IgG index
   equal to $\frac{CSF\text{-}IgG}{serum\ IgG} : \frac{CSF\text{-}albumin}{serum\text{-}albumin}$, compared to the IgG
   quotients, i.e. IgG/total protein and IgG/albumin which are
   commonly used for demonstration of IgG synthesis within the
   CNS in neurological patients.

CSF AND BLOOD LYMPHOCYTE FUNCTION IN MS AND ACUTE ASEPTIC
MENINGITIS

     The effect of PWM has been investigated on CSF and blood
lymphocytes obtained from patients with acute viral meningitis (5).
A microculture technique was used and the lymphocyte transformation
was measured by registration of radioactive thymidine incorporation
into DNA. PWM is considered to stimulate B-cells but also T-cells.
     Fig. 1 shows that PWM induced a vigorous proliferation of CSF
lymphocytes in the four patients with acute viral meningitis. The
proliferation was, however, even more pronounced when blood lymphocytes were stimulated.
     According to unpublished observations by Kam-Hansen et al.
CSF lymphocytes obtained from MS patients respond only very weakly
or not at all when stimulated with PWM. In contrast, blood lymphocytes from MS patients did not differ from control blood lymphocytes
regarding the response to stimulation with PWM.

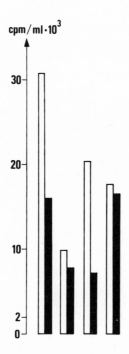

Fig. 1. Effect of PWM on blood and CSF lymphocytes from four
patients with acute viral meningitis. The results are expressed
as mean net counts per minute (cpm) per ml/culture x 10^3. White
bars represent blood lymphocytes and dark bars CSF lymphocytes.

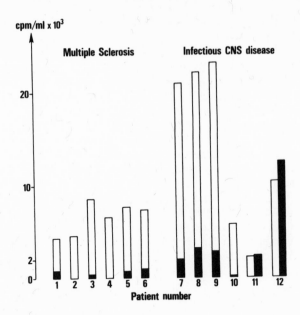

Fig. 2. Effect of PHA on blood lymphocytes (white bars) and CSF
lymphocytes (dark bars) from six patients with MS (patients 1-6)
and from six patients with acute viral meningitis (patients 7-12).
Results are expressed as mean net counts per minute (cpm) per ml/
culture x 10^3.

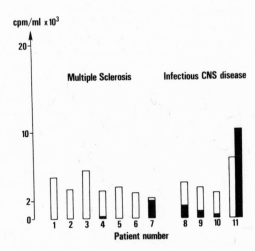

Fig. 3. Effect of Con A on blood lymphocytes (white bars) and CSF
lymphocytes (dark bars) from seven patients with MS (patients 1-7)
and from four patients with acute viral meningitis (patients 8-11).
Results are expressed as mean net counts per minute (cpm) per ml/
culture x 10^3.

The reactivity of CSF and blood lymphocytes to PWM in acute viral meningitis and MS is similar to the effects registered when PHA and Con A were used as mitogens. These two mitogens are considered to stimulate mainly T-lymphocytes. Fig. 2 shows that PHA induced a more or less vigorous proliferation of CSF lymphocytes from the meningitis patients (7). When identical numbers of CSF lymphocytes from MS patients were stimulated with PHA, only a low proliferation or no proliferation at all was registered. Similar results were obtained with Con A (Fig. 3).

The cause for the lower response of CSF lymphocytes to mitogens when compared with the response of blood lymphocytes is not known. The cell death as measured by trypan blue dye exclusion and applied on unstimulated lymphocytes could not account for this finding. It can be argued that the total effect of the cell death in the stimulated cultures has not been established, but this was not possible to perform. Other possible explanations for the reduced DNA-synthesis induced by mitogens in CSF lymphocytes compared to blood lymphocytes are that a helper cell required is lacking, or that more lymphocytes are already activated in the CSF than in the blood and therefore made unresponsive to mitogens.

B-AND T-LYMPHOCYTES IN CSF AND BLOOD IN MS AND ACUTE ASEPTIC MENINGITIS

The distribution of lymphocyte subpopulations in normal individuals has not been established, due to the low cell count. Quantitation of B-lymphocytes by counting immunoglobulin-bearing lymphocytes and of T-lymphocytes by the capacity to bind sheep red blood cells to form rosettes (SRBC-rosettes) has been performed in patients with MS (Fig. 4) and revealed significantly ($p < 0.01$) lower B-cell and higher T-cell values in CSF compared to blood (7). These findings are consistent with the observations by Sandberg-Wollheim and Turesson (23) on four MS patients. As can be seen from Fig. 4 similar deviations of B-and T-lymphocyte values have also been found in mumps meningitis. The values for B-and T-cells in blood in the two patient groups were approximately the same as in 39 healthy blood donors, who had mean values of 10% for B-cells and 72% for T-cells.

It is at present not known whether the decreased B-cell and elevated T-cell values in CSF, compared to blood in MS and aseptic meningitis, represent abnormal findings, or are consistent with the normal distribution of lymphocyte subpopulations in CSF. The finding of lower B-cell values in CSF compared to blood in MS as well as aseptic meningitis is surprising, since elevated immunoglobulin levels and oligoclonal immunoglobulins observed in CSF in these two disorders indicate B cell activation within the CNS. The low B-cell count may be due to loss of surface-bound immunoglobulin when B-cells are triggered to antibody synthesis.

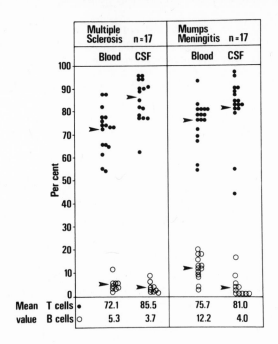

Fig. 4. Percentage of T-and B-lymphocytes in blood and CSF in multiple sclerosis and mumps meningitis. Arrows indicate mean values.

IMMUNOGLOBULIN SYNTHESIS WITHIN THE CNS

It is an axioma that the IgG concentration in CSF may be increased in human demyelinating disorders, and that this increase is due to IgG synthesis within the CNS. Table 1 summarizes some of the data, which indicate that IgG synthesis within the CNS occurs in MS.

The selective CSF-IgG elevation in the presence of normal serum IgG has been well known since the report by Kabat et al. (6), and the demonstration of this abnormality has been of value in the diagnosis of MS. Indirect evidence for IgG synthesis within the CNS has been brought forward by Frick and Scheid-Seydel, who already in 1958 (4) investigated the origin of CSF-IgG by intravenous injection of ^{131}I-labelled IgG into a variety of patients. In those patients whose blood-brain-barrier was judged as normal, and who had a normal CSF-IgG value, they found that the IgG penetrated into the CSF slower than albumin; a steady-state equilibrium of unity was established between serum and CSF in 100 hours. Further, all the CSF-IgG was derived exclusively from the serum. On investigation of 5 MS patients with normal CSF-total protein, indicating a normal blood-brain barrier, and elevated CSF-IgG values, the authors found

Table 1. Evidence for IgG synthesis within the CNS in multiple
sclerosis.

---

1. Selective elevation of CSF-IgG (6).
2. Abnormal exchange of ^{131}I-IgG between blood and CSF (4).
3. Occurrence of oligoclonal immunoglobulins in CSF and brain
    tissue (10, 11).
4. Elevation of antibody-immunoglobulins in CSF (2).
5. In vitro synthesis of IgG in mononuclear cells from CSF (22).

---

that 16-92% of the CSF-IgG was derived from some other sources than
serum - they suggested that it was locally produced in the CNS.
Final proof for intrathecal immunoglobulin synthesis has been de-
livered by Sandberg-Wollheim (22) who demonstrated that CSF lymphocytes from MS patients were capable of synthesizing IgG as well as
IgA in vitro. CSF lymphocytes synthesized more IgG than the same
number of blood lymphocytes obtained from the same patient. More
IgG was synthesized during exacerbations of the disease.

The source of IgG synthesis in the CNS in MS patients has been
clarified by Adams (1), who found that nearly all active MS cases
showed the feature of a lymphocytic meningitis, which was particularly severe in the depth of the cerebral sulci. This meningitis
was characterized by focal dense infiltrates of small lymphocytes
around veins and venules and by more diffusely spread lymphocytic
and monocytic infiltrates, usually enmeshed in a fibrin network.
The presence of fibrin suggests that a local inflammatory exsudate
has been formed in the meningeal membranes, as a response to either
an infective or an allergic process.

Better known than the lymphocytic meningitis is the perivascular
cuffing by large numbers of mononuclear cells, mainly lymphocytes,
which can be found in about 70% of plaques with evidence of recent
activity and in approximately 30% of chronic plaques (1). Adams
(1) has put forward evidence that perivenous cuffing may precede
the formation of a perivenous plaque. In addition, about 60% of
active MS cases displayed perivenular casts of lymphocytes outside
plaques in areas of relatively intact or sometimes oedematous
myelin. By serial sections some of these casts have been shown to
have no continuity with plaques and must be presumed to be independent satellite lesions.

The lymphocytes involved in the meningitis process as well as
the perivenular cuffs of lymphocytes within plaques and in apparently
normal myelin may be presumed to synthesize most of the CSF-IgG in
MS, while the contribution by the lymphocytes present in CSF is of
minor importance at least quantitatively.

Tourtellotte (25) has devised a formula for estimation of the
CNS IgG synthesis. The average MS patient's CNS is producing 29 mg
of IgG per day, with a range of 0-207 mg in 127 cases. Immuno-

suppressive treatment with ACTH and steroids stops IgG synthesis
within the CNS. The CSF-IgG pool in MS may be related to the
average adult total body pool of IgG, which is 66 g with a turnover
rate of 6% per day. The production by the CNS of 100 mg per day
in MS could add to it about 2%. This may be the explanation for the
modest hypergammaglobulinaemia observed in about 15% of MS patients.

IMMUNOGLOBULIN LEVELS IN CSF

It is possible to choose from several different analytical
techniques for quantitation of individual CSF immunoglobulins
without prior concentration of the fluid. Most popular are the
radial immunodiffusion (Mancini), electroimmunoassay (rocket), and
automatic immunoprecipitation (AIP) technique which utilizes
nephelometric analysis of antigen-antibody complexes in a flow
system. The Mancini technique is useful for a small number of
samples and the other techniques for a large series of samples.
All three methods yield results with sufficient accuracy for
clinical work. The choice of a method depends primarily on the
work load and access to instrumental equipment.
Elevated IgG levels in CSF may reflect IgG synthesis within
the CNS. An increase of e.g. CSF-IgG may, however, also occur in
the presence of a damaged blood-brain barrier or an elevated
serum-IgG. The effect of a damaged blood-brain barrier may be com-
pensated for by calculation of either the IgG/total protein ratio
or the IgG/albumin ratio of CSF. However, an increased serum-IgG
level or a decreased serum-albumin level will also cause a rise of
any of these two IgG quotients, which therefore may become mis-
leading. Correction of the variation of serum-IgG and serum-
albumin can be made by calculating the CSF-IgG index equal to

$\frac{\text{CSF-IgG}}{\text{serum-IgG}} : \frac{\text{CSF-albumin}}{\text{serum-albumin}}$ (24). The two ratios included in this
index vary proportionally with age, and the CSF-IgG index will
therefore not change with age. Furthermore, in the presence of a
slight to moderate blood-brain barrier damage both ratios will increase simultaneously, which is in accordance with the high
correlation found between them, and the CSF-IgG index will again
remain constant. Therefore, an abnormally high CSF-IgG index will
merely indicate IgG synthesis within the CNS. Similarly, the CSF-
IgA index equal to $\frac{\text{CSF-IgA}}{\text{serum-IgA}} : \frac{\text{CSF-albumin}}{\text{serum-albumin}}$ can be calculated
in order to demonstrate the occurrence of IgG synthesis within the
CNS.
Elevated serum-IgG is frequently observed in neurological
patients (15). Among 118 subjects, where neurological examination
made the existence of an organic neurological disorder unlikely,
25 (21%) displayed serum protein abnormalities (group I in Table 2).
The remaining 93 subjects have been used in order to establish

Table 2. Frequencies of abnormally high CSF-IgG quotients in three groups of patients with neurological diseases except MS.

Group Neurology Serum proteins	I (n=25) Normal Abnormal		II (n=38) Abnormal Normal		III (n=53) Abnormal Abnormal	
IgG quotient (> +2SD)	No.	Per cent	No.	Per cent	No.	Per cent
CSF $\dfrac{IgG}{total\ protein}$ (> 0.079)	7(7)	28	1(0)	3	21(13)	40
CSF $\dfrac{IgG}{albumin}$ (> 0.154)	11(8)	44	1(0)	3	27(17)	51
CSF-IgG index (> 0.58)	2(0)	8	4(0)	11	8(1)	15

Figures in the parentheses denote the number of patients with the simultaneous occurrence of abnormal serum-IgG concentration and abnormal IgG quotients.

reference values for IgG and albumin in CSF. Among 91 consecutive patients with various neurological disorders except MS, only 38 displayed normal serum proteins (group II in the Table) while the remaining 53 patients (group III) revealed serum protein abnormalities indicating an inflammatory lesion.

Between 28 to 51% of the patients in groups I and III in the Table, who all displayed serum protein abnormalities including elevated IgG levels as an indication of a general inflammatory lesion, revealed abnormally high IgG/total protein or IgG/albumin ratios of CSF. In contrast, an abnormally high CSF-IgG index was found about equally often in the three groups of patients presented in the Table.

The values of the CSF-IgG index in 59 consecutive MS patients are graphically presented in Fig. 5 (16). It is obvious that the increase of the CSF-IgG index, when present, is substantial in most MS patients. This is in contrast to the degree of elevation of the CSF-IgG index sometimes encountered in patients with other neurological disorders. In this group of MS patients, an elevated CSF-IgG index was obtained slightly more frequently when compared with the IgG/total protein or IgG/albumin ratios of CSF.

The CSF-IgG index value reflects at least to a certain extent the amount of IgG synthesized within the CNS. Determination of the CSF-IgG index as well as the CSF-IgA index and the IgM content of CSF should be of value in the follow-up of patients with CNS disorders where immunological reactions are presumed to be involved.

$$\frac{\text{CSF -ALBUMIN} \times 10^3}{\text{Serum-ALBUMIN}}$$

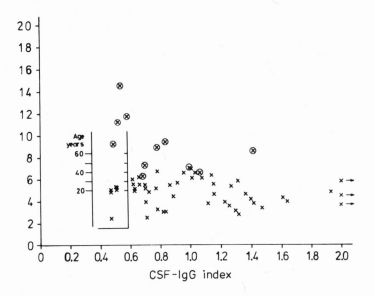

Fig. 5. Graphical presentation of results for the evaluation of the presence of IgG synthesis within the CNS by the CSF-IgG index and the blood-brain barrier function by the CSF/serum albumin ratio in 59 consecutive MS patients. The 95% confidence limits for a reference group are given. Since the CSF/serum albumin ratio is age dependent, this is marked in the figure for the upper confidence limits. Patients with elevated CSF/serum albumin ratios are encircled.

CSF-IgG IN RELATION TO CLINICAL PARAMETERS IN MS

Analysis of the CSF-IgG level in relation to various clinical parameters of MS, e.g. exacerbation of symptoms or the presence of a malignant or benign course of the disease, should yield information about the involvement of immune reaction in the pathogenesis of the disease. Elevated IgG levels have been reported in exacerbations, although this was by no means a consequent finding, not even in the single MS patient who was followed during more than one exacerbation (20). High CSF-IgG values are also more common in severely disabled MS patients when compared with MS patients without disability due to the disease (13, 28). In a recent investigation, disability, duration and onset of the disease were correlated to IgG levels in CSF and serum (21). Significantly higher mean CSF-IgG values were found in disabled MS patients. However, abnormal CSF-IgG levels

were registered more often and were more pronounced in the patients
with the most malignant course of the disease, e.g. in those with
severe disability after a short duration of the disease (< 10 years)
and also in severely disabled patients with an early age at onset
of the disease (< 25 years). On the contrary, normal mean CSF-IgG
values were found in MS patients without disability after a duration
of the disease for 10 years or more, i.e. in benign cases, and
particularly in patients with a benign course of the disease as
well as an early age at onset (< 25 years). MS patients with a
late age at onset (> 35 years) showed a less pronounced immune
response within the CNS, irrespective of the degree of disability.

THE OCCURRENCE OF OLIGOCLONAL IMMUNOGLOBULINS IN CSF AND BRAIN
TISSUE

     Instead of quantitation of individual immunoglobulins, electro-
phoretic analysis of concentrated CSF is carried out, and most
laboratories only report electrophoretic fractions as percentages
or scanning diagrams which show albumin and three or four globulin
fractions. The application of agar gel and agarose gel electrophoresis to the separation of CSF and brain proteins has considerably broadened our knowledge of CNS immunoglobulins. Bands
in the gamma globulin region, in addition to those observed in the
serum gamma globulin area and consisting of immunoglobulins, have
been observed in about 90% of MS patients and in about 50% of
patients with virus infections of the CNS (8, 13). Most patients
with subacute sclerosing panencephalitis (SSPE) also display
extra immunoglobulin bands on CSF electrophoresis, and also in
serum due to increased passage from CSF. In contrast, the occurrence
of immunoglobulin bands on CSF electrophoresis in some patients with
Guillain-Barré syndrome may be due to passage of immunoglobulins
from plasma to CSF, in the same way as may be seen in patients with
myeloma (12).
     The introduction of newer support media and buffer systems for
electrophoresis has resulted in techniques with improved resolution
but there has not been parallel increase in the amount of useful
information. Polyacrylamide gel electrophoresis and isoelectric
focusing give protein patterns with even higher resolution, but
clinically these techniques are not as useful as conventional
patterns or zone electrophoresis on agar gel or agarose gel, or
even on cellulose acetate (9).
     The extra immunoglobulin bands visible on agar gel or agarose
gel electrophoresis of CSF in MS (10) and SSPE (14) have been shown
to consist of IgG. It may be anticipated that a few clones of
activated B-lymphocytes present in the CNS acquire the capacity of
intense IgG synthesis, each clone of cells giving rise to IgG
appearing as one single band on electrophoresis. The immunoglobulins
have been labelled "oligoclonal". It is possible that each

Table 3. Evidence for the presence of oligoclonal IgG in CSF in MS.

1. Discrete IgG bands visible on electrophoresis (10).
2. Restricted electrophoretic heterogeneity of heavy chain bands
    from IgG (10).
3. Abnormal distribution of the ratio of kappa/lambda light chain
    antigenic determinants (17).
4. In vitro synthesis in mononuclear cells from CSF of IgG which
    appears as discrete bands on electrophoresis (22).
5. IgG subclass restriction (26).

homogeneous IgG band is characterized by some microheterogeneity
because more than one B-lymphocyte clone is involved.

     Table 3 summarizes the available evidence for the presence of
oligoclonal CSF-IgG in MS. Of the techniques mentioned, electrophoresis on agar gel or agarose gel and determination of the kappa/
lambda light chain ratio of CSF have become valuable diagnostic
instruments. The determination of the kappa/lambda ratio is based
on the observation that about a half of MS patients display an abnormal predominance of CSF-IgG with light chains of type kappa (17).

                    VIRUS-SPECIFIC ANTIBODIES IN CSF

     It may be postulated that the oligoclonal IgG present in CSF
and brain tissue in various neurological disorder indicates B-
lymphocyte stimulation within the CNS and synthesis of specific
antibodies.

     The type of antibodies present in the oligoclonal CSF-IgG in
MS has not been elucidated, in contrast to the situation in SSPE,
where the bands have been shown to consist of measles virus antibodies (14). Indirect evidence for the synthesis of measles virus
antibodies has also been obtained in about 50% of MS patients by
analyses of serum and CSF for the presence of measles virus antibody
activity and subsequent calculation of the ratio between measles
virus antibodies in serum/CSF. When this ratio showed a fourfold
or higher difference from the corresponding ratio of reference antibodies (adenovirus antibodies and poliovirus antibodies), it was
considered to be significantly reduced and indicating measles virus
antibody synthesis within the CNS (18, 19). The measles virus
antibody titers found in CSF in MS are, however, low, especially
when compared with the titers in CSF in SSPE, and only minimal
amounts of measles antibodies have been recovered from oligoclonal
CSF-IgG in MS (27).

     Further studies regarding this type of antibody present in
oligoclonal IgG in CSF and serum in MS is of fundamental importance
in order to elucidate the pathogenesis of this disorder. Oligoclonal
CSF immunoglobulins are only rarely found in neurological disorders

when MS and infectious CNS diseases are excluded (13). The transient appearance of oligoclonal CSF-immunoglobulins in about 20% of patients with mumps meningitis coincides with a transient mumps virus antibody response including mumps virus antibody synthesis within the CNS (Frydén et al., unpublished observations). It may be assumed that the occurrence of these antibodies may influence the course of the disease.

Acknowledgement. This work has been supported by the Swedish Medical Research Council (Project no. 3381).

REFERENCES

1. Adams, C.W.M., Pathology of multiple sclerosis: progression of the lesion, Brit. Med. Bull. 33 (1977) 15-20.
2. Brown, P., Cathala, F., Gajdusek, D.C. and Gibbs, C.J., Measles antibodies in the cerebrospinal fluid of patients with multiple sclerosis, Proc. Soc. Exp. Biol. Med. 137 (1971) 956-961.
3. Felgenhauer, K., Protein size and cerebrospinal fluid composition, Klin. Wschr. 52 (1974) 1158-1164.
4. Frick, E. and Scheid-Seydel, L., Untersuchungen mit J^{131}-markiertem γ-Globulin zur Frage der Abstammung der Liquorei-weisskörper, Klin. Wschr. 36 (1958) 857-863.
5. Frydén, A. and Link, H., Mitogen stimulation of cerebrospinal fluid lymphocytes in aseptic meningitis, Acta Neurol. Scandinav. submitted for publication (1977).
6. Kabat, E.A., Moore, D.H. and Landow, H., An electrophoretic study of the protein components in cerebrospinal fluid and their relationship to the serum proteins, J. Clin. Invest. 21 (1942) 571-577.
7. Kam-Hansen, S., Frydén, A. and Link, H., Lymphocyte subpopulations and the effect of mitogen stimulation in multiple sclerosis, Acta Neurol. Scandinav., submitted for publication (1977).
8. Laterre, E.C., Callewaert, A. and Heremans, J.F., Electrophoretic morphology of gammaglobulins in cerebrospinal fluid of multiple sclerosis and other diseases of the nervous system, Neurology 20 (1970) 982-990.
9. Laurell, C.B., Determination and interpretation of plasma proteins, Austr. Fam. Phys. 5 (1976) 36-41.
10. Link, H., Immunoglobulin G and low molecular weight proteins in human cerebrospinal fluid: Chemical and immunological characterisation with special reference to multiple sclerosis, Acta Neurol. Scandinav. 43, Suppl. 28 (1967) 1-136.
11. Link, H., Oligoclonal immunoglobulin G in multiple sclerosis brains, J. neurol. Sci. 16 (1972) 103-114.
12. Link, H., Demonstration of oligoclonal immunoglobulin G in Guillain-Barré syndrome, Acta Neurol. Scandinav. 52 (1975) 111-120.

13. Link, H. and Müller, R., Immunoglobulins in multiple sclerosis and infections of the nervous system, Arch. Neurol. 25 (1971) 326-344.

14. Link, H., Panelius, M. and Salmi, A.A., Immunoglobulins and measles antibodies in subacute sclerosing panencephalitis, Arch. Neurol. 28 (1973) 23-30.

15. Link, H. and Tibbling, G., Principles of albumin and IgG analyses in neurological disorders. II. Relation of the concentration of the proteins in serum and cerebrospinal fluid, Scand. J. Lab. Clin. Invest., in press.

16. Link, H. and Tibbling, G., Principles of albumin and IgG analyses in neurological disorders. III. Evaluation of IgG synthesis within the central nervous system in multiple sclerosis, Scand. J. Lab. Clin. Invest., in press.

17. Link, H. and Zettervall, O., Multiple sclerosis: disturbed kappa:lambda chain ratio of immunoglobulin G in cerebrospinal fluid, Clin. exp. Immunol. 6 (1970) 435-438.

18. Norrby, E., Link, H. and Olsson, J.-E., Measles virus antibody titers in cerebrospinal fluid and serum from patients with multiple sclerosis and controls, Arch. Neurol. 30 (1974) 285-292.

19. Norrby, E., Link, H., Olsson, J.-E., Panelius, M., Salmi, A. and Vandvik, B., Comparison of antibodies against different viruses in cerebrospinal fluid and serum samples from patients with multiple sclerosis, Infection and Immunity 10 (1974) 688-694.

20. Olsson, J.-E. and Link, H., Immunoglobulin abnormalities in multiple sclerosis. Relation to clinical parameters. Exacerbations and remissions, Arch. Neurol. 28 (1973) 392-399.

21. Olsson, J.-E., Link, H. and Müller, R., Immunoglobulin abnormalities in multiple sclerosis, J. neurol. Sci. 27 (1976) 233-245.

22. Sandberg-Wollheim, M., Immunoglobulin synthesis in vitro by cerebrospinal fluid cells in patients with multiple sclerosis, Scand. J. Immunol. 3 (1974) 717-730.

23. Sandberg-Wollheim, M. and Turesson, I., Lymphocyte subpopulations in the cerebrospinal fluid and peripheral blood in patients with multiple sclerosis, Scand. J. Immunol. 4 (1975) 831-836.

24. Tibbling, G., Link, H. and Öhman, S., Principles of albumin and IgG analyses in neurological disorders. I. Establishment of reference values, Scan. J. Clin. Invest., in press.

25. Tourtellotte, W.W., Multiple sclerosis research, in Proceedings of a joint conference held by the Medical Research Council and the Multiple Sclerosis Society of Great Britain and Northern Ireland, 17-18 October 1974 (A.N. Davison, J.H. Humphrey, L.H. Liversedge, W.J. McDonald and J.S. Porterfield, eds.) HMSO, London (1975) pp. 9-26.

26. Vandvik, B., Natvig, J.B. and Wiger, D., IgG, subclass restriction of oligoclonal IgG from cerebrospinal fluids and brain

extracts in patients with multiple sclerosis and subacute encephalitides, Scand. J. Immunol. 5 (1976) 427-436.

27. Vandvik, B., Norrby, E., Nordal, H.J. and Degré, M., Oligo-clonal measles virus-specific IgG antibodies isolated from cerebrospinal fluids, brain extracts, and sera from patients with subacute sclerosing panencephalitis and multiple sclero-sis, Scand. J. Immunol. 5 (1976) 979-992.

28. Yahr, M.D., Goldensohn, S.S. and Kabat, E.A., Further studies on the gamma globulin content of cerebrospinal fluid in multiple sclerosis and other neurological disorders, Ann. N.Y. Acad. Sci. 58 (1954) 613-624.

ISOELECTRIC FOCUSING AND ISOTACHOPHORESIS FOR INVESTIGATION OF

CSF AND SERUM PROTEINS IN DEMYELINATING AND INFECTIOUS NEUROLOGICAL

DISEASES

K.G. Kjellin and Å. Sidén[+]

Department of Neurology, Karolinska Hospital

S-10401 Stockholm 60, Sweden

SUMMARY

Isoelectric focusing (IEF) and isotachophoresis (ITP), two methods with excellent separation capacities, have been adapted during recent years for the analysis of CSF proteins. The fractions separated by these techniques can be further studied by e.g. immunological methods. ITP has besides its high separation capacity several valuable advantages: very small samples are needed, unconcentrated CSF can be examined, the analyses are quickly performed and the results are immediately obtained on a recorder.

Examinations by thin-layer IEF in a series of about 2,000 patients have afforded much new information about the CSF and serum proteins in many neurological diseases. Different complex CSF protein aberrations have been found in the gammaglobulin range as well as in more anodal positions in MS, infectious neurological diseases and Guillain-Barré syndromes. These aberrations are probably the result of several interacting factors, e.g. the temporal and spatial characteristics of the disease, the release of decomposition products from destroyed tissues, the genetically determined reactivity of the individual and the type of etiological agent.

[+]Supported by grants from the Swedish Multiple Sclerosis Society.

INTRODUCTION

Using an electrophoretic technique Kabat et al. (8) found an increase of cerebrospinal fluid (CSF) gammaglobulins in multiple sclerosis (MS). Many of the important studies of CSF proteins in MS have recently been reviewed by Thompson (26). On agar gel electrophoresis, the most frequent finding has been that of a relatively uniform aberration with a few abnormal bands in the gammaglobulin range. Abnormalities of the CSF proteins, e.g. due to blood-CSF barrier damages and abnormal gammaglobulins, are frequently found in infections of the nervous system and Guillain-Barré syndromes (17-20, 27).

During recent years the introduction of isoelectric focusing (IEF) and isotachophoresis (ITP), techniques with separation capacities superior to those of conventional electrophoretic methods, has provided a very valuable tool for further analysis of the CSF protein aberrations in neurological diseases.

IEF has been adapted for analytical studies of many proteins (1, 21). The protein molecules are separated according to their isoelectric points (pI) in a pH-gradient formed by carrier ampholytes. Evidence has accumulated favouring the performance of IEF in thin layers of polyacrylamide gel (2, 28). After the potentialities of the method for the separation of CSF proteins had been pointed out by Fossard et al. (6) thin-layer IEF procedures used to examine CSF proteins were reported (3, 4, 9). This technique has afforded much new information about the CSF and serum proteins in many neurological diseases (5, 10, 13-15, 23).

ITP is a self-concentrating electromigration technique. The different sample molecules, arranged according to their different mobility characteristics, migrate at the same speed and are kept in order by a discontinuously increasing field strength from a leading to a terminating electrolyte, and the fractions can be detected by UV-densitometry and/or thermal registration. Introduction of spacer substances, e.g. carrier ampholytes and amino acids, strongly increases the possibilities to detect the different fractions. The first application of ITP for the analysis of CSF proteins was given by Kjellin et al. (11, 12).

The CSF and serum of about 2,000 patients with different neurological disorders, including demyelinating and infectious diseases and Guillain-Barré syndromes, have hitherto been examined with IEF in our laboratory. So far ITP has been performed only in a limited number of cases. In MS different complex CSF protein aberrations are found on IEF. The most frequently occurring abnormalities are regional increases of gammaglobulins and isolated bands of slight to conspicuous intensity and different positions in the gammaglobulin range. In addition, aberrations are observed in regions anodal to the gammaglobulin range. There seems to be a correlation between the patterns of conspicuous gammaglobulin bands and the duration and course of the disease as well as the probable sites of the CNS lesions (14). Numerous CSF protein abnormalities have also been observed on IEF in infectious neurological diseases.

These aberrations seem to be influenced not only by temporal but also by spatial factors (15). Factors related to the genetically determined immunological reactivity of the individual, the activity of etiological agents and the release of decomposition products from destroyed tissues may also influence the findings on IEF in demyelinating and infectious diseases.

EXPERIMENTAL

The number of patients and the diagnoses are given in Table 3. The Schumacher-Kurtzke diagnostic criteria for MS were used (16). A verifiable or probable etiological diagnosis was found in about a third of the patients with (meningo-)encephalitis, meningo-myelitis and meningitis.

IEF and ITP were performed as previously described (7, 10-12). The CSF protein fractions found by IEF were divided into 10 numbered regions as shown in Fig. 1 and the corresponding pH intervals are given in Table 1. Region '2' corresponds to albumin and region '1' includes more acidic proteins, e.g. prealbumins. The main fractions of transferrin and the tau-fraction are found in region '3' and '5', respectively. Region '4' exhibits three to six bands. Usually, no distinct fractions are found in region '6'. The normal gamma-globulin range is divided into three equal parts termed regions '7-9', and region '10' corresponds to the most alkaline range where normally no fractions are found. The abnormal findings of the gamma-globulin range were classified into mean patterns (Table 1) indicating regional ('a' - 'e modified' patterns) or uniform ('f' pattern) increases of proteins.

Table 1. The pH intervals corresponding to regions '1-10' (13) and the mean patterns of the CSF gammaglobulin range. Sample application = s.a.

Region	pH interval	Pattern	Relative increase of proteins in regions '7-10'
1	2.5-4.6	a	8-10, especially 9-10
2	4.6-5.0	b	8-10, rather uniformly
3	5.0-5.4	c	7-10, especially 8-10
4	5.4-5.8	d	8-9, rather uniformly
5	5.8-6.0	e	7-9, especially 9
6	6.0-6.2	e modified	7-9, especially 8-9
s.a.	6.2-6.4	f	7-9, rather uniformly and
7	6.4-7.4		usually very similar to a
8	7.4-8.2		'finger-print' of the corre-
9	8.2-8.9		sponding serum gammaglobulin
10	8.9-11.0		range

Table 2.   CSF protein abnormalities found by IEF.

Number	CSF protein abnormality
1	Abnormally prominent fraction in region '4'
2	Double fraction in region '5'
3	Single fraction in the middle of region '7'
4	Highly alkaline fraction (HAF)
5	Abnormal mean pattern ('a' - 'f')
6	Abnormal gammaglobulin bands other than those numbered 3 and 4

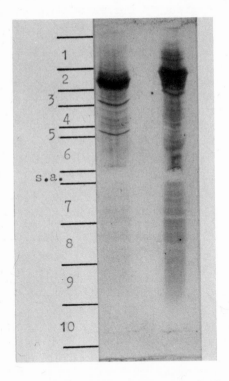

Fig. 1.   IEF of normal CSF. The anode was at the top and the
cathode at the bottom. Serum sample from the same patient to the
right. The division of the CSF protein fractions is given to the
left (s.a. = sample application). Note the weakly stained CSF
gammaglobulin range.

Table 3. Occurrence of the abnormalities numbered 1-5 in Table 2. In group B the examinations were, with the exception of the patients with 'sequelae' and some subjects with (meningo-)encephalitis, performed within 8 weeks after the symptomatic onset of the disorder.

Diagnosis, number of cases in parentheses+	Abnormalities numbered 1-4 in Table 2				Abnormal mean patterns		
	1	2	3	4	a - c	d - e modified	f
A.							
MS (125)	5 (4%)	25 (20%)	16 (13%)	50 (40%)	33 (26%)	86 (69%)	4 (3%)
MS (?) (105)	13 (12%)	24 (23%)	14 (13%)	59 (56%)	15 (14%)	69 (66%)	11 (10%)
ON (20)	-	3	1	7	2	4	2
B.							
(Meningo-)encephalitis (34)	6	9	1	12	9	14	11
Meningo-myelitis (11)	-	1	-	3	2	3	4
Meningitis (16)	3	2	4	7	1	2	13
'Sequelae' (10)	-	5	1	6	-	1	9
Guillain-Barré (22)	2	4	1	11	1	3	18

+MS: Clinically verified MS; MS (?): Probable MS; ON: Optic neuritis; (Meningo-)encephalitis: Encephalitis and meningoencephalitis; 'Sequelae': Objective or subjective sequelae after acute CNS infections months or years earlier.

Table 4. Occurrence of abnormal CSF gammaglobulin bands. Results from the same examinations as in Table 3.

Diagnosis, number of cases in parentheses		Positions of abnormal bands			
		Region 7-9 or 7-10	Region 8-9 or 8-10	Region 9 or 9-10	Region 8
A.MS	(125)	19 (15%)	50 (40%)	40 (32%)	1 (1%)
MS(?)	(105)	7 (7%)	34 (32%)	21 (20%)	4 (4%)
ON	(20)	1	1	2	–
B.(Meningo-) encephalitis	(34)	5	10	6	–
Meningo-myelitis	(11)	–	2	3	–
Meningitis	(16)	1	–	1	–
'Sequelae'	(10)	–	–	1	–
Guillain-Barré	(22)	–	–	2	–

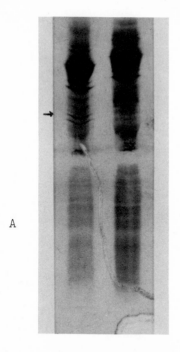
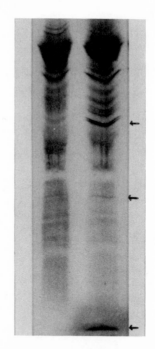

Fig. 2. A: An abnormally prominent fraction in region '4' indicated
by the arrow. The CSF gammaglobulin range exhibits an 'f' pattern.
B: A double fraction in region '5', a single fraction in region '7'
and a HAF indicated by arrows.

RESULTS

The CSF protein abnormalities found by IEF are listed in Table
2 and Figs. 2 and 3 give examples of these abnormalities. One or
more of these aberrations were found in 99% of patients with clinically verified MS, in 98% of subjects with probable MS, in 70% of
patients with optic neuritis, and in 99% of the subjects with infectious neurological diseases or Guillain-Barré syndromes.

The occurrence of the abnormalities numbered 1-5 (Table 2) is
given in Table 3. Ninety-five per cent of patients with clinically
verified MS, 80% of subjects with probable MS, and 30% of patients
with optic neuritis exhibited mean patterns with regional increases
of CSF gammaglobulins; the 'c', 'e' and 'e modified' patterns domi-
nated. Among the remaining abnormalities a double fraction in region
'5' and a highly alkaline fraction (HAF) were most frequent. Mean
patterns with regional increases of CSF gammaglobulins were observed
in 62% of patients with (meningo-)encephalitis and meningomyelitis.
Subjects with meningitis, 'sequelae' and Guillain-Barré syndromes
generally exhibited an 'f' pattern and a HAF occurred in 50% of

these patients. A double fraction in region '5' was found in one half of the subjects with 'sequelae'.

Table 4 gives the occurrence of abnormal bands other than a single fraction in region '7' and a HAF in the CSF gammaglobulin range. Such abnormal bands were observed in 88 and 63% respectively of patients with clinically verified and probable MS and in 20% of subjects with optic neuritis; the most frequent positions were region '8-9' and '9'. A comparison between the clinical data and the band abnormalities in patients with clinically verified MS gave the following results. The abnormalities tended to be more restricted in females than in males. A distinctly higher incidence of bands in region '7' was found in patients with active brain-stem lesions than subjects with active spinal lesions. Among patients with a duration of the disorder of less than one year abnormal bands predominantly occurred in region '8-9', while subjects with a longer duration of the disorder more frequently tended to exhibit more extensive or restricted changes. Abnormal bands in the CSF gammaglobulin range were found in 58% of patients with (meningo-) encephalitis and meningomyelitis, while such changes occurred in only 10% of subjects with meningitis, 'sequelae' and Guillain-Barré syndromes. The largest number and widest extension of bands were observed in subchronic and chronic meningoencephalitis. With the exception of one patient with a monilial meningitis all subjects with extension of the abnormal bands into region '7' had meningoencephalitis with brain-stem/cranial nerve disturbances.

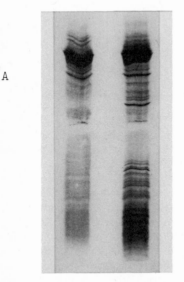
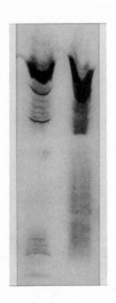

A   B

Fig. 3. Abnormal CSF gammaglobulin bands within a wide range of pI-values (A) and restricted to the cathodal range (B).

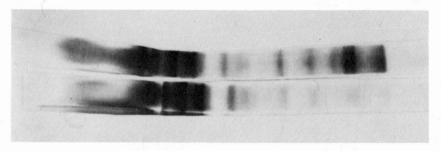

Fig. 4. ITP in polyacrylamide gel. The anode was to the left and the cathode to the right. CSF sample from a patient with MS (above) exhibiting prominent low-mobility gammaglobulin bands in the cathodal range when compared to the findings in a control subject (below).

Two or more CSF examinations (2 weeks to 4 years apart) have been performed in 60 patients with MS or optic neuritis. A double fraction in region '5' was least influenced by the temporal course of the disorder, the mean patterns and the abnormal gammaglobulin bands showed an intermediate degree of variation and the remaining abnormalities exhibited a high degree of influence by the temporal course. In 28 patients with infectious neurological diseases or Guillain-Barré syndromes repeated CSF examinations have been performed; the interval between the initial and last examination ranged from 1 week to 2,5 years and was in three quarters of the cases 6 months or shorter. The abnormal bands in the gammaglobulin range tended to first appear in region '9' and later be followed by bands mostly in more anodal positions; the disappearance of the bands generally occurred before that of the blood-CSF barrier damage. The abnormalities of the gammaglobulin range tended to 'peak' 4 to 8 weeks after the symptomatic onset of the disorder. A double fraction in region '5' remained unchanged, while the other aberrations showed moderate to pronounced degrees of variation during the temporal course of the disease.

The ITP systems used were especially designed for studying the gammaglobulin range. An example of the results on ITP in poly-acrylamide gel is given in Fig. 4. ITP in capillary tubes was performed by the use of either anionic or cationic systems and examples of the findings are given in Figs. 5 and 6. The serum gammaglobulin range may reveal changes similar to but less pronounced than those of the CSF from the same patient. Albumin,transferrin and IgG were detected by a micro-preparative procedure for immunological identification, and an example of the findings with such a procedure is given in Fig. 7.

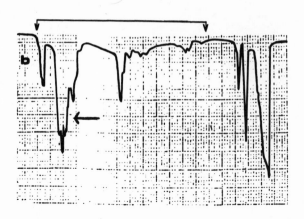

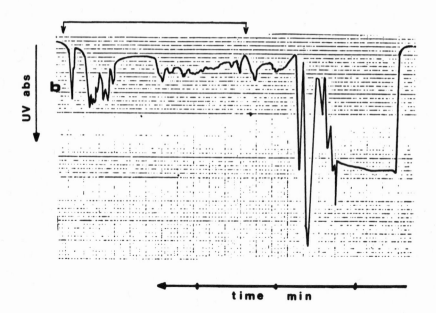

Fig. 5. CSF (above) and serum (below) from a patient with MS
examined by ITP in capillary tubes; an anionic system was used.
The gammaglobulin range is indicated by bar-connected arrows.
Note the prominent peak (arrow) in the CSF gammaglobulin range.
In this patient similar but less pronounced aberrations can be ob-
served in the corresponding parts of the serum gammaglobulin range.

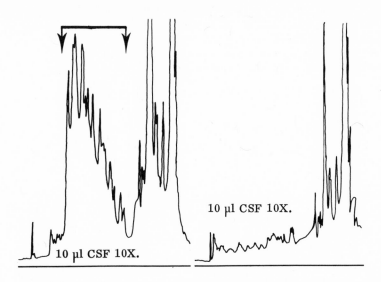

Fig. 6. CSF from a patient with MS (left) and a control subject (right) examined by ITP in capillary tubes; a cationic system was used. Note the multiple prominent peaks (bar-connected arrows) in the gammaglobulin range of the MS patient.

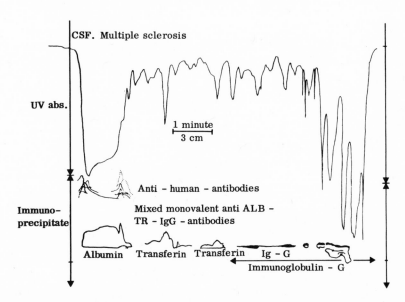

Fig. 7. CSF protein fractions found by ITP and examined by a micro-preparative procedure for immunological identification.

DISCUSSION

The CSF protein aberrations found on IEF can be grouped into
two main categories. The first group of abnormalities includes
oligoclonal bands and mean patterns with regional increases of
gammaglobulins. Such findings are compatible with intrathecal
synthesis of immunoglobulins and are generally found only in demyelinating and infectious neurological diseases. These abnormalities were the predominant finding in MS and occurred in about one
half of subjects with (meningo-)encephalitis and meningomyelitis.
The second group of aberrations, i.e. an 'f' pattern and the abnormalities numbered in 1-4 in Table 2, also occurs in varying
frequencies in other neurological diseases. The 'f' pattern
generally indicates a predominant blood-CSF barrier damage, although
in a few patients it appeared to indicate a polyclonal increase of
CSF immunoglobulins. The occurrence of a double fraction in region
'5', a single fraction in region '7' and a HAF in degenerative and
cerebrovascular disorders might promote the suggestion that these
fractions arise from decomposition products of destroyed tissues,
including myelin breakdown products. Abnormal fractions in region
'4' have previously been described in other neurological disorders
(23). Aberrations in this region have also been found in cerebrovascular diseases and the 'empty sella syndrome', and the abnormality might at least partly be related to affections of intracranial
meningeal and parenchymatous structures.

The different complex patterns of CSF protein aberrations
found by IEF illustrate the great value of the technique for CSF
examinations. Analytical ITP has besides its high separation capacity several valuable advantages for CSF protein studies (11, 12).
The analyses are quickly performed and the results are immediately
obtained on a recorder. Very small samples (μl quantities)are
needed, and biological fluids with very low protein contents can
be examined without prior concentration. Low and high molecular
weight compounds can be analysed. Among the different ITP systems
cationic gammaglobulin separations seem to give more distinct results than anionic separations.

The protein fractions found by IEF can be studied further by
different identification methods, e.g. immunoelectrophoresis. One
crossed immunoelectrofocusing technique (25) has been found appli-
cable to examinations of non-immunoglobulin CSF proteins with acidic
pI-values (24). CSF immunoglobulins can be studied by modified
crossed immunoelectrofocusing techniques (22) and Fig. 8 gives an
example of the findings with such a procedure. The fractions found
by ITP can be further examined by a micro-preparative method, e.g.
for immunological identification of proteins (7).

Several factors may influence the CSF protein findings on IEF.
Not only the temporal course of the disorder, but also the position
of lesions and the release of decomposition products from destroyed
CNS tissues may be of importance; further influencing mechanisms

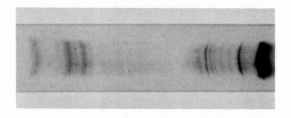

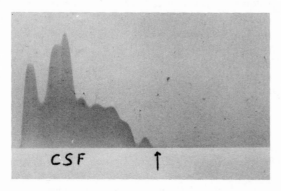

Fig. 8. Crossed immunoelectrofocusing of CSF gammaglobulins;
the corresponding IEF findings are shown above. The immunoelectrophoretic step was performed in a gel containing rabbit antiserum
to human IgG. The arrow indicates the sample application on the
IEF procedure.

might be factors related to the etiological agent and the genetically determined reactivity of the individual. Further CSF protein
studies using analytical and preparative IEF and ITP, including
techniques combining these methods with e.g. immunological identification tests, must obviously be of interest. Important objectives
of such examinations are to study the properties of the abnormal
fractions, their relationships to clinical data and their possible
prognostic signification, and such studies are presently in progress.

REFERENCES

1. Arbuthnott, J.P. and Beeley, J.A. (Eds.): Isoelectric focusing,
    London, Butterworths (1975).
2. Davies, H., Thin-layer gel isoelectric focusing, in Isoelectric
    focusing (J.P. Arbuthnott and J.A. Beeley, eds.) London,
    Butterworths (1975) pp. 97-113.
3. Delmotte, P., Gel isoelectric focusing of cerebrospinal fluid
    proteins: A potential diagnostic tool, Z. klin. Chem. u. klin.
    Biochem. 9 (1971) 334-336.

4. Delmotte, P., Comparative results of agar electrophoresis and
    isoelectric focusing examination of the gammaglobulins of the
    cerebrospinal fluid, Acta neurol. belg. 72 (1972) 226-234.
5. Delmotte, P. and Consette, R., Isoelectric focusing of the
    CSF gamma globulins in multiple sclerosis (262 cases) and
    other neurological diseases (272 cases), J. Neurol. 215 (1977)
    27-37.
6. Fossard, C., Dale, G. and Latner, A.L., Separation of the pro-
    teins of cerebrospinal fluid using gel electrofocusing followed
    by electrophoresis, J. clin. Path. 23 (1970) 586-589.
7. Hallander, L.B. and Kjellin, K.G., Isotachophoresis for in-
    vestigation of cerebrospinal fluid proteins, in Abstracts of
    the 6th International Meeting of the ISN, Copenhagen, August
    1977.
8. Kabat, E.A., Moore, D.H. and Landow, H., An electrophoretic
    study of the protein components in the cerebrospinal fluid
    and their relationship to serum proteins, J. clin. Invest.
    21 (1942) 571-577.
9. Kjellin, K.G. and Vesterberg, O., Thin-layer isoelectric
    focusing of cerebrospinal fluid proteins. A preliminary report
    with special reference to the diagnostic significance in
    multiple sclerosis. In Proceedings of the 20th Congress of
    Scandinavian Neurologists, Oslo 1972, pp. 379-380.
10. Kjellin, K.G. and Vesterberg, O., Isoelectric focusing of CSF
    proteins in neurological diseases, J. neurol. Sci. 23 (1974)
    199-213.
11. Kjellin, K.G., Moberg, U. and Hallander, L., Analytical
    isotachophoresis of cerebrospinal fluid proteins - a prelimi-
    nary report, Sci. Tools 22 (1975) 3-7.
12. Kjellin, K.G., Hallander, L. and Moberg, U., Analytical
    isotachophoresis: a new method for analysis of cerebrospinal
    fluid proteins, J. neurol. Sci. 26 (1975) 617-622.
13. Kjellin, K.G. and Stibler, H., Isoelectric focusing and electro-
    phoresis of cerebrospinal fluid proteins in muscular dystrophies
    and spinal muscular atrophies, J. Neurol. Sci. 27 (1976) 45-57.
14. Kjellin, K.G. and Sidén, Å., Aberrant CSF protein fractions
    found by electrofocusing in multiple sclerosis, Eur. Neurol.
    15 (1977) 40-50.
15. Kjellin, K.G. and Sidén, Å., Electrofocusing and electrophoresis
    of cerebrospinal fluid proteins in CNS disorders of known or
    probable infectious etiology, Eur. Neurol., in press.
16. Kurtzke, J.F., Diagnosis and differential diagnosis of multiple
    sclerosis, Acta Neurol. Scand. 46 (1970) 484-492.
17. Laterre, E.C., Callewaert, A., Heremans, J.F. and Sfaello, Z.,
    Electrophoretic morphology of gammaglobulins in cerebrospinal
    fluid of multiple sclerosis and other diseases of the nervous
    system, Neurology 20(1970) 982-990.
18. Link, H. and Müller, R., Immunoglobulins in multiple sclerosis
    and infections of the nervous system, Arch. Neurol. 25 (1971)
    326-344.

19. Link, H., Immunoglobulin abnormalities in the Guillain-Barré syndrome, J. neurol. Sci. 18 (1973) 11-23.
20. Lowenthal, A., Agar Gel Electrophoresis in Neurology, Amsterdam, Elsevier Publishing Company(1964).
21. Righetti, P.G. (Ed.), Progress in Isoelectric Focusing and Isotachophoresis. Amsterdam, North-Holland Publishing Company (1975).
22. Sidén, Å., Crossed immunoelectrofocusing of cerebrospinal fluid immunoglobulins, J. Neurol., in press.
23. Stibler, H. and Kjellin, K.G., Isoelectric focusing and electrophoresis of the CSF proteins in tremor of different origins, J. neurol. Sci. 30 (1976) 269-285.
24. Stibler, H., Crossed immunoelectrofocusing for identification of normal and abnormal cerebrospinal fluid proteins, J. neurol. Sci. 32 (1977) 331-336.
25. Söderholm, J. and Smyth, C.J., Crossed immunoelectrofocusing for studies on protein microheterogeneity, in Progress in Isoelectric Focusing and Isotachophoresis (P.G. Righetti, ed.) Amsterdam; North-Holland Publishing Company (1975) pp. 99-114.
26. Thompson, E.J., Laboratory diagnosis of multiple sclerosis: immunological and biochemical aspects, Br. Med. Bull. 35 (1977) 28-33.
27. Ursing, B., Clinical and immunoelectrophoretic studies of cerebrospinal fluid in virus meningoencephalitis and bacterial meningitis, Acta Med. Scand. suppl. 429 (1965).
28. Vesterberg, O., Some aspects of isoelectric focusing in polyacrylamide gel, in Isoelectric Focusing (J.P. Arbuthnott and J.A. Beeley, eds.) London, Butterworths (1975) pp. 78-96.

PROLIFERATING CELLS IN DEMYELINATING STATES

M.I. Reunanen, J. Ilonen and K. Järvenpää

Departments of Neurology and Radiotherapy, University
    of Oulu, and Public Health Laboratory
Oulu, Finland

SUMMARY

Proliferation of mononuclear cells was examined with an auto-radiography method in the CSF and peripheral blood of 13 patients with multiple sclerosis (MS), serially during activation of disease in one patient with subacute sclerosis panencephalitis (SSPE), and in some control patients with various neurological conditions. High cerebrospinal fluid (CSF) cell labelling indices, up to 1.7%, which could not be directly related to the clinical activity of the disease, were found in some MS patients. During activation of SSPE there was marked increase in labelled cells of CSF, up to 4.3%. In controls, corresponding CSF indices ranged from < 0.1% to 0.4%. Mononuclear cells in CSF and peripheral blood behaved as clearly different cell populations.

INTRODUCTION

In demyelinating diseases, such as multiple sclerosis (MS), there are signs of active immunological processes in the central nervous system (CNS), including elevated immunoglobulins in the cerebrospinal fluid (CSF) and perivascular cuffing of lymphocytes (for a review, see 5, 6).

A characteristic feature of the immune response is proliferation of immunocytes. This is an initial event in both cell-mediated and humoral response. The cell proliferation can be measured with incorporation of 3H-thymidine into replicating DNA. The number of active proliferating cells can be counted with autoradiography. In this study, proliferating cells in CSF and peripheral blood were examined by autoradiography in 13 MS patients, in one SSPE patient during an activation of the disease, and in some controls with various neurological conditions.

EXPERIMENTAL

Patients. Thirteen patients with confirmed MS, 5 males and 8 females, were included in the study. The age of the patients ranged from 26 to 53 years and duration of the disease from 0.5 to 27 years.

The SSPE patient first presented in 1966, at an age of 6 years, with typical picture of SSPE, including clonic jerks, EEG changes, and high measles antibody levels in serum and CSF. After partial recovery with moderate intellectual defect there were   no signs of disease activity until January 1977, when the patient was admitted to hospital because of right progressive hemiparesis. Within 6 weeks severe encephalitic phase developed, with marked increase in measles antibody titres in serum and CSF.

The control patients had various neurological conditions without any suspicion of demyelinating disease.

Methods. CSF specimens were obtained by lumbar puncture and immediately centrifuged at 1,200 rpm for 5 min. The cells were suspended in RPMI 1640 tissue culture medium (Gibco, Bio-Cult Ltd., Scotland) containing 20% pooled human male serum.

Heparinized peripheral blood was layered on Ficoll-Isopaque gradient and mononuclear cells were separated and washed with Hank´s salt solution (1). The peripheral blood mononuclear cells were then suspended in tissue culture fluid as above.

Cells of the CSF and peripheral blood were incubated for 2 h at 37°C in 5% CO_2 atmosphere with 3H-thymidine (The Radiochemical Centre, Amersham, England) at a concentration of 2 μCi/ml. Cell preparations were then made using a Shandon Scientific cytocentrifuge. The slides were fixed, gelatinized and covered with photographic film (Kodak autoradiographic stripping plates AR 10). They were exposed for 6 days at 4°C, developed and stained with Giemsa.

Labelling indices were determined by counting 1,000 mononuclear cells. Labelled cells were easily recognized because of the heavy accumulation of silver grains over their nuclei (Fig. 1).

RESULTS

The labelling indices (LI) of mononuclear cells in the CSF and peripheral blood of 13 MS patients are presented in Table 1. The number of cells in the CSF and description of the patients are included in Table 1. The data on control patients are presented in Table 2.

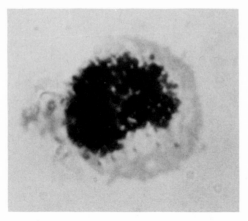

Fig. 1. Autoradiograph of a DNA synthesizing CSF cell from a patient with multiple sclerosis.

Among the MS patients the highest LI´s were 1.4 and 1.7 in patients IJ and SA, respectively. Peripheral blood contained 0.4% proliferating mononuclear cells in these patients. Both patients had the chronic progressive type of MS. The LI´s of two patients with acute stage MS were 0.1 and 0.6 in CSF, 0.1 and 0.1 in blood. In control patients the labelling indices varied from ⋜ 0.1 to 0.4 in CSF. In peripheral blood the values were from ⋜0.1 to 2.0.

Serial investigations of these parameters during a relapse of SSPE are presented in Table 3 with description of clinical changes.

DISCUSSION

In this study we simultaneously examined both CSF and peripheral blood mononuclear cells with autoradiography. These cell populations clearly behaved differently; there was strong proliferation of CSF cells without marked increase of DNA synthesizing cells in blood and also vice versa.

Large numbers of DNA synthesizing cells have been reported in the peripheral blood of patients with a variety of disorders in which involvement of lymphoid tissue is a prominent feature, for example viral infections, autoimmune diseases and drug hypersensitivity states (7, 8). This phenomenon can be considered as a sign of a widespread immune response in the patient. In demyelinating diseases, such as MS and SSPE, immunological factors seem to be important. In the peripheral blood of these patients, however, increased numbers of proliferating cells are not found (2).

Table 1. Autoradiography of CSF and blood mononuclear cells in MS patients. Labelling index: per cent of mononuclear cells.

Patients Code	Age (years)	Date of investigation	Clinical classification of MS	Duration of disease (years)	Cells/µl CSF	Labelling index CSF	Labelling index Blood
PO	32	10/01 77	Acute	4.5	11	0.6	0.1
HP	36	20/01 77	Acute	0.5	3	0.1	0.1
MR	47	29/11 76	Chronic progressive	19	48	0.2	0.1
SA	26	10/12 76	Chronic progressive	5	4	1.7	0.4
KK	33	06/01 77	Chronic progressive	4	4	0.1	< 0.1
MK	30	14/01 77	Chronic progressive	11	9	< 0.1	0.1
EK	53	03/02 77	Chronic progressive	9	10	0.4	0.2
NP	43	17/02 77	Chronic progressive	14	20	0.2	1.1
IJ	30	08/03 77	Chronic progressive	14	10	1.4	0.4
OK	30	23/05 77	Chronic progressive	6	5	0.3	0.4
RB	45	13/12 76	Static	20	9	0.5	0.1
AP	51	07/01 77	Static	27	3	0.2	0.1

Table 2. Autoradiography of CSF and blood mononuclear cells in control patients. Labelling index: per cent of mononuclear cells.

Patients Code	Age (years)	Date of investigation	Diagnosis	Cells/µl CSF	Labelling index CSF	Blood
SJN	26	20/01 77	Cephalalgia tensiva	<1	<0.2	0.3
AR	66	02/02 77	Encephalopathia vascularis seu paraneoplastica	1	<0.2	<0.1
AP	42	03/02 77	Cephalalgia Arthritis rheumatoides	1	0.1	2.0
SJ	28	03/02 77	Migraine	4	<0.1	<0.1
RL	36	17/02 77	Migraine	2	0.4	0.1
AK	47	23/02 77	St.post meningoencepha- litidem (herpes simplex)	4	0.1	1.6
TS	16	06/05 77	Chorioretinis oculi sin.	11	<0.1	0.3

Table 3. Autoradiography of CSF and blood mononuclear cells in one SSPE patient with activation of the disease. Labelling index: per cent of mononuclear cells.

Date of investigation	Cells/µl CSF	Labelling index CSF	Labelling index Blood	Clinical stage
20/01 77	2	0.9	0.1	Relapse of SSPE with right
26/01 77	4	1.2	0.1	progressive hemiparesis
01/03 77	11	4.3	0.9	Severe encephalitic phase with
07/03 77	109	3.5	0.5	unconsciousness, fever, generalized
17/03 77	13	1.0	6.7	increase of muscle tone, increased
24/03 77	5	1.5	5.9	intracranial pressure and
12/04 77	7	0.2	1.0	profound EEG-changes
19/04 77	7	<0.1	0.6	Recovery with permanent severe dementia,
09/05 77	5	0.2	0.3	spastic tetraparesis and totally in need
				of care

Recently Dommasch et al. (3) published a study of various inflammatory conditions of the CNS in which they found a great number
of proliferating mononuclear cells in the CSF by the autoradiography
method. Labelling indices rose up to 0.5-8.0% in various inflammatory processes.

In our study some MS patients had a large number of DNA synthesizing cells in their CSF. This could not be directly related
to the clinical activity of the disease; one patient with an
apparent acute relapse had a labelling index of only 0.1% in the
CSF. This disagrees with the findings of Dommasch et al. who
found two acute phase MS patients with elevated numbers of DNA
synthesizing cells in the CSF. In their chronic progressive MS
patients, as in most of the non-inflammatory neurological controls,
there were <0.1% labelled cells. Yamakawa et al. (9) also reported
rather small numbers of proliferating cells in their control
patients. Earlier this group examined various neoplastic diseases
of the CNS in which they also found DNA synthesizing cells in CSF
(4).

The number of proliferating cells in CSF seemed, however, to
be a measure of specific activity in the CNS. Two controls and one
MS patient had a rather high labelling index in the peripheral
blood. This activity was not reflected in the CSF. One control
had a verified, active rheumatoid arthritis, the other had had
viral meningoencephalitis six months earlier.

There was a strong proliferation response in the CSF of the
SSPE patient during activation of the disease and during the
worsening of the clinical condition. After the disease again stabi-
lized to a new stage the activity of the CSF cells disappeared.
In the blood there was also a proliferating response but this occurred after the activation of the disease and the CSF cell reaction
and could be due to hypersensitivity reactions to antibiotics.

The appearance of proliferating cells in the CSF and blood
should be followed in MS patients to determine the importance of
this activity marker in the clinical course of the disease. It
would also be interesting to study the correlation of proliferation
with various other immunological parameters.

REFERENCES

1. Bøyum, A., Isolation of mononuclear cells and granulocytes
    from human blood, Scand. J. clin. Lab. Invest. 21, suppl.
    97 (1968) 77-89.
2. Cook, S.D. and Dowling, P.G., Neurologic disorders associated
    with increased DNA synthesis in peripheral blood, Arch. Neurol.
    19 (1968) 583-590.
3. Dommasch, D., Grüninger, W. and Schultze, B., Autoradiographic
    demonstration of proliferating cells in cerebrospinal fluid,
    J. Neurol. 214 (1977) 97-112.

4. Fukui, M., Yamakawa, Y., Yamasaki, T., Kitamura, K., Tabira, T. and Sadoshima, S., 3H-thymidine autoradiography of CSF cells in primary reticulum cell sarcoma of the brain, J. Neurol. 210 (1975) 143-150.

5. Haire, M., Significance of virus antibodies in multiple sclerosis, Brit. Med. Bull. 33 (1977) 40-44.

6. Knight, S.C., Cellular immunity in multiple sclerosis, Brit. Med. Bull. 33 (1977) 45-50.

7. Lalla, M., Proliferation of circulating human white cells in health and in non-neoplastic disorders. Academic dissertation, University of Helsinki, Helsinki (1974).

8. Wood, T.A. and Frenkel, E.P., The atypical lymphocyte, Amer. J. Med. 42 (1967) 923-936.

9. Yamakawa, Y., Fukui, M., Ohta, H. and Kitamura, K., 3H-thymidine autoradiography of the CSF cells in cases of non-neoplastic disease, J. Neurol. 211 (1976) 195-202.

TOPOGRAPHIC ANALYSIS OF MS AND CONTROL BRAINS

M. Röyttä, H. Frey, P. Riekkinen and U.K. Rinne

Department of Pathological Anatomy and Department of
  Neurology, University of Turku
Turku, Finland

SUMMARY

Autopsy specimens from five MS and six control cases were
subjected to morphological and biochemical investigations including
protein electrophoresis. On the basis of this study individual
differences between the enzyme activities and the effect of storage
must be taken into consideration when studying autopsy material.
Furthermore, good morphological controls are required when biochemical changes are studied, especially in diseases like MS where
local changes are found.

Biochemical and morphological studies showed that multiple
protein bands, possibly GFA, may be noticed in gliotic areas. The
activity of β-glucuronidase seemed to correlate with gliosis but
the increase of this enzyme did not seem to be the first change in
the plaque areas. It was suggested that the activation of carboxylic
acid esterase preceded the activation of β-glucuronidase. The
activities of lysosomal hydrolases seemed to decrease to a normal
level in morphologically normal brain areas outside the plaques.
In light microscopy, cells resembling plasma cells and containing
Russel bodies were found.

INTRODUCTION

The participation of acid proteinase in the pathogenesis of
plaque formation in MS is commonly found (7, 17), and the breakdown of basic protein (BP) has been shown to take place by the
action of acid proteinase (6, 19). However, Cuzner et al. (4) have
shown that this action of acid proteinase, especially at the rim
of plaques, rather indicates the chronic nature of plaques than

recent changes. The same authors have also shown that the activity
of β-glucurodinase, together with high activity of acid proteinase,
indicates recent plaque formation.

Using electrophoresis both Einstein et al. (7) and Riekkinen
et al. (18) reported that BP is missing from the plaque areas.
Riekkinen et al. (18) have also shown that BP may be missing from
normal-appearing white matter taken from MS brains. However,
Suzuki et al. (20) and Wolfgram et al. (21) reported that normal-
appearing white matter from MS patients did not differ from the
white matter taken from controls. Althaus et al. (2)   observed
only a decreased amount of BP in the plaque areas. An effort has
been made to correlate these findings with morphological results,
and a correlation with demyelination and myelin loss has been found
(17). It has been suggested that the lysosomal reac tion is also
seen in glial cells (astrocytes) but the origin of acid proteinase
and other enzymes related to demyelination is unknown.

The purpose of the present study was to further clarify the
neurochemical and morphological changes in MS on the basis of a
topographic survey of autopsy material.

EXPERIMENTAL

The material consisted of five MS brains taken 6-60 h after
death. From these, 94 samples were analysed. These samples were
taken from plaques near the plaques (border zone areas), from normal-
appearing white matter outside the plaques, and from normal-appearing
white matter without any macroscopically visible plaque nearby. The
size of the sample taken from the plaques varied according to the
area of the plaque, but the samples taken from other places had a
diameter of about 10x5x5 mm. The samples for chemical and electrophoretical analyses were homogenised and stored at -24°C until
analysed (1-4 months). The samples for morphological studies were
fixed in a buffered formaldehyde solution. The control material
consisted of six brains (90 samples) taken from patients without
any neurological disease. The samples from control brains were
taken 6-28 h after death and processed as above. Their anatomical
location is shown in Fig. 1.

All enzyme analyses were performed at 37°C. Acid proteinase,
acid phosphatase and β-glucuronidase were analysed according to the
method of Riekkinen and Clausen (15). The ac tivity of carboxylic
acid esterase was measured according to Naclas et al. (14), 2',3'-
cyclic nucleotide 3'-phosphohydrolase (CNP-ase) by the method of
Kurihara and Tsukada (11), and leucine aminopeptidase according to
Frey et al. (9). Protein electrophoresis was carried out by the
method of Eng et al. (8).

For morphological study the following stains were used: Hematoxylin-Eosin (HE), the Holzer method for glia fibers, Luxol fast
blue (LFB), Methyl green pyronin (MGP) (1), and PAS, which was also
used after incubation in diastase solution.

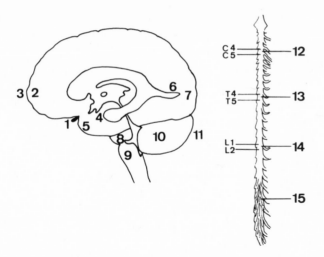

Fig. 1.   The anatomical location of control samples: 1. Optic
chiasma;   2. White matter, frontal lobe;   3. Gray matter, frontal
lobe;   4. White matter near the inferior horn, temporal lobe;
5. White matter, the temporal lobe;   6. White matter near the
posterior horn, occipital lobe;   7. White matter, occipital lobe;
8. Pons;   9. Upper part of medulla oblongata;   10. White matter,
cerebellum;   11. Gray matter, cerebellum;   12. Spinal cord,
cervical IV-V;   13. Spinal cord, thoracic IV-V;   14. Spinal cord,
lumbar I-II.

RESULTS

Controls

    The morphological findings were similar in all controls. Some
vacuolisation due to autolysis was found, but no perivascular inflammatory cells. Rare perivascular inflammatory cells were sometimes noticed. Myelin stained homogenously. The results from biochemical analyses are presented in Table 1. The activities of
acid proteinase, acid phosphatase, carboxylic acid esterase, and
leucine aminopeptidase were highest in the gray matter as well as
in areas containing nerve cells. The activities of β-glucuronidase
and CNP-ase were highest in the white matter.
    In protein electrophoresis, BP was present in all samples
taken from the white matter. In samples taken from the gray matter
the band containing histones moved slightly more rapidly than BP.
Acidic proteins were present in all samples but below them no
distinct bands were noted in samples taken from the brains. In
samples taken from the spinal cord, a thick band was seen in the
middle of the protein bands.

Table 1. The results of chemical analysis of the control patients. The mean ($\pm$ SEM) from five cases are presented. For further details see the text.

Region	Acid proteinase	Acid phosphatase	Carboxylic acid esterase	CNP-ase	β-glucuro-nidase	Leucine amino-peptidase
Optic chiasma	172$\pm$47(4)	19.5$\pm$1.6(4)	21.7$\pm$2.9(3)	10.8$\pm$0.9(4)	14.6$\pm$1.6(4)	2.9$\pm$0.4(4)
White matter, frontal lobe	146$\pm$23(6)	15.7$\pm$0.5(6)	34.3$\pm$1.6(4)	19.6$\pm$0.8(5)	12.5$\pm$0.6(6)	2.9$\pm$0.1(6)
Gray matter, frontal lobe	419$\pm$43(6)	39.2$\pm$3.4(6)	180.4$\pm$13.6(4)	4.3$\pm$0.2(6)	7.8$\pm$0.3(6)	5.1$\pm$0.5(6)
White matter, near the inferior horn, temporal lobe	146$\pm$33(5)	16.3$\pm$0.5(5)	36.9$\pm$2.3(4)	19.3$\pm$0.8(5)	12.7$\pm$0.9(5)	3.5$\pm$0.2(5)
White matter, temporal lobe	155$\pm$23(6)	17.1$\pm$0.7(6)	34.1$\pm$2.7(4)	20.3$\pm$2.7(6)	13.7$\pm$1.0(6)	3.4$\pm$0.2(6)
White matter, near the posterior horn, occipital lobe	136$\pm$19(6)	15.0$\pm$0.8(6)	30.4$\pm$2.0(4)	16.3$\pm$1.0(6)	12.0$\pm$0.7(6)	3.2$\pm$0.2(6)
White matter, occipital lobe	133$\pm$21(6)	15.8$\pm$0.7(6)	27.9$\pm$0.8(4)	15.3$\pm$0.8(6)	11.8$\pm$1.0(6)	3.3$\pm$0.2(6)

Table 1 continued on the next page.

Table 1, continued.

Region	Acid proteinase	Acid phosphatase	Carboxylic acid esterase	CNP-ase	β-glucuronidase	Leucine aminopeptidase
Pons	301±27(6)	20.5±1.3(6)	58.8±3.6(4)	13.9±0.7(6)	11.4±0.6(6)	3.5±0.3(6)
Upper part of medulla oblongata	319±30(6)	22.8±1.2(6)	45.0±3.2(4)	11.0±0.4(6)	13.0±0.6(6)	3.7±0.3(6)
White matter, cerebellum	151±27(6)	17.3±0.4(6)	37.2±1.5(4)	16.4±1.5(6)	14.2±1.1(6)	3.9±0.4(6)
Gray matter, cerebellum	414±46(6)	39.9±2.0(5)	104.7±6.3(4)	2.5±0.2(5)	9.7±0.7(6)	6.1±0.7(6)
Spinal cord, cervical IV-V	207±34(5)	19.3±0.4(5)	30.8±3.1(4)	8.3±0.4(5)	13.2±0.7(5)	3.8±0.4(5)
Spinal cord, thoracic IV-V	175±28(5)	18.5±0.3(5)	25.2±1.5(4)	8.1±0.5(5)	12.4±0.6(5)	3.6±0.3(5)
Spinal cord, lumbar I-II	266±63(5)	22.4±0.9(5)	34.4±4.0(4)	8.9±0.7(5)	14.6±0.7(5)	3.0±0.7(5)

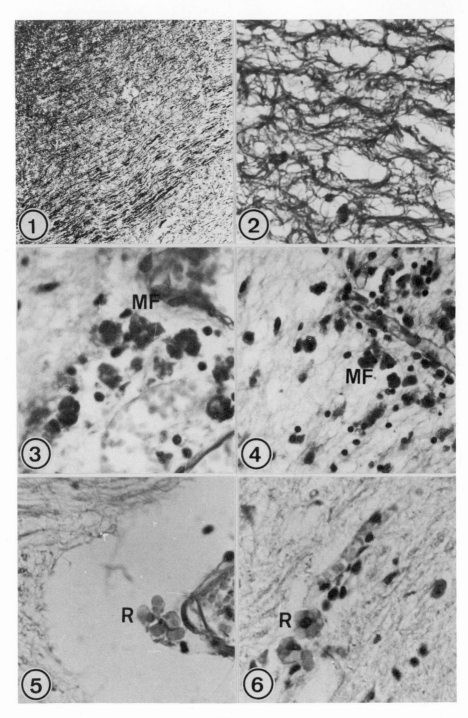

Fig. 2a

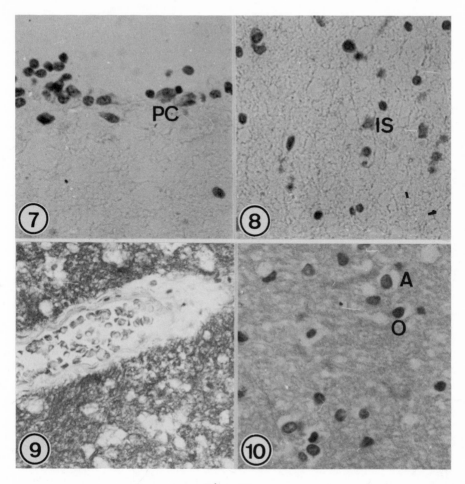

Fig. 2b

Fig. 2. Typical morphological results. Samples 1-8 were taken from MS cases and 9-10 from control cases. 1. Diffuse demyelination at the borderzone area, LFB x 64; 2. Gliosis at the demyelinated area, Holzer x 640; 3. Macrophages (MF) at the perivascular space, PAS after diastase digestion x 640; 4. Macrophages (MF) around the blood vessel, PAS x 320; 5. and 6. Cells containing Russel body-like granules (R), HE x 640; 7. Perivascular inflammatory cells and a plasma cell (PC), MGB x 640; 8. Intensively staining cells (IS), MGB x 640; 9. Normal myelin, LFB x 640; 10. Normal glial cells; astrocyte (A) and oligodendrocyte (0), HE x 640.
Fig. 2a: Samples 1-6; Fig. 2b: Samples 7-10.

MS-samples

Morphology. Typical morphological results are presented in
Fig. 2. Demyelination and gliosis were commonly present in the
plaque areas, although in some samples only neurons could be seen.
Perivascular inflammatory cells were commonly found in the plaque
areas and also in the samples taken from the borderzone areas.
Some samples taken from normal-appearing white matter showed, in
addition to marked demyelination, an increased number of small
round cells, the origin of which could not be determined.
     Cells containing Russel body-like granules were mainly seen
in perivascular areas. These granules were PAS-positive also after
diastase incubation and stained bright red in HE-staining. The
granules within the macrophages were also PAS-positive but stained
negatively after diastase incubation.
     Intensively staining cells were noticed with MGB staining in
the plaque and borderzone areas. The morphology of these cells did
not resemble that of plasma cells and the intensity of the cyto-
plasmatic material varied to some degree.
     Enzyme analyses. The activity of acid proteinase was highest
in the plaques and it decreased towards the normal-appearing white
matter (Table 2). However, the activity was sometimes highest in
the borderzone area. Morphologically these changes seemed to be in
correlation with demyelination and gliotic changes. In one case
light microscopic evidence of demyelination and increased activity
of acid proteinase could be found in all specimens. Even macroscopically normal-appearing white matter outside the topographically
analysed plaque had a higher activity than the borderzone are. In
another case part of the enzyme activity was probably due to neuronal
contamination of some samples.
     The findings on acid phosphatase were similar to that of acid
proteinase in three cases but in two cases some variation was found
in the activities between these two enzymes. In some samples, especially in those from gray matter, the activity of acid phosphatase
was at a normal level or slightly decreased despite the increased
activity of acid proteinase. In these cases, the activity of acid
phosphatase was highest in the plaques.
     The activity of carboxylic acid esterase was in all cases
highest in the plaque area, although with some exceptions. In one
case a sample from normal-appearing white matter had a high activity
despite an almost normal morphology. In one case (Table 2) variation
was also found in about one-half of the topographically analysed
areas, and in one topographical area the highest activity was found
in normal-appearing white matter. However, the activity was nearly
normal in this area.
     The activity of CNP-ase was usually lowest in the plaques and
increased towards the normal-appearing white matter although some
variation could be found in different areas. The activity was sometimes decreased despite normal morphology. Very high activity of

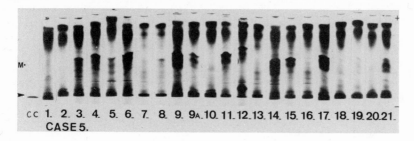

Fig. 3. Results of the protein electrophoresis from case 5. The numbers of the samples correspond to those presented in Table 2. M indicates the location of multiple bands and the arrow the location of BP. 9A is the borderzone sample not subjected to chemical analysis. Cytochrome C (CC) was used as a reference protein.

CNP-ase, despite light microscopic evidence of demyelination, was found in two samples from different cases. In this area numerous small, round cells were also seen.

The activity of β-glucuronidase seemed to correlate with gliosis. However, in one case decreased activity was seen in the plaque areas but this could partly be due to the neuronal content. In other cases increased activity was commonly seen in the plaques as well as in samples from normal-appearing white matter which showed demyelination and gliosis. The activity was very low or normal despite gliosis in some plaque samples from case 5. These samples showed a very high carboxylic acid esterase activity; in other cases this phenomenon also seemed to be the rule and no exceptions were found in samples taken from the white matter of other cases.

The activity of leucine aminopeptidase was highest in the plaques. It decreased towards the normal-appearing white matter.

Protein electrophoresis. In samples taken from the plaques or borderzone areas of two patients BP was sometimes clearly degraded and even lost. In three cases BP was present in all samples analysed, although the band located in the area of BP was sometimes broadened, possibly due to degradation. The most interesting finding was the presence of extra bands below the acidic proteins (= glial fibrillar acidic protein). These consisted of two to three bands and, occasionally, even a fourth band was noticed. These bands were commonly seen in samples which showed gliosis in Holzer staining. In case 5, where six plaques could be accurately analysed in their surroundings, the amount of these proteins decreased towards the normal-appearing white matter and only one sample from the normal-appearing white matter showed these bands (Fig. 3). This sample was the one outside the plaque which contained the very high activity of carboxylic acid esterase.

Table 2. The chemical results and summaries of light microscopic findings from MS case 5. The patient was autopsied 6 h after death. For other details see the text.

Sample	Acid proteinase	Acid phosphatase	Carboxylic acid esterase	CNP-ase	β-glucuro-nidase	Leucine amino-peptidase
1. Gray matter, left frontal lobe	515	33.8	182.9	4.6	8.1	3.5
2. White matter, left frontal lobe	198	16.9	32.1	14.7	14.7	2.0
3. Periventricular plaque, right frontal lobe	354	23.0	167.9	10.5	7.5	3.3
4. Border zone area of the previous plaque	174	16.7	63.0	14.9	11.5	1.7
5. Normal-appearing white matter outside the previous plaque	150	16.3	33.0	16.8	15.2	1.6
6. Periventricular plaque, left parietal lobe	342	30.9	100.9	3.4	15.4	3.6
7. Borderzone area of the previous plaque	171	18.2	31.9	11.3	13.2	2.4
8. Normal-appearing white matter outside the previous plaque	162	17.8	30.9	14.4	15.0	1.9
9. A plaque and borderzone area, right parietal lobe	382	26.9	32.0	7.7	24.6	2.1
10. Normal-appearing white matter outside the previous sample	191	16.4	30.0	15.2	16.7	1.6

Table 2 continued.

Sample	Acid proteinase	Acid phosphatase	Carboxylic acid esterase	CNP-ase	β-glucuronidase	Leucine aminopeptidase
11. Periventricular plaque above the posterior horn	331	30.7	31.2	3.7	29.8	3.1
12. Borderzone area of the previous plaque	268	25.2	28.9	10.0	20.2	2.3
13. Normal-appearing white matter outside the previous plaque	168	17.4	31.4	15.1	15.5	1.8
14. A plaque above the right posterior horn	279	30.0	35.8	0.7	34.6	2.3
15. Borderzone area of the previous plaque	345	25.6	38.1	9.2	24.5	2.3
16. Normal-appearing white matter outside the previous plaque	168	15.6	32.9	19.2	14.0	1.6
17. Periventricular plaque behind the right posterior horn	410	34.0	46.0	2.2	32.9	2.7
18. Borderzone area of the previous plaque	350	25.5	29.9	9.1	24.4	2.1
19. Normal-appearing white matter outside the previous plaque	178	17.4	25.7	13.5	14.4	1.9
20. Cerebellar white matter	215	18.6	40.6	11.1	15.6	1.9
21. Pons (fibrotic)	435	23.7	106.4	8.4	15.3	2.8

Table 2 continued.

Morphology

1. Normal morphology.
2. Some perivascular inflammatory cells, otherwise normal.
3. Almost total demyelination. Numerous perivascular inflammatory cells, a few plasma cells. Gliosis. Intensively staining cells in MGB-staining.
4. Clear demarcation with normal area, some gliosis. A few macrophages. Possibly an increased number of small, round cells.
5. Normal myelin staining, no gliosis. No perivascular inflammatory cells.
6. No myelin, marked gliosis. Some perivascular inflammatory cells, rare plasma cells. Numerous intensively staining cells in the stroma.
7. Diffuse demyelination, gliosis. Some perivascular inflammatory cells.
8. Normal myelin. No gliosis. Some perivascular inflammatory cells.
9. Diffuse myelin in plaque area, and loss of myelin in the border-zone area. Numerous perivascular inflammatory cells in the plaque area and borderzone area, a few plasma cells. In the stroma   the number of small, round cells seemed to be increased. Macrophages in the borderzone area.
10. Diffuse loss of myelin, no gliosis. Perivascular inflammatory cells, rare plasma cells.
11. Almost total demyelination. Gliosis. Numerous perivascular inflammatory cells, rare plasma cells.
12. Some demyelination, macrophages in the stroma. Perivascular inflammatory cells, a few plasma cells.
13. Diffuse demyelination. A few plasma cells and lymphocytes perivascularly.
14. No myelin, marked gliosis. Perivascular inflammatory cells, a few plasma cells. Brightly staining cells in MGB-staining.
15. Macrophages in the stroma. Perivascular inflammatory cells, a few plasma cells. Diffuse demyelination.
16. Normal myelin staining, a few perivascular inflammatory cells.
17. Almost total demyelination. Marked gliosis. Perivascular inflammatory cells, a few plasma cells which are also seen in the stroma. Numerous intensively staining cells of red colour.
18. Diffuse demyelination. Marked gliosis. No macrophages. Perivascular inflammatory cells.
19. Focal slight demyelination and gliosis, where perivascular inflammatory cells and macrophages. Numerous small, round cells in demyelinated area.
20. Few perivascular inflammatory cells, otherwise normal.
21. Slight demyelination around the aqueduct of Sylvii. Some perivascular inflammatory cells. Gliosis around the neurons.

DISCUSSION

Five MS cases and six controls were analysed in the present study. Post mortem changes and possible individual variation must be taken into serious consideration. The results of the control study showed a clear variation in the enzyme activities between individual cases. The duration of storage should also be considered. In another series of studies (Riekkinen et al., unpublished results) the activity of acid proteinase showed marked changes during storage, and the activities of acid phosphatase and leucine aminopeptidase also changed during the six months of preservation. Only the activity of β-glucuronidase was rather stable.

Morphological control is required in a study of biochemical changes. Despite macroscopically normal areas, demyelination could be seen as well as increased activities of lysosomal hydrolases. In areas where the morphological picture was normal the activities of lysosomal hydrolases were usually normal. This finding can at least partly explain why Riekkinen et al. (17) found a loss of BP from normal-appearing white matter.

Cuzner et al. (5) have suggested that the increased activity of acid proteinase, together with an increased activity of β-glucuronidase, is a marker of a recent plaque. In addition to this, the present work showed plaques where the activity of β-glucuronidase was low or normal. In these plaques the activities of lysosomal hydrolases were also increased. Horrocks (10) has suggested that the activity of plasmalogenase, present in oligodendroglial cells, precedes the activation of lysosomal hydrolases as indicated by β-glucuronidase, acid proteinase and neutral proteinase. The high activity of carboxylic acid esterase could thus be explained in a similar manner and thus these plaques could perhaps be considered as very recent ones.

Multiple bands present in protein electrophoresis can be regarded as glial fibrillar acidic protein (GFA) on the basis of reports published by Eng et al. (8). The morphological findings of the present study support this conclusion. The presence of gliosis did not seem to contradict the earlier assumption of a very recent plaque because the glial reaction seems to be rather fast (13). The effect of autolysis on the results of protein electrophoresis can be regarded minimal because the samples were lyophilized after freezing (3).

The presence of Russel bodies is an interesting feature and, according to the knowledge of the authors, not earlier reported. The significance of this finding is obscure but these cells are commonly found in rheumatoid arthritis and are considered as a marker of chronic infection, probably caused by a transport failure of light chains. Therefore, this finding may possibly be connected with the CSF findings in MS (22) although Link (12) could not find this abnormal kappa/lambda relation in MS brain.

MGB staining was used as a marker for plasma cells because it

is known to stain positively the cells containing a large amount
of ribosomal material. In addition to plasma cells numerous cells
which stained positively were noticed mainly in the plaque areas.
The significance of this finding is still open.

Acknowledgement. This investigation was supported by the
Medical Research Council of Finland.

REFERENCES

1. Ahlquist, J. and Andersson, L., Methyl green-pyronin staining:
   Effects of fixation: Use in routine pathology, Stain. Technol.
   1 (1972) 17-22.
2. Althaus, H.H., Pilz, H. and Müller, D., The protein composition
   of myelin in multiple sclerosis (MS) and orthochromatic leukodystrophy (OLD), Z. Neurol. 205 (1973) 229-241.
3. Ansari, K.A., Hendrickson, H., Sinha, A.A. and Rand, A., Myelin
   basic protein in frozen and unfrozen bovine brain: A study of
   autolytic changes in situ, J. Neurochem. 25 (1975) 193-195.
4. Cuzner, M.L. and Davison, A.N., Changes in cerebral lysosomal
   enzyme activity and lipids in multiple sclerosis, J. Neurol.
   Sci. 19 (1973) 29-36.
5. Cuzner, M.L., Barnard, R.O., MacGregor, J.L., Borshell, N.J.
   and Davison, A.N., Myelin composition in acute and chronic
   multiple sclerosis in relation to cerebral lysosomal activity,
   J. Neurol. Sci. 29 (1976) 323-334.
6. Einstein, E.R., Csejtey, J. and Marks, N., Degradation of encephalitogen by purified brain acid proteinase, FEBS Letts.
   1 (1968) 191-195.
7. Einstein, E.R., Dalal, K.B. and Csejtey, J., Increased protease
   activity and changes in basic proteins and lipids in multiple
   sclerosis plaques, J. Neurol. Sci. 11 (1970) 109-121.
8. Eng, L.F., Bond, P. and Gerstl, B., Isolation of myelin
   proteins from disc acrylamide gels electrophoresed in phenol-
   formic acid-water, Neurobiology 1 (1971) 58-63.
9. Frey, H.J., Riekkinen, P.J., Rinne, U.K. and Arstila, A.U.,
   Peptidase activity of myelin during the myelination period in
   guinea pig brain, Brain Res. 22 (1970) 243-248.
10. Horrocks, L.A., Plasmalogenase is elevated in early demyelinat-
    ing lesions due to canine distemper virus, in Myelination and
    Demyelination, Recent Chemical Advances, Satellite Symposium
    of the ISN, Helsinki, August 1977.
11. Kurihara, T. and Tsukada, Y., The regional and subcellular
    distribution of 2',3'-cyclic nucleotide 3'-phosphohydrolase
    in the central nervous system, J. Neurochem. 14 (1967) 1167-
    1174.
12. Link, H., Oligoclonal immunoglobulin G in multiple sclerosis
    brains, J. Neurol. Sci. 16 (1972) 103-114.

13. Lumsden, C.E., The neuropathology of multiple sclerosis, Clin. Neurol. 9 (1970) 217-309.
14. Nachlas, M.M. and Seligman, A.M., Evidence for the specificity of esterase and lipase by the use of three chromogenic substrates, J. biol. Chem.181 (1949) 343-355.
15. Riekkinen, P.J. and Clausen, J., Proteinase activity of myelin, Brain Res. 15 (1969) 413-430.
16. Riekkinen, P.J., Clausen, J., Frey, H.J., Fog, T. and Rinne, U.K., Acid proteinase activity of white matter and plaques in multiple sclerosis, Acta neurol. scand. 46 (1970) 349-353.
17. Riekkinen, P.J., Palo, J., Arstila, A.U., Savolainen, H., Rinne, U.K., Kivalo, E. and Frey, H.J., Protein composition of multiple sclerosis myelin, Arch. Neurol. 24 (1971) 545-549.
18. Riekkinen, P.J., Rinne, U.K., Arstila, A.U., Kurihara, T. and Pelliniemi, T.T., Studies on the pathogenesis of multiple sclerosis, J. Neurol. Sci. 15 (1972) 113-120.
19. Röyttä, M., Frey, H., Riekkinen, P.J., Laaksonen, H. and Rinne, U.K., Myelin breakdown and basic protein, Exp. Neurol. 45 (1974) 174-185.
20. Suzuki, K., Kamoshita, S., Eto, Y., Tourtellotte, W.W. and Gonatas, J.O., Myelin in multiple sclerosis, Arch. Neurol. 28 (1973) 293-297.
21. Wolfgram, F., Wallace, W. and Tourtellotte,W., Amino acid composition of myelin in multiple sclerosis, Neurology 22 (1972) 1044-1046.
22. Zetterwall, O. and Link, H., Electrophoretic distribution of kappa/lambda immunoglobulin light chain determinants in serum and CSF in multiple sclerosis, Clin. exp. Immunol. 7 (1970) 365-372.

BIOCHEMICAL STUDY ON MYELIN IN ADRENOLEUKODYSTROPHY

Tadashi Miyatake[1,2], Toshio Ariga[2], Tetsushi Atsumi[1],
and Yoshiaki Komiya[3]
1) Department of Neurology, Jichi Medical School,
   Yakushiji, Tochigi, Japan
2) Tokyo Metropolitan Institute of Medical Science,
   Honkomagome, Tokyo, Japan
3) The Biochemical Division, Institute of Brain Research,
   Faculty of Medicine, University of Tokyo,
   Hongo, Tokyo, Japan

SUMMARY

Two myelin fractions, heavy and light, were isolated from
white matter of a patient with adrenoleukodystrophy. Morphologically, heavy myelin fraction showed compact lamellar structures, and
light myelin fraction consisted of loose lamellar structures and
rod-like clear space. Analytical studies demonstrated that the
chemical composition of heavy myelin fraction was almost the same
as that of normal myelin and that light myelin fraction consisted
mainly of cholesterol. Long chain saturated fatty acids, $C_{25:0}$
and $C_{26:0}$, were increased and $C_{24:1}$ was decreased in sphingoglycolipids of heavy myelin fraction of the patient.

INTRODUCTION

Adrenoleukodystrophy (ALD) is a hereditary fatal demyelinating
disease and transmitted as an X-linked recessive trait. This
disease is well documented pathologically as a systemic disorder of
lipid metabolism by Schaumburg et al. (19). Recently, abnormal
cholesterol esters with long chain fatty acid were reported to
accumulate in the white matter and adrenal glands of patients with
ALD and similar fatty acid abnormalities were found in sphingoglycolipids of brain of the patients (10, 11). However, the
mechanism of demyelination in this disorder remained unanswered.

To clarify this mechanism, it is important to ascertain whether those abnormalities exist in the myelin of a patient. Komiya et al. (12) reported a decrease of 2',3'-cyclic nucleotide 3'-phospho-hydrolase activity in myelin of a patient with ALD. In this paper, we describe the results of a detailed analytical study on the chemical composition of purified myelin of the same patient.

EXPERIMENTAL

Specimens. The patient, a Japanese boy, was healthy until 4 years of age. The initial findings were visual disturbance and behavioral changes. These symptoms were accompanied by disturbed hearing and gait. Spastic tetraparesis and mental retardation gradually progressed. The patient showed decorticate posture at a late stage, and he died of pneumonia at age 6. He had no signs of adrenal insufficiency and there was no indication of past illness or similar disease in the family.

The diagnosis of ALD was made by histo-pathological examination of the brain which was stored at $-20^{\circ}C$ until biochemical analysis. The control brain was that of a 5-year-old boy who had no neurological symptoms and who died in a traffic accident. The control brain was stored at $-80^{\circ}C$ until used.

Preparation of myelin. Myelin was prepared by the method of Autilio et al. (3) with slight modifications. A 10-per cent 0.32 M sucrose homogenate of cerebral white matter was layered on an equal volume of 0.656 M sucrose and centrifuged at 40,000 g for 30 min (Hitachi Ultracentrifuge Model 65P). Myelin layer at the interface was removed and diluted with distilled water to make 0.32 M in sucrose. The solution was layered on 0.656 M sucrose and centrifuged under the same conditions.

The myelin layer was diluted with an equal volume of distilled water and centrifuged at 77,000 g for 30 min. The precipitate was subjected to hypotonic shock by suspending it in cold distilled water for 20 min, and then centrifuged at 77,000 g for 30 min. The precipitate (crude myelin fraction) was resuspended in 0.32 M sucrose and layered on a continuous 0.32 M - 0.8 M sucrose density gradient and centrifuged at 53,000 g for 12 h. The crude myelin was purified by this step to one or two fractions (light and heavy myelin fractions). The purified myelin was washed four times with distilled water and lyophilized.

Determination of specific gravity. The crude myelin, suspended in 0.32 M sucrose was layered on a continuous 0.32 M - 0.8 M sucrose density gradient and centrifuged at 53,000 g for 12 h. After centrifugation, 20 drops of the sucrose solution were collected from a hole at the bottom of the tube. Specific gravity of the fraction was measured by Abbe refractometer 3L and turbidity was measured by spectrophotometer at 280 nm.

Extraction and fractionation of lipids and lipoproteins. Myelin was homogenized with chloroform-methanol (2:1, v/v) and the homogenate was filtered to remove insoluble materials. The filtrate was evaporated to dryness and dissolved in chloroform-methanol (2:1, v/v). The insoluble fraction was removed by centrifugation. This procedure was repeated three times. Total lipids were fractionated by the method of Folch et al. (8). The lower phase was fractionated and purified by TLC and silicic acid column chromatography. Each phospholipid was separated by TLC in chloroform-methanol-acetic acid-water (25:10:3:2, by volume) and measured by determining phosphate (1). Glycolipids were separated by TLC in chloroform-methanol-water (65:24:4, by volume) and purified further by Florisil column chromatography. Purified glycolipids were measured by the method of Vance et al.(22) and sterol compounds by the method of Zak (23).

Fatty acid determination. Purified glycolipids and phospholipids were methanolyzed in 3% methanolic hydrochloride at 100°C for 2 h. After evaporation of the solution, fatty acid methyl esters were separated into non-hydroxy and hydroxy fatty acids by TLC in the solvent system of n-hexane-ether-acetic acid (90:10:1, by volume). Non-hydroxy fatty acid methyl esters were analyzed by Shimadzu Model 5A gas chromatograph equipped with 1.5 m x 3 mm glass column packed with 10% EGSS-X on Gas-Chrom RP at 200°C isothermally. Hydroxy fatty acid methyl esters were converted into trimethyl-silyl derivatives, followed by analysis in same conditions. The samples were also analyzed in a glass column of 1% OV-17 on Chromosorb W at a programmed temperature of $170-320^{\circ}$C and at a rate of 3°C/min.

Determination of sterol compound. The purified sterol was converted into trimethylsilyl derivatives by the method of Carter et al. (5). The derivatives were analyzed by gas chromatograph (Shimadzu 5A) and Shimadzu-LKB 9,000A gas chromatograph (GC)-mass spectrometer combined system attached with a chemical ionization (CI) source. Gas chromatograph was operated at 250°C by 3 mm x 2 m glass column, packed with 1% OV-1 on Gas-Chrom Q. The conditions for GC-CI-Mass spectrometer were as following. The accelerating voltage was 3.5 KV, electron energy was 500-eV, and emission current was 500 μA. The ion source was held at 290ºC and molecular separator was at 270°C. Isobutane was used as the reagent gas at 0.8 torr. The conditions for gas chromatography were the same as described above.

Estimation of protein. Protein was determined by the method of Lowry et al. (13) with some modification. Dried myelin fraction was dissolved in chloroform-methanol (2:1, v/v). Aliquot of this solution was added to N NaOH and the mixture was heated to evaporate chloroform and methanol. This solution was used as sample solution.

Electron microscopy. The pelleted myelin fractions were fixed in 2.0% (w/v) glutaraldehyde in phosphate buffer, pH 7.4 for 2 h. After washing in the same buffer, the fractions were fixed in 1.0% (w/v) OsO_4 for 2 h and embedded in Araldite-Epon.

RESULTS

Myelin fractions. Two myelin fractions, heavy and light myelin, were obtained from the frontal white matter of the patient, and only one myelin fraction, light myelin, was taken from the occipital white matter, where severe demyelination was observed in neuro- pathological examination. Only one myelin fraction, heavy myelin, was obtained from the occipital white matter of the control brain (Fig. 1). Specific gravities of the light myelin fractions of the frontal and occipital white matter of the patient were very similar. Heavy myelin fraction of the frontal white matter of the patient was slightly heavier than that of the occipital white matter of the control brain (Table 1). The yield of myelin fraction was reduced in the white matter of the patient. The amount of heavy myelin fraction from the frontal white matter of the patient was 17% of normal control (Table 2).

Table 1. Specific gravity of myelin fraction.

	Light	Heavy
Normal occipital lobe	–	1.0735
ALD frontal lobe	1.0517	1.0843
ALD occipital lobe	1.0502	–

Table 2. Yield of myelin fraction.

	Total myelin (mg dry wt/g wet wt)	Ratio light		heavy
Normal occipital lobe	90	0	:	100
ALD frontal lobe	29	43	:	53
ALD occipital lobe	11	100	:	0

Electron microscopic findings of myelin fractions. Electron micrographs of the heavy myelin fraction showed relatively compact lamellar structures (Fig. 2-a). At a higher magnification, the distinction between the period and interperiod line was not seen as clearly as in the normal myelin. The lamellar period was 110 Å. Separations of lamellae were observed, but it could not be deter- mined whether the site of separation was in the period or inter- period line (Fig. 2-b).

Electron micrographs of the light myelin fraction demonstrated two types of lamellar structure and rod-like clear spaces. One lamellar structure were small myelin lamellae with many loosely

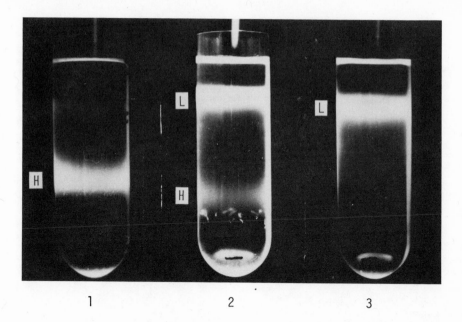

Fig. 1. Photograph of continuous sucrose density gradient centrifugation of crude myelin fraction. 1: Occipital white matter of
normal control; 2: Frontal white matter of the ALD patient;
3: Occipital white matter of the patient. H: Heavy myelin fraction;
L: Light myelin fraction.

arranged separations (Fig. 2-a). In a high power field, some separations in lamellae were found at the interperiod line. Periodicity of the period line was 110 Å at unseparated regions. The
other membrane structure were multilayered membrane whorls which
were considered to be completely separated myelin lamellae. Thickness of the unit membrane was 55 Å. A third component were rod-
like clear spaces surrounded by a membranous structure which were
supposed to be easily soluble material in an organic solvent (Fig.
2-b).

Chemical composition of heavy myelin fraction. Slight abnormalities were observed in the chemical composition of ALD heavy
myelin fraction (Table 3). There was slight decrease in the chloroform-methanol insoluble residue and total lipid, and slight increase
in the proteolipid protein. Individual phospholipids also showed
slight abnormalities. Phosphatidyl ethanolamine was decreased and
phosphatidyl choline increased. The ratio of cerebroside to
sulfatide was the same in the patient and control. Esterified
cholesterol was not detected in the heavy myelin fraction.

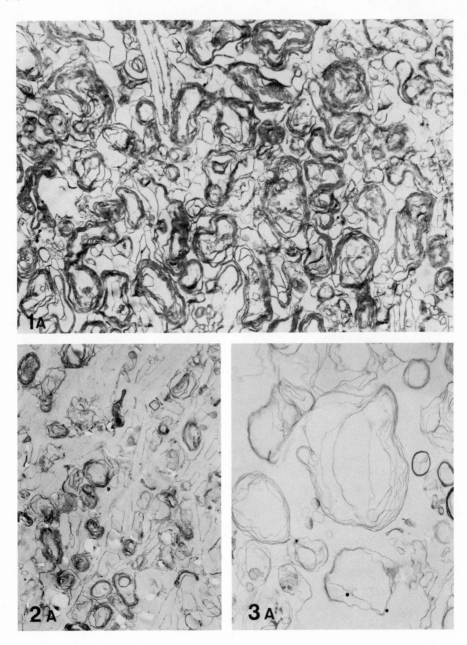

Fig. 2-a

Fig. 2. Electron micrographs of the myelin fractions from the
cerebral white matter of the patient. 1: Heavy myelin fraction;
2 and 3: Light myelin fraction. A (x12,000), Fig. 2-a; B (x48,000)
and C (x180,000), Fig. 2-b.

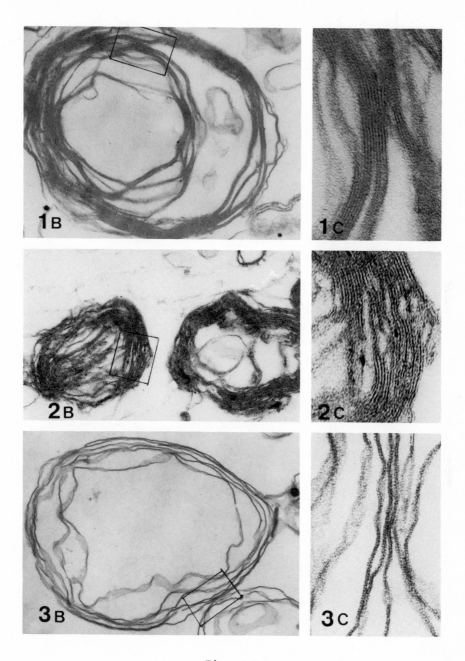

Fig. 2-b

Table 3. Chemical composition of the myelin fractions.

	Normal occipital lobe Heavy	ALD frontal lobe Heavy	ALD frontal lobe Light	ALD occipital lobe Light
	% of dry weight			
$CHCl_3:CH_3OH$ insoluble residue	9.0	3.0	0.8	2.3
Protéolipid protein	20.3	27.7	3.5	3.7
Total lipid	74.3	67.7	90.9	95.8
Sterol (% of total lipid)	23.5	20.1	82.6	91.8
Free	100	100	100	99.0
Ester	0	0	0	1.0
Phospholipid (% of total lipid)	41.2	46.4	8.4	8.6
p-ethanolamine	35.2	30.1	18.6	12.9
p-serine	19.4	16.7	10.1	4.5
p-inositide	2.8	4.1	6.3	2.9
Lecithin	27.5	33.5	45.6	50.1
Sphingomyelin	13.4	13.4	17.0	22.3
Lys-lecithin	1.7	2.2	2.5	2.4
Galactolipid (% of total lipid)	21.7	26.0	3.1	3.0
Cerebroside	18.4	21.8	n.d.	n.d.
Sulfatide	3.3	4.2	n.d.	n.d.

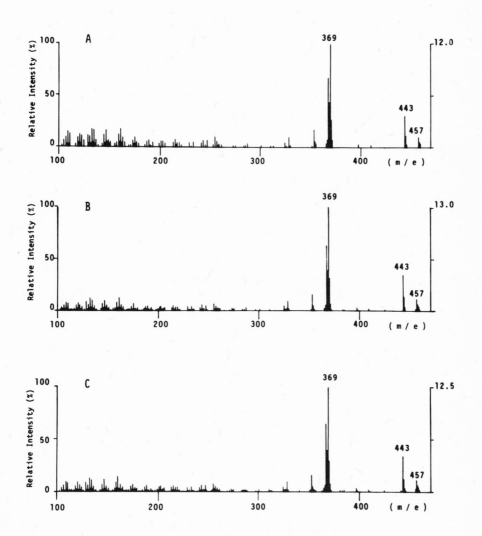

Fig. 3. Mass spectrum of trimethylsilyl derivatives of sterol compounds. A: Standard cholesterol; B: Sterol compound of normal myelin; C: Sterol compound of light myelin fraction from occipital white matter of the patient.

Table 4. Composition of non-hydroxy fatty acids in sphingoglycolipid of purified heavy myelin.

Fatty acids	Cerebroside		Sulfatide	
	Normal	ALD	Normal	ALD
16:0	7.4	3.6	2.7	7.8
16:1	1.6	1.3	–	–
18:0	9.2	3.6	7.8	7.3
18:1	2.4	4.6	3.4	4.4
20:0	7.8	7.4	0.5	0.7
22:0	2.9	2.8	2.8	2.2
23:0	4.9	6.2	7.3	3.4
24:0	18.7	22.5	21.2	19.9
24:1	31.7	17.6	29.4	19.6
25:0	5.4	14.2	7.6	10.9
25:1	6.6	8.5	5.5	8.1
26:0	2.1	5.5	1.6	8.7
26:1	6.2	8.9	10.1	7.0

Table 5. Composition of alpha-hydroxy fatty acids in sphingoglycolipid of purified heavy myelin.

Fatty acids	Cerebroside		Sulfatide	
	Normal	ALD	Normal	ALD
16h:0	0.4	0.5	1.0	2.4
18h:0	0.5	0.9	2.5	12.0
20h:0	0.3	0.3	0.6	–
22h:0	5.5	5.3	4.1	9.6
23h:0	14.1	11.9	9.6	10.8
24h:0	43.7	43.7	52.1	37.3
24h:1	16.7	7.7	12.9	6.4
25h:0	8.9	16.9	8.7	10.8
25h:1	3.8	3.6	2.1	1.7
26h:0	1.4	6.5	3.7	6.5
26h:1	4.7	3.2	2.9	2.6

 Chemical composition of light myelin fraction. The light myelin fraction from frontal lobe showed similar chemical composition to that from occipital lobe of the patient (Table 3). Eighty to ninety-five per cent of the dry weight of this fraction were lipids which consisted mainly of sterol compound. Compared with the heavy myelin fraction, phospholipid decreased to 20% and glycolipid decreased to less than 20% of the heavy myelin fraction. In individual phospholipids, phosphatidyl ethanolamine and phosphatidyl serine were decreased and phosphatidyl choline was increased. Esterified cholesterol was practically not present in this fraction.

 Determination of chemical structure of sterol compound. Trimethylsilyl derivatives of the purified sterol compound in ALD light myelin fraction showed a single peak on gas chromatogram. Mass spectrum of the peak demonstrated quite the same mass pattern as authentic cholesterol (Fig. 3). The main fragment ions were m/e 369, 443 and 457. The ion at m/e 457, corresponding to $(M-1)^{+}$, was dehydrate ion, m/e 443 was fragment ions which appeared as a result of loosing CH_3 radical from molecular ion, and m/e 369 was fragment ions resulting from elimination of trimethylsilyl alcohol from a protonated molecular ion. The sterol compound in the light myelin fractions was identified as cholesterol by those data.

 Fatty acid composition of sphingoglycolipids and glycerophosphatides in heavy myelin fraction. Non-hydroxy fatty acids of sphingoglycolipids in the heavy myelin fraction were demonstrated in Table 4. Long chain saturated fatty acids, $C_{25:0}$ and $C_{26:0}$, were increased in both cerebroside and sulfatide of ALD myelin. However, long chain unsaturated fatty acids, $C_{25:1}$ and $C_{26:1}$, were slightly increased in cerebroside, but $C_{26:1}$ was decreased in sulfatide. Generally, saturated long chain fatty acids, $C_{25:0}$ and $C_{26:0}$, were increased in both cerebroside and sulfatide, but $C_{24:1}$ was decreased in those glycolipids of the patient. Similar changes were observed in hydroxy fatty acids of sphingoglycolipids in myelin (Table 5).

 No remarkable changes were found in the fatty acid pattern of glycerophospholipids in ALD myelin (Table 6).

DISCUSSION

 Extensive pathological investigations on ALD have been recently carried out and the similar morphological changes in brain, adrenal and testis of the patients have suggested that ALD is a systemic metabolic disorder (19).

 The present case had typical neurological symptoms, signs and clinical course of ALD without adrenal failure. The diagnosis of ALD was based on histopathological findings in the brain and on the biochemical demonstration of accumulation of cholesterol esters with saturated long chain fatty acids in the cerebral white matter (2) reported to be characteristic to ALD (10). The relative increase of long chain saturated fatty acids was also found in sphingolipids

Table 6. Composition of fatty acids in glycerophospholipid in purified heavy myelin.

Fatty acids	Phosphatidyl choline		Phosphatidyl serine		Phosphatidyl ethanolamine	
	Normal	ALD	Normal	ALD	Normal	ALD
14:0	1.0	0.8	tr	0.1	1.2	tr
15:1	tr	tr	tr	tr	1.5	2.4
16:0	32.8	36.4	2.5	3.4	4.7	3.6
16:1	1.5	2.8	tr	0.3	1.3	tr
18:0	17.0	11.7	54.2	52.7	25.1	21.5
18:1	42.5	37.1	30.1	28.6	36.8	39.4
18:2	0.6	1.1	1.6	0.4	0.1	tr
20:1	0.4	0.4	4.6	2.3	7.5	6.1
20:2	0.7	0.8	2.0	1.5	2.6	1.9
20:3	0.9	0.7	1.6	1.1	2.3	2.1
20:4	1.9	4.9	1.8	2.0	7.2	7.6
22:4	0.5	2.0	1.3	1.8	2.0	3.1
22:5	tr	tr	0.9	1.0	2.3	2.4
22:6	tr	tr	1.2	1.8	4.8	4.6

of cerebral white matter of the patient (2). An attempt to clarify the problem that those lipid abnormalities could exist in myelin of the patient led us to the present investigation.

Gerstl et al. (9) isolated two myelin fractions, heavy and light, from a patient with sudanophilic leukodystrophy and found that both fractions contained higher proportions of lecithin and lower proportions of phosphatidyl ethanolamine than a normal control. Suzuki et al. (20) found an increase of cholesterol and a remarkable decrease of galactolipids in two cases of Schilder's disease.

We obtained two myelin fractions, heavy and light, by using the continuous sucrose gradient method of Autilio et al. (3). The heavy myelin fraction had a slightly heavier specific gravity but a compact lamellar structure, similar to that of normal myelin.

Contrary to the results of Gerstl et al. (9) and Suzuki et al. (20), no remarkable changes could be found in the chemical composition of ALD heavy myelin fraction. Cholesterol was slightly decreased and glycolipids were slightly increased. Their technique of myelin isolation by discontinuous sucrose gradient could not eliminate light myelin fraction with a specific gravity of about 1.05. This light myelin fraction contained a high proportion of free cholesterol and may have given high proportion of cholesterol to their myelin fraction.

Constant changes were observed in the fatty acid composition of sphingolipids in ALD heavy myelin. Long chain saturated fatty acids, $C_{25:0}$ and $C_{26:0}$, were increased and $C_{24:1}$ was decreased in cerebroside and sulfatide. The degree of fatty acid abnormalities in cerebroside was the same in white matter and myelin. However, the abnormalities in sulfatide were more severe in white matter.

There are only a few reports on fatty acid analysis of sphingolipids in myelin. Eto et al. (6) found a relative decrease of nervonic acid and an increase of lignoceric acid in myelin glycolipids in globoid leukodystrophy, and they also reported that $C_{16:0}$ and $C_{18:0}$ were increased, with proportional decrease of $C_{24:0}$ and $C_{24:1}$ in cerebroside in multiple sulphatase deficiency (7). In the brains of patients with demyelinating diseases, such as SSPE (21) and sudanophilic leukodystrophy (14), relative depletion of nervonic acid in glycolipids was observed. The same change was found in myelin sphingolipids of our patient and this finding is considered to be a secondary manifestation of demyelination. As mentioned above, saturated long chain fatty acids increase in sphingoglycolipids of ALD white matter and myelin. Recently, Ramsey et al. (18) reported the same fatty acid abnormalities in ALD myelin sphingoglycolipids and regarded the increase of long chain fatty acid as the result of depletion of $C_{24:1}$. In the white matter of our patient, cholesterol esters with long chain fatty acids, predominantly $C_{25:0}$ and $C_{26:0}$, were accumulated (2). Considering those facts, further studies are needed to decide whether the fatty acid abnormality in sphingoglycolipid is unique to this disorder.

Light myelin fraction consisted mainly of two components, electron-lucent rods and loose membrane structures. Chemically, this fraction consisted exclusively of sterol which was identified as cholesterol. Free 3β-hydroxysterol, suggested to be present in cytoplasmic lamellae (15), could not be detected histologically. Cholesterol was supposed to be located in electron-lucent rods.

Similar loose membrane structures as observed in light myelin fraction were separated from the brains of patients with SSPE (16) and adreneoleukodystrophy (17) into the fraction lighter than 0.32 M sucrose. Banik et al. (4) obtained lipid-rich low-density membranes by trypsin treatment of myelin in vitro. Those loose membrane structures in light myelin fractions could appear as the result of a demyelinating process.

Acknowledgement. This study was supported by a research grant from the Intractable Diseases Division, Public Health Bureau, Ministry of Health and Welfare, Japan.

REFERENCES

1. Ames, B.N. and Dubin, D.T., The role of polyamines in the neutralization of bacteriophage deoxyribonucleic acid, J. Biol. Chem. 235 (1960) 769-775.
2. Ariga, T., in preparation.
3. Autilio, L.A., Norton, W.T. and Terry, R.D., The preparation and some properties of purified myelin from the central nervous

system, J. Neurochem. 11 (1964) 17-27.

4. Banik, N.L. and Davison, A.N., Lipid and basic protein interaction in myelin, Biochem. J. 143 (1974) 39-45.

5. Carter, H.E. and Gaver, R.C., Improved reagent for trimethyl-
   silylation of sphingolipid bases, J. Lipid Res. 8 (1967) 391-
   395.

6. Eto, Y., Suzuki, K. and Suzuki, K., Globoid cell leukodystrophy
   (Krabbe's disease): isolation of myelin with normal glycolipid
   composition, J. Lipid Res. 11 (1970) 473-479.

7. Eto, Y., Meier, C. and Herschkowitz, N.N., Chemical compositions
   of brain and myelin in two patients with multiple sulphatase
   deficiency (a variant form of metachromatic leukodystrophy),
   J. Neurochem. 27 (1976) 1071-1076.

8. Folch, J., Lees, M. and Sloane-Stanley, G.H., A simple method
   for the isolation and purification of total lipids from animal
   tissues, J. Biol. Chem. 226 (1957) 497-509.

9. Gerstl, B., Rubinstein, L.J., Eng, L.F. and Tavaststjerna, M.,
   A neurochemical study of a case of sudanophilic leukodystrophy,
   Arch. Neurol. 15 (1966) 603-614.

10. Igarashi, M., Schaumburg, H.H., Powers, J., Kishimoto, Y.,
    Kolodny, E. and Suzuki, K., Fatty acid abnormality in adreno-
    leukodystrophy, J. Neurochem. 26 (1976) 851-860.

11. Igarashi, M., Belchis, D. and Suzuki, K., Brain gangliosides
    in adrenoleukodystrophy, J. Neurochem. 27 (1976) 327-328.

12. Komiya, Y. and Kasahara, M., 2',3'-Cyclic nucleotide 3'-
    phosphohydrolase activity in myelin fractions from one patient
    with Schilder's disease, J. Biochem. 70 (1971) 371-374.

13. Lowry, O.H., Rosebrough, N.J., Farr, A.L. and Randall, R.J.,
    Protein measurement with the Folin phenol reagent, J. Biol.
    Chem. 193 (1951) 265-275.

14. Ogino, T. and Yokoi, S., Studies on sphingoglycolipid of the
    brain of three adult cases of leukodystrophy, Folia Psychiatr.
    Neurol. Japon. 28 (1974) 207-215.

15. Powers, J.M. and Schaumburg, H.H., Adrenoleukodystrophy (sex-
    linked Schilder's disease), a pathological hypothesis based
    on ultrastructural lesions in adrenal cortex, peripheral nerve
    and testis, Am. J. Path. 76 (1974) 481-500.

16. Ramsey, R.B., Banik, N.L., Bowen, D.M., Scott, T. and Davison,
    A.N., Biochemical and ultrastructural studies on subacute
    sclerosing panencephalitis and demyelination, J. neurol. Sci.
    21 (1974) 213-225.

17. Ramsey, R.B., Banik, N.L. and Davison, A.N., Neurochemical
    findings in adreno-leukodystrophy, J. neurol. Sci. 29 (1976)
    277-294.

18. Ramsey, R.B., Banik, N.L. and Davison, A.N., Galactolipid fatty
    acid composition in adrenoleukodystrophy, J. neurol. Sci. 32
    (1977) 69-77.

19. Schaumburg, H.H., Powers, J.M., Raine, C.S., Suzuki, K. and
    Richardson, E.P., Adrenoleukodystrophy. A clinical and

pathological study of 17 cases, <u>Arch. Neurol</u>. 32 (1975) 577-591.

20. Suzuki, Y., Tucker, S.H., Rorke, L.B. and Suzuki, K., Ultra-structural and biochemical studies of Schilder´s disease. II. Biochemistry, <u>J. Neuropath. exp. Neurol.</u> 29 (1970) 405-419.

21. Svennerholm, L., Haltia, M. and Sourander, P., Chronic sclerosing panencephalitis. II. A neurochemical study, <u>Acta neuropath</u>. 14 (1970) 293-303.

22. Vance, D.E. and Sweeley, C.C., Quantitative determination of the neutral glycosyl ceramides in human blood, <u>J. Lipid Res</u>. 8 (1967) 391-395.

23. Zak, B., Simple rapid microtechnic for serum total cholesterol, <u>Am. J. Clin. Path</u>. 27 (1957) 583-588.

METABOLIC STUDIES OF ADRENOLEUKODYSTROPHY

Tadashi Ogino, Herbert H. Schaumburg and Kunihiko Suzuki

The Saul R. Korey Department of Neurology, Departments
   of Neuroscience and Pathology, and the Rose F.
   Kennedy Center for Research in Mental Retardation
   and Human Development, Albert Einstein College
   of Medicine, Bronx, New York 10461, U.S.A.

Yasuo Kishimoto and Ann E. Moser

The John F. Kennedy Institute, and Departments of
   Neurology and Pediatrics, Johns Hopkins University
   School of Medicine, Baltimore, Maryland 21205, U.S.A.

SUMMARY

Two series of metabolic studies were prompted by the previous
finding that the brain and adrenal tissues of patients with
adrenoleukodystrophy, an X-linked genetic disorder, contain unusually
long-chain (C_{22} - C_{32}) fatty acids in cholesterol esters and
gangliosides. Postmortem brain tissues from three patients were
assayed for activities of the three distinct cholesterol ester
hydrolases, using [4-^{14}C]cholesterol oleate, lignocerate and
cerotate as the substrates. No deficiency of the crude mitochondrial (pH 4.2), the microsomal (pH 6.0), or the myelin-
localized cholesterol ester hydrolases was detected, although
the activities of the myelin-localized cholesterol ester hydrolase
against cholesteryl lignocerate and cerotate were too low for reliable assays. The activities of the microsomal and myelin-
localized hydrolases were actually higher in adrenoleukodystrophy
than in controls. Uptake and exclusion by cultured fibroblasts
of [1-^{14}C]stearic, [1-^{14}C]lignoceric and [1-^{14}C]cerotic acids were
also examined. All fatty acids were avidly taken up by the fibroblasts. Stearic acid was excluded from the cells much more rapidly
than lignoceric or cerotic acid. No difference was observed in the
uptake and exclusion of fatty acids between the controls and

adrenoleukodystrophy, except that cells from some cases of adrenoleukodystrophy consistently took up the very long chain fatty acids
at greater rates than the control cells. Neither did the distribution of the label among individual lipids reveal differences
between the controls and adrenoleukodystrophy, although there were
interesting and dramatic differences in the metabolism of lignoceric
acid and cerotic acid. Cerotic acid appeared largely inert with
90-95% remaining intact over eight days, while lignoceric acid was
mostly incorporated into complex lipids. This series of studies
did not uncover the fundamental genetic defect underlying adrenoleukodystrophy.

INTRODUCTION

Adrenoleukodystrophy (ALD) is an X-linked genetic disorder
which affects the cerebral white matter, adrenal and testis of
primarily young boys but occasionally of adult males (1). In many
cases, the neurological symptoms and signs may be the only clinical
manifestations. Such cases have in the past been diagnosed as
Schilder's disease or sudanophilic leukodystrophy. However, a
series of clinical and morphological studies, initiated by Schaumburg, Powers and Richardson, demonstrated that the characteristic
histological abnormalities are consistently present in the adrenal
and testis even in patients without apparent systemic symptomatology (for reference, see (22)). Their idea that most, if not all,
cases of so-called Schilder's disease or sudanophilic leukodystrophy
are cases of adrenoleukodystrophy, has been gaining acceptance in
recent years.

The analytical abnormalities reported earlier by many laboratories regarding the composition of the brain, including isolated
myelin, were largely nonspecific changes reflecting the histopathological abnormalities (for literature review, see (23)).
However, in 1976, Igarashi et al. reported what appears to be a
unique abnormality in fatty acids in the white matter and adrenal
of several patients (12). Cholesterol esters in the brain and
adrenal contained substantial proportions of unusually long-chain
fatty acids ($>C_{22}$), which showed a bell-like distribution with
C_{25} or C_{26} at the peak. These very long-chain fatty acids were
mostly saturated in cerebral cholesterol esters, but adrenal
cholesterol esters contained some unsaturated very long-chain
fatty acids. Gangliosides from patients' white matter also
showed varying proportions of very long-chain saturated fatty acids
up to 50% of total. Such abnormal fatty acids were fairly evenly
distributed among different gangliosides in the usual amide-linked
form (11). This fatty acid abnormality was not uniform in that the
fatty acid composition was not abnormal in brain glycerophospholipids, and in serum cholesterol esters. Besides being apparently
unique, cholesterol esters containing very long-chain saturated

fatty acids appear to be responsible for the characteristic birefringent materials in the brain and the adrenal of patients (16). This correlation of pathology and analytical chemistry encouraged our present working hypothesis that this unique fatty acid abnormality somehow reflects the fundamental genetic defect of ALD.

Only a few metabolic studies on ALD have been reported in the literature. Using cultured fibroblasts, Burton and Nadler (4) reported findings suggestive of abnormal cholesterol metabolism in ALD. Another group of investigators, however, were unable to confirm the observation (24). Prompted by the above finding of the long-chain fatty acids, we have carried out two series of metabolic studies of ALD, one concerning cholesteryl ester hydrolase activities of brains of patients with ALD with cholesteryl lignocerate ($C_{24:0}$) and cholesteryl cerotate ($C_{26:0}$) as the substrates, and the other, metabolism of lignoceric and cerotic acids in cultured ALD fibroblasts. The results of these experiments to date have failed to uncover metabolic abnormality specific for ALD.

EXPERIMENTAL

Cholesterol Ester Hydrolases

Enzyme source. Postmortem brains from two neurologically normal patients and from three ALD patients, verified clinically, histologically and analytically, had been stored at $-90°C$ until the enzymatic assays. Gray and white matter were carefully dissected and homogenized in 9 vol of ice-cold 0.32 M sucrose in a Potter-Elvehjem homogenizer with a Teflon pestle (A.H. Thomas, Philadelphia, Pa.). The homogenate was centrifuged at 900 g x 10 min to remove cell debris and capillaries, and the supernatant was used for the enzyme assays. Gray matter samples were used for assays of the pH 4.2 (crude mitochondrial) cholesterol ester hydrolase and the pH 6.0 (microsomal) cholesterol ester hydrolase. For assays of the myelin-localized cholesterol ester hydrolase, white matter samples were utilized. Protein determination was done according to Lowry et al. (17).

Substrates. [4-^{14}C]Cholesteryl oleate (55.5 mCi/mmole) was purchased from New England Nuclear Corp., Boston, Mass. It was diluted with unlabelled cholesteryl oleate (Sigma Chemical Co., St. Louis, Mo.) to a specific activity of 0.56 mCi/mmole. [4-^{14}C]Cholesteryl lignocerate was synthesized from [4-^{14}C]cholesterol (54 mCi/mmole, New England Nuclear Corp., Boston, Mass., diluted to 2.7 mCi/mmole) and lignoceroyl chloride (Nu-Check Prep Inc., Elysian, Minn.) according to Pinter et al. (19). [4-^{14}C] Cholesteryl cerotate was synthesized from the same labelled cholesterol above and unlabelled cerotic acid (Pfaltz & Bauer, Inc., Stamford, Conn. or Applied Science Labs. State College, Pa.) through cerotyl chloride, essentially according to Prabhudesai (20).

All labelled cholesteryl esters were purified by silicic acid
column chromatography (9). Chemical and radioactive purity of the
synthesized cholesteryl esters were ascertained by gas-liquid
chromatography after base hydrolysis (12), and by thin-layer
chromatography in hexane-ethylether-acetic acid (80:20:1, v/v/v),
scraping and counting.

Assays of cholesterol ester hydrolases. The three distinct
cholesterol ester hydrolases of the brain (5-8) were assayed essentially as described previously (5-8, 13-15) but with some minor
modifications (Table 1). The only substantial modification involved
the assay system for the pH 4.2 hydrolase: The substrate and phosphatidylserine were dried together, suspended in 0.1 ml ethanol by
mild sonication and then the buffer was added. The procedure after
the enzymatic reaction was also slightly modified from the original
(13). The reaction was stopped by the addition of 5 ml of hexane-
ethanol (2:1, v/v). After mixing and centrifugation the hexane
phase was transferred to another tube. Free cholesterol was then
precipitated by adding 0.5 ml of 1% digitonin in ethanol-water
(1:1, v/v). The precipitated digitonide was washed sequentially,
twice with 5 ml of hexane-ethylether (1:1, v/v) and once with 5 ml
of ethylether-acetone (2:1, v/v). The final washed digitonide was
counted in a scintillation counter as described previously (13-15).
Sodium taurocholate (crude),Triton X-100 and phosphatidylserine were
from GIBCO (Grand Island, N.Y.), Sigma Chemical Co. (St. Louis, Mo.)
and Koch-Light Ltd. (Colnbrook, England), respectively.

Fatty Acid Metabolism in Fibroblasts

Fibroblasts. Established lines of fibroblasts from control
individuals and ALD patients were maintained in Eagle's minimal
essential medium plus Earle's salts and 13% fetal calf serum in
5% CO_2 atmosphere (Baltimore) or in McCoy's medium with 15% fetal
calf serum in 5% CO2 atmosphere (Bronx).

Radioactively labelled fatty acids. [1-^{14}C]Stearic acid was
purchased from New England Nuclear Corp., Boston, Mass. (54 mCi/
mmole). [1-^{14}C]Lignoceric acid was synthesized as described previously (10). [1-^{14}C]Cerotic acid was customsynthesized by Applied
Science Labs, State College, Pa. (55 mCi/mmole). All of the
labelled fatty acids were appropriately tested for their chemical
and radiochemical purity.

Experimental designs. The experiments involving [1-^{14}C]
stearic acid and [1-^{14}C]cerotic acid were carried out in the Bronx,
and those with [1-^{14}C]lignoceric acid were done in Baltimore.
Since the experimental designs differ in some minor details in the
two laboratories, they are described separately.

[1-^{14}C]Stearic acid was used as a control compound to be compared with the very long-chain fatty acids, lignoceric and cerotic.
[1-^{14}C]Stearic acid, 54 mCi/mmole, 0.25 mCi total, was dried and

Table 1. Assay mixtures for cholesterol ester hydrolases of postmortem human brain.

Constituents	Cholesterol ester hydrolases		
	Crude mitochondrial	Microsomal	Myelin
Whole homogenate, 10%	0.2 ml	0.2 ml	0.2 ml
Substrate	3.8 μmoles	3.8 μmoles	3.8 μmoles
Detergent	-----	Triton X-100 1.5 mg	Na-taurocholate 2 μmoles
Phosphatidylserine	200 μg	-----	200 μg
0.2 M Na-phosphate buffer	-----	pH 6.0, 1 ml	pH 6.8, 1 ml
0.1 M Na-citrate-Phosphate buffer	pH 4.2, 0.9 ml	-----	-----
Ethanol	0.1 ml	-----	-----
Total volume	1.2 ml	1.2 ml	1.2 ml
Incubation at 37°C	120 min	60 min	120 min

neutralized with the addition of 0.5 ml of 10 mM NaOH. Then 25 ml of 1% fatty acid-free bovine albumin (Miles Labs, Inc., Elkhart, Ind.) in saline was added and the mixture shaken gently for several hours. It was sterilized by filtration through a Millipore filter. After filtration, 10 μl of the solution gave 1.80×10^5 cpm. This represented approximately 90% recovery of the total [1-^{14}C]Stearic acid in the Millipore filtrate in the albuminconjugated form. For the chase experiment, non-radioactive stearic acid was similarly processed but at a concentration 50 times that of the radioactive preparation.

Two ALD and two control cell lines were used for this experiment. Cells were grown in 30-ml flasks with 5 ml of the medium. At the stage half-way to confluency, the medium was changed and then 0.2 ml of the above [1-^{14}C]stearic acid preparation (approximately 33 nmoles) added to each flask. Cells were harvested immediately after the addition of the radioactive stearic acid (0-time) and at 3 h, 6 h, 12 h and 24 h thereafter. These samples constituted the short-term uptake study. Twenty-four hours after the addition of the isotope, the medium was removed from all of the remaining flasks, flasks rinsed with the minimum essential medium twice, and 5 ml of fresh medium plus 0.1 ml of the non-radioactive stearic acid was added. These flasks were used to examine exclusion from the cells of once taken up radioactive stearic acid. The 24-hour samples for the short-term uptake study also served as the 0-day sample for the exclusion study. Other flasks were then harvested at 2 days, 4 days, 6 days and 8 days, counted from the time the radioactive stearic acid was removed from the medium. During the experimental period, the medium was changed twice weekly according to the standard schedule, each time with additional 0.1 ml of the nonradioactive stearic acid suspension. The cells were harvested in the following manner. The medium was decanted, and the flask rinsed twice with 2 ml of the minimum essential medium and the cells trypsinized. Trypsinized cells were suspended in 10 ml of saline and centrifuged at 2,000 g x 10 min. The cell pellets were resuspended in 10 ml of saline and re-centrifuged. In one experiment, the medium was changed every day during the chase experiment instead of adding the non-radioactive stearic acid. The results did not differ significantly from the standard experiment.

Attempts to conjugate [1-^{14}C]cerotic acid with fatty acid-free albumin were unsuccessful. [1-^{14}C]Cerotic acid, 100 μCi, 1.82 μmole, in benzene-ethylether (1:4, v/v) was evaporated in the bottom of a sterile bottle at 37°C overnight, the standard culture medium, 20 ml, added and cerotic acid suspended by repeated sonication. This procedure yielded a finely dispersed suspension, which, however, was not as stable as albumin-conjugated stearic acid. Upon standing, cerotic acid slowly precipitated. In two experiments, [1-^{14}C]cerotic acid was diluted ten times with non-radioactive cerotic acid so that a greater amount of cerotic acid can be added to each flask.

Four ALD cell lines and four controls were included in three separate experiments. The experimental designs were essentially identical to that for stearic acid, except that the cells for the long-term (0-day to 8-day) experiments were grown in 250-ml flasks with 12 ml of the medium so that the experiment can start at the beginning of the linear growth phase and finish before the stage of overgrowth is reached. Preliminary experiments indicated that trypsinization and subculture during the experimental period introduced sudden reduction of the cell numbers and retardation of cell growth that were difficult to control. Each flask received 0.2 ml of the cerotic acid suspension; 18.2 nmoles, or 182 nmoles when diluted cerotic acid was used. In one experiment in which 18.2 nmoles of $[1-^{14}C]$cerotic acid was added, 50 nmoles of non-radioactive cerotic acid was added to each flask during the period of the chase experiment, in the manner similar to the experiments with $[1-^{14}C]$stearic acid.

Several experiments were carried out with $[1-^{14}C]$lignoceric acid. The original $[1-^{14}C]$lignoceric acid had a specific activity of 100,000 cpm/mmole (approximately 51 mCi/nmole). For some experiments, it was used undiluted, and for some others, it was diluted progressively with non-radioactive lignoceric acid so that the specific activity would be 200,000 cpm/5 nmoles, 10 nmoles or 20 nmoles. $[1-^{14}C]$Lignoceric acid was dried under nitrogen and dissolved with sonication in a very small volume of ethanol. Then nine volumes of heat-inactivated fetal calf serum was added, mixed vigorously, and allowed to stand at $37^{o}C$ for 10 min. In some experiments, this suspension was added to the culture flasks which already contained the medium. In other experiments, the above suspension was pre-mixed with the medium to give the final calf serum concentration of 5%, and added to the flasks.

A total of five ALD and five control cell lines were used for the experiments with $[1-^{14}C]$lignoceric acid. $[1-^{14}C]$Lignoceric acid was added to the 250-ml flasks at 0-time, and cells were harvested at 48 h and 72 h for the uptake studies. At 72 hours, the radioactive medium was removed from the remaining flasks, which were then rinsed with 10 ml of Eagle's minimum essential medium containing 10% heat inactivated fetal calf serum, and finally 10 ml of the same medium added. The cells for the chase experiments were harvested at 72 hours after the removal of the radioactive lignoceric acid from the medium. Cells were harvested in these experiments by scraping without trypsin. The radioactive medium was decanted and the flask rinsed twice with 5 ml of the minimum essential medium containing 5% fetal calf serum and once with 5 ml of 0.9% NaCl. The flasks were broken and the cells were scraped by a rubber policeman three times, each time with 1 ml of saline and transferred to a centrifuge tube. The cells were centrifuged at 600 g x 5 min. Protein determination for these samples was done by the method of Miller (18) which is a modified Lowry procedure.

Procedures for harvested cells. The cell pellets from the experiments with radioactive stearic or cerotic acid were suspended
in 1.0 ml of distilled water and disrupted to a uniform suspension
by sonication. An aliquot of 0.1 ml was removed for protein determination, and 0.1 ml was used to determine radioactivity in
duplicate. The samples for counting were placed in the scintillation vial, 1 ml of Soluene 350 (Packard Instr., Downers Grove,
Ill.) added, and dissolved by warming to 60°C for 30 min with
loosely screwed caps. The radioacitivity was determined after
addition of 12 ml of a scintillation solvent containing 6 g of
Permablend (Packard Instr.) in a liter of toluene.

The distribution of radioactivity in different chemical
fractions was examined in pairs of ALD and control cell lines fed
with $[1-^{14}C]$cerotic acid in the following manner, using 0.2 ml
each of the remaining cell suspensions. Lipids were extracted by
adding 2 ml of chloroform-methanol (1:1, v/v). The tubes were
centrifuged and the extract transferred to another tube. To the
extract was added 0.2 ml of 5mM sodium citrate buffer, pH 4.2,
and the tubes shaken and centrifuged. The clear "upper phase"
was transferred to the scintillation vial and radioactivity
determined after addition of 12 ml of a scintillation solvent which
contained 6 g of Permablend and 100 ml of Bio-Solv BBS-3 (Beckman
Instr., Fullerton, Calif.) per liter of toluene. The chloroform-
methanol-insoluble cell residue was extracted once more with a
mixture of 1 ml hexane, 0.25 ml chloroform and 0.25 ml methanol.
After centrifugation this extract was added to the lower phase of
the first extraction above. Both the insoluble residue and the lipid
fractions were dried under nitrogen. The entire insoluble residue
was dissolved in 0.1 ml water and 0.9 ml Soluene-350 and the radioactivity determined with 12 ml of the above scintillation solvent
without Bio-Solv. The lipid phase was dissolved in 1.0 ml of
chloroform-methanol (1:1, v/v) and radioactivity determined on 0.1
ml aliquots. Up to this step, data had been obtained for radioactivity in the whole cells, the organic solvent-insoluble residue,
the upper phase solids, and the total lipid fraction.

The distribution of the label among different lipids was examined by Silica gel G thin-layer chromatography, scraping and
counting. Since the amounts of lipid in the samples were insufficient to localize the spots on the plate, standard cholesteryl
oleate, tripalmitin, oleic acid, and cholesterol were added to the
sample for examination of non-polar lipids with the solvent system
of hexane-ethylether-acetic acid (90:10:1, v/v/v). A total brain
lipid mixture was similarly added to the sample for chromatography
of more polar lipids in chloroform-methanol-water (70:30:4, v/v/v).
The TLC plates were exposed to iodine vapor to localize the spots,
appropriately marked, and scraped into the scintillation vial. The
non-polar TLC plates were divided into 5 areas: cholesterol esters,
glycerides, fatty acids, cholesterol, and the rest. The polar
plates were divided into regions of cholesterol and above, fatty
acids, cerebrosides, ethanolamine phospholipids, sulfatide +

lecithin, sphingomyelin, and monophosphoinositide + phosphatidylserine. The scraped silica gel powder was wetted with 0.5 ml of water and 12 ml of the scintillation solvent containing Bio-Solv added. Recovery of radioactivity was essentially 100% and reproducibility was within a few percent errors.

The cell pellets from the experiments with $[1-^{14}C]$ lignoceric acid were processed differently. To each pellet was added 2 ml of chloroform-methanol (1:1, v/v). It was sonicated until all of the pellet was disrupted. After centrifugation at 600 g x 5 min, the extract was transferred and the residue extracted once more. Aliquots of the combined extracts were counted to obtain total lipid radioactivity. TLC separation of lipid was in principle identical with the procedure described above. For nonpolar solvent, a mixture of hexane-benzene-acetic acid (8:2:0.4, v/v/v) was used, and the polar solvent was chloroform-methanol-water (24:7:1, v/v/v). Radioactivity in the separated lipids was estimated by radioscanning with a Berthold LB-2760 TLC scanner and radioautography.

RESULTS

Cholesterol Ester Hydrolases

The activity of the pH 4.2 cholesterol ester hydrolase, which is localized in the crude mitochondrial fraction and is activated most effectively by phosphatidylserine, was detectable in the gray matter of the postmortem human brains using either cholesteryl oleate, lignocerate or cerotate as the substrate (Table 2). The measurable activities, however, were much lower against the very long-chain cholesterol esters. In the normal controls, the activity against cholesteryl lignocerate was approximately 1/50 and that against cholesteryl cerotate was 1/1000 of the activity against cholesteryl oleate. All specimens of the ALD brains gave essentially normal activities of the pH 4.2 cholesterol ester hydrolase against either of the three substrates.

The activity of the microsomal cholesterol ester hydrolase, which shows the pH optimum of 6.0 and is most efficiently activated by Triton X-100, was detectable only with cholesteryl oleate and lignocerate (Table 3). Activity against cholesteryl lignocerate was only a few percent of that against cholesteryl oleate. The microsomal cholesterol ester hydrolase was on the average twice more active in ALD gray matter than in the control gray matter.

The myelin-localized cholesterol ester hydrolase, which is most efficiently activated by the mixture of sodium taurocholate and phosphatidylserine, could not be measured in any of the control or ALD white matter specimens with either cholesteryl lignocerate or cerotate, although detectable with cholesteryl oleate as the substrate (Table 4). Therefore, it was not possible to examine

the activities of the myelin-localized cholesterol ester hydrolase
against the substrates with the very long-chain fatty acids found
in the ALD white matter. However, with cholesteryl oleate as the
substrate, the activity of this enzyme in ALD white matter was more
than twice that in the control white matter. This finding was somewhat unexpected in view of the less than normal amounts of myelin
present in the white matter of the ALD brains.

Fatty Acid Metabolism in Fibroblasts

Several experimental parameters were examined using $[1-^{14}C]$-
lignoceric acid. Cultured fibroblasts took up added $[1-^{14}C]$ligno-
ceric acid avidly, and the uptake was dependent on the concentration
of the lignoceric acid added initially to the flask at least up to
10 nmoles in 10 ml of the medium (Fig. 1). Although less systemat-
ically examined, similar phenomena were observed with $[1-^{14}C]$cerotic
acid. However, the concentration necessary to saturate the system
appeared much greater for cerotic acid. Essentially no difference
in the uptake per mg protein was observed when the amount of cells
seeded for each flask was either 0.1 mg or 0.2 mg protein per flask.
With either stearic acid or cerotic acid as the experimental
compound, trypsinization and subculture during the experimental
period caused a sudden reduction in both cell protein and radioactivity and a subsequent slowed growth rate that were difficult to
control. Therefore, trypsinization and subculture were avoided
in all subsequent experiments.

Table 2.   Crude mitochondrial cholesterol ester hydrolase (pH 4.2)
in adrenoleukodystrophy gray matter.

| | Substrate | | |
Specimen	$C_{18:1}$	$C_{24:0}$	$C_{26:0}$
Control	2640	44.0	4.62
Control	3380	57.2	3.79
ALD	3840	84.4	8.57
ALD	3180	60.4	3.07
ALD	4740	73.1	2.85

Activities are expressed in picomoles/h/mg protein. They are
averages of two separate experiments using separate pieces of
specimens from the same set of brains, each assayed in duplicate.

Table 3. Microsomal cholesterol ester hydrolases (pH 6.0) in adrenoleukodystrophy gray matter.

| Specimen | Substrate | |
	$C_{18:1}$	$C_{24:0}$
	(pmol/h/mg prot.)	
Control	83.9	2.73
Control	92.8	4.78
ALD	229	7.53
ALD	175	4.75
ALD	124	6.42

Activities are averages of two separate experiments using separate pieces of specimens from the same brains, each assayed in duplicate. Hydrolytic activities against cholesteryl cerotate ($C_{26:0}$) (S.A. 6000 dpm/nmole) were undetectable.

Table 4. Myelin-localized cholesterol ester hydrolase (pH 6.8) in adrenoleukodystrophy white matter.

Specimens	Substrate $C_{18:1}$
	(pmol/h/mg prot.)
Control	35.8
Control	44.7
ALD	94.6
ALD	128
ALD	78.0

Activities are averages of two separate experiments using separate pieces of specimens from the same brains, each assayed in duplicate. Hydrolytic activities against cholesteryl lignocerate ($C_{24:0}$) and cerotate ($C_{26:0}$) were undetectable.

Fatty acid uptake. Cultured fibroblasts took up any of the
three fatty acids added to the medium. The uptake was active and
prolonged (Fig. 2). At least with lignoceric acid, continuing
uptake was observed at least up to 72 hours. Almost half of the
total stearic acid added was recovered in the cell pellet at 24
hours. Since the amounts of fatty acids added were different in
these experiments, the capacity of the cells to take up fatty acids
with respect to chain length cannot properly be assessed from these
experiments. No difference was observed in the uptake of $[1-^{14}C]$-
stearic acid by ALD and normal control fibroblasts. While the
general conclusion was the same for the uptake of $[1-^{14}C]$lignoceric
or $[1-^{14}C]$cerotic acid, it was noted that some ALD cell lines
consistently took up the added very long-chain fatty acids more
actively than the control cell lines. This intriguing phenomenon
was observed both with lignoceric acid in Baltimore and with cerotic acid in the Bronx. Repeated experiments consistently showed
higher uptake by the same ALD cell lines, suggesting that the difference was not due to slight differences in the growth phase or
other cell biological variables. In all instances, radioactivity
recovered from the 0-time samples was negligible (less than 1% of
samples), indicating adequate washing.

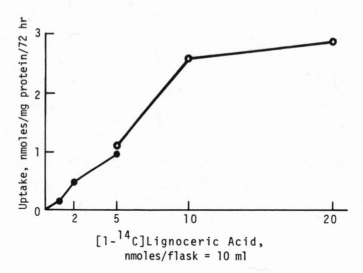

Fig. 1. Uptake of $[1-^{14}C]$lignoceric acid by cultured fibroblasts.
The uptake at 72 hours was dependent on the amount of lignoceric
acid initially added to the flask. This graph is a composite of
two separate experiments represented by closed and open symbols,
respectively. The closed symbols represent averages of the results
from two ALD and two control cell lines. The open symbols represent
averages of one control and one ALD cell line.

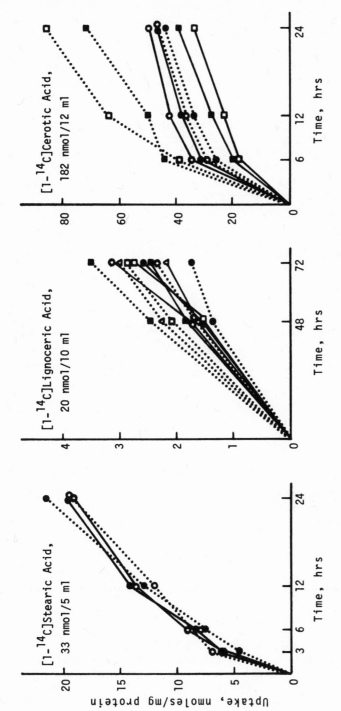

Fig. 2. Uptake of fatty acids by cultured fibroblasts. Uptake of stearic, lignoceric and cerotic acids was studied according to the experimental designs described in detail in the text. Since the amounts of added fatty acids were different, the results are not comparable among different fatty acids. Solid lines represent the control cell lines and dotted lines the ALD cell lines. Some ALD cell lines consistently took up the very long-chain fatty acids at greater rates than controls. Note the different time scale for the experiment with lignoceric acid.

 Exclusion of fatty acids. The behaviors of radioactivity once
taken up by fibroblasts were quite different depending on the chain
length of the fatty acids (Fig. 3). The radioactivity from [1-^{14}C]
stearic acid was relatively rapidly excluded from the cells, reaching approximately 20% of the 0-day value by 8 days. In contrast,
lignoceric acid and cerotic acid were excluded from fibroblasts
at a much slower rate, if at all. In fact, exclusion of cerotic
acid from the cells could not be observed within the experimental
errors, which were much greater for experiments with cerotic acid
than those with stearic acid. At 72 hours after the chase, approximately 80% of the radioactivity from [1-^{14}C]lignoceric acid was
retained by the cells. No significant difference could be detected
in the rate of radioactivity exclusion from the ALD and normal
control cell lines with any of the three fatty acids.
 Distribution of radioactivity. In an experiment with cerotic
acid, two cell lines each for ALD and controls were examined in
detail for the distribution of incorporated radioactivity among
different constituents, at 6 h, 12 h, 24 h, 0-day (start of the
chase experiment after 24-hour uptake), 2 days, 4 days, 6 days,

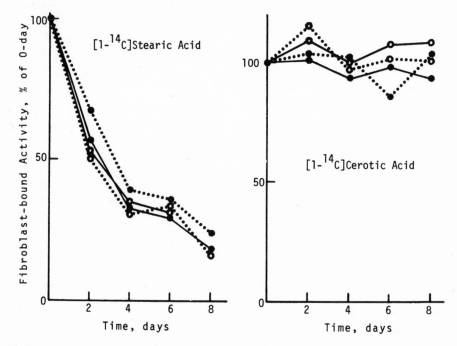

Fig. 3. Exclusion of fatty acids by cultured fibroblasts. Exclusion of the radioactivity from the cells was determined for
eight days after 24-hour uptake. Refer to the text for experimental details. Stearic acid was rapidly excluded from cultured
fibroblasts but cerotic acid appeared to remain cell-bound once
taken up. Solid lines represent the control cell lines and dotted
lines the ALD cell lines.

and 8 days. Throughout the experimental period, the organic sol-vent-insoluble residue never contained more than 0.5% of the total radioactivity, and the radioactivity recovered in the "upper phase solids" was generally less than 2% of the total, except for the 6 h samples, all of which showed 7-10% of total activity in the "upper phase solids". The remainder of the radioactivity was in the lipid fraction. The incorporated $[1-^{14}C]$cerotic acid appeared to be largely inert metabolically in that generally 90-95% of the total lipid radioactivity was recovered from the fatty acid regions of the chromatograms without substantial changes. The region of sulfatide-lecithin always contained the second largest amounts of radioactivity, which increased from approximately 2% of total at 6 h to 4-6% of total at 24 h. The activity of this fraction, how-ever, decreased to 1-2% level during the chase period despite the persistent presence of labelled cerotic acid within the cell. Fractions corresponding sphingomyelin, and monophosphoinositide-phosphatidylserine never contained radioactivity greater than a few percent of the total, and other fractions contained even lower activity. The regions of either cholesterol or cholesterol esters were essentially radioactivity-free throughout the experimental period. Throughout this experiment, no differences were detected in the distribution of radioactivity between the ALD and normal cells.

Interestingly, the behavior of incorporated $[1-^{14}C]$lignoceric acid was quite different from that of $[1-^{14}C]$cerotic acid. This experiment, carried out in Baltimore, examined the radioactivity distribution among individual lipids during the uptake period at 48 h and 72 h, and during the chase period at 72 h. The bulk of radioactivity was associated with sphingomyelin, and to a lesser extent with lecithin and an unknown compound remaining at the origin. Free fatty acids contained 10-30% of the total radio-activity. Approximately 10% of the radioactivity was recovered in the Folch upper phase, and is presumed to be associated with gan-glioside. No radioactivity was detected in the cholesterol ester or triglyceride fractions. The relative distribution of radio-activity among the lipid fractions appeared to be approximately the same in the ALD and control cell lines.

DISCUSSION

The presence of the unusually long-chain fatty acids, primarily in cholesterol esters and gangliosides, in the brain and adrenal of ALD patients (12) appears to be the unique analytical characteristic of this disorder. We have taken two different approaches in order to examine the possible metabolic cause for this abnormality: direct assays of cholesterol ester hydrolases in postmortem brain tissues, and the metabolism of very long-chain fatty acids in cultured fibro-blasts.

Three cholesterol esters with different fatty acids, oleic

($C_{18:1}$), lignoceric ($C_{24:0}$), and cerotic ($C_{26:0}$) were used for the assays of cholesterol ester hydrolases, because separate enzymes might be involved for hydrolysis of cholesterol esters with fatty acids shorter than C_{20} and those with fatty acids longer than C_{22} and because only the latter might be pathologically involved in ALD. The results presented here appear to exclude conclusively that the crude mitochondrial pH 4.2 cholesterol esterase and the microsomal pH 6.0 hydrolase are both not defective in ALD, regardless the specificity with respect to the chain length of fatty acids. The activities were normal in ALD brain with all three substrates for the pH 4.2 enzyme, and were moderately increased with either cholesteryl oleate or lignocerate for the microsomal cholesterol ester hydrolase. The results were less conclusive with respect to the myelin-localized cholesterol ester hydrolase because the activity could not be detected with either cholesteryl lignocerate or cerotate. Its activity against cholesteryl oleate was higher in ALD white matter than in the controls. If we assume only one myelin-localized cholesterol ester hydrolase, then we can conclude that this hydrolase is also not defective in ALD. However, we cannot exclude deficiency of a hypothetical additional cholesterol ester hydrolase in myelin, specific for the very long-chain esters, the activity of which is below the reliable detection limit with the specific radioactivity of our substrates. The higher than normal activity in ALD white matter of the myelin cholesterol ester hydrolase was unexpected. This enzyme appears to be almost exclusively localized in myelin and its activity in whole tissue generally parallels the amount of myelin present (6-8). Since the amounts of myelin in ALD white matter were less than normal, the increased activity indicates considerable activation of this enzyme per unit amount of myelin. This cholesterol ester hydrolase may or may not be a part of the nonspecific esterase reported in myelin histochemically or biochemically (1-2, 15, 21), and its physiological significance is unclear. The increased activity in ALD white matter deserves further exploration.

The fibroblast studies were designed to obtain ideas as to what areas of very long-chain fatty acid metabolism might provide the clue for further studies, if ALD is indeed caused by abnormal metabolism of the very long-chain fatty acids. The presence of such abnormal fatty acids in both cholesterol esters and gangliosides appears to favor the primary abnormality in fatty acid metabolism. Since there is no particular clue, the question we asked in these experiments was, " Do ALD fibroblasts handle added fatty acids, particularly of very long chain, in any way differently from normal fibroblasts?" We clearly failed to detect any specific abnormality attributable to ALD in the fatty acid uptake, exclusion, or the distribution of the incorporated radioactivity among different chemical constituents. The only tantalizing exception was that certain ALD fibroblast lines consistently took up very long-chain fatty acids at appreciably greater rates than normal cells. This phenomenon was observed independently in the two laboratories with different cell lines and different fatty acids. Additional work is required to determine whether or not this finding has any significance because it raised a question, "Does so-called ALD possibly consist of two metabolically distinct diseases?"

Both $[1-^{14}C]$lignoceric acid and $[1-^{14}C]$cerotic acid were retained within the cell much longer than $[1-^{14}C]$stearic acid, although we must be aware that stearic acid was taken up in the albumin-conjugated form while other two fatty acids were added to the medium largely as free suspensions. Unexpected and dramatic differences were observed in the metabolism of lignoceric acid and cerotic acid. Cerotic acid appeared largely inert metabolically in fibroblasts. No appreciable exclusion of $[1-^{14}C]$cerotic acid occurred during the 8-day chase period, and 90-95% of the radioactivity remained as free fatty acid. Since the label was on the carboxyl carbon, it is likely that it remained cerotic acid. On the other hand, $[1-^{14}C]$lignoceric acid was more rapidly metabolized and incorporated into complex lipids. Since very little radioactivity appeared in cholesterol, it is likely that $[1-^{14}C]$-lignoceric acid was incorporated as such, perhaps through acyl-CoA.

It should be cautioned that our findings on fatty acid metabolism in cultured fibroblasts do not necessarily exclude abnormal fatty acid metabolism as the fundamental genetic cause of ALD. We used fibroblasts because these cells are the most readily available sources for this type of metabolic studies which cannot be done with postmortem tissues. However, we may well be studying a "wrong tissue". ALD selectively affects the CNS white matter, adrenal and testis. Therefore, the fundamental genetic defect must involve the metabolic pathway which is common and uniquely important for these organs. Although the genetic defect is expected to be present in all somatic cells, it may not be detectable by the type of experiments we have carried out, if the affected pathway is not important for the general metabolism of fibroblasts.

Acknowledgements. This investigation was supported by grants NS-13578, NS-10885, NS-03356, HD-01799, and NS-13513 from the United States Public Health Service, and a grant from the Alfred P. Sloan Foundation. The authors thank Mrs Olga VanDamme and Mrs Catherine Rappe for their excellent technical assistance.

REFERENCES

1. Barron, K.D., Bernsohn, J. and Koeppen, A., Esterases of human CNS and PNS and myelin fractions, J. Histochem. Cytochem. 18 (1970) 683.

2. Barron, K.D., Bernsohn, J. and Mitzen, E., Nonspecific esterases of human peripheral nerve and centrum ovale: A comparison and observation on esteratic activity of myelin fractions, J. Neuropath. Exp. Neurol. 31 (1972) 562-582.

3. Bernsohn, J., Barron, K.D., Doolin, P.F., Hess, A.R. and
    Hedrick, M.T., Subcellular localization of rat brain ester-
    ases, J. Histochem. Cytochem. 14 (1966) 455-472.
4. Burton, B.K. and Nadler, H.L., Schilder's disease: Abnormal
    cholesterol retention and accumulation in cultivated fibro-
    blasts, Pediat. Res. 8 (1974) 170-175.
5. Eto, Y. and Suzuki, K., Cholesterol ester metabolism in the
    brain: Properties and subcellular distribution of cholesterol
    esterifying enzyme and cholesterol ester hydrolases in adult
    rat brain, Biochim. Biophys. Acta 239 (1971) 293-311.
6. Eto, Y. and Suzuki, K., Cholesterol ester metabolism in rat
    brain: A cholesterol ester hydrolase specifically localized
    in the myelin sheath, J. Biol. Chem. 248 (1973) 1986-1991.
7. Eto, Y. and Suzuki, K., Enzymes of cholesterol ester metabo-
    lism in the brain of mutant mice, quaking and jimpy, Exp.
    Neurol. 41 (1973) 222-226.
8. Eto, Y. and Suzuki, K., Developmental changes of cholesterol
    ester hydrolases localized in myelin and microsomes of rat
    brain, J. Neurochem. 20 (1973) 1475-1477.
9. Horning, M.G., Williams, E.A. and Horning, E.C., Separation of
    tissue cholesterol esters and triglycerides by silicic acid
    chromatography, J. Lipid. Res. 1 (1960) 482-485.
10. Hoshi, M. and Kishimoto, Y., Synthesis of cerebronic acid from
    lignoceric acid by rat brain preparation. Some properties and
    distribution of the α-hydroxylation system, J. Biol. Chem. 248
    (1973) 4123-4130.
11. Igarashi, M., Belchis, D. and Suzuki, K., Brain gangliosides
    in adrenoleukodystrophy, J. Neurochem. 27 (1976) 327-328.
12. Igarashi, M., Schaumburg, H.H., Powers, J., Kishimoto, Y.,
    Kolodny, E. and Suzuki, K., Fatty acid abnormality in adreno-
    leukodystrophy, J. Neurochem. 26 (1976) 851-860.
13. Igarashi, M. and Suzuki, K., Effect of exogenous lipids on rat
    brain cholesterol ester hydrolases, Exp. Neurol. 45 (1974)
    549-553.
14. Igarashi, M. and Suzuki, K., Effect of exogenous lipids on
    activities of the rat brain cholesterol ester hydrolase local-
    ized in the myelin sheath, J. Neurochem. 27 (1976) 859-866.
15. Igarashi, M. and Suzuki, K., Solubilization and characteriza-
    tion of the rat brain cholesterol ester hydrolase localized in
    the myelin sheath, J. Neurochem. 28 (1977) 729-738.
16. Johnson, A.B., Schaumburg, H.H. and Powers, J.M., Histochem-
    ical characteristics of the striated inclusions of adreno-
    leukodystrophy, J. Histochem. Cytochem. 24 (1976) 725-730.
17. Lowry, O.H., Rosebrough, N.J., Farr, A.L. and Randall, R.J.,
    Protein measurement with the Folin phenol reagent, J. Biol.
    Chem. 193 (1951) 265-275.
18. Miller, G.L., Protein determination for large numbers of
    samples, Analyt. Chem. 31 (1959) 964.

19. Pinter, K.G., Hamilton, J.G. and Muldrey, J.E., A method for rapid microsynthesis of radioactive cholesterol esters, J. Lipid Res. 5 (1964) 273-274.

20. Prabhudesai, A.V., A simple method for the preparation of cholesteryl esters, Lipids 12 (1976) 242-244.

21. Rumsby, M.G., Riekkinen, P.J. and Arstila, A.V., A critical evaluation of myelin purification. Nonspecific esterase activity associated with central nerve myelin preparations, Brain Res. 24 (1970) 495-516.

22. Schaumburg, H.H., Powers, J.M., Raine, C.S., Suzuki, K. and Richardson, E.P., Adrenoleukodystrophy, A clinical and pathological study of 17 cases, Arch. Neurol. 33 (1975) 577-591.

23. Suzuki, K., Biochemistry of myelin disorders, in the Physiology and Pathology of Axons (Waxman, S.G., ed.), Plenum Press, New York (1977) in press.

24. Yavin, E., Milunsky, A., DeLong, G.R., Nash, A.H. and Kolodny, E.H., Cholesterol metabolism in cultured fibroblasts in adrenoleukodystrophy, Pediat. Res. 10 (1976) 540-543.

DEMYELINATION

The Possible Viral Etiology of
Multiple Sclerosis

VIROLOGICAL ASPECTS OF MULTIPLE SCLEROSIS

V. ter Meulen

Institute for Virology and Immunobiology,
 University of Würzburg
8700 Würzburg, G.F.R.

Multiple sclerosis (MS) is considered to be a leading candidate among human diseases of the central nervous system (CNS) which may be associated with a viral infection. From a virological point of view the following circumstantial evidence is available: Many studies have compared the frequency of antibodies against all common viruses in the serum and cerebrospinal fluid (CSF) specimens of MS patients to matched controls and patients with other CNS diseases. Although results vary, these studies generally indicate that more patients with MS tend to have a slightly higher antibody titer against measles than the control groups. However, an increase of antibody titers against other common viruses, such as herpes simplex, vaccinia, varicella zoster, adeno viruses, influenza C, parainfluenza 3, mumps and rubella have also been reported in MS cases. Moreover, in some MS patients part of the detectable oligoclonal IgG in the CSF could be identified as viral antibodies suggesting a local hyperimmune reaction against a viral antigen (2).

Electron microscopical investigations described a variety of particles in MS brain material which were associated with virus structures. These structures consist of either ovoid membrane-bound bodies which are now thought to represent myelin breakdown products or dense intracytoplasmic osmiophilic granules of 60 to 83 nm in diameter, which probably represent non-specific changes of reactive astrocytes. More recently, many investigators have found paramyxovirus nucleocapsid-like structures in cellular elements of probably hematogenous origin. However, at present these structures could not be identified as being of viral nature (1).

Many attempts have been made to transmit the disease or to isolate the causative agent from MS material. Viruses such as rabies, herpes simplex, parainfluenza, MS-associated agent or measles have been isolated and their relationship to the disease analyzed. However, at present none of these agents could be etiologically linked to this disease (2).

Besides these virological findings, other indirect evidence supports the notion of a viral process in this CNS disorder. Epidemiological studies indicate a common exposure factor suggesting that an exogenous agent is acquired during childhood or early adolescence which after a long incubation period contributes to the disease. Experimental studies in animals have shown that viruses can cause demyelinating diseases with long incubation periods. Moreover, other viral diseases are known which have a remitting and relapsing course similar to MS. However, one should keep in mind that from a clinical and neuropathological point of view MS seems to be a heterogenous disease which might be related to different agents (3). From studies of other viral diseases it is known that different viruses can cause similar diseases, for example, Epstein-Barr virus or cytomegalo virus leading to infectious mononucleoses, measles and rubella viruses inducing subacute sclerosing panencephalitis, and hepatitis A, B virus or some additional virus cause acute hepatitis.

This aspect certainly complicates investigations on this disease and demonstrates that Koch´s postulates cannot be applied directly. Hopefully, the understanding of the pathogenetic mechanisms in other related CNS disorders such as visna, subacute sclerosing panencephalitis or progressive multifocal leukoencephalopathy will provide experimental tools in unraveling the etiology and pathogenicity of this disease.

REFERENCES

1. Dubois-Dalcq, M., Schumacher, G. and Sever, J.L., Acute multiple sclerosis. Electron microscopic evidence for and against a viral agent in the plaques, Lancet 2 (1973) 1408-1411.
2. Johnson, R.T., The possible viral etiology of multiple sclerosis, in Advances in Neurology, vol. 13 (W.J. Friedlander, ed.) Raven Press, New York (1975).
3. McAlpine, D., Lumsden, C.E. and Acheson, E.D., Multiple sclerosis: a reappraisal (2nd ed.) Churchill-Livingstone, Edinburgh and London (1972).

THE ROLE OF VIRUSES IN THE PATHOGENESIS OF DEMYELINATIVE DISORDER

William Sheremata[+]

Montreal Neurological Institute

Montreal, Canada

Encephalitis is not infrequently a sequel to measles and other paramyxovirus infections. Almost a quarter of such cases of post-infectious encephalomyelitis followed for 18 years by van Bogaert were a prelude to relapsing neurological disease and were diagnosed as multiple sclerosis (MS). This is surprisingly similar to the proportion of animals with experimental allergic encephalomyelitis (EAE) that develop relapsing signs. Recently, Wisniewski et al. and Raine et al. have shown that the neuropathology of these animals is strikingly similar to that of MS.

However, MS might represent chronic or recrudescent viral infection. The finding of impaired immunity to this group of viruses by Jersild et al. and by Utermohlen and Zabriskie seems to offer support for this concept. We also have observed a statistically significant reduction in the cell-mediated immune (CMI) response to measles using two different cell migration assays. Recently, using a highly purified measles virus preparation, even more significant results have been obtained in Dr. Zabriskie's laboratory and in our own. However, this impairment is present in only about half of patients early in their clinical course. Moreover, in serial studies over a period of months to years most of these patients lose their CMI to measles.

Chronic distemper is associated with demyelination. Immunity against distemper is even more effectively induced by measles immunization than by distemper. Sazant in our laboratory has performed migration inhibition factor (MIF) assays using distemper and measles antigens, and myelin basic protein on normal and distemper dogs, their keepers, MS patients and on normal humans. Only dogs

[+]Present address: Department of Neurology, University of Miami, School of Medicine, Miami, Florida, U.S.A.

with distemper, and their human keepers, but not normals, or MS
patients responded to distemper antigen. The distemper animals also
responded to measles and to myelin basic protein. One of the keepers with his first known exposure to distemper was ill with head-
ache only. He responded to myelin basic protein whereas his control,
who was well, did not. These findings suggest that antibody studies
alone may not be sufficient in the search for evidence of animal
virus infection of humans. We may be dealing with a number of
antigenically similar but different viruses with differing potentials for affecting humans. The apparent increased risk of MS with
small dog ownership underlines this question.

Orleans, a small village outside Ottawa, Canada, has provided
over 20 cases of subacute sclerosing panencephalitis (SSPE) to the
Montreal Neurological Institute. Dr. Preston Robb has mused that
the only thing that distinguished Orleans was that horses were the
majority of citizens; and, in the absence of equine encephalitis,
that perhaps the SSPE virus was a "horse distemper". As urban
sprawl has forced the riding stables to leave, so has the risk of
SSPE disappeared, despite a marked increase in population.

The uniform salutory response to long-term immunosuppression
observed by Ring et al., Lance, Delmotte et al., and by ourselves
raises reservations regarding the role of virus in MS. Regardless
of the means employed, stabilization of disease has been observed,
independent of the severity of affection. The observations that
many different viral antibody titres are elevated (Baringer and
others) suggest that no one virus is specifically involved in the
pathogenesis of MS. Alter's recent findings in the Israeli migration studies is that the age of risk of exposure to environmental
factors leading to MS is probably under the age of 6. This suggests
that viral infection may alter the development of normal immune
responsiveness rather than result in chronic or slow virus infection.
We must therefore address ourselves to the factors involved in the
normal immune response and how they are affected by environmental
factors. The observation by McFarlin that while a quota of adult
Lewis rats develop relapsing EAE following sensitization, half of
juvenile animals do. In Wisniewski's experiments juvenile guinea-
pigs have been shown to be more likely to develop relapsing disease.
These observations suggest that in the juvenile animal, and perhaps
also in the human, the factors that regulate immune responses may
result in phasic clinical expression of such sensitization. It is
possible, for example, that depriving a human child during very
early life of infectious experience (or alternatively, suffering
unusual recurrent viral infection) may result in an aberration in
the normal immune responses. To extend this example, immunosuppression may occur secondary to a viral infection that results in
damage in the central nervous system. The period of heightened
immune responsiveness normally following immunosuppression could
lead to hypersensitivity to brain antigens. In turn, this response
may not be held in control in a child. This hypothesis can only be
tested after gaining much more knowledge regarding the acquisition
of an immune response and its regulation.

JEJUNAL VIRAL ANTIGEN IN MULTIPLE SCLEROSIS AND AMYOTROPHIC

LATERAL SCLEROSIS

Albert W. Cook
 Department of Neuroscience, Long Island College
 Hospital, and Downstate Medical Center, State University
 of New York
Louis P. Pertschuk
 Downstate Medical Center, State University of New York
Jagdish K. Gupta
 Department of Medicine, Division of Gastroenterology,
 Long Island College Hospital
Dong S. Kim
 Downstate Medical Center, State University of New York,
 Brooklyn, New York 11203, U.S.A.

Statistical data is presented regarding the identification of viral antigen in the jejunum of patients with multiple sclerosis (MS) and other neurological disease, in particular amyotrophic lateral sclerosis (motor neuron disease). The viral antigens were identified using fluorescent antibody techniques previously described (1-3). Jejunal specimens were obtained by conventional passage of a small peroral tube with an attached capsule. The position of the capsule was identified radiographically to be in the proximal jejunum. In some instances, particularly in patients with amyotrophic lateral sclerosis (ALS), impairment of swallowing necessitated the use of a fiber-optic jejunoscope.

The predominant findings have been measles viral antigen in MS and poliovirus antigen in most patients with motor neuron disease. The concentration of antigen as shown by immunofluorescence was variable as was the presence of complement and distribution of immunoglobulins. Figure 1 illustrates positively stained lamina propria cells in a patient with MS after incubation with specific measles antiserum. In this case there was no staining of either epithelium or epithelial basement membrane although this was commonly observed in other specimens from patients with MS. Figure 2 illustrates poliovirus antigen within lamina propria cells from a patient with motor neuron disease. In Figure 3 a heavy concentration

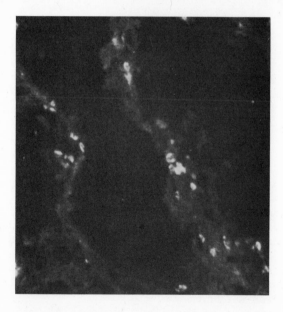

Fig. 1. Jejunal mucosa from patient with multiple sclerosis after incubation with bovine anti-measles serum and rabbit antibovine fluorescein conjugate. Positive lamina propria cells exhibit bright cytoplasmic fluorescence (immunofluorescence microscopy, original magnification x 100).

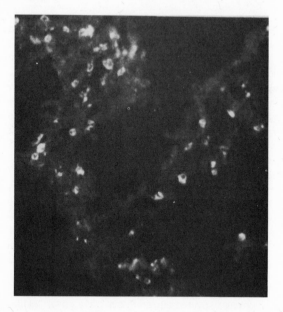

Fig. 2. Lamina propria cells in jejunal mucosa from a case of motor neuron disease containing poliovirus antigen (immunofluorescence microscopy, original magnification x 100).

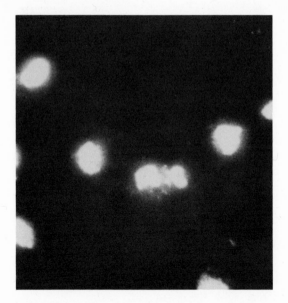

Fig. 3. Jejunal mucosa from an autopsied case of amyotrophic
lateral sclerosis after treatment with fluorescein conjugated anti-
herpesvirus hominis (bivalent) serum. The lamina propria cells
contain large quantities of viral antigen (immunofluorescence
microscopy, original magnification x 500).

of herpesvirus hominis antigen can be seen in lamina propria cells
of another patient with motor neuron disease.

Table 1 portrays our experience with jejunal biopsies from MS
cases. In only 2 were we unable to detect measles virus antigen.
One of these 2 patients had a repeat biopsy which was also antigen-
negative. The clinical features of this patient were reassessed
and it was felt unequivocally that they were those of MS. Despite
the failure to detect measles antigen by immunofluorescence in the
other patient, paramyxovirus, probably measles, was recovered by
co-cultivation of the patient's jejunal tissue and antigen identified by fluorescent antibody studies.

Table 2 illustrates our findings in 40 non-neurologic controls.
One biopsy from a patient diagnosed as ulcerative colitis demonstrated measles antigen. Measles antigen was also present in
specimens from 2 children (ages 18 and 30 months) who died from
non-neurologic disease. In the latter instance it was felt that
this probably reflected persistent viral protein from recent, prior
immunization.

Our experience with motor neuron disease is summarized in
Table 3. In 5 cases, poliovirus antigen was detected, accompanied
by measles virus in one specimen, while large amounts of herpesvirus
antigen were seen in a sixth case. In 2 of these cases the

Table 1. Results of immunofluorescence (IF) examination of jejunal mucosa in clinical multiple sclerosis (78 cases).

Measles antigen only	9 cases
Measles antigen and complement	15 cases
Measles antigen, complement and abnormal immunoglobulins	38 cases
Measles antigen and abnormal immunoglobulins	14 cases
No measles antigen detected, only complement and abnormal immunoglobulins	2 cases

Table 2. Results of IF examination of jejunal mucosa of non-neurologic controls (40 cases).

Measles antigen negative	37 cases
Measles antigen positive	3 cases
A. Two children:	
1.5 years (sudden death)	
2.5 years (nephrosis)	
with isolated positive lamina propria cells	
B. Ulcerative colitis	1 case

Table 4. Results of IF examination of jejunal mucosa in patients with neurologic disease other than multiple sclerosis and amyotrophic lateral sclerosis (7 cases).

Measles antigen negative	6 cases
Ataxia	2 cases
Huntington's chorea	1 case
Parkinsonism	1 case
Cerebral palsy	1 case
Encephalitis	1 case
Measles antigen positive	1 case
Friedreich's ataxia	1 case

Table 3. Results of IF examination of jejunal mucosa in patients with ALS (motor neuron disease).

Case	IgG		IgM		IgA		Complement		Antigen present
	Labeled cells	B.M.*	Labeled cells	B.M.	Labeled cells	B.M.	Labeled cells	B.M.	
1	Increased	Yes	Decreased	No	Average	Yes	C3	Yes	Poliovirus 1,3 Measles
2	Increased	No	Average	Yes	Average	No	C3	No	Poliovirus 1,3
3	Average	No	Average	No	Decreased	Yes	C3,C4	No	Poliovirus 1,3
4	Increased	No	Average	No	Average	Yes	C3,C4	No	Herpesvirus
5	Increased	Yes	Increased	No	Decreased	No	C3,C4	Yes	None detected
6	Increased	No	Increased	No	Average	No	C3A**	No	Poliovirus 3
7	Average	No	Average	No	Average	No	C3	No	------
8	Increased	Yes	Increased	No	Average	Yes	C3,C4,C3A**	No	Poliovirus 1,2
9	Increased	Yes	Increased	No	Decreased	No	No	No	None detected

*B.M. = Deposits in the epithelial basement membrane; C3A** = C3 Activator.

diagnosis of motor neuron disease was established at autopsy. Poliovirus antigen was not detected in any other specimen. In a small number of specimens from patients with other neurologic disease (Table 4), no measles or poliovirus antigen was seen except in one specimen from a patient with Friedreich's ataxia.

These findings do not specifically relate the presence of viral protein to the disease in question. However, there is indication of a fairly constant association between clinical MS and measles viral protein in the jejunum.

REFERENCES

1. Pertschuk, L.P., Cook, A.W. and Gupta, J., Measles antigen in multiple sclerosis: identification in the jejunum by immuno-fluorescence, Life Sci. 19 (1976) 1603-1608.
2. Pertschuk, L.P., Cook, A.W., Gupta, J.K., Broome, J.D., Vuletin, J.C., Kim, D.S., Brigati, D.J., Rainford, E.A. and Nidsgorski, F., Jejunal immunopathology in amyotrophic lateral sclerosis and multiple sclerosis, Lancet I (1977) 1119-1123.
3. Pertschuk, L.P., Cook, A.W., Gupta, J.K., Broome, J.D., Vuletin, J.C., Kim, D.S., Stanek, A.E., Brigati, D.J., Rainford, E.A. and Nidsgorski, F., Measles antigen in the jejunum in multiple sclerosis, Lancet II (1977) 300-301.

ASPECTS OF THE VIRAL ANTIBODY RESPONSE IN MULTIPLE SCLEROSIS

B.R. Ziola and A.A. Salmi

The Neurovirology Study Group, Department of Virology,
    University of Turku
Turku, Finland

It has been suggested that the intrathecal synthesis of viral
IgG antibodies indicates the presence of the corresponding viral
antigen(s) in the central nervous system (CNS) of MS patients (6).
Although measles virus has predominantly been implicated in such
studies, intrathecal IgG synthesis to rubella, mumps and vaccinia
virus has also been detected (4, 7). Intrathecal viral IgG antibody synthesis may, however, be a secondary, non-specific phenomenon
in the pathogenesis of MS. Support for this idea comes from the
fact that IgG antibodies against more than one virus are synthesized
in the CNS of some MS patients (4). Moreover, not all MS patients
have CNS IgG synthesis to a single virus i.e., measles virus (4)
and of the oligoclonal IgG found in the CNS of MS patients, only a
minor fraction is against a given virus i.e., measles virus (9).

Recently, we have analyzed MS patients for CNS IgG antibody
synthesis to the human coronavirus OC43. A sensitive solidphase
radioimmunoassay (RIA) was used (11). RIA determinations of respiratory syncytial virus-specific IgG were concurrently used to
evaluate the integrity of the patients' blood-brain-barriers. Two
MS patients, of 20 studied, were found to have CNS IgG synthesis
to coronavirus OC43. Table 1 presents the data of some of the MS
and control patients analyzed. A serum/CSF ratio of <80 is considered to be a clear indication of intrathecal antibody synthesis
of a specific IgG (5). This demonstration of CNS IgG synthesis to
yet another virus supports the contention that such antibody synthesis to viruses in MS patients may be more general than hereto-
fore expected, and that the bulk of the oligoclonal IgG found in
the CNS of MS patients is secondary to the MS disease process.
This does not exclude, however, that some of the observed CNS
oligoclonal IgG antibodies may have a pathological role in MS.

Table 1. Analysis of viral IgG, total IgG, and albumin in paired
serum (S) and cerebrospinal fluid (CSF) specimens.

Patient (diagnosis)[*]	Coronavirus RIA IgG ($\log_2$)		S/CSF ratio (virus IgG)		CSF/S ratio ($\times 10^{+3}$)	
	S	CSF	Coronavirus	Respiratory syncytial virus	Albumin	IgG
MR (MS)	11.6	5.9	55	220	5.7	17.6
OP (MS)	9.3	4.2	35	335	3.6	4.2
RH (MS)	10.7	4.0	110	870	4.8	4.6
RB (MS)	11.2	2.6	385	205	8.0	21.1
VJ (MS)	10.2	1.7	360	230	3.5	5.9
KP (ALS)	9.6	<1.0	>500	1025	2.4	1.8

[*]MS = Multiple sclerosis; ALS = Amyotrophic lateral sclerosis

Virus specific IgM antibodies generally decline to undetectable
levels following the convalescent phase of viral infections. Thus,
the continued production of IgM antibodies long after convalescence
may indicate a persistence of the viral infection. The human
disease subacute sclerosing panencephalitis (SSPE) is known to occur
months to years after a measles infection. Consequently, studies
of measles IgM persistence in SSPE can be expected to provide useful background information for similar studies with MS patients,
given the association of measles virus with most MS patients.

An immunofluorescence study (8) and an RIA study (13) have
reported finding measles-specific IgM in SSPE patients. Studies
conducted in our laboratories, also with an RIA designed to detect
measles IgM antibodies (1), appeared to confirm that measles IgM
is produced in at least some SSPE patients (2). Possible complica-
tions posed by IgM-class rheumatoid factor (RF), however, were not
thoroughly taken into account in these studies. Therefore, in
order to more fully investigate the possible persistency of measles
IgM in SSPE patients, we developed a sensitive solid-phase RIA to
test for low levels of RF. The RF RIA utilizes natural human IgG:
antigen complexes on a solid-phase to bind RF which is then detected
with ^{125}I-labeled antihuman-mu indicator antibodies (10). With the
availability of the measles IgM RIA and the RF RIA, we then undertook an extensive study of sera and cerebrospinal fluid (CSF) from
19 SSPE patients. It was determined that what was originally believed to be measles IgM in the serum and CSF from some patients
was, in fact, RF interference in the measles IgM RIA. No true
measles IgM was found in the serum and CSF specimens from these
19 SSPE patients.

Similar techniques were then used to study 70 MS patients for
the possible persistence of measles-specific IgM and not a single

patient with genuine measles IgM antibodies was found. These
results indicate that, if there is continued production of measles
IgM antibodies in the serum or CSF of MS patients, the levels are
very low. It is not known at this time whether or not persisting
IgM against other viruses is present in MS patients. Any such
study, however, must clearly take into account low levels of RF
which may be present.

REFERENCES

1. Arstila, P., Vuorimaa, T., Kalimo, K., Halonen, P., Viljanen,
    M., Granfors, K. and Toivanen, P., A solid-phase radioimmuno-
    assay for IgG and IgM antibodies against measles virus, J. gen.
    Virol. 34 (1977) 167-176.
2. Halonen, P., Matikainen, M.-T., Salmi, A., Vuorimaa, T. and
    Ziola, B.R., Antibody response to measles virus in subacute
    sclerosing panencephalitis, Lancet I (1977) 1201.
3. Kiessling, W.R., Hall, W.W., Yung, L.L. and ter Meulen, V.,
    Measles-virus-specific immunoglobulin-M response in subacute
    sclerosing panencephalitis, Lancet I (1977) 324-327.
4. Norrby, E., Link, H., Olsson, J.-E., Panelius, M., Salmi, A.
    and Vandvik, B., Comparison of antibodies against different
    viruses in cerebrospinal fluid and serum samples from patients
    with multiple sclerosis, Infect. Immun. 10 (1974) 688-694.
5. Reunanen, M., Arstila, P., Hakkarainen, H., Nikoskelainen, J.,
    Salmi, A. and Panelius, M., A longitudinal study on antibodies
    to measles and rubella viruses in patients with multiple scle-
    rosis. A preliminary report. Acta neurol. Scand. 54 (1976)
    366-370.
6. Salmi, A.A., Panelius, M., Halonen, P., Rinne, U.K. and Pentti-
    nen, K., Measles virus antibody in cerebrospinal fluids from
    patients with multiple sclerosis, Brit. Med. J. I (1972) 477-
    479.
7. Thompson, J.A., Glasgow, L.A. and Bray, P.F., Evaluation of
    central nervous system vaccinia antibody synthesis in multiple
    sclerosis patients, Neurology 27 (1977) 227-229.
8. Thompson, D., Connolly, J.H., Underwood, B.O. and Brown, F.J.,
    A study of immunoglobulin M antibody to measles, canine dis-
    temper, and rinderpest viruses in sera of patients with sub-
    acute sclerosing panencephalitis, J. clin. Path. 28 (1975)
    543-546.
9. Vandvik, B., Norrby, E., Nordel, H.J. and Degré, M., Oligo-
    clonal measles virus-specific IgG antibodies isolated from
    cerebrospinal fluids, brain extracts, and sera from patients
    with subacute sclerosing panencephalitis and multiple sclerosis,
    Scand. J. Immunol. 5 (1976) 979-992.
10. Ziola, B.R., Meurman, O., Matikainen, M.-T., Salmi, A. and
    Kalliomäki, L., in preparation.
11. Ziola, B.R., Salmi, A. and Hovi, T., in preparation.

AUTOIMMUNITY TO RECEPTORS AS A POSSIBLE CAUSE OF MULTIPLE SCLEROSIS

P.R. Carnegie

School of Biochemistry, University of Melbourne

Parkville, Victoria 3052, Australia

The concept that chronic disease could result from an immune response to cell surface receptors (3) has been supported by the demonstration of an immune response to acetylcholine receptor in myasthenia gravis, thyroid stimulating hormone receptor in Graves' disease, insulin receptor in insulin resistant diabetes, prolactin receptor in animals immunized with the receptor (for references, see review, 2). While binding assays have been used to demonstrate antibody to receptors, more definitive results were often obtained with physiological assays.

In 1971 Carnegie (1) suggested that an immune response to serotonin receptors could explain the clinical symptoms in experimental autoimmune encephalomyelitis (EAE) in guinea-pigs. The idea received only tenuous support (2) until recently when Weinstock et al. (5) clearly demonstrated that the degree of paralysis in EAE correlated with a malfunctioning of the serotonin receptor in the guinea-pig ileum. As EAE has been established as being a disease of the central nervous system it is surprising to find such an abnormality in peripheral serotonin receptors.

Many of the clinical features of multiple sclerosis could be explained by a fluctuating level of an antibody directed against a cell surface receptor on the oligodendrocyte. A virus lodged in the cell membrane adjacent to a receptor could induce an immune response which could interfere with the functioning of that receptor and possibly similar receptors on other cells. There is a need for the development of physiological and biochemical assays to investigate the serum factors, which are present in a high percentage of patients with multiple sclerosis and which block the neuroelectrical activity in frog spinal cord preparations (4).

REFERENCES

1. Carnegie, P.R., Properties, structure and possible neuro-
    receptor role of the encephalitogenic protein of human myelin,
    Nature 229 (1971) 25-28.
2. Carnegie, P.R. and Mackay, I.R., Vulnerability of cell surface
    receptors to autoimmune reactions, Lancet 2 (1975) 684-686.
3. Lennon, V.A. and Carnegie, P.R., Immunopharmacological disease:
    a break in tolerance to receptor sites, Lancet 1 (1971) 630-
    633.
4. Schauf, C.L., Davis, F.A., Sack, D.A., Reed, B.J. and Kesler,
    R.L., Neuroelectric blocking factors in human and animal sera
    evaluated using the isolated frog spinal cord, J. Neurol.
    Neurosurg. Psych. 39 (1976) 680-685.
5. Weinstock, M., Shoham-Moshonov, S., Teitelbaum, D. and Arnon,
    R., Inactivation of neurogenic 5-hydroxytryptamine receptors
    in guinea pigs with experimental allergic encephalomyelitis
    (EAE) induced paralysis, Brain Res. 125 (1977) 192-195.

IMMUNOGLOBULINS IN MULTIPLE SCLEROSIS

Hans Link

Department of Neurology, University Hospital

S581 85 Linköping, Sweden

Data have accumulated indicating that the human brain with its extracellular space, i.e. the cerebrospinal fluid (CSF), must be regarded from an immunological point of view as a separate entity. For example, the reaction of the lymphocytes present in the CSF in multiple sclerosis (MS) is different from that of blood lymphocytes in the same patient. Consequently, immunoglobulin abnormalities may be found in CSF and brain tissue, e.g. elevated immunoglobulin levels and oligoclonal IgG. These immunoglobulins which are synthesized within the CNS consist of specific antibodies in subacute sclerosing panencephalitis and acute viral meningitis. The antibody character of intrathecally synthesized IgG in MS in unknown.

It is not clear whether the immune response which occurs within the central nervous system (CNS) in MS has any protecting effect, or is the cause of demyelination. Additional characterization of the cell-mediated as well as humoral immune response within the CNS in MS during different phases of the disease is of greatest importance and should yield a better rationale for the use of immunomanipulatory therapy in the form of immunosuppression and immunostimulation, which are at present used liberately in this disorder.

Adequate methods for demonstration of immunoglobulin synthesis within the CNS and of oligoclonal IgG should be used. The groups of patients should be meticulously defined regarding clinical parameters. The immune response within the CNS seems to be most pronounced in the majority of MS patients before severe disability has developed, and studies regarding the immune response should be performed in these immunologically active cases. It should be kept in mind that clinical exacerbations of MS represent the top of the iceberg. Postmortem findings as well as CSF investigations indicate that disease activity, as reflected by an inflammatory reaction, occurs continuously in MS at least during the years up to severe

disability. Plaques may also be located in clinically silent zones
of the white matter. Therefore, not too much emphasis should be
laid on the investigation of patients with exacerbations of symptoms,
but of immunologically active patients. More effort should be concentrated to characterize the antibody activity of oligoclonal IgG
present in CSF and brain tissue in MS.

SUMMARY OF THE GENERAL DISCUSSION ON THE POSSIBLE VIRAL ETIOLOGY OF MULTIPLE SCLEROSIS

A. Salmi

Department of Virology, University of Turku

Turku, Finland

The available evidence for and against a viral etiology of multiple sclerosis (MS) was evaluated. It was agreed that, at the present time, no strong virological data are available which would support the notion of a viral etiology of MS.

The 6/94 variant of Sendai virus has been proposed as a candidate for causing MS. Extensive studies have not, however, confirmed that this virus is etiologically related to MS. Nonetheless, it was noted that this virus belongs to the paramyxoviruses, among which may be the best candidates for an infectious agent which triggers the immunological reactions leading to MS.

The MS-associated agent (Carp agent) aroused recently much interest and publicity. Several speakers reported negative results in experiments designed to confirm the original data. Consequently, the conclusion was that no definitive evidence exists for this agent at the moment. It was also concluded that a much more reproducible testing system is needed for demonstration of this type of agent than depression of circulating polymorphonuclear leukocytes in mice or other animals.

The recent finding of measles antigen in jejunal biopsies of MS patients and the isolation of a paramyxo-like virus from these biopsies was discussed in detail. The specificity of the antisera used in these studies was questioned and Dr. A.W. Cook stressed the importance of the proper antisera selection. He stated that not all measles antisera were useful in the measles virus antigen demonstration; for example, serum from a patient with subacute sclerosing panencephalitis could not be used, whereas a batch of measles antiserum made in goats functioned well. It was agreed that jejunal biopsy and other studies of MS tissue with fluorescence antibody techniques are of importance. It was stressed, however,

that careful analysis should be made of the specificity of the
antisera used in such work.

Research necessary for resolving the question of the possible
viral etiology of MS was discussed. It was concluded that work
should be continued on attempts to demonstrate the presence of
viruses or defective viral infections in tissue material of MS
patients, in so far as viruses are still considered to be candidates
for causing MS. The development of special methods for demonstration
of viral "footprints" will be necessary for demonstration of virus-
specific antigens or nucleic acids in human brain material; e.g.,
competitive radioimmunoassays for demonstration of specific viral
antigens and nucleic acid hybridization techniques for demonstration
of specific viral genetic material.

It was suggested that virologists could further contribute to
MS research by studying persistent virus infections in vitro and in
vivo (animal models), by studying virus-induced demyelination in
animal models, and by studying functional changes in cells persistently infected with viruses. Finally, it was stressed that viruses
known to cause disturbances in the immunological system should be
carefully studied, measles virus being one example. In studies on
the pathogenesis of persistent viral infections in animals not only
is the lytic effect of importance, but the immunologically mediated
damage must be taken into consideration as well.

acetylcholine, 148, 637
acetylcholinesterase, 119, 390
acid-base balance, 56
action potential, 218
adenovirus, 540, 623
adrenoleukodystrophy (ALD), 515, 585, 601
albumin, 21, 89, 312, 331, 357, 368, 530, 547, 606, 634
alkylating agent, 497
alkylnitrosourea, 487
alloxan, 484
Alzheimer's disease, 427
amino acid, as spacer substance, 546
ampholyte, 10, 546
amyotrophic lateral sclerosis, 503, 627, 634
antibody, against
  brain, 501
  enzyme, 46
  glial cell, 89
  myelin, 22, 433
  myelin basic protein, 3, 97, 280, 502, 514
  receptor, 637
  virus, 384, 396, 623, 626, 633
antigen
  in experimental allergic encephalomyelitis, 280, 290, 330, 348, 366
  in experimental allergic neuritis, 472
  in multiple sclerosis, 501, 623, 626, 627
  stimulation, 3
  viral, 399, 627
antiserum, against
  galactocerebroside, 89
  JHM-virus, 396
  measles virus, 627
  myelin, 433
  myelin basic protein, 515
  oligodendroglia, 87

arachnoiditis, 408
astrocyte, astroglia, 56, 77, 386, 400, 425, 570, 623
atrophy, cerebral, 427
autoimmunity, 218, 277, 303, 366, 530, 563, 637
autolysis, 426, 571
automatic immunoprecipitation (AIP), 536
axon, 44, 84, 96, 173, 218, 236, 366, 386, 397, 464, 484, 488
axonal transport, 439

bacteriorhodopsin, 202
basement membrane, 627
basic protein of CNS myelin (MBP)
  action in rat brain, 147
  aggregation, 213
  amino acid sequence, 208, 289, 303
  antibodies, 377, 414, 514
  binding to β-lipoprotein, 508
  binding to probe, 190
  cellular response, 501, 530
  in cerebrospinal fluid, 148, 513
  clearance from blood, 329
  conformation, 207
  cross-linking to lipid bilayers, 221
  degradation, 2, 347, 365, 569
  desensitization, 330
  electrophoresis, 118
  encephalitogenecity, 281, 289, 303, 345, 501
  encephalitogenic determinant, 303
  and glial myelin, 79
  HNB-treatment, 3
  humoral response, 501
  hypersensitivity, 508
  inhibition of hydrolysis, 362
  isoelectric point, 229

basic protein of CNS myelin (MBP)
(cont'd)
  large basic protein, 122, 137,
    162, 194
  location in myelin, 241
  and migration inhibition
    factor, 625
  monomer, dimer, 212, 231
  oligomer, 208, 231
  peptides, 2, 22, 111, 148,
    208, 232, 241, 281, 290, 303,
    309, 330, 351, 414, 508, 522
  phosphorylation, 159
  preparation, 149, 209, 222,
    502, 522
  radioimmunoassay, 414, 513
  small basic protein, 20, 118,
    137, 162, 194
  synthesis, 21
blood-brain barrier, 8, 375,
  412, 432, 534, 546, 633
blood coagulation, 375

cancer, 362, 389, 487, 503, 567
canine distemper, 384, 429, 625
carbohydrates, 111, 191
carbonic anhydrase, 55, 128
carboxylic acid esterase, 570
"Carp-Henle agent", 419, 641
casein, 357, 375
catecholamine, 440
cathepsin
  A, 3, 308
  B, 308
  D, 232, 308, 348
cell fusion, 385
central pontine myelinolysis,
  515
ceramide, 79, 271
cerebroside, 20, 77, 84, 171,
  199, 236, 263, 310, 457,
  489, 589, 608
cerebrospinal fluid (CSF)
  in multiple sclerosis, 530,
    561, 634
  myelin basic protein, 148,
    513
  plasmalogenase, 432

cerebrospinal fluid (CSF)
(cont'd)
  protein fragments of myelin,
    377
  proteins, 8, 545
  proteolytic activity, 521
  in subacute sclerosing pan-
    encephalitis, 387
chaotropic force, 216
DL-p-chlorophenylalanine, 455
cholesterol, 29, 77, 172, 190,
  236, 266, 454, 493
cholesterol esters, 489, 585,
  602
cholesterol ester hydrolase, 603
choline-acetylcholine-trans-
  ferase, 390
choline phosphatides, 20, 77,
  216, 237, 609
chromatography
  column, 11, 45, 97, 258, 316,
    488, 587
  gas-liquid, 29, 172, 266, 456,
    587, 604
  paper, 292
  thin-layer, 29, 79, 193, 223,
    252, 268, 488, 587, 604
chromosomal aberration, 185
chymotrypsin, 294
citraconic anhydrase, 294
co-cultivation method, 386
colitis, 629
collagenase, 376
complement, 627
complement fixation test, 8,
  433, 501
conduction velocity, 444
copper deficiency, 412
corona-virus, 395, 633
counterimmunodiffusion, 502
cuprizone, 21
cyanide sensitive factor, 50
2',3'-cyclic nucleotide-3'-
  phosphohydrolase (CNP), 3, 20,
    66, 78, 119, 172, 180, 411,
    480, 570, 586
cytochrome, 44, 148, 357
cytochrome c reductase, 78
cytomegalo virus, 624

dansyl chloride, 250
Debye length, 215
dementia, 427
demyelination
  and adrenoleukodystrophy, 585
  and autoimmunity, 218
  and cerebrospinal fluid and
    serum proteins, 545
  and cerebrospinal fluid factors,
    521
  and diphtheria toxin, 439
  and enzymes, 2, 351, 423, 570
  in experimental allergic en-
    cephalomyelitis, 473
  histology, 99
  and immune response, 529
  inflammatory, 365
  and myelin basic protein,
    148, 514
  pathogenesis, 19, 236
  and proliferating cells, 561
  and proteolysis, 310
  relation to myelination, 171
  and toxic agents, 488
  and virus infection, 383, 396,
    625
denervation, 450
deoxycholate, 222
desaturase, 46
diabetes, 479, 637
differential scanning calorimetry,
  190
diphtheria toxin, 21, 439
DM-20, see intermediate protein
dopamine, 148
dysmyelination, 135

edema, in brain, 56, 427
Ehrlich ascites cell, 44
elastase, 348
electrophoresis
  of cerebrospinal fluid proteins,
    539, 546
  of myelin proteins, 2, 79, 97,
    118, 136, 161, 193, 209, 223,
    309, 488, 504, 570
  of peptides of myelin basic
    protein, 290, 332, 349, 368

encephalitis, 384, 502, 522,
  547, 562, 625
encephalitogen, see basic
  protein of CNS myelin
encephalomyelitis
  with canine distemper, 385, 429
  with corona virus, 396
  postvaccinal, 7
  subacute demyelinating, 402
endoplasmic reticulum, 19, 78,
  119
endothelial cell, 44, 530
ependymitis, 397
Epstein-Barr virus, 624
equine infectious anemia (EIA),
  391
erythrocyte membrane, 191, 237
ethanolamine phosphatides, 20,
  77, 236, 252, 264, 424, 608
ethylnitrosourea, 487
experimental allergic
  encephalomyelitis, 3, 21, 95,
    108, 147, 279, 289, 303, 308,
    329, 347, 366, 433, 502, 515,
    530, 625, 637
  neuritis, 95, 108, 308, 471

fatty acids
  in fibroblasts, 610
  in human brain, 27, 585, 602
  in human myelin, 32, 199, 454,
    585
  in rat brain, 45
fatty alcohol, 44
fibrin, 535
fibrinolysis, 367
fibroblast, 603
fluorodinitrobenzene (FDNB), 250
Fourier transform method, 209
freeze-fracture method, 237, 325
Freund's adjuvant, 3, 89, 97,
  281, 290, 330, 348, 433, 472,
  515, 530
Friedreich's ataxia, 630

galactocerebroside, see
  cerebroside
galactolipid, 29, 77, 174, 493,
  596
galactose, in cerebroside,
  244, 264, 457
galactose
  oxidase, 192, 238, 250, 264
  periodate, 238
galactosyltransferase, 128
ganglioside, 77, 155, 203, 602
gitter cell, 386, 402
glial cell, 5, 19, 22, 43, 56,
  72, 160, 177, 179, 389, 397,
  497, 570
glial fibrillary acidic protein
  (GFA), 3, 331, 577
gliosis, 405, 575
globoid leukodystrophy, 597
glucose-6-phosphatase, 45, 78,
  481
β-glucosaminidase, 481
β-glucosidase, 481
β-glucuronidase, 3, 426, 480,
  570
glycerol, 245
glycerophosphatide, 44, 595, 602
glycolipid (see also cerebroside),
  99, 172, 191, 236, 250, 264,
  489, 587
glycoprotein
  in CNS myelin, 118, 160, 191
  in glial myelin, 79
  in PNS myelin, 100
gnotobiotic dog, 429
Golgi apparatus, 78, 400
granulomatous disease, 389
Graves' disease, 637
guanidinium hydrochloride, 209
Guillain-Barré syndrome, 433,
  471, 505, 539, 546

hemoglobin, 357, 375
hepatitis, 384, 624
herpes, 384, 623, 629
hexachlorophene, 66
histone, 150, 213, 232, 333,
  357, 571

HNBr-protein, 6
hybridization, 385
hydrocephalus, 405
hypersensitivity, delayed, 7,
  366
hypomyelination, 464
hypothyroidism, 412

imidazole, 66
immunity
  cell-mediated, 6, 281, 289,
    366, 387, 413, 507, 521,
    529, 561, 625, 639
  humoral, 387, 529, 561, 639
immunoabsorption, 505
immunodeficiency, 389, 412, 625
immunodiffusion, 97, 318, 344,
  388, 504, 536
immunoelectrophoresis, 10, 388,
  505, 536, 556
immunofluorescence, 87, 396,
  433, 627, 634
immunoglobulin
  IgA, 631
  IgG, 8, 24, 311, 386, 433,
    508, 533, 546, 561, 623, 627,
    633, 639
  IgM, 387, 433, 631, 634
immunoradiometric assay (IRMA),
  8, 331
immunosuppression, 280, 385,
  536, 626, 639
inclusion body, 386, 397
infarction, in CNS, 518
influenza, 391, 623
inositol phosphatides, 77, 237,
  489, 609
insulin, 637
intermediate protein (DM-20),
  118, 137, 164, 194, 368
intoxication, 487
ion movement, 56
irradiation, 179
ischemia, in CNS, 426, 556
isoelectric focusing, point,
  10, 539, 545, 546
isotachophoresis, 545

jejunal viral antigen, 627, 641
JHM-virus, 396
jimpy mouse, 425

kappa/lambda ratio, 540, 581
ketone bodies, 465

lactic dehydrogenase, 57, 450
lactoperoxidase, 202, 250,
   322, 522
LCM-virus, 390
lecithin, see choline phosphatides
leucine aminopeptidase, 570
L-leucyl-2-naphthylamidase, 172
light scattering, 222
lipase, 45
lipids
   in adrenoleukodystrophy, 585
   in brain, 179
   in CNS myelin, 160, 190
   in oligodendroglia, 77
lipolysis, 2, 425
lipophilin, 324
lipoproteins, 586
liposome, 255, 269, 324
liver, in viral infection, 402
lymph node, 3, 348, 375
lymphocyte
   in canine distemper, 386
   B-cell, 502, 521, 530
   T-cell, 4, 281, 367, 391, 413,
      521, 530
   in cerebrospinal fluid, 639
   culture, 502
   in diabetes, 480
   in experimental allergic en-
      cephalomyelitis, 347
   in experimental allergic
      neuritis, 472
   from sensitized donor, 3, 280
   transformation, 531
   in visna, 384
lymphoid cell, 397
lymphokine, 521
lysolecithin, 425, 493
lysophospholipase, 425

lysosome, 4, 78, 308, 355, 366,
   425, 472, 521, 570
lysozyme, 345, 368

macrophage, 4, 312, 365, 384,
   386, 473, 503, 521, 575
malnutrition, 179, 411, 464
measles, 384, 540, 562, 624,
   625, 627, 633, 641
membrane
   components, 189
   glial plasma membrane, 20, 72,
      355, 425
   lipids, 222, 497
   potential, 155
   probe, 190
   proteins, 117, 384
membrane (M) protein, of virus,
   388
meningitis, 384, 397, 522, 530,
   547, 567, 639
metachromatic leukodystrophy, 515
methylnitrosourea (MNU), 488
microfilament, 191
microglia, 376
microsome, 20, 45, 56, 78, 119,
   136, 425, 603
microtubule, 75, 191, 404
migration inhibition factor,
   index, 502, 504, 625
mitochondria, 3, 44, 75, 100,
   140, 148, 355, 425, 440, 485,
   603
mitogen, 386, 530
mixed lymphocyte culture (MLC),
   530
monoamine oxidase, 78
monocyte, 375, 502
mononeuritis, 502
mononuclear cell, 348, 376, 399,
   535, 562
motor neuron disease, 408, 522,
   627
multiple sclerosis (MS)
   autoimmunity, 277, 330, 637
   autopsy findings, 570
   cerebrospinal fluid, 412, 513,
      530, 546, 561, 581, 623, 639

multiple sclerosis (MS) (cont'd)
  diagnostic criteria, 547
  CNS enzymes, 569
  exacerbation, 9, 22, 377, 502,
    513, 522, 535, 639
  immune response, 530, 561
  lipids in CNS, 2
  loss of myelin basic protein,
    2, 308, 480
  myelin basic protein in CSF,
    148, 513
  neuropathology, 569
  neurotoxic serum factor, 19,
    24, 506
  neutral proteinase in lympho-
    cytes, 359, 366
  neutral proteinase in macro-
    phages, 366
  particles in brain, 623
  plasmalogenase activity, 427
  possible virus etiology, 411,
    623, 625, 627, 633, 641
  proteins in CNS, 2
  remission, 9, 502, 514, 522
  response to myelin basic
    protein, 501
  serum, 89, 177, 412, 537, 623,
    637
  spleen, 412
  transmissible agents, 412
mumps, 384, 530, 541, 623, 633
muscle cell, 444
mutation, 388
myasthenia, 502, 637
myelin, of the CNS,
  action of trypsin, 307
  in adrenoleukodystrophy, 585,
    603
  cerebrosides, 263
  cholesterol ester hydrolase,
    609
  degradation, 3, 163, 308, 348,
    396, 480, 556, 623
  dehydration, 66
  in experimental phenylketo-
    nuria, 453
  fatty acids, 32, 199, 236, 264,
    454, 585
  fluid mosaic model, 190

myelin, of the CNS (cont'd)
  formation, maintenance, 19,
    71, 160, 207
  fractionation, 21, 56, 72, 118
  glycoproteins, 79, 160, 191,
    244, 250, 265
  heavy myelin, 56, 75, 588
  in intoxication, 487
  in vitro, 171
  lamellar structure, 2, 20, 75,
    130, 160, 172, 191,215, 236,
    250, 264, 311, 348, 376, 588
  light myelin, 56, 75, 588
  lipids, 19, 27, 160, 172, 190,
    221, 236, 250, 264, 309, 454,
    488, 586
  lipoproteins, 586
  molecular organization, 189,
    208, 235, 249, 323
  preparation, 28, 57, 160, 172,
    193, 310, 367, 456, 488, 586
  preparation, small-scale, 11,
    135
  proteins, 20, 78, 117, 136,
    160, 196, 236, 258, 303, 349,
    488, 571
  sheath, 20, 44, 56, 137, 172,
    192, 218, 236, 250, 263, 348,
    383, 440, 494, 526
  specific gravity, 586
  staining, 571
myelin, of the PNS,
  action of trypsin, 307
  amino acid composition, 97
  antigenic activity, 97
  basic proteins, 96
  demyelination, 425, 473, 480
  glycoproteins, 96, 309
  lamellar structure, 100, 270
  neutron diffraction, 216
  preparation, 96
  proteins, 95, 293, 309
  proton magnetic resonance
    spectra, 190
myelination
  abnormal in vitro, 171
  and enzymes, 43, 56, 129, 411
  in experimental phenylketo-
    nuria, 459

myelination (cont'd)
  incomplete, 7
  and malnutrition, 179
  mechanism, 19, 85, 135, 233
  and myelin lipids, 27
"myelin-like" fraction, 20, 56,
  75, 140, 176
myelitis, 515, 547
myosin, 442

neuron
  and axonal transport, 440
  and diabetes, 480
  and enzymes, 43, 65, 119,
    425, 576
  and firing, 218
  and infective agent, 19, 386,
    397
  in vitro, 73
  and myelin basic protein, 148
neurotransmitter, 52, 148
neutron activation, 172
neutron diffraction, 216
p-nitrophenylphosphatase,
  472
noradrenaline, 49, 148
nuclear magnetic resonance,
  190, 208, 222
nucleic acid, 77, 384, 497,
  531, 561, 642
nucleocapsid, 386, 623
5'-nucleotidase, 78, 355
nude allele, in mouse, 412

oligodendroglial cell
  and infectious agent, 412
  isolation, 45, 71
  maintenance, 71
  and myelin structure, 233,
    237, 250, 396
  and myelin synthesis, 71,
    130, 192, 208
  and myelination, 19, 66
  and plasmalogenase, 424
  and receptors, 637
  and toxic agents, 497
  and virus infection, 377, 396

oncogenic properties
  of toxins, 487
  of viruses, 389
oncorna virus, 384, 408
onion bulb formation, 484
opiate receptor, 149
optic nerve, tract, 20, 136,
  402, 502, 513, 549, 571
ovalbumin, 312

panencephalitis, 397
papova virus, 389
parainfluenza, 384, 623
paramyxovirus, 385, 623, 625,
  629, 641
parvalbumin, 214
pepsin, 294, 348
pepstatin, 350
peptidase, 4, 362
peptides, of myelin basic
  protein, 2, 22, 111, 148,
    208, 232, 241, 281, 362,
    522
peripheral nerve
  and axonal transport, 440
  in experimental allergic
    neuritis, 471
  protein synthesis, 22
pertussis vaccine, 303
phagocyte, phagocytosis, 366,
  375, 473, 480, 521
phenylalanine, 5
  hydroxylase, 454
  metabolites, 453
phenylketonuria, experimental,
  453
phosphatase
  acid, 3, 78, 355, 481, 570
  myelin-bound, 160
phospholipase, 3, 44, 425
phospholipids
  of fibroblasts, 608
  of myelin, 20, 29, 43, 165,
    172, 190, 215, 236, 264,
    424, 456, 493, 587
  of oligodendroglia, 77
Piracetam, 46

plaque
  in canine distemper, 386
  in multiple sclerosis, 2,
    308, 366, 484, 521, 535,
    569, 640
plasma cell, 387, 530, 575
plasmalogen, 29, 44, 245,
  424, 489
plasmalogenase, 386, 423, 581
plasmin, 370
plasminogen activator, 4, 366
poliovirus, 540, 627
polylysine, 357, 376
polymerase, DNA, 384
polymorphonuclear leukocyte,
  397, 412, 473, 502, 521, 641
polyneuropathy, 502, 530
prealbumin, 547
probe, membrane, 190, 238,
  249, 264, 311
progressive multifocal leukoencephalopathy (PML), 388,
  624
prolactin, 637
proliferating cells, in
  demyelinating disease, 561
prostaglandin, 425
protamine sulfate, 357, 376
protease, see proteinase
protein, axonal transport, 440
protein deficiency, 184
protein kinase, 160
proteinase
  acid, 2, 308, 348, 375, 426,
    472, 480, 521, 569
  basic, 4
  neutral, 3, 308, 333, 348,
    365, 426, 480, 521, 581
  participation in the break-
    down of myelin basic protein,
    148, 232
proteolipid protein, of myelin,
  20, 79, 118, 137, 163, 190,
  239, 258, 309, 349, 368
proteolysis, 2, 231, 308, 347,
  369, 521
proton magnetic resonance, 190
proton T_1 experiment, 209
protozoal infection, 391

provirus, 384
Purkinje cell, 148, 173, 399
puromycin, 21
pyridoxal phosphate, 250

Quaking mouse, 135, 159

rabbit eye model, 376, 507
rabies, 7, 384, 623
radioimmunoassay
  for CNS proteins, 8, 93
  for myelin basic protein,
    331, 377, 414, 513
  for virus-specific IgG, 633
radio-immunoelectrophoresis,
  507
Ranvier's node, 218
receptor, 637
remyelination, 484
respiratory syncytial virus,
  633
reticuloendothelial disease,
  389
retina, 21
retravirus, 391
rheumatoid arthritis, 581
rheumatoid factor (RF), 634
ribonuclease, 357
ribosome, 75, 582
rinderpest virus, 385
rosette formation, 533
rubella, 391, 623, 633
Russel body, 575

S-100 protein, 8, 331
Schilder's disease, 411, 596,
  602
Schwann cell, 440, 473, 484,
  497
sciatic nerve, 439, 480
scrapie, 428
segmental demyelination, 484
seizure, 56
Sendai virus, 641
sensitization, to myelin basic
  protein, 282, 348, 626

serine phospholipids, 77, 237, 252, 264
serotonin, 637
serum proteins, in neurological diseases, 545
sialic acid, 77
slow virus infection, 384, 626
sodium periodate, 264
Solomon-Bloembergen equation, 209
sphingomyelin, 27, 77, 191, 236, 252, 489, 585, 609
spongioblast culture, 389
spongy state, of white matter, 399, 488
sterol, 239, 587
"sticky tube" assay, 331
streptozotocin, 480
stroke, 503
subacute sclerosing pan-encephalitis (SSPE), 387, 411, 503, 539, 562, 597, 624, 626, 634, 639
substance P, 148
succinic dehydrogenase, 355, 442, 481
sudanophilic leukodystrophy, 596, 602
sulfatide, see cerebroside
sulfotransferase, 128
synaptic cleft, 400
synaptic transmission, 50
synaptosome, 140, 148

tau-fraction, 547
Theiler's virus, 413
thiamine pyrophosphatase, 78
thioglycollate, 367
thymocyte, 385
thymus, 354, 412, 530
thyroid stimulating hormone (TSH), 637
transferrin, 547
trauma, 434
triethyltin (TET), 66, 494
trinitrobenzene sulphonic acid (TNBS), 250
trypsin, 72, 89, 294, 307, 348, 375, 597, 606

tumor virus, 385

urokinase, 372

vaccinia virus, 633
varicella-zoster, 384, 623
virus, 19, 192, 366, 383, 396, 522, 531, 563, 623, 625, 627, 633, 639
visna, 384, 624
vitamin, vitamin deficiency, 184, 427

van der Waals attraction, 216
Wallerian degeneration, 324, 476
Wolfgram protein, 20, 118, 137, 164, 194, 310, 368

X-ray diffraction, 190, 233, 237

zinc deficiency, 412
zwitterion, 231